# HUMAN SEXUALITY:

## Psychosexual Effects of Disease

# HUMAN SEXUALITY:
## Psychosexual Effects of Disease

EDITED BY

## Martin Farber, M.D.
Professor and Chairman, Department of Obstetrics and Gynecology
Albert Einstein Medical Center
Philadelphia, Pennsylvania

**Macmillan Publishing Company**
NEW YORK

Collier Macmillan Canada, Inc.
TORONTO

Collier Macmillan Publishers
LONDON

Copyright © 1985, Martin Farber, M.D.

Printed in the United States of America

All rights reserved. No part of this book may be reproduced or transmitted in any form or by any means, electronic or mechanical, including photocopying, recording, or any information storage and retrieval system, without permission in writing from the Publisher.

Macmillan Publishing Company
866 Third Avenue, New York, New York 10022

Collier Macmillan Canada, Inc.

Collier Macmillan Publishers • London

**Library of Congress Cataloging in Publication Data**

Main entry under title:

Human sexuality.

   1. Sick—Psychology.  2. Sick—Sexual behavior.
3. Sexual disorders.  4. Generative organs, Female—
Diseases—Psychological aspects.  I. Farber, Martin,
1940–   . [DNLM: 1. Disease—psychology.  2. Psychosexual Development.  3. Psychosexual Disorders.
4. Surgery, Operative—psychology.  WM 611 H918]
R726.5.H86   1985        616.6′9        84–29490
ISBN 0–02–336190–5
ISBN 0–02–336200–6 (pbk.)

Printing: 1 2 3 4 5 6 7 8     Year: 5 6 7 8 9 0 1 2 3 4

*Dedicated to
Judith, Jason, and Adam,
my wife and two sons,
without whose continued encouragement
this textbook would not have been possible.*

# PREFACE

Seventeen years ago when I was Chief Resident in Gynecology, a 77-year-old woman presented herself to my Clinic at the Boston Dispensary with a complaint of uterine prolapse. After thorough evaluation of the patient, I requested that the Professor and Chairman of the Department, Dr. George W. Mitchell, Jr., assist me in the performance of a LeFort colpocleisis: surgically closing the vagina and reducing the prolapsed organ. The evening prior to surgery Dr. Mitchell carefully explained that, postoperatively, coitus would not be possible, whereupon the patient exclaimed, "But Doctor, I am a married woman."

As with most medical students and resident physicians today, up to that point in my training no one had bothered to emphasize the importance of the psychosexual effects of disease processes and surgical procedures. This important educational omission persists to the present, although currently resident physicians and nursing students are expected to metamorphose into mature, sentient health care providers, possessed of the wisdom of the ages, capable of anticipating the effects of disease processes on the quality of life, the day after their training is completed.

This textbook is an attempt to fill an obvious informational void. Twenty-four chapters contributed by authorities in their respective disciplines address normal psychosexual development (Unit I), the psychosexual effects of major organic diseases (Units II and III), and psychosexual dysfunction pursuant to drug abuse, rape, and gender identity disorders (Unit IV). Hopefully, patients and health care providers will use this textbook as an easily readable source of current information pertinent to a very important topic, and it is my hope and anticipation that this textbook will have a positive impact on the quality of health care

MARTIN FARBER, M.D.

# ACKNOWLEDGMENTS

I sincerely appreciate the kind cooperation of all the contributing authors, the guidance of Ms. Edith Craft, Senior Editor of the Macmillan Publishing Company, and the technical assistance of my secretary Ms. Linda Zimmer.

M. F.

# CONTRIBUTORS

**Eli Y. Adashi, M.D.**
Associate Professor
Obstetrics and Gynecology and Physiology
  and Director
Division of Reproductive Endocrinology
University of Maryland School of Medicine
Baltimore, Maryland

**Barrie Anderson, M.D.**
Associate Professor
Department of Obstetrics and Gynecology
and Director of Gynecologic Oncology
University of Iowa Hospitals
Iowa City, Iowa

**Elaine P. Bencivengo, M.A.**
Executive Director
Joseph J. Peters Institute
Philadelphia, Pennsylvania

**Jane Berry, R.N., M.S.N.**
Head Nurse—High Risk/Obstetrical Unit
Hospital of the University of Pennsylvania
Philadelphia, Pennsylvania

**Jerry G. Blaivas, M.D.**
Associate Professor of Urology and Director
  of Neurourology
College of Physicians and Surgeons
Columbia University
New York City, New York

**David Charles, M.D.**
Professor and Chairman
Department of Obstetrics and Gynecology
Marshall University School of Medicine
Huntington, West Virginia

**Arnold W. Cohen, M.D.**
Director
Division of Maternal and Fetal Medicine
Department of Obstetrics and Gynecology
Albert Einstein Medical Center
Northern Division
and Associate Professor of Obstetrics and
  Gynecology
Temple University School of Medicine
Philadelphia, Pennsylvania

**Michael J. Daly, M.D.**
Professor and Chairman
Department of Obstetrics and Gynecology
Temple University School of Medicine
Philadelphia, Pennsylvania

**Alan DeCherney, M.D.**
Professor
Department of Obstetrics and Gynecology
  and Director
Division of Reproductive Endocrinology
Yale University School of Medicine
New Haven, Connecticut

**Martin Farber, M.D.**
Chairman
Department of Obstetrics and Gynecology
Albert Einstein Medical Center
Northern Division
and Professor and Deputy Chairman
Department of Obstetrics and Gynecology
Temple University School of Medicine
Philadelphia, Pennsylvania

**Martin Freedman, M.D.**
Director—Section of In Vitro Fertilization
Department of Obstetrics and Gynecology

Albert Einstein Medical Center
Northern Division
and Assistant Professor
Department of Obstetrics and Gynecology
Temple University School of Medicine
Philadelphia, Pennsylvania

**Steven G. Gabbe, M.D.**
Professor
Department of Obstetrics and Gynecology, Pediatrics
and Director of the Jerrold R. Golding Division of Fetal Medicine
Department of Obstetrics and Gynecology
University of Pennsylvania School of Medicine
Philadelphia, Pennsylvania

**Ned L. Gaylin, Ph.D.**
Professor and Director of Marriage and Family Therapy Education and Training
Department of Family and Community Development
University of Maryland
College Park, Maryland

**Douglas D. Glover, M.D.**
Associate Professor
Department of Obstetrics and Gynecology
Marshall University School of Medicine
Huntington, West Virginia

**Robert C. Goodlin, M.D.**
Professor
Department of Obstetrics and Gynecology
and Director of Maternal–Fetal Medicine
University of Nebraska School of Medicine
Omaha, Nebraska

**Dorothy A. Greenfeld, M.S.W.**
Clinical Social Worker
Department of Obstetrics and Gynecology
Yale New Haven Hospital
New Haven, Connecticut

**Edward T. Heck, Ph.D.**
Clinical Instructor of Pediatrics, Neuropsychology
Tufts University School of Medicine
Boston, Massachusetts

**Richard I. Katz, M.D.**
Attending Neurologist
Albert Einstein Medical Center
Northern Division
and Clinical Associate Professor—Neurology
Temple University School of Medicine
Philadelphia, Pennsylvania

**Leonardo Magran, M.D.**
Chairman
Division of Child Development and Child Psychiatry
Department of Psychiatry
Albert Einstein Medical Center
Northern Division
and Clinical Associate Professor of Psychiatry
Department of Mental Health Sciences
Hahnemann University
Philadelphia, Pennsylvania

**George W. Mitchell, Jr., M.D.**
Professor
Department of Obstetrics and Gynecology
and Director of Gynecologic Oncology
University of Texas Health Science Center, at San Antonio
San Antonio, Texas

**Harris M. Nagler, M.D.**
Assistant Professor of Urology
College of Physicians and Surgeons
Columbia University
and Assistant Attending Urologist
Presbyterian Hospital
Columbia Presbyterian Medical Center
and Director of the New York Male Reproductive Center
Columbia Presbyterian Medical Center
New York City, New York

**Bertrand L. New, M.D.**
Clinical Associate Professor of Psychiatry
Cornell University Medical Center
New York City, New York

**Maria New, M.D.**
Professor and Chairman
Department of Pediatrics
Cornell University Medical Center
New York City, New York

**Joel Noumoff, M.D.**
Director
Division of Gynecologic Oncology
Department of Obstetrics and Gynecology
Albert Einstein Medical Center

and Associate Professor
Department of Obstetrics and Gynecology
Temple University School of Medicine
Philadelphia, Pennsylvania

**Bruce Parsons, Ph.D.**
Post Doctoral Fellow
Department of Pharmacology
University of Pennsylvania
Philadelphia, Pennsylvania

**Ira B. Pauly, M.D.**
Professor and Chairman
Department of Psychiatry and Behavioral
 Sciences
University of Nevada School of Medicine
Reno, Nevada

**Mary Lake Polan, M.D., Ph.D.**
Assistant Professor
Department of Obstetrics and Gynecology
Section of Reproductive Endocrinology
Yale University School of Medicine
New Haven, Connecticut

**John S. Rinehart, M.D., Ph.D.**
Assistant Professor of Obstetrics and
 Gynecology
University of Wisconsin Medical Center
Madison, Wisconsin

**Joseph J. Romero, M.A.**
Research Associate
Joseph J. Peters Institute
Philadelphia, Pennsylvania

**Isaac Schiff, M.D.**
Associate Director of Reproductive
 Endocrinology
Department of Obstetrics and Gynecology
Brigham and Women's Hospital
and Associate Professor of Obstetrics and
 Gynecology
Harvard Medical School
Boston, Massachusetts

**Jay S. Schinfeld, M.D.**
Associate Professor
Department of Obstetrics and Gynecology
and Director of Gynecologic Endocrinology
 and Infertility
University of Tennessee College of Medicine
Memphis, Tennessee

**Elisabeth C. Small, M.D.**
Associate Professor of Psychiatry and
 Obstetrics and Gynecology
University of Nevada School of Medicine
Anderson Medical Science Building
Reno, Nevada

**Marjorie Seltzer Stanek, M.D.**
Co-Director Cardiac Rehabilitation Program
Albert Einstein Medical Center
Northern Division
and Assistant Professor of Medicine
Temple University School of Medicine
Philadelphia, Pennsylvania

**George E. Tagatz, M.D.**
Professor
Department of Obstetrics and Gynecology
and Director
Reproductive Endocrinology
University of Minnesota Medical School
Minneapolis, Minnesota

**Roger C. Toffle, M.D.**
Fellow—Reproductive Endocrinology
Instructor—Department of Obstetrics and
 Gynecology
University of Minnesota Medical School
Minneapolis, Minnesota

**Ralph de Vere White, M.D.**
Associate Professor of Urology
Columbia Presbyterian Medical Center
and Associate Attending Urologist
Presbyterian Hospital
New York City, New York

**Thomas Wolman, M.D.**
Clinical Assistant Professor of Psychiatry and
 Human Behavior
Jefferson Medical College
Philadelphia, Pennsylvania

**Ruth York, Ph.D., B.S.N.**
Assistant Professor in Health Care of Women
University of Pennsylvania
Philadelphia, Pennsylvania

# CONTENTS

*Preface* vii
*Acknowledgments* ix
*Contributors* x
*Contents* xiii

## Unit I  PSYCHOSEXUAL DEVELOPMENT — 1

Chapter 1. History of Psychosocial Medicine — 3
*Michael J. Daly, M.D.*

Chapter 2. Prepubertal and Pubertal Psychosexual Development — 10
*Leonardo Magran, M.D.*

Chapter 3. The Educational Process — 28
*Edward T. Heck, Ph.D.*

Chapter 4. Marriage — 40
*Ned L. Gaylin, Ph.D.*

Chapter 5. Human Sexuality During Normal Pregnancy — 55
*Arnold W. Cohen, M.D.*

Chapter 6. Sexuality and the Menopause — 77
*John S. Rinehart, M.D., Ph.D., and Isaac Schiff, M.D.*

## Unit II  PATHOPHYSIOLOGY OF HUMAN SEXUALITY IN OBSTETRIC AND GYNECOLOGIC DISEASE — 85

Chapter 7. External Genital Ambiguity — 87
*Bertrand L. New, M.D. and Maria I. New, M.D.*

Chapter 8. Anomalous Female Genital Duct Development — 96
*Martin Farber, M.D., Joel Noumoff, M.D., and Martin Freedman, M.D.*

Chapter 9. Endocrine Correlates and Ontogeny of Feminine Sexual Behavior: Basic and Clinical Considerations — 113
*Eli Y. Adashi, M.D., and Bruce Parsons, Ph.D.*

| | | |
|---|---|---|
| Chapter 10. | Contraception and Psychosexual Function<br>*Roger C. Toffle, M.D., and George E. Tagatz, M.D.* | 128 |
| Chapter 11. | Psychosexual Dysfunction and Infertility<br>*Jay S. Schinfeld, M.D.* | 141 |
| Chapter 12. | Pelvic Relaxation<br>*George W. Mitchell, Jr., M.D.* | 154 |
| Chapter 13. | Psychosexual Problems Related to Pelvic Pain<br>*David Charles, M.D., and Douglas D. Glover, M.D.* | 159 |
| Chapter 14. | Human Sexuality and Benign Neoplasia<br>*Alan H. DeCherney, M.D., Dorothy A. Greenfield, M.S.W., and Mary Lake Polan, M.D., Ph.D.* | 169 |
| Chapter 15. | Malignant Neoplasia<br>*Barrie Anderson, M.D.* | 178 |
| Chapter 16. | Breast Disease<br>*Elisabeth C. Small, M.D.* | 189 |
| Chapter 17. | Psychosomatic Aspects of High Risk Pregnancy<br>*Robert C. Goodlin, M.D.* | 201 |
| Chapter 18. | The Puerperium<br>*Ruth York, Ph.D., B.S.N., Jane Berry, M.S.N., R.N., and Steven G. Gabbe, M.D.* | 213 |

## Unit III  PATHOPHYSIOLOGY OF HUMAN SEXUALITY IN MAJOR MEDICAL AND SURGICAL DISEASE — 229

| | | |
|---|---|---|
| Chapter 19. | Cardiovascular Disease<br>*Marjorie Seltzer Stanek, M.D.* | 231 |
| Chapter 20. | Impotence: Diagnosis and Treatment<br>*Harris M. Nagler, M.D., Ralph deVere White, M.D., and Jerry G. Blaivas, M.D.* | 240 |
| Chapter 21. | Neurologic Disease and Sexual Function<br>*Richard I. Katz, M.D.* | 264 |

## Unit IV  PATHOPHYSIOLOGY OF HUMAN SEXUALITY IN PSYCHOSOCIAL DISEASE — 275

| | | |
|---|---|---|
| Chapter 22. | Drug Addiction<br>*Thomas Wolman, M.D.* | 277 |
| Chapter 23. | Rape<br>*Elaine P. Bencivengo, M.A., and Joseph J. Romero, M.A.* | 286 |
| Chapter 24. | Gender Identity Disorders<br>*Ira B. Pauly, M.D.* | 295 |

*Index* — 317

# HUMAN SEXUALITY:
## Psychosexual Effects of Disease

# UNIT 1 Psychosexual Development

# CHAPTER 1  HISTORY OF PSYCHOSEXUAL MEDICINE

*Michael J. Daly, M.D.*

## INTRODUCTION

Probably no area of human behavior has been subjected to as many different influences as human sexuality. The history of these influences and the changing attitudes they have produced has resulted in diversified patterns of sexual behavior. At the outset, civilization was concerned with sexuality as a means of propagating the human species, and tribal customs, religious practices, and laws were developed to foster human reproduction.

Human sexual behavior was basically initiated when man learned to use his hands. Coitus became possible at all times, not just when the female was ovulating or when pregnancy was possible. Thus human sexuality differed from other mammalian sexual behavior. Cultural, religious, and political pressures further molded human sexuality. Only recently has medicine attempted to bring a more scientific approach to the understanding and management of sexual problems. The involvement of physicians and other interested professionals in human sexual life and practices has been met with a great deal of resistance, misunderstanding, and hostility. In spite of these attitudes, significant advances in the study of human sexuality have been made in the last 75 years through meaningful research, the education of physicians, and improved therapeutic methods. This chapter will trace these developments from the time of the early physicians to the current state of psychosexual medicine.

## THE PHYSICIAN AND SEX

### ANCIENT TIMES

Scientific medicine began with the Greeks, although the art of healing was practiced long before the time of the Greek physician. Certainly, the Egyptians and others practiced a form of medicine. Circumcision, for example, was performed in a number of ancient societies. However, the basic study of anatomy, physiology, and pathology began with the Greeks. The Father of Medicine has been designated as Hippocrates, who was born in 460 B.C., the son of a Greek physician.

Norman Sussman (1976) has pointed out that most physicians, when being conferred the degree of Doctor of Medicine, take the Hippocratic Oath. In taking this oath, physicians are singled out from others for sexual prohibition. "Whatsoever house I enter. There will I go for the benefit of the sick, refraining from all wrong doing or corruption, and especially from any act of seduction, of male or female, of bond or free." Thus, physicians from ancient times were cautioned about matters of sex. Their role in matters of reproduction were not only limited by knowledge, but also by creed. Although barrier contraceptives were known to be used as early as 1850 B.C., early medical men had little to do with reproductive control. However, as is clear from the Prohibition in the text of the Hippocratic Oath, "I will not give a woman an abortive remedy," some may have performed abortions. Soranus, another Greek physician, recommended the use of pessories, vaginal plugs, and chemicals as contraceptive measures (Sciarra, 1979).

The Roman sexual mores were somewhat different from the Greek. Galen (200 A.D.), a respected teacher of medicine, had a great curiosity concerning contraceptives and sexual activity. He may well have been the first proponent of sex education for physicians. Galen suggested exercise, moderate eating, and the use of body oils before coitus, and bathing afterwards. He hypothesized that hysterical symptoms resulted from the lack of a sexual outlet and felt that masturbation would relieve these symptoms. He reasoned that lack of orgasm in the male and the female led to anxiety and psychic imbalance. If Hippocrates was the father of medicine, Galen was the father of psychosomatic medicine (Sussman, 1976).

Ancient Oriental sexual practices are depicted in art, which has been preserved to the present. Although the role of Oriental medicine men is not fully known, it is reasonable to conclude that they were concerned with problems of human sexuality, but were limited by their lack of knowledge, as well as by the prevalent mores.

## THE MIDDLE AGES

During the Middle Ages (500 A.D. to 1500 A.D.) the primary influence on sexuality in Western Europe was the Roman Catholic church. Roman civilization had been destroyed, and a new civilization, based on the ideals of love, charity, and virtue, came into being. As asceticism and chastity were encouraged, sex was devalued and separated from other spiritual and social activities. In the *Confessions,* St. Augustine wrote about his struggle with his own sexual drive, while another influential cleric, St. Paul, argued for the suppression of passion. Celibacy was required of the clergy, and recommended for the general population. It was proclaimed that sexual activity should occur only for the purpose of procreation. During that period, physicians were forbidden to provide contraceptives or to perform abortions. However, this strong prohibition against the enjoyment of sexuality failed not only with the masses, but also, frequently, with the clergy.

## THE RENAISSANCE, REFORMATION, AND PURITAN PERIOD

During the Renaissance, syphillis had a more profound effect upon sexual practices in Europe than religion. Syphillis was thought to have been brought from the New World, and at the beginning of the Renaissance it was epidemic in Western Europe. Hospitals were built solely to treat the disease. Guaracum was a drug used to treat patients diagnosed as having secondary syphillis, and the Roman physician Fallopius (1523–1563) fabricated the first condom from linen to prevent sexual transmission of the infection. The Reformation, Puritanism, and Calvinism were significant factors in bringing about sexual repression (Sussman, 1976).

## THE EIGHTEENTH AND NINETEENTH CENTURIES

Despite the social restraints of sexuality in the eighteenth century, two French physicians, Drs. Dennis Diderot and Choderlos de Laclos, accurately described human sexual drives as well as some mental illnesses. Their work really laid the foundation for research in psychosexual medicine. Unfortunately, few national leaders paid any attention to their findings.

During the first half of the nineteenth century, the cultural ideal was to pursue love without sex. By the middle of the century Victorianism had given way to Romanticism, which embraced sexual feelings and passion.

However, during the Victorian era, physicians supported the control of sexual activities. In the latter part of the eighteenth century, Dr. Samuel Auguste Andre David Tissot had theorized that the loss of semen through masturbation was physically debilitating (Breecher, 1976). Another prominent physician, Charles Drysdale, theorized that nocturnal emission was a disease, which he called spermatorrhea. These concepts resulted from theological concern over masturbation, and physicians spent a great deal of time and effort attempting to develop methods for its prevention. It was not until the latter half of the Victorian period that psychosexual medicine became more realistic with contributions from Drs. Sigmund Freud, Henry Havelock Ellis, and Charles Knowlton.

In America, Knowlton wrote that sexual desire was a normal bodily appetite to be reasonably fulfilled in the interest of one's health. In this way it was like hunger. He strongly supported contraception, and in his writings he described the so called vaginal tent or diaphragm. A layman, Francis Place, is credited with founding the Population Control Movement which sought to further separate sexual enjoyment from reproduction. However, a Dr. William Acton, followed the teaching of Tissot, and promulgated more misconceptions concerning the harmful effects of masturbation, coitus during pregnancy, and other touching of the pregnant woman.

In 1898, George M. Beard wrote about sexual neurasthenia which was of great concern not only on the European continent, but also in America. He suggested that the body had a given amount of energy, and that this energy could be depleted through sexual activity. Electrodes were developed to be inserted into the rectum and urethra to restore this vital energy. Beard felt that masturbation and nocturnal emissions were the etiology of neurasthenia. However, he thought that coitus did not drain the body's vital energy significantly. Although this idea would seem to be a logical contradiction, many physicians accepted the theory. It is interesting that prostitution, pornography, and sexual affairs flourished throughout the various social levels of Victorian society.

Sigmund Freud's (1856–1939) concept of psychosexual development from infancy to adulthood was another major contribution to the understanding of human sexuality. His description of the oral, anal, and genital stages in the first five years of life was revolutionary and only recently has been seriously questioned. During the 1890s and early 1900s, Freud published the *Psychopathology of Everyday Life, The Interpretation of Dreams, Three Essays on the Theory of Sex, Wit and Its Relation to the Unconscious, Totem and Taboo,* and *The History of the Psychoanalytic Movement.* In these books, Freud theorized that sexual deviations (including homosexuality) were a form of disease, that they represented immature sexual development, and that they should be so treated. Freud also theorized that masturbation and nocturnal emissions were signs of immaturity and needed therapeutic intervention. (Because of Freud's beliefs the American Psychiatric Society (APA) initially classified homosexuality as a disease state in its *Diagnostic and Statistical Manual,* although it has recently changed this classification.)

At first, Freud was interested in patients who suffered from hysteria. He attempted to demonstrate the relation of hysteria in women to early sexual abuse (Freud, 1917). His concept that a clitoral orgasm was immature, and that only a vaginal orgasm, occurring upon male penetration, was a mature sexual response has been bitterly attacked, and rightly so. Obviously Freud was not correct in all his conclusions, but he brought a new dimension to psychosexual medicine, and he opened the door to understanding many of the emotional problems that might affect normal sexual response.

While Freud concentrated on the psyche of his patients, other early twentieth century physicians concentrated their studies on genital anatomy, the effects of castration and clitoridectomy, and the utilization of mechanical devices to curb masturbation. Richard von Krafft-Ebing, a German psychiatrist who was a contemporary of Freud, chaired the initial presentation of the latter's thesis on hysteria. Krafft-Ebing had a very distasteful view of many sexual practices. As a forensic psychiatrist he became involved with the investigation of sexual crimes, and he viewed any sexual practice other than a procreative one as perversion. He equated voyeurs, fetishists, and homosexuals with rapists and sex murderers. He also believed that transvestites were part of the same matrix. He insisted masturbation was a major factor in the etiology of the horrible crimes he studied, and he presumed that sexual desires in the elderly led to senile dementia. Krafft-Ebing probably did more disservice to the development of psychosexual medicine than any other single physician. Unfortunately, his publication *Psychopathia Sexualis* is still being read and used as a reference book today.

A second contemporary of Freud was Henry Havelock Ellis, who believed that each individual has a unique sexual behavior. He thought that an individual's sexuality was the result of personal attitudes and experiences. His concept of homosexuality and other less common sexual practices was that they were an extension of individual needs forged by the social environment. Thus, he expanded the parameters of so-called normal behavior. Ellis' major contributions were his strong support for sexual education, his support of equal sexual rights for women, his interest in normal sexual responses, and his acceptance of childhood sexuality. Edward Breecher (1975), in summarizing this era, states that those interested in psychosexual medicine today should review the ruthless sexual atrocities reported by von Krafft-Ebing, the psychotherapeutic approaches to the sexual problems advocated by Freud, and the relatively liberal acceptance of unusual sexual practices fostered by Ellis.

In 1899, at the 50th Annual Meeting of the American Medical Association in Columbus, Ohio, Dr. Denslow Lewis presented a paper entitled "The Gynecological Consideration of the Sexual Act." In his presentation, Lewis, a professor of gynecology from Chicago, attempted to encourage his colleagues to learn more about the normal sexual response of women and to help those with marital problems and sexual dysfunction (Lewis, 1893). His paper covered a description of the sexual act, anatomical interference with coitus, sexual education, marital incompatibility, and the sexual response of women. Dr. Howard A. Kelly of the Johns Hopkins Medical School discussed the paper. He strongly opposed any discussion of sexual matters in public. He also stated that he did not believe mutual pleasure in the sexual act had any bearing on the happiness of life. His final statement was that the discussion should be considered filth. Dr. Sherwood Dunn of Boston also commented on Dr. Lewis' presentation, but fully supported it, expressing his opinion that the information would be beneficial to the medical profession as well as to the public. Nevertheless, Dr. George H. Simmons, editor of the *Journal of the American Medical Association*, refused to publish the manuscript.

### THE TWENTIETH CENTURY—THE SEXUAL REVOLUTION

With the beginning of the twentieth century, information concerning sexuality moved out quickly from under the shrouded cover of the Victorian period into an open and conscious arena. Gradually concepts based on ignorance, guilt, and fear began to give way to a more realistic, knowledgeable, and humanistic approach. In Europe the gynecologist Theodor Van de Velde, wrote a book entitled *The Ideal Marriage* in which he frankly described sexual techniques, including oral–genital stimulation. This work brought to light different forms of sexual behavior heretofore practiced in secrecy. Van de Velde also stressed the importance of sexuality as a form of communication between a man and a woman. In 1933 Dr. Robert Dickinson published an *Atlas of Human Sex Anatomy,* but felt that sexual attitudes had precedence over anatomy.

Twenty years later in America, the first truly in-depth scientific study of human sexual behavior was reported by Alfred Kinsey and his colleagues. They toured the country acquiring data from individuals of all ages and from all social strata. Their findings were published in two volumes, *The Sexual Behavior of the Human Male* (1948) and, later, *The Sexual Behavior of the Human Female* (1953).

During the following years various other aspects of human sexual behavior were elucidated. Evidence was found that transvestitism existed in earlier societies in compliance with a desire for cross-gender identity, but it was only in the middle of the twentieth century that surgical procedures for transsexuals were performed. In the early 1950s operative procedures together with steroid hormones were utilized to physically change a person's sex. Major programs were developed initially at the University of Minnesota and the Johns Hopkins University to manage transsexuals, and subsequently programs arose in New York, Philadelphia, and Los Angeles. At first the results were encouraging, but as disappointing evaluations of larger groups of these individuals over a longer period of time were found, interest in performing "sex-change" operations began to wane.

In 1944, Dr. Helene Deutsch, a psychiatrist trained by Freud, published a psychoanalytic essay entitled, *The Psychology of Women*. She wrote that at the core of womanhood were three basic elements: feminine eroticism, feminine passivity, and feminine masochism. It was Deutsch's contention that the attitude, behavior, and sexuality of a woman reflected the degree to which each of these elements prevailed. The normal woman had an equal balance of these three characteristics. Her conclusions have been challenged by many, especially by the women's movement whose leaders emphasize the role of educational and cultural factors that influence a woman's behavior and minimize the part played by anatomical, biological, and psychological factors as suggested in Freud's *Anatomy Is Destiny* and reinforced by Deutsch. It should be noted that psychoanalysts had never denied the importance of the social milieu, but stressed that culture and society are not the only forces in psychological development. It is only fair to point out that Deutsch was reporting what she had observed in women in the Boston area during the first part of this century—women whose psychosexual development occurred during a specific era with a defined sexual morality. In light of this fact, it would be foolish to disregard her findings totally.

The discovery, by a Catholic gynecologist, of a contraceptive pill was a dramatic development in the 1950s. Dr. John Rock of Boston raised the hopes of many that the ideal form of population control had been found with the ability to control ovulation. This pill freed many women; women could now enjoy sexual relations without the fear of pregnancy. The "pill" was the springboard that launched the so-called copulation explosion. With the development of newer plastic materials, other methods of contraception, such as the intrauterine device (IUD), were also improved.

As a result of better means to prevent the unwanted pregnancy, a dramatic change developed in sexual attitudes. Expectations for sexual gratification resulted in many individuals seeking help from practicing physicians for their sexual problems. Unfortunately, too few physicians were willing or able to help. Dr. Harold Lief, a psychiatrist, undertook a study of the sexual knowledge and attitudes of physicians and medical students. Lief (1963) found that most physicians were less knowledgeable about human sexuality than most other adults, and that their sexual attitudes were more rigid. He further found that in medical schools, education about human sexuality was inadequate.

Today, because of the efforts of Lief and others to improve sex education for physicians, most medical schools offer a course in human sexuality, whereas in the 1960s only a few medical schools, such as those of the University of Pennsylvania, Temple University, and Wake Forest University, had such programs.

Interest in marital and sexual counseling developed throughout the United States. Publications in these areas were numerous, and by such authors as Dr. D. Wilfred Abse (Abse, Nash, and Louden, 1974), Ethel M. Nash (Nash, Jessner, and Abse, 1964), and Professor Richard A. Klemer (1965). More importantly, national professional organizations that aided in sharing knowledge about human sexuality developed, such as the American Association of Sex Education in Medicine (AASEM), Sex Information Education Council of the U.S. (SIECUS), and the American Society for Psychosomatic Obstetrics and Gynecology (ASPOG). All of these societies have made considerable contributions to education and research in human sexuality. A few outstanding examples of individuals in the field were: Dr. Mary Calderone, who provided leadership in educating men and women about contraceptives; Dr. Lewis Helman, who brought acceptable contraceptive help to New York City; and Drs. William Kroger and Charles Freed, who published the book, *Psychosomatic Obstetrics and Gynecology* (1951).

## TWENTIETH CENTURY RESEARCH

Masters and Johnson's studies (1960) of the normal sexual responses of men and women, from which developed the behavioral approach in treating sexual dysfunction, was a giant step forward in sexual research. Initially, Masters (1959) presented his data on the physiological response of the vagina to adequate sexual stimulation at the New York Academy of Science. Although this research was of a most revolutionary type, it elicited very little interest from the medical community. Later Drs. Masters and Johnson sought to have their work published in obstetrical and gynecological literature, but to no avail. Finally it was accepted and published in the *Western Journal of Surgery* (Masters and Johnson, 1960). Their difficulty was the persistent taboo prohibiting physicians from investigating human sexuality. However, unlike Dr. Denslow Lewis who, at the turn of the century, failed to have his research published, Masters and Johnson succeeded in publicizing their ideas. Five principal developments resulted:

1. The Freudian concept that only a vaginal orgasm was a mature response was questioned. An orgasm was recognized as such no matter what the sexual stimulation—homosexual stimulation, heterosexual stimulation, masturbation, or fantasy.
2. Physicians could now engage in sex research without being ostracized from their medical and social communities.
3. Short-term behavioral therapy for the treatment of sexual dysfunction was developed and learned by many health care professionals.
4. The importance of not only genital stimulation, but total body stimulation in achieving sexual gratification was substantiated.
5. The concept that sexuality is a form of communication between two people developed, and the concept of the uninvolved partner was rejected.

Most strategies of sexual therapy used today are based on the work of Masters and Johnson. Utilizing their techniques results in an 80 percent success rate and a more rapid response to therapy, often obviating the necessity for expensive traditional psychotherapy.

While Masters and Johnson were obtaining information regarding the physiological responses to adequate sexual stimulation, Drs. John Money and Anke Erhardt were studying the development of sexual identity and the importance of hormonal stimulation during fetal development. Their work has largely dispelled the fetal unisex concept. The effects of fetal androgens, which ultimately influence adult sexual behavior, on the developing brain are continuing to be elucidated. During the same period the effects of neonatal deprivation of affection in the monkey were demonstrated to result in abnormal sexual function in these primates by adulthood.

Recently Ernest Borneman, Ph.D., (1983) presented data based on 30 years of research on the sexual behavior of children. His conclusions are that:

1. prior to the anal, oral, and genital periods, there is a "Cutaneous Phase" that stems from stimulation of the infant's

skin and allows adult sexuality to be transgenital
2. separation anxiety of infants occurs only when there is inadequate love between their parents or when there is unfulfilled commitment by their parents
3. the Oepidus complex need not be developed as it is not seen in children from Kibbutzim or extended families
4. sexual behavior is the manifestation of psychosexual development which is independent of genital maturity.

His revolutionary findings contest the earlier observations of Freud and are indicative of the continuing need to question old theories concerning human psychosexual development.

## REFERENCES

Abse, D. W.; Nash, E. M.; and Louden, L M. R.: *Marital and Sexual Counseling in Medical Practice.* Harper and Row, Hagerstown, Md, 1974.

Borneman, E.: Progress in empirical research on children's sexuality. *SIECUS Rep.,* 12/Nov.: , 1983.

Breecher, E. M.: History of human sexual research and study. In Freedman, A. M.; Kaplan, H.; Sadock, B. J.: (eds.): *Comprehensive Textbook of Psychiatry/II,* 2nd ed. Williams and Wilkins, Baltimore, 1975.

Breecher, E. M.: History of human sexual research and study. In Sadock, B. J.; Kaplan, H.; Freedman, A. M.: (eds.): *The Sexual Experience,* 1st ed., Williams and Wilkins, Baltimore, 1976, pp. 71–78.

Deutch, H.: *Psychology of Women.* Grune and Stratton, New York, 1944.

Dickinson, R. L.: *Atlas of Human Sex Anatomy.* Williams and Wilkins, Baltimore, 1933.

Klemer, R. H.: *Counseling in Marital and Sexual Problems.* Williams and Wilkins, Baltimore, 1965.

Krogen, W. S., and Freed, S. G.: *Psychosomatic Obstetrics and Gynecology.* Saunders Company, Philadelphia, 1951.

Lewis, D.: The gynecologic consideration of the sexual act. *JAMA,* 250:222–227, 1983.

Lief, H. I.: What medical schools teach about sex. Bull. *Tulane U. Med. Faculty,* 22: 1963.

Masters, W. H.: The sexual response cycle of the human female: Vaginal lubrication. *Ann. NY Acad. NYAS,* Sci. 83:301–317, 1959.

Masters, W. H.: The sexual response of the human female. I. Gross anatomic considerations. *Western J. Surg. Obstet. Gynecol.* 68:57–62, 1960.

Nash, E. M.; Jessner, L.; and Abse, D. W.: *Marriage Counseling in Medical Practice.* University of North Carolina, Chapel Hill, 1964.

Sciarra, J. J.: Vaginal contraception: Historical perspective. In Zatuchni, G. I.; Sobrero, A. J.; Speidel, J. J.; and Sciarra, J. J.: (eds.): *Vaginal Contraception: New Developments,* 1st ed. Harper and Row, Hagerstown, Md, 1979.

Sussman, N.: Sex and sexuality in history. In Sadock, B. J.; Kaplan, H.; Freedman, A. M.: (eds.): *The Sexual Experience,* 1st ed. Williams and Wilkins, Baltimore, 1976, pp. 7–70.

# CHAPTER 2  PREPUBERTAL AND PUBERTAL PSYCHOSEXUAL DEVELOPMENT

*Leonardo Magran, M.D.*

## INTRODUCTION

In the sequential phases of human development, puberty is a period of rapid physical and psychological growth, matched only by the early years of childhood (Daniel, 1983). In some ways puberty replicates that earlier period at a more advanced level of integration and functioning. In observing the behavior and attitudes of the teenager, one is impressed by the return of the repressed oral, anal-sadistic, phallic expression of instinctual drives, conflicts over infantile dependency and overly assertive autonomy, Oedipal issues and concomitant guilt, as well as by the heroic attempts by the ego to maintain an unstable balance between the unswerving demands of the id, the policing superego, and an often confusing and contradictory outer world, itself baffled by the young person's needs (Blos, 1962).

In this process of acclimation to a new, revolutionary development, culminating with the capacity to procreate, the individual shapes and reshapes in the psyche the introjected representations of self and object that started early in life and progress at a hectic rate during puberty. The qualitative and quantitative changes in instinctual forces, based on the neuroendocrine activation at puberty and efforts by the ego to muster these biological forces as it searches for a sense of personal identity, occur against a background of continued and progressive disengagement from the family of origin. Mainly, in the present, these are the parents, but most significantly they are the introjects of the remote past.

This author considers the effort at disengagement from the parental images, with accompanying reaction to object loss and restitutional attempts, to be the most trying, desperate and conflictual dilemma of the teenage years. Its vicissitudes, manifestations, and resolution depend greatly on the manner in which the original separation–individuation process of early childhood was worked through, assisted by the loving, supportive, understanding parent(s) (Mahler, Pine, and Bergman, 1975).

In this chapter the nouns "puberty" and "adolescence" will be used interchangeably, although puberty is preferred to signify the biological growth leading to sexual maturation and reproduction, while adolescence, as a more inclusive term, is extended to cover the psychosocial aspects of this stage of development (Shonfeld, 1971).

In the reciprocal interaction between the individual and the environment, as well as in the reciprocal interaction among the different agencies of the mind (ego, superego, and id), conflicts are unavoidable and involve psychological functions aimed at controlling, managing, and, if possible, resolving them. Assisted in these mechanisms of defense, other functions operating outside the areas of conflict, that is, the conflict-free ego sphere, facilitate the adaptation of individuals to the required tasks of their social groups. During adolescence the development of cognitive functions attains the highest level of operation—abstract thinking—promoting in the young person the capacity to reason, judge, evaluate *a priori* the consequences of personal actions and alternatives to problems (Dulit, 1983). The achievement of this stage of cognitive development results in the phasing out of the adolescent period and the attainment of adulthood. Consequently, a multiplicity of phenomena characterize this period and will be examined separately in the following subsections. They do not occur independently from one another, but in intimate interaction and interrelationship.

## PHYSICAL CHANGES AND EMOTIONAL REACTIONS ASSOCIATED WITH PUBERTY

### THE ENDOCRINOLOGY OF PUBERTY

The onset of puberty is triggered by the maturation of the brain, more specifically, the activity of the hypophysiotropic cells of the median eminence of the hypothalamus, which at that time exhibits a decreased sensitivity to the negative feedback effects of the circulating sex hormones and increases the production of luteinizing hormone-releasing hormone (LHRH) acting upon the pituitary gland. This change in the gonadostat, that is, the response of the hypothalamic cells to the gonadal steriods, initiates a cascade effect whereby LHRH will stimulate the secretion by the anterior pituitary gland of two gonadotrophins: follicle stimulating hormone (FSH) and luteinizing hormone (LH), which in turn activate the testes and ovaries to produce androgens and estrogens.

In the male, the Sertoli cells of the testes and certain cells of the epididymis respond to the influence of FSH by producing an androgen-binding protein and inhibin, a protein that by negative feedback inhibits the release of FSH by the pituitary. FSH also stimulates the opening of the seminiferous tubules leading to the enlargement of the testes in early puberty. The luteinizing hormone (LH), acts on the Leydig cells causing them to secrete testosterone, the main male hormone, and small amounts of estradiol, the equivalent female hormone. Testosterone reaches the seminiferous tubules directly from the interstitial spaces where the Leydig cells are located, and promotes the maturation of spermatozoa. It is also secreted into the blood stream, by which conduit it reaches the target organs initiating and supporting the development of the secondary sex characteristics. It exerts an inhibitory effect upon the release of LHRH and LH on the hypothalamus and pituitary respectively (Bardin and Paulsen, 1981; Federman, 1984b).

Similar developments in the female lead to the maturation of ovarian follicles and the unfolding of secondary sex characteristics. As in the male, LHRH is transported to the anterior pituitary via the pituitary portal system where it stimulates the secretion of FSH and LH, but different from the male in whom the secretion is maintained at a pulsatile tonic, sustained level, the pulses follow a cyclic pattern with a marked midcycle increase FSH begins to rise in the last few days of the preceding menstrual period leading to the ripening of follicles and increased secretion of estradiol. One of the follicles overtakes the rest and will rupture halfway into the cycle following a sudden increase in FSH and LH, resulting from a positive feedback of estrogen, presumably upon the pituitary. As suddenly as this rise occurs, it drops when the oocyte is released and the corpus luteum is formed. Progesterone, the primary hormone of the corpus luteum, begins to rise together with estradiol. Both levels fall at the end of two weeks, and endometrial shedding and a menstrual period ensues unless pregnancy has occurred. Initially and for the following year or two only about 10 percent of the cycles are ovulatory.

It takes from three to five years after menarche for the cycles to become consolidated, that is, more regularly ovulatory (Federman, 1984a; Ross, Vande Wiele, Frantz, 1981).

In sum, the orderly interplay of the hypothalamic–pituitary–gonadal system, whose operation is primarily determined by genetic factors, but influenced by environmental and psychological forces, will—around the age of 10 in the female and 12 in the male—initiate the process that will culminate in full reproductive capacity, physical and psychological maturity, and the social rank of adulthood.

## Physical Changes Associated with Puberty

The age of onset, rate, and range of physical changes during puberty varies with different individuals, but once initiated follows a relatively set pattern. This has facilitated the development of diagnostic criteria in the evaluation of pubertal progress and maturational level (Tanner, 1962).

Females mature earlier than males. This has been the trend all along since birth, and by puberty the age difference averages two years. The female growth spurt also starts before the male, about age 9 or 10 and reaches its peak shortly before menarche, usually by age 12, at which point it begins to decline. The male growth spurt begins around age 12 and does not peak until 14 or 15 while the development of secondary sex characteristics is in full bloom (Shonfeld, 1971; Vaughan, 1983). In the majority of adolescents full physical maturity is achieved by the age of 16 in the sense that both sexes are now capable of procreation.

Puberty starts in the female with the budding of the breasts and the skeletal growth spurt followed by the appearance of pubic hair, at first downy and later on progressively coarser, pigmented, and curled. The contour of the body acquires the classical feminine shape of broad, rounded hips due to the remolding of the bony pelvis and the deposition of fat. During this period, there is also an enlargement of the uterus, vagina, labia, and clitoris. Axillary hair begins to grow when the girl begins to menstruate but does not reach its full thickness until late adolescence or early adulthood.

In males the beginning of puberty is less noticeable than in females and starts at age 10 or 11 with a slight enlargement of the testes, due to increased spermatogenetic activity and the opening of the seminiferous tubules, and of the penis, and the appearance of straight downy pubic hair, which progressively increases in thickness, pigmentation, and curliness. With the acceleration of skeletal growth, the speed of growth in size of the testes and the penis, and the pigmentation of the scrotum increases. Seminal emission follows and with it the skeletal growth spurt slows down though it continues for a longer period of time than in the female due to the continuous presence of testosterone. Final height may not be reached until 18, by which time axillary hair has grown almost to adult thickness, the deepening of the voice due to the enlargement of the larynx and vocal chords has occurred, as well as increased muscular development and physical strength. The appearance and multiplication of sebaceous and sudorific, odorific glands in the facial skin, axilla, genitals, and anus, causes changes in body odor, and the possible development of acne. Seminal emissions, which mark the increased activity of the testes and prostate gland, are sterile for some time but after a couple of years, as in the female, acquire the full capacity for impregnation and consequently procreation.

## Emotional Reactions to the Physical Changes in Puberty

Before the secondary sex characteristics, the growth spurt, and reproductive functions make their appearance, the activation of the endocrine system results in an increase in energy, restlessness, instability, distractibility, forgetfulness, and a myriad of vague symptoms. These are often interpreted as emotional rather than physiological and are ignored, discounted, or examined with too much consideration, since they are of passing significance at this stage of development (English and Pearson, 1955; Group for the Advancement of Psychiatry, 1975).

Some youngsters are excited at the prospect of puberty, others are worried; some appear indifferent, and many take it in their stride. The reactions described here refer primarily to the response the child experiences in perception, interpretations, and behavior to the actual changes in body size, shape, and functions during this period. Obviously, these reactions will be highly influenced by the child's personality make-up, ongoing intrapsychic changes, and family responses, but will center primarily on what the child sees and feels at the more concrete level of physical maturation. Youngsters worry about their height, the contour of their body, pimples, and appearance. Their concerns are mainly physical which, in the extreme, may become obsessive and hypochondriacal.

Those youngsters who mature earlier may have difficulties in adjustment based on the discrepancy between their chronological age and physical development. They feel alienated from peers their age and draw toward older teenagers who, by this time, may be intensively involved heterosexually and in activities for which the younger child is ill-suited and of which the parents disapprove. The child's excitement and anxieties associated with these activities are often reflected in a loss of interest in school, excessive daydreaming, and a drop in academic performance. Judged lazy by parents and irresponsible by teachers, the youngster, who really cannot help feeling this way, has to contend now with the problem of disappointing parents, teachers, and a personal ego ideal. The youngster may become angry and defiant, demanding more freedom to associate with the older children, or depressed and despondent by failure. Despite these problems, the early maturers seem to overtake their peers in emotional, cognitive, and social maturity. The late maturer, on the other hand, may show greater insecurity, sensitivity, and awkwardness. Although physical maturity eventually keeps pace, the latecomer remains restless, irritable, and immature.

Boys during this period are concerned with the size and shape of their penis, the appearance and distribution of pubic hair, and then facial and body hair. Acne may be a source of considerable distress at this time, not only because of blemishes, but for the misconception that acne betrays sexual interest and masturbatory activities. Also of concern is fat distribution which, other than in obesity, may suggest femininity. Concerns about this can produce an aversion to going to school and participating in physical activities. A transient enlargement of the breasts, gynecomastia, if not handled properly may turn into a traumatic disorder by affecting the youngster's sense of self-esteem, gender identity, and sexual orientation. Because adolescents are exquisitely sensitive to their appearance, these concerns should not be treated lightly by adults. Otherwise, what started as a resistance to attend classes may develop into a full-blown phobia, hindering the child more seriously.

The most common focus for girls is the development of the breasts and the onset of menstruation. Breasts, as the most visible secondary sex characteristic, attract the most attention. As a source of erotic pleasure, they also betray the girl's interest in sex, about which she may have some conflicts. Consequently, those who are inhibited will feel ashamed and try to hide their breasts; others, in rebellious assertiveness, will throw the chest out in denial of any apprehension or self-consciousness. In those whose breasts develop late, strong feelings of inadequacy may appear, leading to social isolation and depression.

Menses and seminal emissions trouble many adolescents, in spite of the information available to them at home and at school because the information received deals mostly with the physical and physiological aspects of copulation and reproduction. Menstruation and ejaculation may be discussed with little attention to feelings, interests and concerns involving other issues, such as parenting and family formation, love, tenderness, caring, responsibilities toward one another. Presentations of this sort reveal the ambivalence of adults toward sexuality, particularly to the young who may have a greater need to learn about relationships than sexuality *per se.*

Despite our present-day freedom to experience and learn, the knowledge acquired does not influence the fantasies on which much of human behavior is based. These fantasies, the normal by-product of psychosexual development, distort the perception and color whichever concepts are learned with the particular affect and assumptions of younger years. Menstruation in fantasy, may represent damage to the genitals as it was perceived in early childhood, or may be associated with excretory activities and conflicts of the anal-sadistic stage, or may be related to fantasies of violence in intercourse linked to the primal scene, incestual wishes, and rape. Seminal emissions may also cause concern because of unconscious fantasies of a similar nature, aggressive as well as erotic, rooted in urinary–anal-sadistic discharge, loss of control and injury, castration anxiety, and fear of loss of potency and the capacity to procreate. The extent to which these unconscious fantasies influence the perceptions, developments, and assimilation of new knowledge will depend on the resolution of the unavoidable conflicts present at every stage of psychosexual development, which involves instinctual drives in interaction with the maturing ego–superego system and the external world.

In dealing with the pubertal child it is important that parents, teachers, and doctors, recognize that physical complaints, diminished scholastic performance, increased or low energy levels with periods of overactivity and periods of lethargy, may be the transitory expression of biological changes and concerns associated with these changes. These concerns will diminish in time as the ego–superego structures regain control over the instinctual drives, and reality testing again supersedes fantasy as the child progresses toward the late phase of adolescence and adulthood.

## PSYCHOLOGICAL DEVELOPMENT FROM BIRTH THROUGH ADOLESCENCE

In the preceding section the physical and physiological changes characteristic of adolescence have stressed the arrival of the individual at biological possibilities at once exciting and feared and of his emotional reactions to these changes. In this section the intrapsychic rearrangements and evolution in interpersonal relations will be examined. The progressive adaptation of the pubertal child to this new role thrust upon him by the dual influence of the increased instinctual urges and societal expectations require three major efforts: (1) learning to control impulses, (2) separating from parents, and (3) establishing independence, while redirecting energy toward the pursuit of new, stable attachments and training to assure financial independence as well (Blos, 1962; Group for the Advancement of Psychiatry, 1975).

The ease or difficulty with which an adolescent will succeed in achieving these goals will depend on the child's upbringing to that point, the ways and means learned to adjust to the ongoing and endless negotiations with the environment to secure the gratification of basic needs and needs for expansion, the response of the caretakers to these needs, any intrapsychic unresolved conflicts affecting present day decisions, and the internal operation of what has become the conscience.

### The Childhood Years: From Birth to Latency

For most of the first year of life, the infant's concerns center around survival. The need for food and shelter, so to speak, overshadows every other consideration and dependency on the caretaker, preferably the mother, is extreme to the point that without her support the infant may die.

Infants are born with different temperaments, as anybody walking through a nursery of neonates can attest. They are different in the intensity of their instinctual demands, their intolerance in the fulfillment of these demands, and the manner in which they extract the necessary responses from the environment. Some react with a smile, some with a frown, some settle down quickly, some take a long time to regain their composure whenever their homeostasis is disturbed by internal (instinctual) or external (sensory) stimulation. Infants are endowed with limited reflex responses and have to learn appropriate actions to obtain favorable reactions from, it is hoped, an accepting and nurturing environment. But the infant needs, wishes, and seeks out more than replenishment of nutrients or preservation of heat. During waking periods, an infant seeks the contact and stimulation of a caretaker without whom, the baby grows detached, lonely, distrustful, and despondent.

The good mother or caretaker in synchrony with the infant, supplies the material goods to satisfy oral needs and the stimulation that will draw the infant's attention away from an almost exclusive preoccupation with himself (primary narcissism), into an outer world where interesting things happen. The caretaker is simultaneously the tamer of the id and trainer of the budding ego. A continuous, predictable, dependable relationship with the mother supports the maturation of the infant through the initial autistic and symbiotic stages, which covers approximately the first six months of the first year, and the differentiating phase of the separation–individuation process, which covers the second half of the first year (Mahler et al., 1975).

By the end of this period, the child has a dim awareness of itself as separated from its mother—of the "me" and the "not me," the self and the object, and if a child's experiences with her have been, on the whole positive, the child will have developed basic trust; that is, a sense of relative certainty that needs will not go unmet indefinitely, causing unnecessary discomfort and despair. A child's sensory and motor intelligence is also progressing to the point where he is now capable of alternatives to trial and error attempts at problem-solving, because of the substitution of a more logical means-to-an-end approach (Piaget and Inhelder, 1969).

Equipped with these new assets of self-delineation, basic trust, and cognitive resources, more stable on their own two feet and uttering words to express wants, children now venture out into an exciting exploration of the world, never too far from the mother, to whom they often return for anchor. In this practicing phase of the separation–individuation process, which lasts for about six months, children achieve greater mastery of mobility and expressive language as they move around investigating whatever strikes their fancy, under the watchful vigilance of the protective adult. This further facilitates the intrapsychic establishment of self and object representations which, in turn, lead to object permanence, the awareness that out of sight does not mean necessarily out of existence, and a different modality of transacting with the environment.

When reaching the rapprochement phase, at about 18 months, a child who in zest for mastery of action and communication has neglected the mother somewhat, now wants her and other members of the family to share in discoveries, play, and investigations. Still omnipotent in their wishes and assumptions, children demand the cooperation of others and resent their indifference or rebuff. As the education of toilet habits is being instituted at this time, a child learns that he must conform to certain requirements to be accepted as a desirable member of the group. But these expectations run contrary to his own anal-sadistic interests, and the transactions that in the early oral stage were negotiated around the kitchen table have now been displaced to the bathroom area.

This displacement in the environment has also taken place in the child's own mind where oral-libidinal and aggressive-instinctual impetus have moved downward to the lower gastrointestinal tract, its contents, the anus, and its surroundings. The child begins to learn more forcefully about discipline, time and place, as well as control over feces. The child decides to withhold them, relinquish them, or smear them for pleasure or revenge for what is perceived as intolerable oppression by adults. Here again, as happened before and will happen over and over again in the future, a compromise is reached where both partners emerge from the struggle reasonably satisfied with the outcome; this occurs in a situation where behavior was learned within the context of a supportive, encouraging, loving, dyadic relationship between the young child and the primary caretaker.

The young child's sense of omnipotence is brought to a sudden halt when that child realizes his power to control the outside world, in reality and fantasy, is limited. This knowledge causes a serious blow to the primary narcissism which may heal, though never completely, if compensatory rewards are bestowed for the mastery of primitive impulses sublimated in behaviors more acceptable by the child's small society. Another observation of this period which brings grief to the child, aside from the realization that he does not stand at the center of the world, is the observation of the anatomical differences between boys and girls. To the loss of infantile omnipotence and its negative impact on nascent self-esteem, the befuddlement, confusion, uncertainty, anxiety, and disappointment resulting from this discovery adds its burden of doubts about physical integrity, competence, and potential for success.

The rapprochement phase, which lasts for about 18 months, is a period of considerable turmoil for the child and the caretaker during which significant developments occur. Under favorable conditions the child is persuaded to control his sphincters and aggression, and he is loved for it. In his exploratory zest he has, now it is hoped, a willing companion who is at one and the same time a peer and a mentor, a facilitator and a protector, who without discounting the child's need for autonomy and self-realization shows new, perhaps more exciting, but always more constructive ways to play as a precursor for work; to react, as a precursor of self-esteem regulation; and to relate, as a precursor of concern and consideration for others. The rapprochement phase, which started with the closing of the sensory–motor stage of cognitive development and achievement of object permanence, comes to a close of its own when object constancy is reached between 3 and 3½ years of age. While object permanence defines the operation of ego function such as perception and memory, object constancy refers to crucial intrapsychic formations of self and object representations with its accompanying affective valences (Kernberg, 1976).

The child who had emerged relatively unscathed from the separation–individuation process will be better equipped to progress through the next stages of growth and development, assimiliating and adapting to the tasks of those stages with ease and self-confidence as well as trust and reliability in the good will of others. The child is now prepared to attend nursery school away from home and mother, without succumbing to separation anxiety and to engage in the Oedipal struggle without being overwhelmed by castration anxiety or the hurt and resentment of the castration complex. This child will have emerged from the quasi-exclusive dyadic relationship with its mother into a wider network of triadic and multiple associations, from the pregenital to the genital instinctual cathexis and ego organization.

The genital stage of psychosexual development with the Oedipal complex at its center lasts roughly from 3 to 6 years of age. Sexual feelings and fantasies combined with affectionate attachment are directed toward the parent of the opposite sex, while ambivalent feelings toward the parent of the same sex typically color the interaction among the members in this family developmental drama and the intrapsychic rearrangement necessary to overcome it. The resolution of the Oedipal complex, the neurophysiological maturation of the brain and the entrance into a new phase of cognitive development mark the beginning of the latency period.

This period represents an interlude between the intense and rapid changes of the preceding years and those which occur during puberty

(Blos, 1962; English and Pearson, 1955). The relative quiescence of this stage results from firmer control that the ego has mustered over the libidinal and aggressive drives, assisted in its efforts by the progressive internalization and definition of the superego. As the early years of childhood culminate in the establishment of object constancy, also implying the establishment of constancy of the self, so will the latency years culminate in the attainment of superego constancy. While before the child needed the presence of the parents to guide and regulate behavior, now the child seems more capable of doing it alone. The child is more interested in learning skills (an ego function) and rules of conduct (a superego function) and requires less parental approval to sustain self-esteem than peer approval through the mastery of competence and fairness.

For the female to negotiate the sublimatory, defensive, and adaptive changes of this period, she will be torn, for a while, between the need to identify with her mother, the object of gratification as well as frustration and disappointment, and regression to the dependent, infantile position of early childhood. For her to progress, she must forcefully repress her pregenital instinctual interests while proceeding relatively free in the direction of heterosexuality, propelled by the undiminished attraction toward the male even though sexual wishes for her father must be relinquished. She does not meet the threat of castration during the genital stage of psychosexual development as the boy does with the resultant effect that her Oedipal conflict does not come to a sudden and stringent halt, but may linger until the time she marries and has her first child.

The male has a more difficult time with these conflicts. He has renounced the genital instinctual urges and incestual wishes toward his mother, but not his early affectionate and dependent love relationship with her. He can proceed to identify with his father while at the same time act in a more immature fashion where the expression of outmoded sexual and aggressive impulses are again reactivated, such as exhibitionistic, voyeuristic, sadomasochistic patterns of behavior. The boy will move away from girls and find respect in his associations with other boys.

This difference in the nature of repression is needed to facilitate identification with the parent of the same sex. Pregenital drives in the female and genital drives in the male explain the earlier psychological maturation of the female in whom sexual interests continue unabated. However, these are centered less in the anatomical aspects of sexuality than in the physiological, such as menstruation, conception, pregnancy, and so on. These dual intrapsychic developments of repression and identification are the trademark of the latency period, one harnessing instincts while the other promotes growth and mastery.

Stability in mood and attitude, the industry with which children apply themselves to work and learning, their awareness of and greater empathy with social situations, their use of logical and methodical reasoning, their adherence to values, ideas, and rules of conduct, are clear indications that a significant shift has occurred within the realms of the mind. Here the ego and superego have gained ascendancy over the id and relationships are less strained and conflicted than in the preceding phases (Blos, 1962).

These transformations and rerouting of cathexis occur within the wider scope of the separation–individuation process, which never ceases but reverberates throughout life, reaffirming and reinforcing at every stage of human development the three most crucial accomplishments of man's strivings object constancy, superego constancy, and identity constancy, manifested at the close of adolescence.

## THE PREPUBERTAL YEARS

The latency years constitute a necessary respite for the ego to gain mastery of the environment and control of the instinctual drives supported by the superego. By this time the child has incorporated and identified with the values, expectations, and attitudes of the parents primarily, as well as of those individuals whom the child has found attractive and worthwhile. The superego has become more firmly established within the intrapsychic structure of the mind.

This relative calm in the child and the surroundings becomes steadily and progressively disrupted by the endocrine changes which begin to occur around 8 or 9 years of age, preceding pubertal bodily changes but nonetheless causing physical discomfort such as vague body sensations, emotional lability, and increased activity (Goldings, 1979; Group for the Advancement of Psychiatry, 1975). Children play more vigorously, but maintain the segregation between the sexes that marked the preceding phase, although there are evidences of an increasing wish to mix, more often in negative ways than in friendly overtures. Boys flaunt their dislike of girls or tease them as they brag about their prowess, while girls reassert their competitive claims in a burst of tomboyish behavior. There is considerable interest and curiosity in siblings or peers who have already reached puberty: the way they act, what they say, the reaction of the parents and other adults to their changes.

As the attitude of society towards sexuality has been, on the whole, ambivalent and the response of the parents to the impending changes of puberty conflicting, the youngsters themselves develop an attitude of anxious anticipation and an obsessive preoccupation for sexual matters. They also demonstrate a relative loss of interest in tasks or activities the parents regard as necessary but for the child are now of lesser priority. In private and among peers there is active self-investigation and mutual exploration, and stimulation of the body and its pleasureable and reproductive functions about which the child may have been informed through conversations with the parents and lectures at school. This information however, may have been insufficient or inadequate to dispel the youngster's misunderstanding of the meaning and expression of sexuality. The lack of certainty based on the ambivalence of the grown-ups, with their conflicting and confusing messages, the intrapsychic conscious and unconscious conflict between the demands of the instinctual drives and their rejection by the superego, and the need to rely on one's limited experience and understanding and those of peers, strain the ego's adaptational resources and causes it to either mobilize its defenses, which will assist it in its efforts, or weaken its controls and proficiency. The child becomes more difficult to reach, to reason with, and to control; just the opposite of the way the child was during the latency period.

The fluidity of drives and defenses causes physical complaints such as headaches, free-floating anxiety or phobias, irritability, sleeping problems, regressive behavior, and the like. Boys show envy of the capacity of women to procreate in their raising and caring for pets, and interest in their mating and reproductive behavior, while girls display envy of the male in their aggressive, forward, overly assertive attitudes and actions. Some children hold on to the more peaceful existence of the latency period and deny that practically any change is taking place; others regress to a more comfortable dependent position, while still others will jump ahead of themselves and join older teenagers in a show of pseudo-adolescence and pseudo-heterosexuality.

In the passage through the prepubertal years, one may be able to identify aspects of the separation–individuation process described in early childhood that become even more accentuated at the onset of puberty. For example, in their increasing insistence to have their own way and in their increasing activity, one may see indications of the differentiating–practicing phases of the separation–individuation process, while at the same time as manifested by their voracious appetite, disorderliness, dirtiness, "bathroom humor," and such, one may see regressive indications of oral and anal instinctual expression. The changes of latency to puberty are akin to walking in quicksand. In abandoning the firmer grounds of latency to arrive at the next station in psychosexual development, the child will need to travel through uncharted territory. Old fears, conflicts, and styles of coping re-emerge with varying resolve and results as he struggles to reach his destination.

## PUBERTY

The psychological balance reached during the latency period of psychosexual development and mildly disturbed during the prepubertal years is handed a jolt at the onset of puberty. The upsurge in the instinctual sexual and aggressive drives tilts the scale in favor of the id and taxes the ego–superego system which, for the next several years (until the midteens) will struggle to re-establish an equilibrium in the functioning of the personality and in the relationship between the individual and the social milieu. The significant difference in the behavior of the young adolescent when compared with that of the older adolescent (from midteens to 18) justifies the separation of this period into two major phases: early adolescence and late adolescence, where the balance of power shifts back to the ego.

**Early Adolescence.** Youngsters react to the onset of puberty in diverse ways based on previous styles of adaptation and the response generated in parents and other significant figures in their lives (Malmquist, 1979). Some react by ignoring the changes and holding on to the prescribed behavior of the latency years when subordination to and cooperation with established regimes were the rule. To attain this posture the individual needs to restrain himself or herself and restrict activities in order to avoid any expression of aggression and sexuality which may meet with disapproval by parents or the superego. An example of this is the youngster who avoids joining his peers in social, athletic, or recreational activities and spends most of his time engaged in intellectual pursuits. Others will do just the opposite: neglect their chores and obligations in a constant search for excitement, rebelling against any attempts by parents and others responsible for their care, as if suddenly all manners of control have dissolved and only, or primarily, the instinctual expression of needs ought to be gratified. These adolescents are demanding and unreasonable, hostile and impulsive, thoughtless and self-centered.

Many youngsters express concerns over the changes taking place in their bodies in hypochondriacal complaints or anxious preoccupations. For the majority, the ebb and flow of instinctual demands remains within acceptable boundaries instituted by the ego–superego and adult control and guidance. Whatever the reaction, close observation and inquiry reveal that the behavior is the result of strong erotic and aggressive impulses which seem to have come from nowhere and clamor for expression. The sudden disequilibrium of the psychic apparatus is evidenced in the unstable and often bizarre conduct of the child who may have been an exemplary model of respect and moderation until then. This adolescent vascillates between a loud assertion of the right to do "his own thing" and succumbing to the wish to be as pampered and indulged as a little child. Breakthroughs of instinctual desires occur in trying to catch a glimpse of the naked parent or sibling, with pangs of guilt, embarrassment, and seclusion to expiate the deed. There is regression to sloppiness, disorderliness, negativism, neglect of personal hygiene, and often a decline in school performance (the "seventh or eighth grade slump"). All these are indicative of the unrest and battering of the old structures by the waves of new, instinctual inputs correlating with the increase in the production of steroid hormones by the gonads.

This stormy initial phase of pubertal changes, not all of it expressed behaviorally, alters course in the midteens. This shift is effected through a combination of factors involving: 1. the hormonal system, which has achieved some homeostatic constancy; 2. the mastery by the ego of the initially unclear, uncertain, and confusing instinctual feelings, fantasies, interests, and interactions promoted by them; 3. the relaxation of parental ties, actual or from the incorporated past; 4. turning away from the family toward a girlfriend or boyfriend in whom to fulfill sexual as well as dependent needs.

A major shift also occurs at this time in cognitive development—from the concrete operational modality to the formal operational style, which implies that the youngster thinks not just about things, but about ideas, concepts, theories, and so on (Dulit, 1983; Piaget and Inhelder, 1969; Rosen, 1977). By moving away from the immediate need to link thoughts to action, an adolescent can utilize this increased capacity for the highest form of abstract thinking; that is, "he thinks before he leaps." Therefore, adolescents will reason things out in their own minds before carrying them out and question by words rather than deed accepted dicta of society, such as religion, politics, morals, and decisions by the ruling classes about matters that affect present needs for autonomy and future opportunities for growth and performance. The acrimonious arguments give way to calmer discussions and negotiations of conflict with increased acceptance of both parties of the inevitability of growth, distancing, and reciprocity if the developing young person is to achieve parity and at some point to replace the adult.

Adolescence is a time when the separation–individuation process of early childhood is reawakened and worked through over and over again. Consequently, in the behavior of the child during the pubertal years, one may be able to identify the phases of this process with emphasis on re-establishing a sense of self separate from the object, now not simply in the physical sense, but in a more expanded sense, incorporating the vastly important aspect of gender identity and opportunities for heterosexual interaction devoid of instinctual underpinning.

It is against this background of early childhood attempts at establishing himself intrapsychically and in reality, *vis à vis* the caretaker (namely the parents), that a young adolescent tests newly acquired functions and potential for action. If the separation–individuation process of the early years proceeded smoothly, one may reasonably expect that the secondary separation–individuation process of adolescence will be equally successful (Blos, 1967). If that was not the case, even though the adolescent process may come to a close, the organization of the personality may lack the stability and maturity in adulthood of those who were more fortunate. It is characteristic of this period that the young person does not remain uniformly level in attitude and behavior but, to the contrary, alternates between disturbed behavior and relative quiescence. These episodes of turmoil and calmness may last minutes or hours or extend over several months. The breakthrough of more primitive instinctual acting out will be restored when the ego regains its equilibrium and returns the functioning of the individual to the competence attained when calm. This variation in adjustment is often disturbing, always befuddling, and aims at testing both the inner resources, defenses, and coping mechanisms and external controls and acceptance. The intervening period following the disruptive episodes can prove productive in learning about the manner in which the episode could have been handled more effectively.

In early adolescence the spurt in physical growth, the growth of the genitalia, and the appearance of secondary sex characteristics cause intense preoccupation in the young person who observes the changes with apprehension and excited anticipation. With the onset of menstruation in the female and ejaculation in the male, the added capability for reproduction increases the concern for what may now happen as a consequence of the loss of control of one's impulses, excitement over the newly acquired functions, and causing considerable doubts as to one's sexual competence. The earlier interest in parents' sexuality is reawakened at this time and incestual wishes and fantasies mobilize defenses against their becoming conscious, since by now the possibility for acting them out is very real. The young girl, who until now did not reject her father's affection, reacts to it with marked aversion. The boy, who until now did not mind shopping for clothes with his mother protests vociferously against it. They downgrade their parents and find them uninteresting, clumsy, unfriendly, and old-fashioned. They recoil at their expression of love for one another. At the same time, they are intensely curious about their parents' sexual behavior or that of older siblings; behaviors which they discuss with friends and occasionally try to watch, albeit discreetly.

The growth in physical size and strength,

the force of the sexual and aggressive drives, the awakening of incestuous desires and fantasies are met first by an attempt to shore up the existing defenses, all aimed at reducing the possibility of acting out with the parents. Rejection of the parents becomes then a necessary means to avoid forbidden taboos for which the severe punishment of castration looms large in the unconscious, but also the unremitting pull toward infantile gratification of narcissistic needs persists, that is, to be dependent on the parents (Freud, 1958; Marohn, 1983). The move towards independence is an imperative which sooner or later will be achieved if the maturational process is to be preserved and continued. The process of disengagement from parents does not imply an actual physical separation as is often suggested, but rather separation in the mind: emotional and psychological separation involving the internal representation of self and objects with the redirection of cathexis away from parents and to others in the outside world. Adolescence brings less dependency on the parents for emotional support and less willingness to abide by their values, judgment, and advice. As a matter of course there is a debasement of parental beliefs, lifestyle, tastes, and choices often expressed by a total disregard for their feelings, as exemplified in the youngster of the affluent family who treasures torn blue jeans and worn-out sneakers.

Youngsters object to parental control even in situations which are relatively unimportant such as what to eat, how to dress, bedtime, and evenings out; or of greater concern, what company they keep, what places they visit, and in what activities they engage. It is a common complaint of the young that their parents do not trust them when, in actuality, parents in their concern simply wish to supervise to some extent their offsprings' whereabouts. What the youngster means is that parents suspect he may be engaging in the kind of behavior (mostly sexual) to which his own superego objects, but is projected on to elders. While parents seek reassurance that the youngster will not take unnecessary risks, the youngster insists that the parents are judgmental and disapproving. This conflict diminishes with the phasing in of late adolescence and its accompanying improved capacity to think abstractly.

It is in this push and pull that one can draw similarities among the different phases of the separation–individuation process of early childhood. The assertiveness, obstinancy, contrariness, and sloppiness; the wish to think, feel, and act differently resembles the "terrible two's" although, of course it is different from the toddler's narrow scope of experience and objects. Still the insistence and persistence in the wish for autonomy reminds and helps one to understand why excesses in actions and reactions, if regressive at some level, signify the reshaping, remodeling, and redefining of the sense of self and others. This process, one hopes, will increase the young person's objectivity, that is the perception of reality by this constant reactivating evaluation of the introject. In rejecting parental judgment young people distance themselves defensively as they repress unacceptable wishes and fantasies, and they also tear down and rebuild more adequate structures—helped by the advancement of the cognitive process to sustain them as they move irrevocably toward adulthood. Disengagement is accompanied by a deep sense of loss; not the actual loss of the parents, but the loss of the parents in their introjected representation and the relationship enjoyed until then between the introjected self and objects. This sense of loss is manifested and worked through in a fashion similar to mourning, and accounts for the moodiness of the adolescent which does not seem to have actual life experience precipitants. In addition to the moodiness, youngsters appear confused, indecisive, and, at times, unintelligent. Withdrawal from the parents has left them without previously provided guidelines and, as not having yet developed their own, they feel in limbo.

Many of these reactions will fade as the youngster begins to feel more familiar and comfortable with both the internal world and the external environment, but until that occurs feelings of loneliness and isolation may stir up strong wishes for self-gratification that could take multiple avenues: masturbation, eating, drug use, and sexual indulgence. If the youngster has a strong, built-in superego, he or she may react to the gratification of erotic or aggressive impulses with guilt, self-deprecation, and worsening of depression. The unhappy combination of sadness over the fantasized loss of the supportive introjects and guilt over the sense of badness for their self-indulgence sometimes leads adolescents to contemplate suicide as a way out of what appears to be an unresolvable dilemma. Equilibrium is restored or there is a swing in the opposite direction when another object for loving is found. Then, elation and excitement replace moodiness, lethargy, and boredom. Adolescence is a time of wide mood swings linked to losses and restitutions, whether real or fantasized.

As part of the restitutional efforts resulting from progressive disengagement from the parents, youngsters divert their interests toward teachers, neighbors, counselors, and, in a more distant (idealized) but equally intense fashion, to celebrities whom they come to emulate and incorporate as accretions to the new emerging self. Those relationships are often short-lived but all-consuming while they last, pointing to an intense need to incorporate, introject, and identify with compatible characteristics of the objects while repelling the unsuitable ones. The "crushes" of the young fall into this category of relationships, causing intense family distress on occasion because in the "practicing" behavior of this period the youngster appears particularly vulnerable to the influence of others, which is not always constructive. Nevertheless, most will return to the script of their past, this time with additions of their own.

The teenager who destroys these relationships does so for two reasons: his perception that the adults to whom he is attached may not provide that for which he seeks, and his fear of losing his budding sense of identity. In disengaging from the subordinate role of the child to the parent, a teen will not readily accept another adult to whom to submit. These are trial identities compared with the primary introjects and are either accepted or rejected with increasing selectivity and discrimination.

Much of the confusing, trying, distressing behavior of the early phase of puberty becomes clearer if one thinks in terms of the agonizing efforts at separation and individuation stemming from the sudden upsurge of sexuality and aggression, physical growth, and maturation, as well as the awareness of the acquisition of a new status—all of which call for a rearrangement of the old modes to accommodate the additional revolutionary changes advanced by puberty. The ambivalence stirred up by these changes is enormous as the demands for independence and autonomy and the rejection of parental or adult control or guidance is contradicted by the need for the love, care, and support of the parent—the wish to remain dependent and tied to the very object from whom the child needs to separate. The conflict is made worse because the rebellion, at first verbal, becomes active as the child grows older, worsening the parents' feelings of helplessness and despair. Although more often than not the conflict remains within manageable limits, it is also true that with the scant support the extended family provides in contemporary society, the nuclear family is left to deal with the conflict alone, straining its emotional endurance and exhausting the family's resources to the breaking point (Katz, 1983). In the same way that the pubertal child needs the physical presence, support, limit setting, and encouragement of the family while experiencing developmental changes, the family benefits from the supportive cushion of an extended family or in its place a community with a clear understanding and a consistent attitude toward the young.

The adolescent is greatly assisted in the plight of growing up by peers. If the attachment to adults other than parents (as transient as they may be) provides the opportunity of reshaping the superego and ego ideals, a teen's relationship with peers will provide occasion to experience, experiment, and learn the common ways in which erotic and aggressive impulses are expressed, conflicts are worked out, and sublimatory avenues are found. The adolescent merges with peers by adapting and conforming to their habits, which will vary according to the group values and interests. They share the choice of attire, hairstyles, language, music, activities, and the like. With friends, a teenager also shares an intense and all-consuming curiosity about sex, which they now begin to practice in increasing, though tentative, contact with members of the opposite sex. With peers a teenager also practices the debunking of parents and others in authority whom they fear, distrust, and resent. Together they evolve a subculture of their own with interests, attitudes, values, and systems where many of the issues of concern can be exposed, explored, and tentatively resolved. It is a world where the young person escapes from the restraints imposed by the parent–superego and where a freer expression of the id is permissible. At the same time the ego tests and tries ways and means of bringing these opposing forces into line with the expectations of the community. In this sense, the peers serve an important function of providing the haven and the testing ground for learning about interpersonal relationships, both homosexual and heterosexual, and the part that intrapsychic operations play in their practice.

Associating with and talking to friends under normal circumstances fulfills such a need in the young adolescent that whenever thwarted from having direct contact, telephoning is a much used substitute. It gives the young boy and girl an open line for playing out their feelings toward one another without the awkwardness felt with physical presence. It puts some restraint on the overt stimulation which otherwise may sweep them away into a more intimate sexual involvement that they seek but may want to avoid. It also allows the young person an instant escape from an otherwise oppressive situation with parents, helps defuse conflicts when they become unbearably intense, and alleviates the loneliness brought about by the loss, real or imagined, of parental ties.

There are many such attitudes and activities that express the uncertainties and conflicts existing between the desire to interact with the opposite sex and the fear and guilt associated with it, stemming from all previous phases of psychosexual development. Aggression is mixed with sexuality to the point that horseplay between a brother and sister or taunting and embarrassing a classmate in front of others can be either aggressive or sexual, and it is often difficult to separate and manage appropriately. Through these activities, the youngster tests his or her own ability to control how far and how safe it is to practice quasi-adult behavior without actually indulging in it. Provocative sensual dancing, seductive exhibitionistic dressing, and peculiar language, aimed at keeping grown-ups off balance and confused (as the youngsters have little trouble understanding the meanings and innuendos) are all manifestations of a common goal: setting themselves apart from the older generation while trying to establish a nascent sense of psychosexual identity by experimenting with themselves and interacting with others with their newly emerged instinctual prowess.

Both boys and girls find a source of release and pleasure in masturbation that may become an organizing focus for later sexual behavior. Fantasies from earlier stages in the development together with fantasies in present-day association, anxieties of retaliations for earlier incestual wishes for the parent of the opposite sex, and ambivalent feelings toward the parent of the same sex are worked through and possibly resolved, as instinctual cathexis leaves the parental introjects in pursuit of actual objects to whom to relate—either adults or peers, homo or heterosexual. Homosexual encounters at this time are not unusual in boys and girls, and they may become extremely distressing if misjudged and mishandled. They are, as other breakthroughs of instinctual impulses (voyeurism, exhibitionism, transvestism) evidence of the disequilibrium of the ego in dealing with the forces of the id and superego pressing from within, and the temptations, restrictions, and retaliations pressing from without.

The mastery of the drives by the overtaxed ego is made more difficult by the process of separation that is taking place simultaneously. The young individual is deprived of the support and guidance that helped to sustain him before. The teenager is wobbling through the initial phase of puberty very much as the young child was wobbling along, learning to walk. The emotional response is often dramatic and so often misinterpreted that further alienation ensues until a new object for love and sustenance is found. During this period the young person tends to be action-oriented and sometimes impulsive, as if some of the controlling powers, which characterized the latency period, have been lost. This tendency to act stems from an increase in physical energy, as a means for the release of tension, as an expression of anxiety, or as a defense against it. An increase in energy as a release of tension is age-appropriate, servicing the ego in its maturational drives; the increase to express or avoid anxiety is symptomatic of imbalance or maladjustment, for which some intervention may be required.

As youngsters mature and the cognitive functions of the ego advance, they will slow down and substitute thinking for action, which means that they will plan and examine options before choosing the action most appropriate for their needs. Unfortunately, before reaching that level of reason and control, a youngster may run into unintended difficulties through a combination of excess physical energy, lack of familiarity with his own body, and concrete operational thinking. The highest level of abstract thinking in the stages of cognitive development first appears at puberty. This formal operational level supersedes the concrete style of the preceding latency and prepubertal years, during which the individual thought mostly in terms of cause and effect as it applied to observable physical objects. Now a teen can think about ideas, theories, and hypotheses, mentally rehearsing associations, relationships, alternatives, possibilities, or trial actions before taking action in reality. This expansion in the cognitive process does not occur equally in all adolescents. Spontaneous stratifications in school populations occur according to operational styles which vary from the concrete, where emphasis and interest are in manual tasks, to the more abstract, embracing the sciences and humanities. What leads one youngster to choose one or another depends on a complexity of causes including native intelligence, identification, ego mechanisms of defense, accessibility to resources.

As the pubertal process progresses, so does the consolidation of heterosexual relationships following the initial period of avoidance and preference for individuals of the same sex. The first encounters are rather crude and with less concern for the feelings of the girl on the part of the boy, who is more intent in proving his sexual prowess and acceptability; and of the boy on the part of the girl, who, in her teasing and derogatory remarks, may be expressing both her envy and resentment for his endowment before turning into a more receptive, soft, and passive partner. Relationships during the early phase of puberty are largely narcissistic, each sex seeking in the other his or her own gratification until, by the midteens, a more subtle, loving, caring attitude engulfs both, marking the end of the early phase and the beginning of the late phase of adolescence. This position solidifies through a confluence of factors: the mastery by the ego of the instinctual drives, the sharing with peers of the same sexual excitement, fear and consternation of the new and awesome functional capability with its mixtures of promise and responsibility, and the awareness of an increasing interest and receptivity of the opposite sex which facilitates the reciprocal wish to get closer to one another. Heterosexual dating has usually become established by the midteens.

**Late Puberty.** (Blos, 1962; Freud, 1958; Offer, 1983; Peterson, 1979). The tumultuous psychophysiologic changes precipitated by the onset of puberty begin to subside, on the average, by the midteens, when the ego reasserts its ascendency over the id and the process of distancing from the family of origin slows down to a less hectic phase. The youngster is, by this time, entering high school or in high school, and interests and associations are directed toward a future course. The teenager is less preoccupied with the self, while turning to outside activities and relationships which reflect both the operation of the reality principle and a heterosexual orientation, less narcissistically bound and experimental. Parents and other grown-ups, until then active contenders in the struggle for autonomy, have developed greater tolerance and respect for the needs of their offspring realizing that with each upcoming generation social and cultural changes are unavoidable and often welcomed. In this reciprocal interaction youngsters become more responsible and dependable, beginning to hold jobs, getting involved in the political system, doing volunteer work and participating with great zeal in social movements aimed at correcting the wrongs which they perceive exist within their social milieu of family, school, community, or society at large.

The social structure, on the other hand, responds very much as the intrapsychic structures do to the forces of the id. It copes with this emerging adult by setting limits that must be respected, rules and regulations that must be followed if teens are to be granted acceptance and participation in the adult world. They have to fulfill set requirements to graduate, get jobs, drive cars, drink, vote, and so on. There are also social conventions to follow regarding attire, appearance, manners, performance, respect for others, values, and property. Great variation exists in this vast area of social conformity. Some rules apply to all, but many are particular to the culture to which the youngster belongs. The enormous variations in behavior that one observes at this age should not distract us from identifying the common forces and functions which promote them. On one side are the institutions, which support adherence to the old, and on the other side are the young people clamoring for changes with increasing awareness of what is feasible and increasing willingness to negotiate rather than control. Peers provide the support system to carry on the struggle in what has been described as the conflict of generations which, in strained circumstances, may lead to alienation from one another resulting in more serious social dislocations. Normally, adolescents want to be integrated, not regarded as mere "puppets" but persons in their own right. The more gifted find a way to achieve their goals assisted by their greater cognitive abilities. Others are less fortunate and keep meeting obstacle upon obstacle in the search for position to the detriment of their self-esteem, and sometimes leading to social maladjustment.

While the young person proceeds with development, a sense of role playing makes the activities in which he is seriously involved feel somewhat unreal, as if he were acting the role of the adult without firmly identifying with the model. The process of incorporation evident in this type of behavior indicates the great receptivity and pliability of the ego at this time in obvious contradistinction to the rejection and rebellion otherwise shown and described before. Remembering that not all experimentation intends to be rebellious as it may appear helps the adult react to the adolescent with greater understanding and empathy. However, this is not always possible, despite good intentions, due to repression of that stage of development.

The vacillation between the opposing wishes for independence and dependence are less pronounced in late adolescence as contact with the parents decreases and as opportunities for self-reliance and self-sufficiency become more tangible. The young person may obtain a job, pay for a car, move out of the home, and be independent. Those who choose to go away to college will need to depend on themselves for many of the chores previously left to the parents, from doing the laundry to opening their own checking accounts. Interesting reactions are shown at the time of physical separation indicative of the unremitting struggle to fight the regressive pull towards dependency. Depressive reactions are not uncommon and the young person may not be able to function at work or at school for a while, sometimes unaware of being homesick—"cryptic nostalgia." Some become physically ill or accident prone and return home for care, while others try to soothe themselves by using drugs excessively, becoming sexually promiscuous, or developing appetite disorders, to mention just a few eventualities.

From the midteens on, the signs of identity-seeking are evident. As the way toward object constancy followed rapprochement in the early years of childhood, so does late adolescence follow a quest for identity constancy. Now the adolescent becomes more interested in cultural and social issues, religious and ethical assertions to reshape the superego built primarily out of the values of the parents and to accommodate the new findings. In the process the teen may become cynical at times, while at other times he may be a deeply committed idealist. The adolescent questions the status quo and is offended by parents and other adults for their actions, particularly when these contradict their stated beliefs. In questioning values and social mores, the adolescent is reshaping the internal representations of the parents into a more realistic and less idealized concept. As this process goes on intrapsychically, the outward behavior supports the impression that the adolescent is now consolidating peer relationships, activities, interests, causes, and ideals. This is partly prompted by the need to fill the vacuum left by the disengagement from parents, thus replacing one ideal for another. However, much of it results from the sexual thrust seeking gratification in love objects other than the parents. Feelings of tenderness and concern for the loved one are added now to the narcissistic desire to obtain satisfaction for oneself, sometimes reaching the extreme devotion or self-sacrifice so characteristic of this age.

Together with this outward movement of cathexis, the young man and young woman begin to relate to one another in ways that indicate a greater desire for reciprocal attention and gratification, tenderness, intimacy, permanence, empathy, and care. This heterosexual drive may lead to any of the current couple arrangements including marriage, although usually the first several romantic involvements do not tend to last. They are important however, to help the young person experience the meaning and feeling of being in love, including the physical aspects of lovemaking. They are the first steps toward success in the adult roles of spouse and parent.

Another expression of the push toward identity-seeking and constancy is the choice of vocation. This choice synthesizes a cluster of multidetermining factors going all the way down to the earliest stages of problem facing and problem solving, instinctual wishes, mastery of skills, identifications, relationships, self-esteem. These factors rest on and are superimposed on a genetic structure and on the individual's special talents. There are always historical precursors and unconscious motivations for the selection of an occupation. A successful choice is often dependent on the ability to assess realistically one's capabilities as well as the social needs and job opportunities.

## CONCLUSION

In summarizing the vicissitudes of the adolescent/pubertal process, the major characteristics of the early phase include: disengagement from the parental ties, present and introjected; intense preoccupation with the body and self (narcissistic cathexis); marked increase in sexual and aggressive drives; intense need for peer relations support; displacement of feelings and needs toward other love objects, replacing the parents as ego ideals; expansion and experimentation, including people and activities further removed from family and home (Group for the Advancement of Psychiatry, 1975).

The extensive reshaping of the personality progressing through late adolescence and culminating with the attainment of adulthood is in turn characterized by: resolution of the dependence–independence issue in relation with the parents, and attainment of a sense of relative equality in transacting with them; the establishment of sexual identity and self constancy, which implies having developed a clear and consistent perception of oneself, one's values, capabilities, interests, and goals; a capacity for empathy with the needs and feelings of others; and finally, the capacity for sustained relationships and heterosexual involvement, comprising both genital sexual love and feelings of tenderness (Berkovitz, 1983; Offer, 1983).

## REFERENCES

Bardin, C. W., and Paulsen, C. A.: The testes. In Williams, R. H.: (ed.): *Williams Textbook of Endocrinology,* 6th ed. Saunders, Philadelphia, 1981.

Berkovitz, I. H.: Emerging from adolescence: I. Theoretical discussion. *Clin. Update Adolesc. Psychiatr.* 1(15):1-11, 1983.

Blos, P.: *On Adolescence: A Psychoanalytic Interpretation,* 1st ed. Free Press, New York, 1962.

Blos, P: The second individuation process of adolescence. In Eissler, R. S.; Freud, A.; Hartmann, H.; Kris, M.: (eds.): *Psychoanal. Study Child.,* Vol. 22. International Universities Press, New York, 1967.

Daniel, W. A.: Evaluation of adolescents. In Behrman, R. E., and Vaughan, V. C.: (eds.): *Nelson's Textbook of Pediatrics,* 12th ed. Saunders, Philadelphia, 1983.

Dulit, E. P.: Cognitive development in adolescence. *Clin. Update Adolesc. Psychiatr.,* 1(6): 5, 1983.

English, O. S., and Pearson, G. H. J.: *Emotional Problems of Living.* 1st ed. Norton, New York, 1955.

Federman, D. D.: Ovary. Endocrinology. *Sci. Am.,* 3(3):1-3, 1984a.

Federman, D. D.: The testis. Endocrinology. *Sci. Am.,* 3(11):1-2, 1984b.

Freud, A.: Adolescence. In Eissler, R. S.; Freud, A.; Hartmann, H.; Kris, M.: (eds.): *Psychoanal. Study Child.,* Vol. 13. International Universities Press, New York, 1958.

Goldings, H. J.: Development from ten to thirteen years. In Noshpitz, J. D.: (ed.): *Basic Handbook of Child Psychiatry,* Vol. I, 1st ed. Basic Books, New York, 1979.

Group for the Advancement of Psychiatry: Normal Adolescence: Its Dynamics and Impact, 6, Report No. 68, New York, 1975.

Katz, P.: The adolescent in a changing society. *Clin. Update Adolesc. Psychiatr.,* 1(3): 5, 1983.

Kernberg, O.: *Object Relations Theory and Clinical Psychoanalysis,* 1st ed. Jason Aronson, Inc., New York, 1976.

Mahler, M. S.; Pine, F.; and Bergman, A.: *The Psychological Birth of the Human Infant,* 1st ed. Basic Books, New York, 1975.

Malmquist, C. P.: Development from thirteen to sixteen years. In Noshpitz, J. D.: (ed.): *Basic Handbook of Child Psychiatry,* Vol. I, 1st ed. Basic Books, New York, 1979.

Marohn, R. C.: Introduction and review of Anna Freud's 1958 article on adolescence. *Clin. Update Adolesc. Psychiatr.,* 1(1):00-00 1983.

Offer, D.: The self-image of normal adolescents: 1962-1982. *Clin. Update in Adolesc. Psychiatr.,* 1(5): 5, 1983.

Peterson, A. C., and Offer, D.: Adolescent development: sixteen to nineteen years. In Noshpitz, J. D. (ed.): *Basic Handbook of Child Psychiatry,* Vol. 1, 1st ed. Basic Books, New York, 1979.

Piaget, J., and Inhelder, B.: *The Psychology of the Child,* 1st ed. Basic Books, New York, 1969.

Rosen, H.: *Pathway to Piaget,* 1st ed. Postgraduate International, Inc., Cherry Hill, New Jersey, 1977.

Ross, G. T.; Vande Wiele, R. L.; and Frantz, A. G.: The ovaries. In Williams, R. H.: (ed.): *Williams Textbook of Endocrinology,* 6th ed. Saunders, Philadelphia, 1981.

Shonfeld, W. A.: Adolescent development: biological, psychological and sociological determinants. In Feinstein, S.; Giovacchini, P. L.; Miller, A. A.: (eds.): *Adolescent Psychiatry,* Vol. I, 1st ed. Basic Books, New York, 1971.

Tanner, J. M.: *Growth at Adolescence,* 2nd ed. Blackwell Scientific Publications, Oxford, England, 1962.

Vaughan, V. C.: Growth and development during adolescence. In Behrman, R. E., and Vaughan V. C.: (eds.): *Nelson's Textbook of Pediatrics,* 12th ed., Saunders, Philadelphia, 1983.

# CHAPTER 3 — THE EDUCATIONAL PROCESS

*Edward T. Heck, Ph.D.*

## INTRODUCTION

In every known human society males differ from females in both developmental patterns and behavioral characteristics. They are also treated differently from infancy through adulthood (Kagan, 1978). The long and complex journey that ultimately results in the development of an adult male or female who functions competently and productively in society begins at the moment of conception and continues well into adulthood. In the most ideal circumstances, healthy, loving, and resourceful parents living in a peaceful and supportive society stand ready and able to guide their child to an adulthood that will both satisfy the individual and benefit society.

On the other hand, an extraordinary gamut of biological, psychological, social, toxic and traumatic possibilities await the developing individual, and each is capable of modifying the outcome of the journey in less ideal ways. It is important to note that the effects of these influences must be inferred from rather fragmentary bits of evidence. The processes of human physical development are complex and not yet fully understood. The processes that govern the functioning of social systems are, perhaps, equally complex and certainly not fully understood. Neither set of processes seems constant and both seem to be changing noticeably over time. In the physical–sexual area, puberty is occurring progressively earlier. In the psychological–behavioral area, schools have become increasingly influenced by political forces. There are also serious methodological complications in most current studies since boys and girls in the same school grade are usually selected for comparison. Since males and females mature at different rates, this arbitrary selection by school-grade placement might account for at least some of the psychosexual differences in school performance reported to date. Consequently, a comprehensive report of the effects of public school attendance on psychosexual development will have to await the completion of large scale, objective, longitudinal studies. This chapter presents but a few of the issues such efforts would address.

## PSYCHOSEXUAL DEVELOPMENT

Psychosexual development involves the processes of maturation as they pertain to the relationship between psychological and sexual phenomena or, in other words, to the development of behavior patterns and attributes typical of males and females in the society. The processes of psychosexual development are determined both by biological factors and by the learning that results from the interaction of the individual with the social environment. In contemporary American society, public schools are a significant part of the social environment, and they can be expected to play a major role in the psychosexual development of the people who attend them.

Much of what we learn in life can be attributed to observing other people and interacting with them. These processes begin at birth and continue throughout life. Through observation and interaction we learn about the world in which we live and the other people who live here with us. We also learn about ourselves and our place in the world. From the very beginning boys and girls are treated differently by the adults who care for them. From earliest infancy, the child begins to develop an awareness that males are different from females. The product of this interaction and learning is the development of a set of abstract constructs, concepts, or schema in the child's mind about what it means to be a man or a woman in the society into which he or she was born. Thus, the psychosexual development of the child involves not only the learning of concepts about gender in society, but it also involves the learning of a set of concepts that enable that child to deal appropriately with members of the complimentary gender. Money and Tucker (1975) state: "If you're a man you use your female schema to anticipate the behavior of girls and women and as a guide to how you will react to them as a male. If you are a woman you use your male schema to anticipate the behavior of boys and men and as a guide to how you will respond to them reciprocally as a woman" (p. 8). The developing set of gender schemas is also important because it forms the cognitive basis for our personal gender identity, our sense of ourselves as either male or female.

The long and complex road to adulthood involves a great deal of learning. The experiences on which that learning is based involve virtually continuous observation of and interaction with other people. As the child matures, the lessons become more varied and complex. In very complex societies, like the American society, a major part of that learning process has become institutionalized in the form of universal public education. While the institutional part of the learning process formally concentrates on the literary and technical skills, it, informally and often unknowingly, teaches lessons about what it means to be male or female and what to expect of males and females—at least as they are represented within the school system. In other words, the public school system has an important and almost universal influence on the psychosexual development of young people because it influences their developing gender schemas and gender identities. This influence is exerted by both the school programs and the people who work in them.

## PUBLIC EDUCATION

Education can be defined as the process by which culture is transmitted to the young and public schools are our society's primary institutions for accomplishing that purpose. In simpler, more homogeneous societies the important elements of the culture could be passed from one generation to the next by family members or, perhaps by members of a larger kinship group or tribe. As society became more hetrogeneous and more technically complex, it became less likely that an individual or a small group of individuals could reliably pass on the increasingly complex culture. As a consequence, children in modern American culture go to school because the home structure alone cannot transmit the culture of our complicated society.

In a society characterized by technical complexity and rapid change, the educational process has been started at increasingly early ages and continued, off and on, well into adulthood. Thus, the educational process has been applied both to the acculturation of the young, who are being introduced to the culture, and to the not-so-young, who are in need of updating or re-education because society and technology are moving so fast.

The passing on of agreed upon and defined elements of any human culture is a formidable task under the best of circumstances, but in a complex, democratic, and pluralistic society it becomes nearly impossible. In relatively homogeneous, stable, and stratified societies the culture is passed from elders to juveniles and from masters to students. Within such a society there is usually a broad consensus about the essential elements of the culture and to whom, by whom, and in what order they should be transmitted. In a democratic and pluralistic society, however, no such consensus exists. Public schools are community service organizations that respond to the myriad political and social forces at work in the communities of which they are parts. Thus, the acculturation service they provide can proceed only in areas where there is consensus and this represents a relatively small subset of all possible cultural values. In the average public school, for example, widespread agreement could be reached among students, parents, teachers, administrators, and community citizens about the appropriateness of physical violence in school, destruction of property, or similar acts. This consensus would probably be significantly reduced if agreement was sought concerning the establishment of standards for promotion or nightly homework. Issues such as morality, decorum, and appropriateness of sex-stereotyped behaviors would probably yield more conflict than consensus among the school's constituents. In the more homogeneous, stratified society, therefore, the culture tends to be passed from the masters to the students largely because the masters have defined exactly what the culture is. In contrast, the constituents of the public school in a democratic society determine by consensus the agreed upon aspects of culture that are to be passed on. Since the masters are dependent upon their constituents for consensus about what aspects of the culture are to be transmitted, the educational process becomes much more political, negotiable, and complex.

## The Public School System

It has become fashionable in the past few years to examine the nation's public primary and secondary school systems critically. To be sure, many of the criticisms are valid and in urgent need of remedial attention. On the other hand, it must be noted that in several ways the public school system of this country has been a remarkable success. It has been both the agent for acculturation and the route of upward social mobility for millions of Americans.

Public school attendance is a virtually universal experience in modern American society. Almost all children attend school in America and about 90 percent attend public schools. Most young people remain in school today, at least until high school graduation. In fact, about 75 percent of students can be expected to complete high school and about 60 percent of these graduates can be expected to enter college. To accomplish this wholesale acculturation, our society devotes nearly 7 percent of its gross national product and the concentrated efforts of millions of its citizens. The National Center for Education Statistics (Grant and Eiden, 1982) reports that nearly one out of every four persons in this nation of 230 million people was directly involved in the educational process in 1981. Almost 18 million students are enrolled in primary and secondary public schools, and almost 2 million people are employed as classroom teachers in elementary and secondary schools (Grant and Eiden, 1982).

The demographic characteristics and behavior of the adults who teach in public schools and the social and political environments in which they work profoundly influence nearly everyone in this country today. The National Center for Education Statistics (Grant and Eiden, 1982) report that in primary and secondary schools, women teachers outnumber men teachers by two to one (66.9 percent to 33.1 percent respectively). In 1981, the average male teacher was 38 years old and the average female teacher was 36 years old. Twenty years earlier (1961) the average male teacher was 34 years old and the average female teacher was 46 years old. Thus, while the ratio of female to male teachers has remained fairly constant over the past 20 years, large numbers of older women have left the teaching profession to be replaced by a group of much younger female teachers.

Formal education has not always been such a major public enterprise. In preindustrial, pretechnical society a person's life work was probably learned during an apprenticeship in close association with a master or expert. The basics of literacy could be mastered at home or in brief periods at school. The most important aspects of the learning process involved on-the-job training, and one of the most important parts of the training was direct association with a competent adult who was routinely performing the duties for which the apprentice was being prepared (Kett, 1977). In contrast, most of today's public school students are subjected to prolonged exposure to the public school environment while, at the same time, they are almost totally isolated from association with competent adults who are working at occupations for which the student is presumably being readied. To compound their isolation from at least half of the adult world further, increasingly large numbers of today's students are being raised by a single, usually female, parent. In reality, most of today's young people are being prepared for their adulthood within the confines of social systems that are very much segregated on the basis of age, sex, and adult occupation.

## SEX DIFFERENCES THROUGHOUT THE EDUCATION PROCESS

### Early Childhood and Preschool Education

We become male or female by stages (Money and Tucker, 1975). Before birth most of the factors influencing our development are biological rather than psychological. While the behavior and habits of pregnant women profoundly influence the development of their unborn children, that influence is usually indirect since it is first mediated by the mother's body before being passed on to the fetus. From the moment of birth however, the newborn infant begins to interact directly with his or her environment and to learn from that interaction.

Sex differences in the behavior of infants have been reported very early in life (Kagan, 1978). From the beginning of life, boys seem to be more variable than girls both physically and behaviorally. Girls tend to cry more, babble more, and be less active than boys. In general, girls seem to be more biologically precocious and to develop more rapidly than boys. And from the beginning, parents seem to treat male and female infants differently. One study reported more physical contact with male infants and more object or material play with female infants by both mothers and fathers. Mothers were described as interacting with infants of both sexes in more social and verbal ways and using more social and verbal attention-getting behaviors than fathers. Fathers, however, seemed to have more effect on the female infants (Landerholm, 1981).

In general, girls tend to adopt family values more strongly than boys (Money and Tucker, 1975). The socioeconomic status of the family is an influential factor too, since it has been reported that the lower the socioeconomic level of the mother, the less likely she will be to stimulate, reward, and encourage her daughter's accomplishments. From the very beginning the cultural environment begins to pass on to the new arrival a set of behavioral expectancies about how to behave as a boy or a girl and what kind of behavior to expect from men and women. The learning that results from these early interactions form the foundations of the child's gender schema or learned concepts about what it means to be a man or a woman in society.

Interaction with other children early in childhood also seems to influence boys and girls differently. Studies reporting the influence of the peer group on the behavior of children as young as 24 months have reported the effectiveness of the male peer group in shaping male sex-typical behavior even when the boys were placed in play groups with other styles of play (Fagot, 1981). These stereotypic, sex-typed behaviors seem to be established quite early and to be resistant to concentrated efforts to change them (Roddy, Klein, Stericker, and Kurdek, 1981).

Some educators have suggested that the formal education of children begins in infancy. White and Watts (1973) contend that the period of life between 10 and 18 months is a critical one for what they call "the foundations of competence." They propose the establishment of formal infant education programs that could be associated with the provision of day-care services for working mothers. While mothers worked, their children would learn social competence, language skills, abstract thinking, and general intellectual development. White and Watts and their colleagues suggest that while attendance at day-care centers does not seem to result in the development of a psychological profile very much different from that resulting from home rearing, formal infant education programs are necessary because our society does not train individuals for parenthood and specifically for the development of "competence" in the very young child. While these studies are based on very small numbers of children who are not representative of the whole population, they do raise interesting issues and proposals. They are also in concert with the trend of beginning formal education at increasingly early ages.

## Primary School and the Early Grades

Even in the absence of infant education programs, the formal education process begins all too soon for many children. By their first day in primary school, boys' and girls' level of maturity and behavior patterns are noticeably different. On that first day of school the average boy will seem less mature than his average female classmate. While the average boy will probably learn best through active manipulation of his environment, which the school program does not emphasize, his average female classmate will probably learn best through verbal communication, which the school program does emphasize. The average little girl will seem much more inclined to comply with the rules of the classroom, attend to the teacher, and imitate the teacher's behavior. The average little boy, on the other hand, will probably find the classroom to be a virtual cornucopia of distractions, and his active and inattentive behavior will probably not escape the critical notice of his female classmates or his teacher. The public school system with which these children will interact will steadily and predictably accelerate the further development of these differences over the next 12 or 13 years.

Throughout the primary grades the average girl is a more successful student than her average male classmate. During these years the girls seem to be more persistent and to earn better grades than the boys (Kagan, 1978). Both the curriculum and classroom activities tend to be female oriented since the public schools are staffed primarily by women and the environment is dominated by female norms of politeness, cleanliness, and obedience (Levine and Ornstein, 1983; Ornstein and Levine, 1982). Sexton (1969) stated that "schools are feminizing institutions that discriminate against males and sometimes subvert his (sic) identity." She suggests that this may explain why three of every four problem children in the public schools are boys, and she concludes that the feminine values of the public elementary school together with boys' behavior and sexual identification problems explain why boys greatly outnumber girls as school dropouts and delinquents. Across the United States the ratio of boys to girls with learning and behavior problems has traditionally been close to six to one.

Several skilled investigators (Sexton, 1969; Ornstein and Levine, 1982) have described the public schools as feminine places, so it is not surprising to learn that young children of both sexes also perceive their schools that way. The odds are two to one that a woman will be in charge of the classroom, orchestrate the various activities, and probably place a premium on obedience and the suppression of restlessness and playful aggression. These are traditional feminine values and the children are likely to recognize them as such (Cuneen and Sloan, 1981). Kagan (1978) observes that if young boys perceive the school as feminine they will tend to resist complete involvement in classroom activities and, predictibly, fall behind their female classmates in academic progress. He suggests that the situation changes as the boys approach adolescence because at that point they begin to equate academic success with the masculine vocational fields to which they aspire.

A recent study reported by the Massachusetts Department of Education illustrates the pattern of differences between the academic achievement levels of male and female students in the state's public schools (Basic Skills Policy, 1983). This statewide summary of student achievement in the basic skills of reading, writing, and mathematics reported test scores for 201,000 public school students; 16,000 additional students were enrolled in special education programs and did not participate in the testing. Since boys outnumbered girls in these special education programs a disproportionate number of lower scoring boys was excluded from the test results. Females outperformed males in all skill areas at both elementary and secondary school levels. The minimum standard criteria for reading and mathematics were set at test scores between 50 and 60 percent—a modest standard indeed. Consequently, about 90 percent of all students evaluated met local minimum standards. Achievement of these modest standards was highest at the elementary level and lowest at the secondary level suggesting that, at least in Massachusetts, students fall steadily behind as they progress up the public school ladder.

It has been popularly assumed that the amount of money spent on public schools is directly related to the achievement level of students. It is also popularly assumed that there is a direct relationship between the wealth of a community and its allocation of funds to public services and education (Basic Skills Policy, 1983). To explore these popular assumptions the Massachusetts Department of Education undertook an examination of the relationship between community wealth and/or fiscal ability and how well students achieve modest standards in reading, writing, and mathematics. Not surprisingly, it was reported that across all grade levels and skills for most comparisons the percentage of students meeting minimum standards was highest in the wealthiest communities and lowest in the poorest communities. Throughout, the girls seemed to do better through all skill areas. It is important to point out, however, that during this same period the expenditure per pupil in Boston was the highest in the nation ($4,111 per pupil per year) and nearly twice the national average for big cities. The average pupil to teacher ratio in Boston (13:1) was much lower than the national average (Grant and Eiden, 1982). Thus, it seems that the steady decline of student achievement in this state public school system cannot be attributed to lack of expenditure or lack of staff alone. These data suggest that important factors are at work across primary and secondary public school environments and that these factors are exerting powerful effects on the basis of sex.

By fourth or fifth grade sex differences begin to count heavily in school and make themselves increasingly felt in reactions to school life (Gesell and Ilg, 1946). Recently, several government and foundation supported publications have readdressed the topic of sexual stereotyping in the schools (Weiner, 1980). The problem addressed by these publications is that the public education system favors males and significantly narrows the life choices available to females. Data supporting this hypothesis include surveys of school books and other materials that cast women in less desirable social roles than their male counterparts. One such publication asserts that by fourth grade "young girls have already learned to limit their horizons to home and family" (Verhyden-Hilliard, 1980). Verhyden-Hilliard identifies the culprit as "sexism" and suggests as a solution that children break free of traditional sexual stereotypes. A "sexist" is defined as "an advocate of sexism, all those attitudes and actions which relegate women to a secondary and inferior status in society"

(Verhyden-Hilliard, 1980). A U.S. Department of Health, Education, and Welfare publication (National Project on Women and Education, 1978) suggests the following criteria to judge school material as sexist:

1. It demeans females by using patronizing language,
2. It omits the actions and achievements of women, and
3. It shows females and males only in stereotyped roles with less than the full range of human interest traits and capabilities.

To support the contention that the public school teachers respond differently to boys and girls with respect to instruction, information, and praise, a study of 15 classrooms was presented. The study reported a disproportionate rate of detailed, step-by-step instruction for boys. The rate of this kind of individualized instruction was more than 8 times greater for boys than for girls. On the basis of these data it was concluded that the girls were the victims of sex-based discrimination in their classrooms. No mention was made of relative immaturity of the boys or their disproportionate learning, attention, and behavior problems in school so it is possible that the boys in this study needed the extra instruction just to keep up with their girl classmates. The ultimate purpose of a scientific experiment is still to rule out competing hypotheses, and in this important respect these publications do little to further our understanding of the effects of public schools on psychosexual development.

While sexism may be a factor, it is almost certainly not the only factor influencing students' career choices and much remains to be learned in this area. A recently reported study of the relationship between career aspirations of girls and prenatal hormone treatment found only an indirect relationship between a pioneering career choice in a currently male-dominated field and prenatal hormone treatment (Erhardt, Ince, Meyer-Bahlburg, 1981). Of perhaps greater interest, however, was the finding that girls who favored pioneering career choices (1) had higher I.Q. scores; (2) were more often persistent tomboys throughout childhood; (3) were several months older than their more traditionally inclined classmates; and (4) had parents who were more highly educated.

If the public school environment treats boys and girls differently with respect to the development of new academic and social skills it seems reasonable to assume that a complementary pattern of effects will exist with respect to the extinction or punishment of behaviors that are considered inappropriate. And indeed it does. While girls appear to be misbehaving more than they did in the past, the boys continue to misbehave more in most types of classroom antics. Some studies have shown that preschool teachers have been more likely to reprimand loudly boys than girls for aggressive behavior. Similarly, elementary school teachers, most of whom were women, tended to be more critical of boys and to overlook girls' misbehavior more than that of boys (Good and Brophy, 1977). A number of studies have suggested that teachers might report girls' misbehavior inaccurately and enforce rules more strictly and more frequently with boys (Serbin and Connor, 1979). Students' social and economic status are also factors in determining if behavior is to be judged as appropriate or inappropriate. In general, the lower the social status of the child the more likely teachers were to accept behavior that would have been judged misconduct for higher status students (Good and Brophy, 1977).

## Adolescence and High School

In preindustrial America adolescence was equated with a period of growth and increasing strength rather than prolonged awkwardness (Kett, 1977). During those earlier times adolescence was also a shorter period of life; young people were often gainfully employed in their life work during the early teen years. In fact, the onset of puberty frequently signaled the onset of the assumption of adult working patterns. Those young people were integrated into adult society rather early in life, at least by modern standards, but several societal factors combined to facilitate the transition. Most occupations were technically simpler, and the pace of life was slower. Competent male and female models of appropriate social and occupational behavior were available for observation and, within the culture of that time, there was a more uniform consensus about what appropriate male and female behavior patterns were supposed to be.

The prolonged transition period between childhood and adulthood we know today as adolescence is shaped and sustained by complex physical, psychological, and social realities that did not exist in preindustrial America. In recent years it has been noted that the onset of puberty has been occuring earlier and earlier—at a rate of about one year per generation. The coincidence of the advent of prolonged adolescence and prolonged schooling has served both to isolate the average young person from the mainstream of adult society for several years and to increase the influence of the school environment and the peer group during this period. Thus, the school has become a cultural workshop of unique power as childhood merges into adolescence (Gesell, Ilg, and Ames, 1956).

The interaction between the student and the public high school continues to be influenced by sexual determinants. Female teachers outnumber their male counterparts in both junior high schools and high schools just as they do in the earlier grades. Several historical reasons have been suggested to explain the feminization of public school teaching, including the increasing demand for public education resulting from the process of state school formation, as well as cultural restraints on women's work participation in other sectors of the economy (Richardson and Hatcher, 1983). In any case, as modern society has become more complex, adolescence has become more prolonged, and the modern adolescent's transition into adulthood is more significantly segregated on the basis of occupation and sex.

Johnson (1978) has pointed out that almost half of all Americans never reach "adolescence" in their capacity to think. In other words, they have not mastered the concrete mental operations of reading, counting, remembering, and organizing. This is a vitally important factor in academic development because individuals who have not mastered these basic skills will be at a disadvantage when it comes to thinking abstractly and doing independent mental work that requires abstract thinking. Because these basic skills are needed to function successfully in high school, it follows that large numbers of young people arrive at the doors of these institutions with seriously compromised prospects for further successful intellectual development.

Since boys exhibited significantly more learning and behavior problems than girls throughout primary school and since they are physically about two years behind the girls through about age 15, one might reasonably expect them to be disproportionately represented in the group whose academic prospects are the least promising on the first day of public high school enrollment. When one considers the girls' superiority on academic achievement tests in primary school that suspicion changes to confident anticipation. Throughout high school, males are much more likely to drop out, act out, and achieve mediocre to poor grades (Dillon, 1982).

The variability that characterizes adolescent males can be seen in their over representation in both the most successful and least successful student groups. Each year college-bound high school seniors take the Scholastic Aptitude Test (SAT) and interesting, sex-related patterns of scores have emerged over the years. In 1966–1967 the SAT verbal scores for males and females were about equal. In that same year males scored significantly higher in mathematics (male 514, female 467). SAT verbal scores have remained about equal for males and females over the years, although both have dropped noticeably. Males have continued to earn SAT mathematics scores about 50 points higher than those earned by their female classmates (Grant and Eiden, 1982).

Why do these differences exist? Presumed differences between males and females in science and mathematics have preoccupied educators for years. A recent study analyzed 298 papers dealing with sex differences in attitudes and achievement in science. The results indicated that sex differences were much smaller than generally assumed (Steinkamp, 1982). Perhaps males and females take different classes in high school? However, males and females take about the same number and level of courses in English, history, mathematics, and science, at least through the intermediate level of concentration (2½ years) in each subject area. Males are slightly more likely to take the advanced courses in trigonometry, calculus, and physics (Grant and Eiden, 1982). Males and females participate about equally in high school class discussions, and no pattern of male dominance has been demonstrated in that area (Dillon, 1982). So it is interesting to note that girls are nearly twice as likely to earn all As in school. The pattern of female overrepresentation holds for A to B grades as well. At the other end of the grade spectrum, males are over 50 percent more likely than females to earn all Cs and over twice as likely to earn all Ds (Grant and Eiden, 1982). It has been reported that academic track position is one of the best predictors of student attitudes and behavior, and the study reporting this result also reported more females enrolled in the higher academic tracks (Kelly, 1976). Male variability alone does not seem to offer a satisfactory explanation for this sex-related pattern of school grades. At least some contribution to this pattern probably derives from the female high school student's generally better behavior, since grades frequently reflect decorum as well as the mastery of academic skill. In addition, stereotyped female patterns of attentiveness and classroom behavior are probably more conducive to learning in the school environment.

While female students seem to get better marks in high school and to experience significantly less school problems than their male classmates, the social environment of the school seems to become increasingly problematic with age for them (Gregg, 1976). A study of the ways in which men and women are distributed in social roles across the society may suggest at least a partial explanation of this situation (Eagly, et al., 1982). It was suggested that the higher status positions in society are perceived as more instrumental or task-oriented and the lower status positions are perceived as more expressive or social–emotional. If a school's program emphasis or staffing pattern encourages female students to seek expressive goals to the exclusion of instrumental goals, the developing gender schema of individuals will be restricted, their life prospects will be limited, and society will be denied the instrumental contributions they might have made. And to the extent that males are encouraged to seek instrumental goals to the exclusion of expressive goals, their developing gender schema will be restricted, their life prospects limited, and society will be denied their potential expressive contributions. It would be very difficult to ascertain the proportional contributions of home, community, and school to the distribution of men and women in social roles across the society. The situation is being partially addressed by efforts to present both males and females in a broader range of activities and roles in school materials. The involvement of greater numbers of female students in intramural and varsity athletics is an important step in this direction. A more comprehensive approach, however, would require major changes in school programs and staffing patterns.

The progressively earlier onset of puberty has been an impediment to the intellectual development of children of both sexes but the adverse effects on females are particularly noticeable. Juvenile sexual activity has resulted in an epidemic of teenage pregnancy and abortion, the tragic effects of which are borne primarily by females. Even the availability of contraceptives to juveniles tends to impede their intellectual development since it encourages the formation of prolonged, exclusive, and intense mini-marriages. These relationships are destructive not only because they limit the opportunity for social experiences with other people, but also because they absorb mental and emotional energy that should be devoted to intellectual development. In our sexually preoccupied adolescent society, young people who are keeping regular company are too often presumed to be sexually active. Even if this is not so, dating more than one person at a time is often seen as a sign of sexual promiscuity and social pressure is exerted in the direction of limiting experience. These social limitations—and the emotional energy they absorb—adversely affect both males and females, although the female high school student seems to pay a particularly dear price for them.

Studies of juvenile delinquents and potential delinquents report poor emotional adjustment and low academic achievement for both males and females. Female delinquents were described as less poised and more moody. Their negative affect differentiated them significantly from their nondelinquent female classmates, but this pattern did not hold true for male delinquents (Conger, 1973). Other studies have described male delinquents as being influenced primarily by such factors as rebellion against female authority that was needed to assert their manhood, lack of opportunity to pursue legitimate goals, and a desire to emulate adult models (Kratkoski and Kratkoski, 1975). If these descriptions are even partially correct, it can be safely predicted that the public high school environment will present the delinquent of both sexes almost unlimited opportunities for self-defeating conflict.

## CONCLUSION

In every known human society males differ from females in both developmental patterns and behavioral characteristics. As the individual progresses from infancy to adulthood, he or she learns what it means to be a man or a woman in the society into which he or she was born. This individual also learns what to expect from and how to react to members of the other gender in that society. The learning of these gender- or sex-related behavior patterns is the essence of psychosexual development.

In contemporary American culture, the public schools are the primary institutional agents for the acculturation of the young and the not so young. Consequently, the social values, organizational characteristics, and staffing patterns of the public schools exert a profound influence on the psychosexual development of their students. This is a matter of great importance because the public schools influence how their students will behave as adult men and women. In this period of rapid social and technical change, the roles of men and women in contemporary society have also been changing. As a consequence of these changes, increasing attention has been focused on the public schools and how they might influence the psychosexual development of students.

The fragmentary data currently available suggest that males are more variable, less mature, and less successful in school than girls. Overall, male students account for a greatly disproportionate share of learning problems, behavior problems, and school failures. This pattern has variously been attributed to the high proportion of female teachers in the school and the "feminization" of the public school environment. Such results may well be spurious since they are based on the grouping of students by age or grade placement. Since boys are generally less mature than girls, the results of studies comparing them would, no doubt, be different if they were grouped so as to be equivalent with respect to physical maturity, ability to pay attention, and ability to regulate activity. The employment of such criteria would do much to facilitate the exploration of the schools' contributions to psychosexual development. It would be of even greater importance to place children in learning environments based on some combination of maturational criteria because to do so would improve chances for their success rather than invite failure.

The data presented in this chapter raise several clinical and public policy issues concerning the role of public schools in psychosexual development. Since boys and girls do not mature at the same rates, how can we expect them to respond uniformly to the same age-graded class rooms? Perhaps boys and girls should be separated for some or all of their educational experience. If coeducation is to be maintained in the public schools, perhaps children should be placed in grades on the basis of their maturity rather than their chronological age. Perhaps the concept of "grade" itself is obsolete and schooling should proceed on the basis of the individual's maturity and academic competence. Mass education, or mass anything, inevitably takes a homogenized view of society, concentrating on the group defined as "average" and experiencing greater conflict with individuals defined as "exceptional." Perhaps schools could be organized differently with smaller, more flexible teaching units than is the case today. Perhaps we should pay more attention to the kinds of people who teach in public schools and make sure that the teaching staffs are more representative of adult males and females and the range of adult occupations that exist in society generally. What we already know about the effects of the public school environment on the psychosexual development of individuals suggests that the answers to these and similar questions are well worth pursuing.

## REFERENCES

*Basic skills improvement policy: 1981–82 statewide summary of student achievement of minimum standards in the basic skills of reading, writing, and mathematics,* 2nd annual report. Massachusetts Department of Education, Boston, 1983.

Conger, J. J.: *Adolescence and Youth.* Harper and Row, New York, 1973.

Cuneen, J., and Sloan, C. A.: *Analysis of the Effect of Teacher Sex on Sex Role Classification of School Related Objects.* U.S. National Institute of Education Research, Report 143, 1981.

Dillon, J. T.: Male–female similarities in class participation. *J. Educ. Res.,* 75(6):350–53, 1982.

Eagly, A.; Steffey, V.; and Izraeli, D.: *Gender and social roles: A distributional theory of gender stereotypes.* Paper presented at the American Psychological Association Convention, Washington, D.C., Sept., 1982.

Ehrhardt, A.; Ince, S. E.; and Meyer-Bahlburg, H.: Career aspiration and gender role development in young girls. *Arch. Sex. Behav.,* 10(3):281–299, 1981.

Fagot, B. T.: Continuity and change in play styles as a function of sex of child. *Int. J. Behav. Dev.,* 4(1):37–43, 1981.

Gesell, A., and Ilg, F. L.: *The Child from Five to Ten.* Harper and Row, New York, 1946.

Gesell, A.; Ilg, F. L.; and Ames, L. B.: *Youth: The Years from Ten to Sixteen.* Harper and Row, New York, 1956.

Good, T. W., and Brophy, J. E.: Changing teacher and student behavior: An empirical investigation. *J. Educ. Psychol.,* 66:390–405, 1977.

Grant, W. V., and Eiden, L. J.: *Digest of Education Statistics 1982.* National Center for Education Statistics, Washington, D.C., 1982.

Gregg, G.: High school—A tough place for girls, *Psychology Today,* 10(7):36–37, 1976.

Hoffman, A. D.: Adolescents in distress. In symposium on adolescent medicine. *Med. Clin. North Am.* 59:1429–37, 1975.

Johnson, E.: *How to Live Through Junior High School.* Lippincott, Philadelphia, 1978.

Kagan, J.: *The Growth of the Child: Reflections on Human Development.* W.W. Norton, New York, 1978.

Kelly, D. H.: Track position, school misconduct, and youth deviance. *Urban Educ.,* 10:379–88, 1976.

Kett, J. F.: *Rites of Passage; Adolescence in America: 1790 to The Present.* Basic Books, New York, 1977.

Kratkoski, P. C., and Kratkoski, J. E.: Changing patterns in the delinquent activities of boys and girls: A self-reported delinquency analysis. *Adolesc.,* 10:83–91, 1975.

Landerholm, E. J.: *Comparison of Mothers' and Fathers' Play with Their Male and Female Infants.* Paper presented at the National Association for the Education of Young Children, Detroit, 1981.

Levine, D. U., and Ornstein, A. C.: Sex differences in ability and achievement. *J. Res. Dev. Educ.,* 16(2):66–72, 1983.

Money, J., and Tucker, P.: *Sexual Signatures: On Being a Man or a Woman,* Little, Brown, Boston, 1975.

National Commission on Excellence in Education: *A Nation at Risk: The Imperative for Educational Reform.* U.S. Government Printing Office, HEW Publication No. 065–000–00177–2, Washington, D.C., April, 1983.

National Project on Women and Education: *Taking Sexism Out of Education.* U.S. Government Printing Office, HEW Publication No. (O.E.) 77–01017, Washington, D.C., 1978.

Ornstein, A. C., and Levine, D. U.: Sex, schools, and socialization, *Educ. Forum,* 46(3):337–341, 1982.

Peterson, D. R.: Behavior problems of middle childhood. *J. Consult. Clin. Psychol.,* 25:205–209, 1961.

Richardson, J. G., and Hatcher, B. W.: The feminization of public school teaching: 1870–1920. *Work and Occupation: An International Journal* 10(1): 81–100, 1983.

Roddy, J. M.; Klein, H. A.; Stericker, A. B.; and Kurdek, L. A.: Modification of stereotypic sex-typing in young children. *J. Genet. Psychol.,* 139(1):109–118, 1981.

Rothenberg, J.: *Classroom Activity Structures and Patterns of Peer Associations.* U.S. National Institute of Education, (N.I.E. 9–79–0079), Washington, D.C., April, 1982.

Serbin, L. A., and Connor, J. M: *Environmental Control of Sex Related Behaviors in the Preschool.* Paper presented at the Biennial Meeting of the Society for

Research in Child Development, San Francisco, March, 1979.

Sexton, P. C.: *The Feminized Male.* Random House, New York, 1969.

Steinkamp, M. W.: *Sex Related Differences in Attitude Toward Science: A Quantitative Synthesis of Research.* American Educational Research Association, New York, 1982.

Verheyden-Hilliard, M. E.: *A Handbook for Workshops in Sex Equality in Guidance Opportunities Project.* American Personnel and Guidance Association, 1980.

Weiner, E. H.: (ed): *Sex Role Stereotyping in the Schools,* 2nd ed. National Education Association, Washington, D.C., 1980.

White, B. L., and Watts, J. C., *Experience and Environment: Major Influences on the Development of the Young Child,* Prentice–Hall, Englewood Cliffs, New Jersey, 1973.

# CHAPTER 4  MARRIAGE

*Ned L. Gaylin, Ph.D.*

## INTRODUCTION

Marriage may be defined as the public and conscious taking of a member of the opposite sex for a life partner. No other social institution is either so indigenous to us or so defining of us as a unique species. Although cross cultural comparisons reveal all manner of variations (including homosexuality) on the typical monogamous unit we have come to know, marriage remains the most basic of all human institutions. For all cultures, marriage serves the universal function of maintaining responsible intimacy. Marriage has thus become one of the few remaining bastions of interpersonal security—the safehouse of love and trust.

In the present period of rapid social change, there is much conjecture about the viability of the institution of marriage. Figures abound to highlight the plight of the modern marriage: two out of every five marriages now end in divorce; illegitimate births have nearly tripled since 1960; 15 percent of American children live in single-parent homes (double the number of 25 years ago) (Glick and Norton, 1977). Certainly one might conclude that the future of marriage is at best uncertain. However, the other half of the story might well lead to some different conclusions. Of the 40 percent of divorced individuals, over three-fourths remarry. Furthermore, the two-thirds of our population who marry for life stay married far longer due to the increase in our life span.

Despite what recently appeared to be a declining marriage rate, but which actually proved to be a delayed marriage trend, America is still the most "marrying" country in the world (Gaylin, 1980).

Thus, to question the viability of marriage is tantamount to questioning the viability of civilization as we know it. The real issue facing us is how the institution of marriage is being modified and employed to help us as a species adapt to our modern world. It is not that we are not marrying; we are marrying, divorcing more frequently, and remarrying. We are continuously seeking the right relationship, the eternal match. A force that impelling—the romantic quest for the ideal state between man and woman—surely speaks to who we are and where we are going.

All mammalian species mate for sexual reproduction, and it belabors the obvious to note that this biological imperative is requisite for species continuance. While some infrahuman species have analogues to monogamous marriage (e.g., certain species of birds tend to mate for life) there is little evidence that any have the special consciousness of the future that the bonds of matrimony imply. Thus, marriage is palpably different from any analogous mating behavior in other animals. Marriage is a conscious contract that has an explicit past as well as an implicit future. Marriage transtemporally bridges the past by recognizing ancestry, the present by joining individuals and families, and the future by anticipating and producing heirs. Marriage, because of its link with the past and its projection into the future, is in fact humankind's attempt to overcome the limitations of the life span. By marrying, one establishes a relationship with ramifications greater than either partner's individual longevity. Thus, conscious transtemporality and generative function enable marriage to bridge and connect individuals, generations, families, communities, even empires. Marriage and its inevitable sequel, the family, are the social paradigm, the keystone in the arch of civilization.

Integral to an understanding of humankind's place in the world is an understanding of ourselves as individuals. Although earlier attempts at self-understanding are replete in our written histories and philosophies, it was Sigmund Freud, who, standing on the shoulders of Darwin, catapulted psychology into the 20th century, at the same time that Einstein launched the physical sciences, thus ushering in "the age of science." Analogously, just as it was necessary to understand the largest concepts of the universe by understanding its smallest, so the study of human interaction needed to begin with the individual.

Joining the biological—more specifically, the sexual—aspects of humankind's nature with the psychosocial, Freud laid the groundwork for a more integrative conceptualization of human motivation and interaction. At the same time he took sex out of its closet and infused it into all areas of life. While his intent was to put human sexuality into perspective, the impact of Freud's work, in many ways, was just the opposite. Sex became ubiquitous. We not only became conscious of sexuality in a different way, we became self-conscious. Thus, psychoanalytic ideation, which dominated psychological thought for the first half of this century, promoted (and we accepted) the notion that we, like our animal ancestors, are dominated by lust, and that our nobler accomplishments were little more than a sublimation of our animal drives

It was at about mid-twentieth century (see Kluckhohn, Murray, and Schneider, 1956) that other branches of the social sciences (*i.e.,* anthropology and sociology) began to weave psychoanalytic ideas with their own in an effort to understand individual behavior in cultural context. Simultaneously, the study of child development began to focus on the importance of the mother–child bond and its ramifications on the developing individual (Bowlby, 1952; A. Freud, 1944; Spitz, 1945). Thus child psychology and child guidance were launched as legitimate professional disciplines. The fields of home economics and social work moved theory out of the university and clinic and into the home and community, and thus gave visibility and credence to the family as a focal unit of social change. As the perspective of the individual in dynamic context evolved, the various behavioral science disciplines separated and stabilized their own identities, thus facilitating a multifaceted perspective of the individual and social interaction. Thus, the last half of this century has witnessed the psychological and sociological birth of the study of marriage and family. The most recent developments are those of marriage and family psychotherapy. The rapid growth of this clinical approach to the amelioration of maladaptive behavior suggests both public and professional recognition of the importance of marriage and family as the most central institution to human adaptation.

## GENERAL THEORETICAL CONSIDERATIONS AND DEFINITIONS

Anthropology, sociology, and psychology all claim the study of marriage and family as their legitimate concern. In an attempt to organize and conceptualize the study of marriage and family within the social sciences, three major frameworks have been developed: structural–functional; symbolic interactional; and developmental. (For a succinct exposition of these frameworks, the reader is referred to Clayton, 1975.) Until recently, each framework has had its devotees and critics. Presently, some convergence of these frameworks seems to be evolving through the integrative perspective of human ecology. Each of the three frameworks contribute somewhat different and necessary dimensions to the study of the complexities of marriage and family. Thus, the identification of societies' structural components, the determination of their functions and interactions, with an awareness of change over time, may yield a more comprehensive picture of how and why individuals behave in a social context.

All fields of inquiry develop a language or nomenclature to describe and discuss certain observable phenomena, and to differentiate concepts. Such nomenclature also lends insight into the manner in which the observed phenomena are conceptualized. A scientific schema requires that the categories be both comprehensive and mutually exclusive so that any observation may fall into only one named category. However, because of pandisciplinary origins, marriage and family terminology tends to overlap and blur distinctions. Nevertheless a brief glossary is presented to facilitate an understanding and discussion of marriage and family within the context of contemporary behavioral sciences.

All studies of marriage deal with the broad distinctions between monogamous and polygamous unions. Virtually all modern Western marriages fall under the category of monogamy: one man married to one woman. Historically, Western marriage is thought to have emanated from one form of polygamy, that is, polygyny: one man wedded to more than one woman. The other form of polygamy, polyandry—one woman married to more than one man—continues to be exceedingly rare.

Once the marital unions are defined they are put into the perspective of larger family units, namely, the nuclear and extended families. Although much of the foregoing terminology is familiar, the following subdivisions tend to be used less commonly. Usually thought of as mother, father, and offspring, the nuclear family can be defined as a family of orientation (the family into which one was born) or the family of procreation (the family one creates by marrying). These two terms use the individual as the reference point, and are longitudinal in nature. Thus, those of us who are married and have children belong simultaneously to a family of orientation (our mother, father and siblings) and to a family of procreation (our spouse and children).

In contrast to the longitudinal terminology presented above, social scientists define extended families in cross-sectional terms. The family may be organized according to either conjugal (marital) or consanguinal (blood line) relationships. The latter include the concepts of: (1) lineage—patrilineal or matrilineal; (2) authority—patriarchal or matriarchal; and (3) place—patrilocal, matrilocal, or neolocal, where the marital pair establishes a new place of residence. Three new terms emerge to describe modern marriage and family phenomena. With regard to authority the term "egalitarian," neither matriarchal nor patriarchal, is commonly employed. In response to the current trend towards more frequent divorce and consequent remarriage, the terms "serial monogamy" and "blended families," have been introduced. With structural changes occuring regularly in the American family, it is likely that more terminology will be created.

Until recently, the American family of the twentieth century might have been described as monogamous, and have emphasized the family of procreation. The monogamy tended to be patrilineal, egalitarian, and neolocal. If we follow recent trends we might refer to the emerging American family as serially monogamous, patrilineal (though this appears to be changing to a bilineal form with the wife frequently retaining her family name and inheritance) more egalitarian in power, nuclear, and neolocal. While experimentation with marriage forms occurs continuously (e.g., group marriages based on communal living) the stability and popularity of these forms in our culture (particularly after the advent of children) is highly questionable, and their viability in contemporary American society seems unlikely.

What has become apparent from studying marriage and family over time and across cultures is that despite the variability in form, the nuclear family, at least, remains relatively similar and universal. This was the conclusion reached by the cultural anthropologist, George Murdock (1949) after studying 250 different cultures. His unequivocal statements regarding family universality continues to be bandied about by social scientists. However, his conclusion remains accepted by virtually all.

Murdock's examination of these societies led him to determine four functional prerequisites for marriage and family grouping. Accordingly, the necessary and sufficient functions of the family in all its permutations in all cultures, are: (1) socialization, (2) economic cooperation, (3) reproduction, and (4) control of sexual relations. In examining contemporary American society, Parsons and Bales (1955) have suggested that the functional prerequisites for marriage and family may be reduced to two: (1) socialization and acculturation of the young, and (2) the stabilization and acculturation of the adult members of that society. In even more reductionistic terms, Ira Reiss (1965) has distilled the prerequisites to one, proffering "nurturant socialization" as the sole universal function of marriage and family. While, perhaps not as clear as one might want it, the developing nomenclature has value, both descriptively as well as heuristically. Furthermore, these new terms are indicative of the development of a growing science.

## WESTERN MARRIAGE AND FAMILY IN HISTORICAL PERSPECTIVE

Western marriage and family as we know them today had their roots in ancient civilizations of the Hebrews, Greeks, and Romans. What little is said about marriage of prewritten history is largely inferred from scanty anthropological clues combined with ethological and biological speculations. Some investigators (Washburn and DeVore, 1961) go so far as to date the origins of marriage within the Middle Pleistocene period (roughly 300,000 years ago). They believe that for even the most primitive of marriage and family forms to have been generated, humankind must have developed distinctly different roles for the sexes: that is, women would have had to have been gatherers, planters, and tenders of the young; men would have had to have been hunters of game. Hunting, particularly large game, would have required bands of men working cooperatively. Such cooperative efforts would have required exogamus (outside the group) mating in order to establish affiliative bonds and enlarge the community. These investigators (among others, see Ardry, 1970; Morris, 1967) assume that this period also saw the inception of the incest taboo which precludes inbreeding as a means of enhancing communal expansion.

The incest taboo, its function, origins and centrality to a concept of human behavior, has been widely discussed and debated by biologists, anthropologists, psychologists, and sociologists. There are some animal behaviorists who observe the tendency for exclusively exogamous behavior in a few infrahuman species, particularly those prone to relatively small close groupings (e.g., lions, certain monkeys, and apes; Wilson, 1980). Despite some rare exceptions (e.g., the ancient royalties of Egypt, Peru, Samaria, and a brief period of Roman history) the incest taboo is universal and is accepted as such by virtually all scholars of marriage and family. There remains wide debate about reasons for the inception of the taboo, but few disagree with the importance of it in the prevention of disruptive sexual rivalry and role confusion, and the enlargement of the marrying group, which thus facilitated survival (Stephens, 1963).

Comprehension of propagation, and the lifelong concern for the physical and psychological well-being of mate and offspring distinguish humankind from all other mammalian species, even its closest infrahuman cousins. The crucial distinction is the idea of lifelong concern. It requires the culmination of a special kind of consciousness: a transtemporal awareness. This includes the cognizance of history, a unique form of memory, as well as an ability to anticipate the future. With this kind of consciousness, the development of complex communication—nonverbal, spoken, and written language—is associated.

With a study of written history, there is firmer support for conjecture that marriage is an institution central to humankind. The period of the ancient Hebrews is the first for which we have appreciable written information (Old Testament; Pritchard, 1955). This historical period introduces the perspective by which we view marriage today, especially with respect to structure and male–female role delineation. Even though it is assumed that the Old Testament patriarchs practiced polygyny, the biblical tracts nonetheless imply a preference for monogamy. The emphasis on primacy of the patriarch–matriarch pair, and the probability that the majority of people were not affluent enough to maintain more than one wife, are both suggestive of this propensity. Though probably idealized and romanticized by the Bibilical poets, these ancient reports also recount a gradual evolution from a nomadic lifestyle to an agrarian and then an urban society.

From the times of the ancient Hebrews, to the Hellenic polis, to the Hellenistic city state, to the Roman Empire, the dual practice of polygyny and monogamy continued. Concubines were not uncommon among the wealthy, but the marital dyad was generally the norm, perhaps because of economic necessity, moral rightness, and/or natural proclivity.

The early writings of the Hebraic, Greek, and Roman cultures make plain the highly defined differences between male and female roles and the superior status of the males, although there is evidence that the premise was at least sometimes questioned. (For example, see the Old Testament, Plato's *Republic,* New Testament.) However, by the time of the Roman Empire, continued urbanization and expansion saw a very gradual shift in gender role designations. Men were sent off to war, leaving women to manage households, thereby giving them greater visibility in governance than they had had earlier. Also a concurrent shift from barter to monetized wealth took place, and probably gave impetus to the codification of the laws of family lineage and inheritance. Separated from the land, wealth and power became symbolized through money, and thereby portable and inheritable.

What the latter part of the Roman period began, Christianity continued. Women were at least nominally accorded a more focal role and greater status than they had previously had. Christianity also intensified the notion that marriage had divine sanctity. Sexuality was considered subservient to parenthood; the main purpose of marriage was procreation. Furthermore, the Medieval Church made divorce (previously a relatively easy option, at least for the male) far more difficult to obtain, and thereby emphasized the morally correct role of the marital dyad. These trends continued through the Middle Ages and the Renaissance (Bardis, 1964). As marriage and extended family ties were solidified by the Church, the economic rules of the feudal manor combined with the rules of inheritance to ensure the consolidation and continuity of family wealth along patrilineality. Thus, in addition to fulfilling religious and moral obligations, marriage (at least for the more prosperous) became as much an economic institution as an affectional one.

These are the historical foundations of marriage which we have inherited. The growth of urbanization, the nation state, and industrialization saw the continuation of those trends developed at the beginning of the Common Era. Men continued to leave the home—not to hunt game but to work in trades. Despite some small change in women's status and visibility, their vocation remained the family: caring for their spouses, the young, and the old. Role delineation was still highly circumscribed. With the emergence of Protestantism, followed by the industrial revolution, the way was paved for dramatic changes in gender role differentiation and economic opportunity.

First, Protestantism extended the concept of vocational "calling" outside of the priesthood or marriage and thus dignified the earthly ambition of earning money (Weber, 1930). Then machinery began to minimize some of the biological differences (primarily brute strength) that had kept women working inside and men working outside the home. Travel for economic, as well as for religious and political, opportunity established the marital pair and its issue as the nuclear family, now a functional and portable unit of civilization. These trends continued into the new world and intensified in posttechnological society (Aries, 1962, 1979).

## A LIFE SPAN OVERVIEW OF MARRIAGE

The identification of social structures and the delineation of their functions and interactions give us a comprehensible picture of society. With its longitudinal perspective, the developmental framework gives a sense of dimension and life to our understanding. Morphology without development is a Galatea without a Pygmallion. Because the focus here is the interpersonal social institution of marriage, discussion of development will be constrained to that context (although drawing upon the affective and cognitive developmental theories of Freud, 1962; Piaget, 1952; and others). In the sense that our interests lie in the continuance of the species, the emphasis is on the more directly observable interpersonal and biological elements. From this perspective, development is divided into those stages which precede and follow marriage. It should be mentioned that all stage theories demarcate the inclined plane of development in discrete comprehensible steps. That theory presented here is no exception. Development is a gradual and continuous process with few easily demarcated points along the way.

### Premarital (Family of Orientation) Stages

Despite a relatively limited range of socioemotional responses at birth (*i.e.*, contentment versus distress) human neonates display a predisposition to empathy. As early as one day of age, infants have been observed to cry empathically to the sound (real or simulated) of other infants' cries (Sagi and Hoffman, 1976), and respond bodily to the adult voice (Condon and Sander, 1974). By as little as 10 days of age, infants will also mimic adult lip and tongue motions (Meltzoff and Moore, 1977). Despite this kind of early responsiveness, the human infant is totally dependent on its caretakers. This complete helplessness and the child's "innocent" physiognomy are highly evocative of parental nurturing and caring (Gaylin, 1976). These factors create an intense symbiosis between mother and child during the first year of life which is crucial to the child's appropriate future psychosocial development. The child's total dependency continues for nearly two years and relative dependence may, in our culture, last for at least another 15 years.

Although the infant's discovery of itself as a separate entity undoubtedly begins somewhere in the first year (through self-exploration of body parts), self-awareness and a sense of a separate identity are probably not really crystalized until about the end of toddlerhood. Since the child under three remains dependent upon the parent for nurturance and security, the child receives love, and looks for approbation but is really not much of a reciprocal actor in the process. It is within this period of total dependency that basic trust is established (Erikson, 1964).

At about 2 to 3 years of age the distinctly human, biosocial phenomenon of toilet training begins and expectations of self-help skills are made of the child. It is this period that Sullivan (1953) regards as the true beginning of the child's self—the "good me, bad me," and "not me." It is the "good me" and its enhancement, which are for Sullivan the beginnings of self-esteem, which, in turn, form the basis for the child's ability to love. The child as reciprocator begins to take social form, first in the bosom of the nuclear family, then in the extended family, and finally with peers. The process is impelled through play: first solitary, then parallel, then cooperative, and finally competitive. In the process, the child ideally learns to imitate, then emulate and identify with others, and eventually develop a true sense of empathy.

While sex cleavage (the exclusive association of boys with other boys and girls with other girls) is commonly observed by virtually all investigators, little is subsequently made of it. For Sullivan (1953), however, it is the establishment of this intense homoaffiliative behavior of the preadolescent that is crucial to the appropriate development of mature love in the well-functioning adult. Sullivan sees this preadolescent homoaffiliative behavior highlighted by a unique relationship: the same sex best friend, or "chum." Few other theorists have attended so carefully to this period and this focal relationship unique to it. The importance of the chum, whose well-being becomes as important as the preadolescent's own, is for Sullivan both the paradigm and precursor of true heterosexual love. Initially, it is the finding comfort with, and caring for another who is like oneself which enables the later caring for another who is different from oneself, which eventually becomes mature heterosexual love. Thus, the transition from preadolescence to adolescence is effected.

Gradually, through socially sanctioned means, such as school dances and sports events, the two gender groups begin comingling, often with the more physically and socially mature females taking leadership in heterosexual pairing. One or two of the more mature couples begin to seek privacy, although for a long period group dating is the norm. The onset of pubescence tends to finalize the move from homoaffiliative to heterosexual patterning.

Perhaps no developmental phase receives as much attention in our culture as adolescence. The term itself is rather new, circa the 15th century. Adolescence means growing up; it is the bridge between immaturity and maturity. It is also the one stage of development experienced by both males and females that is marked by a series of clearly observable biological events which constitute puberty. The onset of puberty (roughly ages 11 to 14) and its occurrence earlier in girls than boys poses a good many problems for our posttechnological society. In other cultures and in other times, social readiness for parenting more closely corresponded to biological readiness. Courtships in those societies were either short or ceremoniously instantaneous, and marriages often were prearranged by parents. On the other hand, the hiatus between biological and social readiness as defined by our society is often half a generation—10 years—or more in length! Until recently, our culture placed heavy sanctions against premarital sexual practice as preparation for taking on the spousal role. Nonetheless, we encouraged ever-increasing intimacy through dating, where privacy is both expected and given. Thus we exacerbated the strain between the individual's biological readiness and our society's sanctions against sexual practice at specific developmental stages, and highlighted a discontinuity in our cultural conditioning (Benedict, 1938). Some mitigation of this discontinuity seems to be occurring of late, undoubtedly as a result of the increased availability, ease, and knowledge of contraceptive techniques.

In this century, before 1960, the reported rates of female premarital intercourse remained at about the 20 percent level. After 1960, this rate more than doubled. While some increase has occured in the frequency of premarital coitus for men, it is not nearly so dramatic as that for women, and the percentage of men entering marriage with no sexual experience still remains lower than that of women (King, Balswick, and Robinson, 1977). With the relaxation of the concept of *"in loco parentis,"* the years of college (in which now the majority of our young participate) would appear to be serving as much a sexual apprenticeship as an educational or vocational one (Clayton and Bokmeir, 1980; Macklin, 1980). It is after the college years that we marry, at about 21 years of age for women and 23 for men (U.S. Department of Commerce, Statistical Abstract, 1980). Because of the manner in which our dating and courtship patterns develop, marriage in America tends to be highly endogamous: we tend to marry those from similar backgrounds, education, and interests (see Rice, 1983).

Unless one wishes to count the procurement of blood tests and a civil license, the practice of prenuptial ritual in our society may vary widely from elaborate to nonexistent. However, ceremonious weddings for first marriages are the rule rather than the exception. That this is so, speaks to the emphasis (and the burden) we as a culture and as individuals place upon the institution most central to our humanity: marriage.

## Postmarital (Family of Procreation) Stages

After the marriage ceremony, our society looks differently upon the married individuals. They now constitute a socially recognized and sanctioned unit. Despite the fact that the couple may have been cohabiting, the public announcement of their commitment to each other makes a difference—not just socially, but to the couple as well. They are now Mr. and Mrs., Mr. and Ms., or sometimes just M/M, although even this is changing somewhat as more and more women are choosing to retain their family of orientation names (viz., "maiden" names). Thus, our etiquette or operating procedures, our conventions built over the years, all speak to the appropriateness of the husband and wife union. But we have as yet, no rules or conventions for dealing with cohabiting couples, and our cultural confusion is evidenced by our social awkwardness. For example, how to make an introduction with reference to the kind of relationship the two individuals share; how to extend a formal invitation to a cohabitation member for an event to which only family relatives are invited, and the like. (It is interesting to note that the same awkwardness occurs in dealing with a formerly married pair.)

In direct contrast to our social ambivalence regarding premarital sexuality, that period immediately following the wedding, the honeymoon, receives our open (although sometimes more subtle) recognition of its sexual nature. Our own romantic fantasies, memories, and humor surrounding the honeymoon are cultural indicators of our (albeit shy) social approbation and recognition of the marriage bed as the right place for sexual activity. Our children are finally adults and are expected (after a sanctioned brief period of experimentation) to produce children of their own. While some may question the validity of pressure towards pregnancy following marriage today, procreational expectations from parents, other family, and society at large are nonetheless present and, to varying degrees, explicit. As the sole tangible means for continuity or immortality, grandchildren represent a sense of completion, and serve as a source of profound gratification to the new couple's parents. Society still tends to look with question, pity, or disdain upon a childless union.

The period of the childless dyad is relatively brief for most marriages. While there are the strains of getting to know the other person, and the corresponding need to accommodate to each other, young marrieds report these years as happy. As might be anticipated, it is this period where sexual activity is reported to be the highest. Newlyweds generally are given social latitude by friends and relatives, and while the blending of the two extended families often requires some fine tuning, the couple's happiness and settling into marriage are considered the priority by everyone, including the new husband and wife (Mace and Mace, 1974).

Furthermore, for nearly all marriages, the childless period is brief because both the biological and social imperatives make the dyad unstable. Although biology sets the lower baseline to nine months, most American marriages extend this childless period to about two to three years (Duvall, 1971; Norton, 1983). With the birth of the first child, the honeymoon seems to be over. The dyad of lovers is now irrevocably transformed into the triad of family. The lovers are now parents with responsibilities, not just to themselves, but to the next generation as well. The new child places severe demands upon the couple's time and economic resources. Child rearing is demanding and absorbing, particularly for the relatively isolated nuclear family of our highly complex world.

Most family developmentalists see the child rearing phase of marriage as anywhere from two to as many as six discreet periods (depending on the children's stage of development) in the progression of the married progenitors' lives (see, Cavan, 1969, Duvall, 1971; Rogers, 1962). In all, the child rearing stage may comprise as many as 25 years of the couple's married history. Increasingly, however, in relation to the marital career, child rearing is proportionately not the longest period. The trend toward fewer children has decreased the child rearing years on the one hand, while simultaneously, life expectancy has increased longevity on the other. Thus, the marital career is now longest at its end for a growing number of couples.

Research on marital satisfaction and adjustment indicates that the middle marital stage (child rearing years) is often the most problematic for many married couples. Indeed, until recently, investigators contended that marital satisfaction and consensus between partners decreased to their lowest ebb during these child rearing years, never to return to their former, early marriage high (Rollins and Feldman, 1970; Spanier, Lewis, and Cole, 1975; Udry, 1971). If the quintessential function of marriage is "nurturant socialization" (i.e., child rearing), the finding that the child rearing years are also the least satisfying period for many couples, certainly seems ironic and deserving of some scrutiny.

Undoubtedly, one of the sources of dissatisfaction during child rearing is that the marital pair has less time to focus on itself and its needs. Sexual relationships decrease in this period relative to the childless years as a result of both familiarity and fatigue (i.e., the greater demands on time and energy, Greenblatt, 1983). Part of the problem seems to arise out of another major discontinuity of cultural conditioning: There is inadequate preparation for the role of parenting and a lack of anticipation of the intensity of its demands (Russell, 1974). The small, relatively isolated nuclear families of orientation of today offer little firsthand exposure, let alone experience with child care. Except for books on the subject and paid child care, there may be few sources of help for the first-time parents. This contrasts sharply with cultures (both past and present) where extended family members are available to help, and communities are smaller and more intimate.

In short, once past the honeymoon and the first few years of marriage, the family of procreation in America today is left alone and has little support in performing its tasks. This strain is exacerbated by the romantic fantasies about love, marriage, and child rearing perpetuated by the popular mythology. Unrealistic expectations create frustration and anguish, particularly when one is tired, money is short, the baby is crying, and one's spouse is angry about something you did or did not do. Yet, despite the child rearing periods being the most frequent stage in which extramarital affairs and divorce may occur, it is perhaps an attestation to the institution of marriage that most marriages (over two-thirds) survive this period. Furthermore, it is also worthy of comment that many couples report that the raising of their children, while perhaps arduous, was the most rewarding of their lifetime activities.

The final stage of marriage, when the children leave home, is often conceptualized in two or three phases, named for the events common to them (i.e., "empty nest," retirement, aging, widowhood, etc.). This period, when the marital dyad finds itself alone again, once used to be considered, basically, as the time of preparation for death. Both members of the dyad were believed to be experiencing growing demoralization over loss of personal generativity: for women menopause was the issue, for men retirement. Loneliness and isolation were often considered typical of the aging marital pair. Recent studies have indicated that these assumptions are baseless, at least for the present generation of middle-aged couples. Indeed, the reverse tends to be true: marital satisfaction appears to increase after the last child is launched (Schram, 1979; Spanier and Lewis, 1980). While adjustment must be made to the aging process (e.g., decreasing vigor, increasing infirmity, and the eventual dying of the marriage partner, other intimates and/or family members), most couples in the early phases of this stage of marriage seem to find pleasure in renewed mutual intimacy, a relaxed attitude about sexuality, and freedom to enjoy each other with fewer demands on their time and economic resources.

## MARITAL STRAIN, DIVORCE, AND REMEDIATION

Marriage is the ultimate form of intimacy between adult members of society. As such it is a primary counteragent to loneliness and isolation—states which are anathema to the human condition. Marriage is a bulwark that serves as a buffer to crises and stresses (both normative and aberrant) which occur during the adult years. Marriage is, however, also a responsive institution that may be positively or negatively affected by life's vicissitudes as well.

One of the first stressors on marriage is the adaptation the newlyweds must make to each other. Within each person's responses to the mundanities of life there are behaviors to which the other of the newly married pair must learn to accommodate. Often individuals are attracted to each other because of their differences and complementary styles. A relaxed person often finds an intense person interesting, a loquacious person may find a taciturn individual fascinating, and vice versa. However, common life stressors can turn healthy complementarity into conflictual polarization. Those attributes considered charming, attractive, or humorous during courtship and even through early marriage may prove to be sources of irritation and conflict later, when the pressures of daily living mount. Even though in intimate personal relationships conflict is inevitable, we are neither educated in its understanding nor trained in methods for its resolution (Bach, 1968). However, with a mutually engendered intimate and loving relationship and a willingness to confront and resolve conflict, most marriages are capable not only of withstanding, but mitigating both the expectable and unexpected stresses and crises that are inevitable in life.

One of the more dramatic accommodations for the newly married is sexual reciprocation. The pleasures of a mutually satisfying sexual life are a major source of joy when successful, and, correspondingly, a source of anguish when not. Sexual satisfaction is also pivotal because it may be affected adversely when the couple is under stress in other areas. As a result, the other problems may be exacerbated rather than resolved (Belliveau and Richter, 1970). While our society affords our maturing members few opportunities to prepare for this aspect of their mature years, both nature and society do offer some time for the newlyweds to accommodate to each other sexually. Furthermore, while greater numbers of young people are entering marriage with some sexual experience, still a large percentage are virtually inexperienced in this most crucial aspect of the marital relationship.

Unlike our animal cousins, our awareness of the importance of sexuality often creates self-consciousness, awkwardness, and a sense of failure during initial interactions. For males in our culture, who are expected to be skilled, sophisticated, and satisfying lovers—and who also must be psychologically and biologically primed—the anguish can be devastating. Likewise, disappointment, hurt, and feelings of failure are not uncommon to the female who now is expected to be orgasmic (often multiply so) to be considered responsive. With a more relaxed attitude about sexuality, as well as greater knowledge, better sexual accommodation leading to increased marital adaptation may be anticipated.

Catastrophic events are rarely anticipated, hardly ever prepared for, and usually devastating to those directly involved. Such events include those indigenous to society (some tragically so, like war or murder) or to life on this planet (like natural disasters, severely debilitating illness, or untimely death). Regardless of origin, when a catastrophe affects one individual in a married pair, the catastrophe also impinges on the marriage itself. Paradoxically, marriage, family, and society in general, are the individual's best source of protection, support, and comfort against such contingencies. One might even go so far as to say that it is in response to these adversitites that marriage and society, in general, came into being.

Some crises and the potential strains they create are both inevitable and therefore expectable. These growth pains which are anticipated throughout the lifespan are also commonly stressful and are often termed normative crises. The impact of crisis and stress upon the institution of marriage, and the manner in which the institution and its members respond and cope with these events have received increasing attention by theorists and researchers (Figley and McCubbin, 1983). Reviewing the investigations of stress and coping during the decade of the 1970s, McCubbin and his associates (1980) summarized the major life events considered sources of stress: "(1) transition to parenthood, (2) child launching, (3) post parental transition (i.e., 'empty nest'), (4) retirement, (5) widowhood," and "(6) relocation and institutionalization," the last category being associated with aging.

Less attended to in the literature, though ubiquitously observed in the popular press and the records of mental health professionals as sources of intense personal stress, are those annual events such as holidays and the changing of the seasons. At these times, an individual's nostalgic fantasies or expectations often contrast sharply with the less than ideal realities experienced. Thus, Christmas and spring are times which are apt to bring on feelings of loneliness and despair, particularly if one's interpersonal relationships are simultaneously found lacking.

Another stressor with more insidious erosive qualities is that of economic insecurity. In our highly monetized society, economic insecurity as a form of stress does not refer just to those experiencing poverty. Any abrupt change in living standards, or an event which is likely to cause the anticipation of such a change (e.g., change of job, temporary or long-term unemployment, illness) can impose strain severe enough to have deleterious effects on the marital relationship. This tends to be particularly true of men, for whom self-esteem is highly dependent upon the ability to provide adequately for their wives and children. Ironically, in its most severe form such strain can lead to aggression and physical abuse of loved ones within the family (Prescott and Letko, 1977).

While marriage is the most basic and perhaps the most resilient of all social institutions, it is not immune to failure. Historically, divorce, the dissolution of the "eternal" bonds of matrimony, has always been recognized as an option, even if an unhappy one. Because of the importance we place upon marriage (even to the point of attributed divine approbation), heavy sanctions have generally been placed against divorce. Even today, with divorce having become a relatively common occurrence, it is nevertheless looked upon with high disfavor, and heavily imbued with the notion of both personal and interpersonal failure.

However, it may be wise to reconsider recent figures on divorce which are often used to attest to the fact that marriage as an institution is somewhat of a failure. Although demographers themselves warn against the cursory examination of census figures and note the difficulty in their interpretation, these figures are often misunderstood and misused (Norton, 1983). For example, the high divorce rate found in the first two years of marriage, often leads to the interpretation that these years are often the hardest (Rice, 1983). This would appear to be in direct contradiction with the results of studies on marital satisfaction that indicate that couples view these as the most satisfying years. The divorce statistics also indicate that teenage marriages are high risks. Considering that the process of divorce takes months, a final decree in the first year or two after marriage suggests that the relationship would have had to have been problematic at its inception. We are also aware that while the figures are difficult to obtain, many teenaged couples marry post pregnancy. Actually, the only reason for the marriage may have been the pregnancy. Therefore, it is likely that a good many of those marriages which fail in the early months had the seeds of failure sown before the union was legalized. Thus rather than attest to the failure of marriage as an institution, these results may indeed, indicate the contrary—that marriage may have been successful as a means to legitimize a child and give it a name.

Divorce, by nearly any standard, must be viewed as a highly negatively charged life event. It certainly qualifies as a discontinuity in cultural conditioning. Although we have cultural tools for facilitating an appropriate entry into marriage (*i.e.*, ceremony, social witnessing, etc.), we have none for easing our exit. If we are to address divorce as a necessary cultural phenomenon, we must comprehend both its rational and nonrational aspects. From an emotional perspective, divorce typically represents an extreme form of personal loss. Like any other such loss, divorce may also require a grieving and mourning period before rehabilitation can be anticipated.

Finally, in a discussion of divorce the possibility of remarriage exists. As noted in the introduction, the increase in the divorce rate seems to have done little to disenchant us with the idea that marriage is the best way for man and woman to live together. Nearly 90 percent of all divorced men and women remarry (Carter and Glick, 1970), and recent figures indicate that nearly one-third of our annual marriage rates are comprised of remarriages for either one or both partners (Price-Bonham and Balswick, 1980). These figures would seem to suggest that it is not the institution of marriage we consider a failure, but rather our abilities at it or our preparation for it.

We do not know much about the quality of life for remarrieds. There are certainly aspects to it that would make it different from first time marriages for the individuals involved. Often the marital pair starts out with a preformed or blended family, that is, one or both spouses enters the new marriage with children from an earlier relationship. This instantly structured new family may pose strains regarding the children's acceptance of the new spouse as parent (decision maker, disciplinarian) and as intimate partner to the child's original parent. The newlyweds often have little time and even less privacy in which to try to accommodate to each other. Moreover, the failure of the first marriage may cause worry and anxiety about the second. On the other hand, the couple is often older, wiser, and probably more realistic with regard to expectations (see Sager, *et al.* 1983).

It would seem that we are becoming aware that marriage is an institution worthy of being worked at, and one not to be taken for granted. While it would be unwise to make an association between this presumption and the observation that marriage and family therapy is now a defined and accepted clinical intervention approach by the mental health community, the fact does remain that in the same generation which has seen a rapid increase in the frequency of divorce, there has been a corresponding increase in marriage and family therapy as a mental health option.

Although marital therapy has its critics (Lasch, 1977) its increased attention from both the public and the mental health community would indicate that it is filling a need. No brief attempt here can do justice to the plethora of theoretical material and growing empirical research produced in this field in little more than a generation (see Gurman and Kniskern, 1981; Levant, 1984). As a specialty, marriage and family therapy had its beginnings at about the middle of this century, with roots in child guidance, mental health, sociology, and home economics—all of which claimed the marriage field as their legitimate heir. Theoretically, marital therapy draws upon not only these disciplines, but also from the newer disciplines of communications, systems theory, and cybernetics (see Keeney, 1983). But simply put, marital and family therapy deals with relationship problems within the context of the relationship. This contextual emphasis represents a departure from individual psychotherapy. This contextual approach also makes marital and family therapy a more pragmatic approach that often deals with immediate problems in living and major life stressors, as well as those of a much more long-standing nature. Because all of individual development may be seen as a preparation for marriage, it is not unusual for individual, personal problems, relating to either or both spouse's premarital history, to surface during the course of marriage therapy. These too, then become available for resolution within the context of the marital relationship.

Like individual psychotherapy, outcome research on the effectiveness of marital therapy is at best equivocal. There is, however, one finding which stands out: For ameliorating marital difficulties, marital therapy is decidedly more effective than no therapy and dramatically more effective than individual therapy, which, indeed, can even be considered deleterious to the marital relationship (Gurman and Kniskern, 1978). While the observation that individual psychotherapy tends to be counterproductive in dealing with marital distress may seem surprising at first glance, it actually makes good sense. In individual therapy, the therapist hears and responds to the individual client's perceptions and in so doing tends to validate and confirm those perceptions. By contrast the marital therapist is presented with the perceptions of both the husband and wife (as each spouse is presented with the view of the other). Although in the case of individual therapy there is no opportunity to clarify misperceptions and misunderstandings regarding given events or feelings, in marital therapy this process is central.

Recently two pragmatic allied counseling approaches have emerged. These are divorce mediation and family financial counseling. Both of these endeavors, as their names suggest, deal with more circumscribed issues within the marital context and have come into being to meet specific needs.

Through the adversarial stance of the judicial system, the anguish surrounding divorce has been exacerbated. Divorce is now too often traumatic and the scars created may have long-term and far-reaching repercussions on the principals and those around them. Divorce mediation, a hybrid of marital, financial, and legal counseling, is an attempt at mitigating the stress of terminating a marriage and often splitting a family. While it is, as yet, too new to predict its effectiveness, some report success in reducing the acrimony surrounding the divorce process (Coogler, 1979; Haynes, 1978).

Our society's heavy emphasis on acquisition and spending, and our less than adequate preparation for responsible consumerism find our modern couples often foundering while in the process of performing those tasks necessary to create and maintain households and raise families. With the ease of credit, and the ability to buy without having adequate resources, couples often find themselves over their heads in debt, and panicked. The overwhelming nature of the problem, so basic to life in America, often affects the totality of the couple's relationship, extending even into the sexual arena and the conjugal bed. Here too, the field of family financial counseling (VanArsdale, 1982) is too new to predict its ability to aid the institution of marriage and us as individuals in our attempts to live productive and satisfying lives.

No form of psychotherapy as yet devised, however, is likely to eliminate many of the problems discussed in this chapter. There are few if any psychotherapeutic cures for poverty, pestilence, or death. Our best armor against the inevitable psychological distress incurred by coming up against the contingencies of life has been marriage (and family) itself. The best that marriage therapy can hope to do is enhance the institution's ability to do what it does best—teach us to care about and help one another through a mutual life course.

## CONCLUSION

The debate with regard to the universality and viability of marriage and family will undoubtedly continue among social scientists and social critics. However, in such debates, the issues are academic. Suffice it to say that for all intents and purposes the idea of marriage—even in cultures where sexual permissiveness is accepted and prevasive—is indigenous to the human species. Thus marriage is perhaps the most satisfactory institution we have fallen heir to, and far more functional than any other we have as yet devised.

# REFERENCES

Ardry, R.: *The Social Contract: A Personal Inquiry into the Evolutionary Sources of Order and Disorder.* Atheneum Press, New York, 1970.

Aries, P.: *Centuries of Childhood: A Social History of Family Life.* (Trans. R. Baldick.) Knopf, New York, 1962.

Aries, P.: The family and the city in the old world and the new. In Tufte, V., and Myerhoff, B.: (eds.): *Changing Image of the Family.* Yale University Press, New Haven, 1977.

Bach, G. R.: *The Intimate Enemy.* Avon, New York, 1968.

Bardis, P.: Family forms and variations historically considered. In Christianson, H.: (ed.): *Handbook of Marriage and Family.* Rand McNally, Chicago, 1964.

Belliveau, F., and Richter, L.: *Understanding Human Sexual Inadequacy.* Bantam, New York, 1970.

Benedict, R.: Continuities and discontinuities in cultural conditioning. *Psychiatry* 1:161–167, 1938.

Bowlby, J.: *Maternal Care and Mental Health.* World Health Organization, Monograph no. 2, Geneva, 1952.

Carter, H., and Glick, P. C.: *Marriage and Divorce: A Social and Economic Study.* Harvard University Press, Cambridge, Mass., 1970.

Cavan, R. S.: The family life cycle. In Cavan, R. S.: (ed.): *Marriage and Family in the Modern World.* Thomas Y. Crowell, New York, 1969.

Clayton, R. R.: *The Family, Marriage, and Social Change.* Heath, Lexington, Mass., 1975.

Clayton, R. R., and Bokmeir, J. L.: Premarital sex in the seventies, *J. Marriage Fam.,* 42:759–776, 1980.

Condon, W. S., and Sander, L. M.: Synchrony demonstrated between movement of the neonate and adult speech. *Child Dev.,* 45:456–462, 1974.

Coogler, O. J.: Divorce mediation: A means of facilitating divorce and adjustment. *Fam. Coordin.,* 28:255–259, 1979.

Duvall, E. M.: *Family Development,* 4th ed. Lippincott, Philadelphia, 1971.

Erikson, E. H.: *Childhood and Society,* Rev. ed. W. W. Norton, New York, 1964.

Figley, C. R., and McCubbin, H. I.: *Stress and the Family. Vol. I: Coping with Normative Transitions; Vol. II: Coping with Catastrophe.* Brunner/Mazel, New York, 1983.

Freud, A.: *Infants Without Families.* International Universities Press, New York, 1944.

Freud, S.: *Three Contributions to the Theory of Sex.* Dutton, New York, 1962. (Originally published, 1910).

Gaylin, N.: Rediscovering the family. In Stinett, N.; Chesser, B.; DeFrain, J.; Knaub, P.: (eds.): *Family Strengths: Positive Models for Family Life.* University of Nebraska Press, Lincoln, 1980.

Gaylin, W.: *Caring.* Knopf, New York, 1976.

Glick, P. C., and Norton, A. J.: Marrying, divorcing, and living together in the U.S. today. *Population Bulletin* 32:1–39, 1977.

Greenblatt, C. S.: The salience of sexuality in the early years of marriage. *J. Marriage Fam.,* 45:289–299, 1983.

Gurman, A. S., and Kniskern, D. P.: Research on marital and family therapy: progress, perspective, and prospect. In Grafieldm S. L., and Bergin, A. E.: (eds.): *Handbook of Psychotherapy and Behavior Change: An Empirical Analysis,* 2nd ed. Wiley, New York, 1978.

Gurman, A. S., and Kniskern, D. P.: (eds.): *Handbook of Family Therapy.* Brunner/Mazel, New York, 1981.

Haynes, J. L.: Divorce mediator: A new role. *Soc. Work,* 23:5–9, 1978.

Keeney, B. P.: *Aesthetics of change.* Guilford Press, New York, 1983.

King, D.; Balswick, J.; and Robinson, I.: The continuing premarital sexual revolution among college females. *J. Marriage Fam.,* 39:455–459, 1977.

Kluchkohn, C.; Murray, H.; and Schneider, D.: *Personality in Nature, Society, and Culture.* Knopf, New York, 1956.

Lasch, C.: *Haven in a Heartless World: The Family Besieged.* Basic Books, New York, 1977.

Levant, R. F.: *Family Therapy: A Comprehensive Overview.* Prentice–Hall, Englewood Cliffs, New Jersey, 1984.

McCubbin H. I.; Joy, C. B.; Cauble, A. E.; Comeau, J. K.; Patterson, J. M.; and Needle, R. H.: Family stress and coping: a decade review. *J. Marriage Fam.,* 42:855–871, 1980.

Mace, D., and Mace, V.: *We Can Have Better Marriages If We Want Them.* Abingdon, Nashville, Tennessee, 1974.

Macklin, E. D.: Nontraditional family forms: A decade of research. *J. Marriage Fam.,* 42:905–922, 1980.

Meltzoff, A. N., and Moore, M. K.: Imitation of facial and manual gestures by human neonates. *Science,* 198:75–85, 1977.

Morris, D.: *The Naked Ape.* McGraw-Hill, New York, 1967.

Murdock, G. P.: *Social Structure.* Macmillan, New York, 1949.

Norton, A. J.: Family life cycle: 1980. *J. Marriage Fam.,* 45:267–275, 1983.

Parsons, T., and Bales, R. F.: *Family, Socialization and Interaction Process.* Free Press, New York, 1955.

Piaget, J.: *The Origins of Intelligence in Children.* Trans. M. Cook. International Universities Press, New York, 1952.

Prescott, S., and Letko, C.: Battered women: a social psychological perspective. In Roy, M.: (Ed.): *Battered Women: A Psychological Study of Domestic Violence.* Van Nostrand Reinhold, New York, 1977.

Pritchard, J. B.: (ed.): *Ancient Near Eastern Texts Relative to the Old Testament.,* 2nd ed. Princeton University Press, Princeton, 1955.

Price-Bonham, S., and Balswick, J. O.: The noninstitutions: divorce, desertion and remarriage. *J. Marriage Fam.,* 42:959–972, 1980.

Reiss, I. L.: The universality of the family: A conceptual analysis. *J. Marriage Fam.,* 27:443–453, 1965.

Rice, P. F.: *Contemporary Marriage.* Allyn and Bacon, New York, 1983.

Rodgers, R.: *Improvements in the Construction and Analysis of Family Life Cycle Categories.* Western Michigan University Press, Kalamazoo, 1962.

Rollins, B., and Feldman, H.: Marital satisfaction over the life cycle. *J. Marriage Fam.*, 32:20–27, 1970.

Russell, C. S.: Transition to parenthood: Problems and gratifications. *J. Marriage Fam.*, 36:294–302, 1974.

Sager, C. J.; Brown, H. S.; Crohn, H.; Engel, T.; Rodstein, E.; and Walker, L.: *Treating the Remarried Family.* Brunner/Mazel, New York, 1983.

Sagi, A., and Hoffman, M. L.: Empathic distress in the newborn. *Dev. Psychol.*, 12:175–176, 1976.

Schram, R. W.: Marital satisfaction over the family life cycle: A critique and proposal. *J. Marriage Fam.*, 41:7–12, 1979.

Spanier, G. B., and Lewis, R. A.: Marital quality: A review of the seventies. *J. Marriage Fam.*, 42:825–839, 1980.

Spanier, G. B.; Lewis, R. A.; and Cole, C. L.: Marital adjustment over the life cycle: The issue of curvilinearity. *J. Marriage Fam.*, 37:263–275, 1975.

Spitz, R.: Hospitalism: An inquiry into the genesis in early childhood. In Freud, A: (ed): *The Psychoanalytic Study of the Child.* Vol. I. International Universities Press, New York, 1945.

Stephens, W. N.: *The Family in Cross-Cultural Perspective.* Holt Rinehart and Winston, New York, 1963.

Sullivan, H. S.: *The Interpersonal Theory of Psychiatry.* W. W. Norton, New York, 1953.

Udry, J.: *The Social Context of Marriage.* Lippincott, Philadelphia, 1971.

U.S. Department of Commerce. Bureau of the Census. *Statistical Abstract of the United States, 1980.* U.S. Government Printing Office, Washington, D.C., 1980.

VanArsdale, M. G.: *A Guide to Family Financial Counseling.* Dow Jones–Erwin, Homewood, Ill., 1982.

Washburn, S. L., and Devore, I.: The social behavior of baboons an early man. In Washburn, S. L.: (ed.): *Social Life of Early Man.* Aldine, Chicago, 1961.

Weber, M.: *The Protestant Ethic and The Spirit of Capitalism.* G. Allen, London, 1930.

Wilson, E. D.: *Sociology.* Harvard University Press, Cambridge, Mass., 1980.

# CHAPTER 5  HUMAN SEXUALITY DURING NORMAL PREGNANCY

*Arnold W. Cohen, M.D.*

## INTRODUCTION

Sexual behavior expresses the totality of one's being. It may express love, caring, affection, aggression, lust, or power. There is strong data to suggest that human beings are different from other animals in that there is an inverse relationship between the advancing phyletic status and the degree to which female sexual behavior is controlled by hormones (Beach, 1947). Certainly testosterone, progesterone, and estrogen have an effect on sexual behavior in human beings, but gonadotropin releasing hormone (GNRH), dopamine, and serotonin, which act in the brain rather than at the genital organ site, are involved to a much greater degree in human sexuality than in other animals (Beach, 1947). Since sexual relations strengthen the ties of caring and mutual respect by providing pleasure and intimacy between two people at the same time (Reamy, et al., 1982), marital success and happiness does depend to a large degree on a high level of sexual satisfaction. Therefore, changes in sexual practices due to sexual inhibitions or restrictions imposed by pregnancy may produce serious consequences for even a stable marriage.

Pregnancy is a time in which many changes and stresses occur. There are many physiological, as well as psychological adjustments that have to be made in both the female and the male. It is a time "when lovers become parents and a couple becomes a family" (Dameron, 1983). These changes in family status stress both the mother and the father. Kumar and colleagues (1981) maintain that maternal personality, childhood relationships, marital conflicts, depression, previous miscarriages, difficulty in conceiving, and fear of harming the fetus all affect maternal sexuality. There are many changes and accomodations that have to be made for both partners during pregnancy. This chapter will explore the factual information available relating to sexuality during pregnancy. It will review the anatomic changes associated with pregnancy, as well as the physiologic changes of the sexual response seen during this time of a woman's life. The sexual response of the female during pregnancy, including libido, coital frequency, and orgasm will be considered in relationship to different stages of gestation. The various alternatives and changes in sexual practices will be considered for both the male and the female. Finally, the effects of coitus, orgasm, and noncoital sexual behavior and their relationship to the outcome of the pregnancy will be reviewed.

## EFFECTS OF PREGNANCY ON SEXUALITY

Most mammalian females do not seek intercourse during pregnancy (Solberg et al., 1973). Sexual activity during pregnancy, whether it be coital or noncoital, therefore, places the human female at a different behavioral level than most other mammals. Because of this different behavior many religious and moral taboos have been adopted through the years. Jewish law prohibits intercourse during pregnancy and lactation. The Catholic Church has stated that since sex during pregnancy is not for procreation, but only for pleasure, it is not good (Sloan and Bing, 1983). Limner (1970), in what has been called a sociologic diatribe concerning sexuality during pregnancy, states that maternal sexual activity has a lasting deleterious effect on the developing fetus from a physiological, as well as a psychological standpoint. He believes that Adam had coitus with a pregnant Eve and this act resulted in the consequences of the "original sin." He states that the "original sin" was a violation of the natural sex taboo appreciated by all other pregnant animals.

Despite these attitudes, no factual data suggests that these statements are true. Information from the Bible mentions that polygamy was a means of avoiding the stresses that a male would be confronted with during pregnancy. In Genesis 4, Lanech had two wives. One was said to be for bearing his children and one for "cavorting" (Holtzman, 1976). Limner (1970) also states that few males of the animal world would ever think of approaching a pregnant female sexually. To the contrary for humans in today's society, there is good evidence that prolonged abstinence may actually threaten the monogamous marital unit by encouraging adultery (Masters and Johnson, 1966). When many different societies have been studied, it was found that 21 out of 60 societies prohibited sex during pregnancy (Ford and Beach, 1951). Of these 21 societies though, 19 of them practiced polygamy so that the husband had access to other legitimate sexual outlets during the pregnancy of one wife. In societies that prohibited sex during pregnancy there was the underlying fear that coitus would harm the fetus and that abstention from sexual activity would prevent the fetus from any injury *in utero*. In today's society, sexuality can be repressed when necessary during pregnancy to promote motherhood. When a problem is found in a gravid patient that would necessitate abstinence from sexual activity, practicing obstetricians find almost total cooperation from the patient, though the male partner's cooperation during this time may be variable.

Sexuality during pregnancy is influenced by the interrelationship of cultural, psychological, religious, sociological, and biological factors (Battacchi, et al., 1978). Swanson (1980) has stated that four factors influence a couple's adjustment during pregnancy. The first factor is the obstetrician's role during pregnancy. In many cases there is a transference of the wife's love during the pregnancy from the husband to the physician. This transference may result in increased jealousy on the part of the husband, which could interfere with instructions or admonitions given by the physician to the woman during the pregnancy. The second factor is the husband's response to the pregnancy. Many men experience an ambivalence. They may be very happy about the pregnancy, but have a great deal of anxiety concerning the changes in their lives that will occur after the birth of a child. The "Couvade syndrome" has been found in the husbands of pregnant women. In a study of 267 mates of pregnant women at a Rochester, New York, Health Maintenance Organization, 60 men (22.5 percent) developed some complaints of pregnancy similar to those their wives were experiencing (*Courier Post,* 1983). It is felt that the complaints represent the husbands' attempt to identify with their wives during the pregnancy. The third factor that influences the couple's adjustment during pregnancy is the wife's emotional response. Her fantasy activity during sexual dreams may increase, and these dreams may actually produce intense orgasmic responses that are uncontrollable by the pregnant woman. The fourth factor is that this uncontrollable activity can produce guilt. Since orgasm does not relieve much of the pelvic congestion associated with pregnancy, the woman has a continued feeling of discomfort and guilt related to sex during pregnancy.

Falicov (1973) found that women with a high level of sexuality prior to pregnancy showed less ambivalence or conflict about sexual relations during pregnancy, experienced fewer and milder changes in their sexuality during pregnancy, and enjoyed sex at this time more than women who had lower sexual ratings prior to pregnancy. Those women who enjoyed sex more prior to pregnancy tended to continue to have sex until later in pregnancy and returned to sexual activity sooner after the pregnancy ended. These findings were confirmed by Perkins (1982) who found that sexually experienced and satisfied women compensate better in changed circumstances (i.e., pregnancy) than inexperienced and unfulfilled women. He found the rewards of sexual satisfaction retarded the rate of decline in sexual interest and activity experienced by most women during pregnancy. Despite this finding, though, the influences of pregnancy are sufficiently potent and pervasive that regardless of prior conditioning and experience almost all pregnant women tend to react similarly with some decrease in sexuality late in pregnancy. Even though coital activity decreases in the majority of pregnant women, there is still an increased desire for close physical contact during pregnancy (Hallender and McGehee, 1974; Tolar and DiGrazia, 1976). These findings show that sexuality during pregnancy can be expressed in many ways, and these will be discussed later in this chapter.

## PHYSICAL CHANGES ASSOCIATED WITH PREGNANCY

The deposition of fat in the truncal areas, as well as the enlarging uterus and breasts, combined with the edema that occurs not only in the legs but in the face, cause a marked change in the physical appearance of the woman during pregnancy. These changes are secondary to increases in estrogen, progesterone, prolactin, and other hormones. The resulting effects of dyspnea, intolerance to heat, frequent urination, nausea, vomiting, gingival hypertrophy with vascular abnormalities, and changes in posture associated with pregnancy may alter the desire for sexual activity in both the male and the female. Women may not be considered a desirable sexual object during pregnancy due to these changes. This results in a decrease in sexual feelings and behavior. The vasocongestion of the sexual organs associated with sexual arousal added upon the vasocongestion of these organs related to pregnancy alone may cause an increased sensitivity of the breasts and the pelvic organs. This congestion, in some women, may cause discomfort while in others it may cause an increased intensity of sexual response. It has been found that in some patients orgasm is only achieved for the first time during pregnancy and multiple orgasm may occur frequently. The increase in vaginal secretions associated with pregnancy may be pleasurable for some, but others find it to be a deterrent to orogenital sex (Solberg, et al., 1973). Since the cervix bleeds with coitus at times during pregnancy this can also cause alarm and fear in both partners (Dameron, 1983).

## SEXUAL RESPONSE DURING PREGNANCY

Despite the fact that sex is probably the most frequently written about subject in the English language, surprisingly few studies actually evaluate the sexual response during pregnancy. We are indebted to the work of Masters and Johnson (1966), which remains the best physiologic account of sexual response during pregnancy. Review of this work is necessary for anyone who is interested in human sexuality at this time in a woman's life. It must be realized that this work was based on the study of six subjects who underwent anatomic and physiologic evaluation at various times in the pregnancy. Four of the six patients had participated in studies prior to pregnancy. These patients therefore are highly selected and may not actually represent normative behavior or response. Despite this drawback, the information provided by this work is the best available to date.

## Breast Changes

The increased size of the breasts seen in early pregnancy is due to both vascular and glandular growth. It may be one of the first signs of early pregnancy in many patients. During the plateau phase of sexual tension 20 to 25 percent of non-pregnant women have an increase in the size of their breasts during the first trimester. The increase in venous congestion that normally occurs in a nulliparous patient is accentuated with sexual stimulation. Because of the severe vasocongestion related to sexual stimuli during pregnancy women may complain of severe breast tenderness during the advanced stages of sexual tension early in pregnancy. The nipples become turgid and are associated with an enlarged areolar area, which may be quite sensitive. During the second and third trimester there is a decrease in the complaint of breast tenderness in the nulliparous woman. Sexual tension does not increase the breast size any longer. The nipples though, do remain erect and areolar tumescence remains. Orgasmic phase sexual tension may result in the "letting down" of milk, which at some times may cause alarm in both the male and the female. This, though, is a normal response.

## Genital Organs

The genital organs during pregnancy have an increase in vascularity both internally, as well as externally. When the physiologic response to sexual stimulation is further superimposed upon the normal changes of pregnancy there may be a feeling of massive pelvic congestion. Falicov (1973) found that 18 of 19 patients appreciated that their vagina felt smaller because of this pelvic congestion. For some patients penile penetration becomes painful. A feeling of vaginal numbness may occur during the first trimester in a minority of patients. Four of the six patients studied by Masters and Johnson (1966) experienced cramping and aching in the middle of the lower abdomen during and immediately after orgasm in the first trimester. Despite this discomfort, none of the women developed bleeding or aborted the pregnancy. During the excitement phase of sexual response the vasocongestion of both the internal and external genitalia to sexual stimulation appears to be more significant than the myotonia that is seen in the non-pregnant woman. The labia majora of the nullipara usually meet in the midline. During the excitement phase they thin out and flatten against the perineum. There is also a slight elevation of the labia majora in the upward and outward direction. In multiparous patients there is an excessive engorgement of these organs. They become edematous and there is an involuntary lateral withdrawal from the vaginal outlet. The elevation and the flattening of the labia majora are absent after the first trimester.

The labia minora are usually markedly engorged. They may be two to three times the normal size. Vasocongestion increases with sex stimulation during the first and second trimester, but during the third trimester these organs are so engorged from the effects of pregnancy that further distention with sex cannot occur. At the end of the first trimester there is an increase in the amount of vaginal transudate that results in increased vaginal lubrication. This appears to develop earlier during sexual stimulation and is more extensive than in non-pregnant patients. The increased lubrication appears to be greater in multiparous than in primiparous women. There is a light mucoid discharge by the end of the first trimester that occurs all the time during pregnancy related to the pelvic congestion and transudation of fluid. This discharge also increases with sexual excitement.

At the end of the first trimester the uterus becomes an intraabdominal rather than an intrapelvic organ. Physiologic distention and elevation, even in the retroverted or retroflexed uterus, occurs during the excitement phase of sexual response early in pregnancy. The vaginal expansion and distention seen in the non-pregnant patients continues to occur during pregnancy, but the tenting of the vagina that increases the transcervical vaginal depth secondary to uterine elevation during the excitement phase cannot be demonstrated after the uterus becomes an intraabdominal organ. Despite the changes in the vaginal secretions there is no evidence of an increase in cervical secretions during the excitement phase of sexual stimulation.

During the plateau phase of sexual stimulation the labia minora retract and there is engorgement of the outer third of the vagina. This is referred to as the orgasmic platform. In the nulliparous patient engorgement is so intense that 75 percent of the vaginal lumen may be obliterated. In multiparous women the orgasmic platform develops and almost completely obliterates the entire vaginal barrel. The more advanced the pregnancy, the more severe the venous engorgement and the more extensive the orgasmic platform becomes. In the plateau phase uterine elevation, as previously stated, cannot be demonstrated after the uterus becomes an intraabdominal organ. In the non-pregnant patient, uterine vasocongestion increases the size of the uterus and broad ligament. In pregnancy this cannot be identified properly because of the insensitivity of the means of measuring these parameters.

During the orgasmic phase of sexual stimulation the orgasmic platform contracts. These contractions continue to occur during the first and second trimester. In the third trimester vasocongestion is so intense that the contractions of the orgasmic platform appear to be minimal, despite the fact that orgasm may be subjectively satisfying and intense. Uterine contractions related to orgasm have been noticed during the last several weeks of pregnancy. These contractions may be tonic rather than intermittent. They may last up to one minute in length and continue for approximately one-half hour after the orgasmic experience.

In pregnancy vasocongestion is not entirely relieved by orgasm. There is continued engorgement of both the labia majora and minora, as well as the vaginal barrel. During the second trimester resolution may take 10 to 15 minutes after orgasm in the primiparous patient and up to 30 to 45 minutes in the woman who has previously had a child. This incomplete resolution may account for the subjectively higher sexual tension levels seen in the second and third trimesters. Despite the incomplete resolution, orgasm may feel subjectively quite satisfying, but it may not entirely relieve all sexual tension.

These physiologic studies on six pregnant patients by Masters and Johnson are the basis for our understanding of sexual response during pregnancy. Most other studies done are concerned with the subjective and quantitative aspects of sexuality during pregnancy or the consequences of sex upon the mother, fetus, or marital unit. These studies will be considered next.

## SEXUAL ACTIVITY DURING PREGNANCY

Sexual relations during pregnancy may invoke guilt and fear. Perkins (1982) found that 34 out of 141 patients studied practiced orgasm suppression because of fear of hurting the baby or starting labor. There is a decrease in the frequency of sexual relations during the first trimester in many patients because of a fear of aborting the pregnancy or harming the fetus (Battacchi et al., 1978; Falicov, 1973; Kumar et al., 1981). Husbands have also expressed a concern that the fetus may act as an observer to the sexual act and that the presence of this "third" person inhibits sexual spontaneity. There can also be a fear that the fetus could harm the man's penis during coitus (White and Reamy, 1982). These fears in both the male and female can produce changes in sexual behavior. With the knowledge that the pregnant patient and her mate go into pregnancy with certain fears—whether they be founded or unfounded—concerning the effect of sexual relations on the fetus, many studies have been undertaken to evaluate the effect of pregnancy on sexual activity, including sexual interests, sexual frequency, sexual satisfaction, orgasm, and changes in position which occur during pregnancy.

## LEVELS OF SEXUAL DESIRE

It is interesting to note that the Kinsey report, published prior to Masters and Johnson's thesis, did not cover any sexual behavior during pregnancy. The first major prospective study to address this issue was by Masters and Johnson (1966) in which 111 pregnant patients were studied regarding sexual behavior. Of the 111 patients, 43 were primigravid. There were ten pregnancy losses during this study period. Of the 101 women who remained pregnant and who were studied throughout the pregnancy the average level of education was nearly three years of college. A great variation in the level of eroticism and sexual satisfaction was found during the first trimester. Of the 43 nulliparous patients, 33 had a decrease in sexual tension as well as a decrease in the effectiveness of sexual performance due to vomiting, sleeplessness, and fatigue. More than half of the patients had a significant fear of injuring the conceptus and abstained from sexual activity to avoid miscarrying. Six of the 43 patients had no change in their sexual interest level or effectiveness and only four of the 43 (10 percent) had an increase in sexual interest. In the multiparous patients, 57 out of 68, or almost 84 percent, had very little change in the level of sexual interest or effectiveness of performance. About 10 percent of the patients had a decrease in sexual interest because of nausea and vomiting and only four of the 68 patients had an increase in their sex drive or improved performance level.

In the second trimester Masters and Johnson found an increase in eroticism and effectiveness of performance regardless of age or parity. Of the 101 patients, 82 had an increase in sexuality over their prepregnancy level, while 19 of 101 had no change in their sexual interests. The researchers found that many of these patients not only had an increased interest in the sexual encounter, but also had an increase in their fantasy and dream content relating to sexuality. There is also an increased demand for satisfaction with sex during this time period. By the third trimester, nulliparous patients once again reported a decrease in coital frequency related to fatigue, irritability, abdominal fullness, pelvic tension, and backache. For 31 out of the 43 nulliparous patients intercourse was prohibited by the physician. In fact, 33 out of these 43 patients actually had lost interest in sex by the last trimester. Two-thirds of the multiparous patients also experienced a decrease in eroticism. This decrease was believed to be due to exhaustion and the physical demands of caring for other children.

These general findings by Masters and Johnson, showing a decrease in sexual activity and sexual satisfaction in the first trimester with an increase in these parameters during the second trimester and then a subsequent fall during the third trimester, have been re-evaluated by many other investigators. Studies done on sexual desire during pregnancy tend to show that 10 to 20 percent of patients have an increased desire during the first trimester while in a third of the patients this desire tends to decrease during this time period. The majority of patients have no change in their libido. The second trimester has similar findings with a slightly increased number of patients having a decrease in sexual desire. The third trimester is marked by a much greater number of patients showing a decrease in sexual desire. It should be noted, though, that anywhere from 8 to 24 percent of the patients studied still show an increase in sexual desire during the third trimester (Battacchi et al., 1978; Kenny, 1973; Kumar and Brant, 1981; Solberg et al., 1973; Tolar and DiGrazia, 1976). These findings are summarized in Table 5–1.

Most of these statistics are obtained from questionnaires that are distributed in the postpartum period. Therefore, the reliability of these data is dependent on patient recall. Reamy (Reamy et al., 1982) followed 52 patients in a prospective fashion from the first trimester and found that there was great varia-

TABLE 5-1 **Level of Sexual Desire during Pregnancy**

| Level | Trimester | | |
|---|---|---|---|
| | 1st | 2nd | 3rd |
| | (% of patients studied) | | |
| Increased | 10–23 | 14–24 | 8–24 |
| Unchanged | 45–57 | 32–72 | 15–34 |
| Decreased | 28–39 | 34–47 | 42–70 |

tion in sexual desire. His conclusion was that in most cases, compared to prepregnancy levels, there is a decrease in sexual desire during the first trimester and a trend toward a reduced desire during the second trimester. There is much individual variation during the second trimester, but a definite decrease in sexual desire occurs during the third trimester in almost all patients. Lumley (1978) in a study of 30 primigravidas found a progressive decline in sexual desire throughout the pregnancy. Falicov (1973) studied 19 primigravidas throughout pregnancy and found a decrease in desire during the first trimester, a relatively slight increase in this parameter during the second trimester compared to the first trimester (but still a decreased desire compared to prepregnancy levels), and a marked fall in sexual desire during the third trimester. In general one can say that studies done from many different societies with multiparous and primiparous patients show a trend toward gradual abatement of sexual desire as pregnancy progresses despite the great individual variation noted (Bartova et al., 1969; Battacchi et al., 1978; Falicov, 1973; Holtzman, 1976; Kenny, 1973; Landes et al., 1950; Lumley, 1978; Masters and Johnson, 1966; Reamy et al., 1982; Solberg et al., 1973; Tolar and DiGrazia, 1976).

## FREQUENCY OF SEXUAL RELATIONS

The frequency of sexual relations during pregnancy, as well as eroticism, has been considered by many authors. Masters and Johnson (1966) found that unmarried patients had little or no eroticism and this resulted in a decreased frequency of sexual relations during the first trimester. It was felt that these patients were overwhelmed by the social aspects of their circumstances as well as their concerns for financial security which the pregnancy imposed upon them. Morris (1975) studied 114 pregnant patients in Thailand and found that the average frequency of coitus was 1.7 times per week. There was a gradual fall in the number of experiences per week until the seventh month, but it was only after the seventh month that a statistically significant decreased frequency was found. In a similar study done by Pongthai (Pongthai et al., 1979), 210 women were studied and the average frequency of coitus was between two and three times per week prepregnancy. This rate continued until the second trimester. In the third trimester it fell to approximately one time per week. This investigator found that if coital frequency was greater than four times per week prior to pregnancy, coitus continued at a similar rate until the third trimester. In those patients who had a baseline rate of coitus of one or less times per week, though, there was a faster decline in coital frequency during the pregnancy than in those patients who had a baseline rate of more than one time per week.

Solberg and colleagues (1973) found that in the United States the average number of coital acts per month in the prepregnant state was 14. This rate declines in a sequential fashion to about six coital acts per month in the ninth month of pregnancy. In a study of 25 women, Holtzman (1976) found a linear decline in coital frequency from 2.8 times per week to 1.7 times per week as pregnancy progressed. Tolar and DiGrazia, (1976) also found that the frequency of coitus prior to pregnancy was 2.1 times per week; this remained stable until the third trimester when it fell to one time per week. Studies that have looked at the distribution of the frequency of sexual relations during pregnancy have found that approximately 10 percent of patients will have coitus at greater than four times per week during all trimesters. The number of patients who have coitus between two and three times per week gradually reduces in a linear fashion from the first to the second to the third trimester. The number of patients who have intercourse about one time per week is about 33 percent in the first and second trimester and declines to about one in five during the third trimester. In these studies total abstinence dramatically increased in frequency during the third trimester (Kumar et al., 1981; Morris, 1975) (Table 5-2). Kumar (Kumar et al., 1981) in London found that 93 percent of patients reduced the frequency of coitus by the third trimester.

There is a gradual drop in the number of patients who have an increased frequency of sexual relations compared to prepregnancy levels when one gets to the third trimester, as there is a gradual increase in the number of patients who have a decreased frequency of sexual relations as one gets to the third trimester (Battacchi et al., 1978; Kenny, 1973; Kumar et al., 1981). These findings of a decrease in the frequency of sexual activity during pregnancy seem to be consistent across many different societies i.e., Czechoslovakia (Bartova et al., 1969; Prochazka and Cernoch, 1970), Thailand (Morris, 1975; Pongthai et al., 1979), London (Kumar et al., 1981), Jerusalem (Mills et al., 1981), Italy (Battacchi et al., 1978), and the United States (Falicov, 1973; Holtzman, 1976; Kenny, 1973; Lumley, 1978; Perkins, 1979; Reamy et al., 1982; Sloan and Bing, 1983; Solberg et al., 1973). Kumar (Kumar et al., 1981) found that a lower level of sexual activity during pregnancy was related to low levels of sexuality before conception, relative infertility, and a fear that sex may harm the fetus. In his study, 25 percent of the patients stated that fatigue interfered with their sex life. Battacchi (Battacchi et al., 1978) found that only 10 percent of women had decreased sexual activity because of physical changes. Mills (Mills et al., 1981) suggests that the frequency of intercourse was decreased in the first and second trimester because patients with previous spontaneous abortions were advised to abstain from intercourse at a greater rate than those who had not had this adverse pregnancy outcome. Morris (1975) states that the finding of a decreased frequency of coitus during pregnancy in all groups studied suggests a cross-cultural process that may be secondary to medical advice, patient discomfort, and an intrinsic biologic process.

In studying other possible causes of decrease in coital frequency, Grudzinkas (Grudzinkas et al., 1979) found that 19 percent of patients were still sexually active in the last trimester and that there was no association between gestational age and incidence of coitus in the final four weeks of pregnancy. In a study of 260 women in the immediate postpartum period, Solberg (Solberg et al., 1973) found no association between coital frequency with race, religion, male or female educational level, negative feelings about pregnancy, or the number of previous pregnancies. He did find, though, that with increasing age or increasing length of time that people had been married there was a decrease in coital frequency. Others have found that the frequency of sexual relations during pregnancy is not related to race, private versus clinic patients, planned versus unplanned pregnancy, educational levels, parity, age, age of first coitus, or means of birth control (Holtzman, 1976; Perkins, 1982). It can be seen from most of these studies that when one looks at the frequency of sexual relations generally there is a decrease in the first trimester probably due to nausea, vomiting, mastalgia, and fatigue that are associated with pregnancy. An increased frequency of sexual relations relative to the first trimester is found during the second trimester and then a marked decrease in the frequency of coitus occurs during the third trimester. These changes appear to be seen in all the different cultures studied. There is

TABLE 5-2 **Frequency of Coitus in Pregnant Patients**

| Frequency | Trimester | | |
|---|---|---|---|
| | 1st | 2nd | 3rd |
| | (% of patients studied) | | |
| 4/week | 10–14 | 8–13 | 5–9 |
| 2–3/week | 24–52 | 18–55 | 0–32 |
| 1/week | 24–55 | 24–36 | 18–26 |
| 0/week | 7–11 | 7–38 | 35–73 |

the possibility that Masters and Johnson's findings of an increased sexuality during the second trimester may relate to the select population they studied, and their findings may not be applicable to the general population that does not participate in prospective sexual experimentation.

If one looks at the number of patients who totally abstained from coitus during pregnancy, one sees that during the first and early second trimester up to 10 percent of the patients do so. As the patient progresses to the third trimester abstention occurs in 33 to 95 percent of the patients studied (Falicov, 1973; Kumar et al., 1981; Mills et al., 1981; Morris, 1975; Pongthai et al., 1979; Solberg et al., 1973). The reasons for abstinence have been elucidated by Solberg (Solberg et al., 1973). About one-half of the patients abstain because of physical discomfort and one-fourth because of fear of injury to the baby or loss of interest. Other reasons for abstention include awkwardness, recommendations by the physician, the feeling of loss of attractiveness, or recommendations by other persons who are not physicians. Other investigators have confirmed these findings (Holtzman, 1976; Perkins, 1979, 1982; Rayburn and Wilson, 1980; Reamy et al., 1982; Semmens, 1971; Sloan and Bing, 1983; Solberg et al., 1973; Steege and Jelovsek, 1982; Swanson, 1980). Husband apprehension was found to be a problem by Holzman (1976) in 4 percent of her patients. Overall researchers found that 52 percent of all patients continued having coitus up until delivery.

LEVEL OF SEXUAL SATISFACTION

The level of sexual satisfaction obtained by most patients during pregnancy decreases as the pregnancy progresses, but the greatest decrease occurs during the third trimester (Battacchi et al., 1978; Falicov, 1973; Kenny, 1973; Kumar et al., 1981; Masters and Johnson, 1966; Perkins, 1982; Reamy et al., 1982; Tolar and DiGrazia, 1976). The changes in sexual satisfaction are noted in Table 5-3. As can be seen, even in the third trimester, there is a small percentage of patients who have

TABLE 5-3 **Change in Sexual Satisfaction During Pregnancy**

| Level of Satisfaction | Trimester | | |
|---|---|---|---|
| | 1st | 2nd | 3rd |
| | (% of patients studied) | | |
| Increased | 10–16 | 12–25 | 3–12 |
| Unchanged | 35–64 | 38–73 | 20–31 |
| Decreased | 24–36 | 9–49 | 20–73 |

an increase in sexual satisfaction despite what most patients find as a time of decreasing levels of sexual satisfaction. Perkins (1982) states that a satisfying sexual experience tends to perpetuate itself even during pregnancy despite apparent adverse influences. Falicov (1973) found that sexual satisfaction was slightly increased during the second trimester compared to the first trimester, but that it never reached prepregnancy levels. He felt that fatigue, breast tenderness, discomfort in the genital areas, and the changing shape of the pregnant patient interfered with satisfaction. Battacchi (Battacchi et al., 1978) found that primigravidas have the greatest decrease in sexual satisfaction and the greater the number of pregnancies in any patient the smaller the change in sexual satisfaction experienced.

Because of anatomic changes associated with pregnancy, techniques used to effect sexual satisfaction change. Solberg (Solberg et al., 1973) found that as pregnancy progressed there was a gradual decrease from the male superior position with an increase in the side by side position and rear entry approach. Other investigators have confirmed these changes (Holtzman, 1976; Reamy et al., 1982).

Maternal orgasm during pregnancy should be viewed from two perspectives: its ability to relieve sexual tension and its possible adverse effects on the pregnancy. The possible adverse effects of orgasm and coitus on the pregnancy will be considered in a subsequent portion of this paper. Masters and Johnson (1966) found that there were usually 8 to 12 uterine contractions and an increase in contractility tension with orgasm during pregnancy as compared to the non-pregnant state. They also found that multiple orgasm was experienced for the first time during pregnancy in some of their patients. The contractions produced by orgasm may last up to one minute and may continue for 30 minutes following the termination of coitus (Masters and Johnson, 1966). Orgasm may be achieved in about 75 percent of pregnant women (Goodlin et al., 1971; Rabach et al., 1968). Masters and Johnson (1966) and others (Goodlin, 1973; Swanson, 1980), have found that orgasm does not relieve the pelvic congestion associated with sexual tension during pregnancy and this lack of relief is especially marked during the third trimester.

Zlatnik and Burmeister (1982) found that there is an increased incidence of orgasm with an increase in formal education of the patient, but this finding was not statistically significant. Orgasm without intercourse though, was more common in those with a higher education. Steege and Jelovsek (1982) found that orgasmic response was increased with maternal age. Goodlin (Goodlin et al., 1971) found that 76 percent of patients were orgasmic during pregnancy: 57 percent with coitus, 20 percent with self-manipulation, and 4 percent with dreams. He found that 73 percent of patients experienced postorgasmic discomfort and only 25 percent of his patients had no discomfort after orgasm. Most patients experienced pelvic pain, pressure, or contractions. About 20 percent of the patients experienced some back pain or thigh pain, and 10 percent had an increase in vaginal discharge. Perkins (1982) found that 34 out of 141 patients practiced orgasmic suppression because of fear of hurting the baby, of starting labor, of pain with orgasm, or because of cautions against having orgasms as counseled by their physicians.

Reamy (Reamy et al., 1982) found, in a study of 52 women followed prospectively, a decrease in orgasmic response as pregnancy progressed. Despite this, he found that orgasmic women who were pleased or who were ambivalent about the pregnancy had a greater satisfaction during the middle and late months of pregnancy as compared to nonorgasmic women. Tolar and DiGrazia (1976) also found that the percentage of patients achieving orgasm decreased in the third trimester. Solberg (Solberg et al., 1973) noted that the number of patients who had orgasm with less than 25 percent of their coital experiences increased as pregnancy progressed and that the strength or intensity of orgasm decreased in almost 50 percent of the patients by the ninth month of pregnancy. In Kumar's 1981 study of 119 primigravid Londoners 74 percent of the mothers were orgasmic with at least one-half of their sexual experiences prior to pregnancy, but only 60 percent continued to have orgasm with the same frequency during the first and second trimester and only 6 percent in the third trimester.

The question of pain during intercourse in the pregnant patient was raised by the original studies of Masters and Johnson (1966) which showed that vasocongestion was not entirely relieved by orgasm. In their study of 1500 patients, Steege and Jelovsek (1982) found that dyspareunia occurred frequently in only about 2.5 percent of patients. It occurred occasionally in 7 percent and rarely in about 10 percent of patients. Almost 81 percent of patients had no complaints of dyspareunia during pregnancy. Even in those who did have dyspareunia the pain did not decrease the frequency of intercourse. It was found that patients who did not lubricate during the excitement of sexual activity had a decrease in responsiveness and decreased libido with a resultant vaginismus.

When one looks at the research on sexual activity related to parity there seems to be general agreement that frequency, as well as desire, enjoyment, and orgasm decrease more in nulliparous patients as compared to multiparous patients (Battacchi et al., 1978; Kenny, 1973; Masters and Johnson, 1966; Reamy et al., 1982; Steege and Jelovsek, 1982). It is felt that the adverse effect on sexual activity is secondary to the primiparous patient's fear of aborting and damaging the fetus with sexual relations. The multiparous patient is usually reassured from a previous successful experience that sexual relations will not harm the fetus. In Thailand, Pongthai and colleagues (1979) found that primigravid patients abstained less frequently during the second trimester than multiparous patients, but Holtzman (1976) found no difference in the number of patients who abstained from intercourse when she compared primigravidas versus multiparous patients. Reamy (Reamy et al., 1982) found that multiparous patients had more enjoyment and more multiple orgasms as compared to primiparous patients.

When looking at sexual activity related to other factors, Battacchi (Battacchi et al., 1978) found that women 14 to 20 years old reduced the number of acts of sexual intercourse less than older women, but there was no effect of parity in this group. In these young patients previous abortion had no effect on the frequency of sexual intercourse, but if the patient had a previous negative obstetrical outcome besides abortion, threatened abortion, or toxemia during this pregnancy, there was a decrease in coital frequency. Pongthai (Pongthai et al., 1979) found that if the male was greater than 30 years old there was an increased incidence of abstinence during the pregnancy, but the higher the education level the less the effect. Maternal age was not related to abstinence (Battacchi et al., 1978; Pongthai et al., 1979). Solberg (Solberg et al., 1973) in a study of 260 patients in Seattle, Washington found that with increasing length of marriage there was a decrease in coital frequency, and this frequency was not associated with race, religion, male or female education level, negative feelings about the pregnancy, or the number of previous pregnancies. Steege and Jelovsek (1982) in studying 1500 patients found that married patients had a greater frequency of coitus than unmarried patients, single parous patients had a greater frequency as compared to single nulliparous patients, and single patients who were above average weight had a greater frequency of sexual relations than those who were of normal weight.

Patients who never had orgasm and were of an advanced educational level were also found to have a significant decrease in the frequency of sexual relations.

Cravitz and Hayes (1979) studied the adolescent pregnant patient and compared her to the sexually active non-pregnant adolescent. When the authors evaluated the subjects for self-esteem, sexual information, sexual activity, grade of school completed, and reported school average, no differences between the two groups were found. They did find though, that sexually active non-pregnant controls were more rational, more assertive, and more oriented toward self-fulfillment than their pregnant counterparts. They also found that the pregnant adolescent perceived her father as viewing her mother as an admirable person less frequently than the non-pregnant adolescent. This study shows that many attitudinal factors determined by the home are important aspects in adolescent sexuality.

## NONCOITAL SEXUAL ACTIVITY

Because of the physical discomforts that occur during pregnancy related to sexual intercourse, many patients turn to noncoital activity for sexual pleasure. Zalor (1976) studied 216 patients and evaluated the techniques used for sexual gratification. The findings of this study are listed in Table 5-4. As can be seen,

TABLE 5-4 **Percentage of Patients Engaging in Noncoital Sexual Activity**

| | Trimester | | |
|---|---|---|---|
| Activity | 1st | 2nd | 3rd |
| | (% of patients studied; total N = 216) | | |
| Breast stimulation | 25 | 26 | 25 |
| Clitoral stimulation | 27 | 30 | 32 |
| Vaginal stimulation | 30 | 22 | 15 |
| Anal stimulation | 3 | 2 | 1 |
| Cunnilingus | 6 | 14 | 13 |
| Fellatio | 4 | 4 | 4 |
| Masturbation | 4 | 0 | 3 |

Source: Zalor, M. K.: Sexual counseling for pregnant couples. Am. J. Matern. Child Nurs., May/June: 176, 1976.

about one-fourth of the patients continued using breast stimulation or clitoral stimulation throughout the pregnancy for sexual gratification. The incidence of noncoital vaginal stimulation fell from about 30 percent during the first trimester to 15 percent during the second trimester. Anal intercourse, masturbation, and fellatio were relatively unchanged. The incidence of cunnilingus increased more than 100 percent from first trimester to the third trimester.

Despite these noncoital techniques for sexual gratification, the percentage of patients achieving orgasm during the third trimester decreased as compared to other trimesters (Tolar and DiGrazia, 1976). Solberg (Solberg et al., 1973) found that not only orgasm and sexual interest decreased, but noncoital behavior decreased linearly in his patient population throughout the pregnancy. He also found that of the approximately 16 percent of the women who used masturbation for sexual gratification prior to pregnancy about two-thirds of them were able to achieve orgasm with manual stimulation. During pregnancy, however, only 40 to 50 percent of those who masturbated continued to do so, but the ability to achieve orgasm did not change because of the pregnancy. He found that 45 percent of patients allowed their partner to use hand stimulation prepregnancy and 57 percent were successful in achieving orgasm; forty percent of those patients using this technique prior to pregnancy did not continue its use during the pregnancy. Reamy (Reamy et al., 1982) found that coitus with or without manual stimulation was used equally during the first and third trimester to produce an orgasmic response, whereas during the second trimester coitus was the preferred method. Holtzman (1976) found that despite the fact that 44 percent of the patients used mutual masturbation as a technique for orgasm prior to pregnancy only about 25 percent did so during pregnancy. She also found that it was more difficult to achieve orgasm with this technique during the pregnancy.

Perkins (1982) found in those patients who said that pregnancy made them feel less attractive, an increase in noncoital sexual behavior. There was also an increased incidence of masturbation in those patients who stated that they experienced a decreased quality of coital sensation. Perkins (1982) also found that all sexual stimulation techniques, including coitus with partner stimulation, coitus with self-manipulation, hand stimulation, oral stimulation alone, masturbation, and other types of stimulation decrease during pregnancy. Tolar and DiGrazia (1976) and Holtzman (1976) also found that there was no increased incidence of orogenital sexual relations or fellatio during pregnancy. In the Solberg study (Solberg et al., 1973), 39 percent of the patients used orogenital stimulation prior to pregnancy and 53 percent of these patients reached orgasm with this technique. Fellatio was practiced in 32 percent of the patients, 17 percent used cunnilingus, and 50 percent used both. Of these patients though, only about 50 percent used prepregnancy techniques during the pregnancy. Oral stimulation by the husband was found to be used more frequently near term than during the other trimesters by Reamy (Reamy et al., 1982). This study, however, is in disagreement with other investigators who have found that the increased secretions associated with pregnancy make this form of sexual stimulation less desirable to the husband, leading to a decreased frequency of its utilization during pregnancy (Dameron, 1983; Holtzman, 1976; Perkins, 1979; Solberg et al., 1973; Tolar and DiGrazia, 1976).

Despite all these other techniques used for sexual gratification during pregnancy, Tolar and DiGrazia (1976) found that being held was the most frequent alternative to sexual intercourse preferred by pregnant women. About 50 percent of the patients said that they just wanted to be held during each of the trimesters, and about one-fifth of the patients had an increased desire to be kissed. There was an increase from 5 to 13 percent in the desire to touch the husband, but there was only a very small percentage of patients who wanted to have their husband touch their sex organs. White and Reamy (1982) also reported that as sexual desire decreases there is a corresponding increase in nonsexual physical contact that occurs as an expression of love.

## EFFECTS OF SEXUAL RELATIONS ON THE PREGNANCY

We have considered the physiological, physical, and psychological changes associated with sexual relations during pregnancy. Now we must consider what effects sexual relations have, if any, on the normal pregnancy. Sexual activity during pregnancy has been implicated in many complications: premature labor, intrauterine fetal demise, chorioamnionitis, fetal distress, abortion, meconium staining of the amniotic fluid, premature rupture of the membranes, antepartum hemorrhage, air embolism, sexually transmitted diseases, and neonatal complications. It has been shown that during the last several weeks of pregnancy, orgasm may result in tonic uterine contractions that can last for as long as one minute and persist for up to 30 minutes after the orgasmic experience (Masters and Johnson, 1966; Zalor, 1976). Masters and Johnson (1966) have also shown that when coitus is prohibited noncoital orgasm frequency increases. There is also an increase in orgasmic intensity in patients who have abstained from intercourse and intense orgasm may occur during dreams. Perkins (1979) found that approximately 10 percent of patients experienced contractions with orgasm during the first and second trimester; this percentage increases to 16.3 in the last trimester.

Speroff and Ramuiell (1970) have postulated that human seminal fluid containing a high level of prostagladins may stimulate the uterus to contract, but there is no evidence that these prostaglandins can initiate premature labor. Goodlin (1976) knowing that orgasm can cause an increase in oxytocin levels, prolactin levels, and catecholamines, postulates that there would be a decrease in uterine blood flow with orgasm. He measured uterine contractions and found them to occur with orgasm. Despite these contractions, labor did not ensue.

Masters and Johnson (1966) found that only 4 of 101 women studied went into labor immediately after orgasm. All of these patients were near term and had normal babies. Perkins (1979) studied 155 patients and found no association between coitus, orgasm, or other sexual experience with the onset of labor. Of the 155 patients, 20 reported the onset of labor within 24 hours of the last sexual experience, but there was no increased incidence of prematurity or rupture of membranes. Perkins actually found that patients, who were orgasmic with masturbation, delivered a significantly greater number of term infants than women who were not orgasmic by this technique. No association was found between the sexual techniques used for sexual gratification or the response of the women and the outcome of the fetus measured by fetal growth. He concurred with the findings of others—that 70 to 80 percent of patients do not feel contractions with sexual activity late in pregnancy. With these physiologic facts in mind we will review sequentially each one of the proposed complications of pregnancy related to sexual relations.

### ABORTION

The fear that sexual relations will cause abortion is ingrained in many societies, intertwined with religious, moral, and social beliefs. Slate (1970) in a study of 1000 cases of spontaneous abortion found only one incident of spontaneous, first trimester loss due to external trauma or psychic shock. He felt that the deep location of the uterus and the cushioning effect of the amniotic fluid appear to protect the fetus from external trauma. In examining the records of over 250,000 pregnant patients Javert (1960) found fewer than .007 percent of abortions were due to factors that could be categorized as major injuries. He did suggest, though without data, that patients who have frequent or multiple orgasms early in pregnancy had a higher incidence of spontaneous abortions. Since the publication of his report in 1960 there have been no further indications that patients who do not have any evidence of threatened abortion or pregnancy complications have a greater chance of abortion due to sexual relations in the first trimester. Therefore, no major indication to date has been found that implicates sexual relations or orgasm with first trimester, spontaneous abortion in the healthy pregnancy; only those admonitions that have been handed down from generation to generation connect the two.

## Premature Labor

Many studies have been done trying to implicate sexual relations or orgasm with the onset of premature labor. Since the vagina contains *Bacteroides fragilis, Peptostreptococcus, Fusobacterium necrophorum* and *Streptococcus viridans,* all of which are high in phospholipase A2 content, it has been postulated that the innoculation with sexual relations of a high number of these bacteria high into the vagina causes a release of the enzyme which stimulates prostaglandin synthesis. Therefore, endocervical or intrauterine contamination with the appropriate bacteria would then initiate premature labor (Bejar et al., 1981). These findings, as well as the findings of orgasm being associated with an increased level of serum oxytocin, are facts that may lead one to believe that coitus and orgasm are etiologic factors in the initiation of premature labor (Fox and Knoggs, 1969).

Goodlin (Goodlin et al., 1971), in his study of 50 women who delivered prematurely, found an increased incidence of orgasm after 32 weeks. Unfortunately, the controls were not matched well. Those who delivered prematurely had a lower weight gain during pregnancy, a greater number of previously delivered prematures, and a higher incidence of LSD consumption than those in the control group. Also, the criterion for considering orgasm as the etiologic mechanism for the onset of premature labor was if labor started within 50 hours after sexual relations. These factors render these data inconclusive (Goodlin, 1969; Goodlin et al., 1971). Naeye and Ross (1982) found a fourfold increase in premature labor when South African mothers were studied.

Most of this increase was related to supposed infection and will be discussed with chorioamnionitis. Many other authors have found no relationship between premature labor and sexual relations (Grudzinkas et al., 1979; Holtzman, 1976; Mills et al., 1981; Perkins, 1979; Pugh and Fernandez, 1955; Rayburn and Wilson, 1980; Sloan and Bing, 1983; Solberg et al., 1973; Wagner et al., 1976; Zlatnik and Burmeister, 1982). Perkins (1979) actually found that pregnant women who were orgasmic had a lower percentage of premature deliveries than did anorgasmic women. He also found that patients who were orgasmic with masturbation delivered a higher number of term infants than those who were nonorgasmic by masturbation.

Rayburn and Wilson (1980) found no association between frequency of coitus or the frequency of orgasm with the onset of premature labor in those patients who had preterm labor versus those who had a term delivery if there were no predisposing factors for the premature delivery. They found that the incidence of coitus within two days of delivery in those who delivered between 26 and 37 weeks was the same (16 percent) as those who delivered after 38 weeks (Rayburn and Wilson, 1980). In the Solberg study (Solberg et al., 1973) of 260 patients, 19 were premature. None of these patients noticed the immediate onset of labor after coitus or orgasm. These same findings were found in 19 prematures studied by Wagner (Wagner et al., 1976). After reviewing this data it appears that, despite the hypothetical postulates that could be presented to relate premature labor with orgasm or sexual activity, no proven relationship exists between these two occurrences in the low-risk patient.

## Premature Rupture of Membranes

Studies by Zlatnik and Burmeister (1982), Pugh and Fernandez (1955), and Perkins (1979) have shown that there is no relationship between sexual relations and rupture of membranes. In fact, in the Pugh study of 155 patients, ruptured membranes was more frequent if orgasm occurred greater than 24 hours prior to admission rather than less than 24 hours prior to admission. Also they found that if the last sexual experience was nonorgasmic there was a greater chance of rupture of membranes on admission. Of those patients who had labor within 24 hours of sexual relations a significantly greater number were admitted with rupture of membranes if orgasm had not occurred. Therefore, their conclusions (analogous to those of other authors) are that sexual relations or coitus are not related to rupture of membranes or the delivery of a premature infant. It does not appear that the physical penetration of the penis into the vagina is capable of producing this complication.

## Chorioamnionitis

A large number of aerobic and anaerobic bacteria are endogenous to the vaginal tract, and it has been postulated that coitus during pregnancy is related to the development of intrauterine infections. In his retrospective study of 26,886 pregnancies between 1959 and 1966, Naeye (1979) seems to confirm this postulate. Placentas were saved from 12 hospitals affiliated with medical schools and studied for signs of infection. It was found that infection occurred in 156 per 1000 patients when coitus occurred greater than one time per week during the month prior to delivery and at a rate of 117 per 1000 patients in those who abstained from coitus. This study also found not only an increase in infection rate, but an increase in the severity of the infections. Eleven percent of the infected infants died if the mother had coitus versus 7.4 percent when no coitus had occurred within a month of delivery. In this study, the interval from coitus to delivery was not determined, although it did not appear that there was an increased incidence of amniotic fluid infection if patients delivered between 33 and 38 weeks of gestation. Also no relationship was found between the number of coital episodes per week and the frequency or severity of infection. This study included an overrepresentation of blacks and lower socioeconomic groups in the coital group as compared to the controls and is weakened because no correction was made for the possibility of poor nutrition when the increased incidence and severity of amniotic fluid infection was considered (Naeye and Peters, 1978). This study is also faulted because the definition of infection is based on a histologic evaluation of the placenta where more than four polymorphonuclear leukocytes per high power field were seen in the subchorionic plate of the placenta. No cultures were taken and only this microscopic criterion was confirmation of the disease (Naeye, 1979).

As shown by Driscoll (1979) leukocyte infiltration of the placenta is highly correlated with prematurity, but it is not necessarily related to sexual relations. Therefore, Naeye's conclusion from this study that sexual relations are related to amniotic fluid infection is suspect. Naeye also postulates that coitus allows a greater number and a greater variety of bacteria to reach the amniotic fluid or the lower uterine segment and that sperm or the proteolytic enzymes in the semen may facilitate bacterial penetration into the amniotic fluid. The increased incidence of infection in his study was only found in patients less than 33 weeks gestation or greater than 38 weeks gestation. The increased infection rate prior to 33 weeks was felt to be due to the inability of the amniotic fluid to protect against infection, and the increased incidence after 38 weeks was related to the shortening of the lower uterine segment that facilitated the spread of the bacteria.

Naeye (1982) also studied a group of patients from Durbon, South Africa, where there was a high rate of infection due to poor nutrition. In this group he found a progression of chorioamnionitis from being confined to the extraplacental membranes when coitus occurred within two days of delivery to infection in the amniotic fluid three to four days after coitus. Infection rate declined to baseline levels if the patient did not deliver until eight days after coitus (Naeye and Ross, 1982). When condoms were used this increased infection rate did not occur; therefore, endogenous bacteria of the vagina could not be implicated in these infections. This study was in an obviously high-risk group and is based on the presumption of total compliance with condom usage. Therefore, it may not be applicable to the low-risk patient.

Other investigators (Grudzinkas et al., 1979; Pugh and Fernandez, 1955; Sloan and Bing, 1983; Zlatnik and Burmeister, 1982) have not found an association of chorioamnionitis with sexual relations or orgasm. Zlatnik and Burmeister (1982) in studying 413 patients postpartum found that the percentage of patients who had orgasm and/or intercourse within seven days prior to delivery was not associated with chorioamnionitis or neonatal sepsis. An uncontrolled study of 6000 couples who were interviewed also showed no relationship of sexual activity with chorioamnionitis (Sloan and Bing, 1983). Therefore, at this time it cannot be concluded that sexual relations at any time during pregnancy in the low-risk, well-nourished patient is associated with a markedly increased risk of infectious morbidity for the mother or the neonate.

## Antepartum Hemorrhage

Masters and Johnson (1966) found that when the presenting part was deep in the pelvis the cervix was brought into the vaginal axis. Because of this, direct penile contact could produce vaginal bleeding, although this did not appear to have any negative effects on the fetus. Naeye (1981) found that antepartum hemorrhage (definition of "hemorrhage" not included in the paper) was found in 30 out of 1000 patients who had had recent coitus (coitus since the last clinic visit) versus 19 per 1000 who did not have recent coitus. He suggested that the frequency of vaginal bleeding increased with the frequency of coitus. This correlation was not strong in pregnancies that ended preterm. The perinatal mortality rates in this study were not corrected for gestational age and all patients who delivered between 20 and 44 weeks of gestation were grouped together. Zlatnik and Burmeister (1982) and Pugh and Fernandez (1955) were unable to find any relationship between third trimester bleeding and coitus in the patients they studied. Therefore, in some patients it may be found that there is some bleeding after sexual relations, but it does not appear that this bleeding significantly affects the outcome of the pregnancy.

## Intrauterine Fetal Demise

Since contractions can compromise uteroplacental blood flow, it has been postulated that orgasm or sexual activity may be related to intrauterine distress or demise. Goodlin (1976) measured uterine contractions and blood flow to the lateral vaginal fornix utilizing a photoelectric plethysmographic probe. With this method he demonstrated that orgasm produced a decrease in the blood volume pulsed to the vagina. The fetus would then become hyperactive in the postorgasmic phase. In one patient studied by Goodlin (Goodlin et al., 1972), seven orgasms were induced in 17 minutes through vulvar and vaginal manipulation by the patient and her husband. Uterine tension was recorded by an external pressure transducer. After three orgasms mild variable decelerations were seen in association with the uterine contractions. It appeared that the uterine contractions increased in intensity with succeeding orgasms, but decelerations were not consistently found with each orgasm, and they did not increase in severity. This patient delivered an 8 lb 5 oz baby six days later who did well. Goodlin also states that on an informal basis he has evaluated patients who have unexplained intrauterine fetal demises and has never been able to associate a fetal death with sexual activity or orgasm (Goodlin, 1976; Goodlin et al., 1972). Mills (Mills et al., 1981) in his study of 10,981 singleton pregnancies found no increased incidence of perinatal deaths in patients who had intercourse late in pregnancy as opposed to those who abstained. He also found no delayed harmful effects of intercourse that occured even as early as one month prior to delivery. Therefore, it can be safely assumed that despite the fact that intercourse and/or orgasm may result in uterine contractions, these do not appear to cause significant

## Fetal Distress

As previously described, Goodlin (Goodlin et al., 1972) found that in a patient who experienced multiple orgasms within a short period of time, mild variable decelerations could be recorded using an external dopler technique. He also had one patient go home with a handheld dopler that was used during orgasm to record fetal heart rate. There was no decrease in the fetal heart rate in this patient. Zlatnik and Burmeister (1982) in studying 413 patients found no association between the Apgar scores of the neonate and the time interval between delivery and sexual relations. Solberg (Solberg et al., 1973) in his study of 260 patients also found that Apgar scores were independent of the frequency of coitus or orgasm. Grudzinkas (Grudzinkas et al., 1979) found though, that there was a greater incidence of Apgar scores less than six at one minute and meconium staining of the amniotic fluid in patients who had had intercourse within four weeks of delivery. Since so many other obstetrical and nonobstetrical factors are involved in producing a low one-minute Apgar score, this data is suspect. Even in this study the low one-minute Apgar scores were not associated with a higher incidence of perinatal mortality. Therefore, at the present time no clear cut data indicates that coitus or orgasm can cause significant fetal distress in the patient who has an intact utero-placental unit.

## Neonatal Morbidity

Naeye has found an increased perinatal mortality rate in the seasons usually associated with increases in coital frequency (Naeye, 1980), but many other investigators (Grudzinkas, et al., 1972; Javert, 1960; Perkins, 1979, Zlatnik and Burmeister, 1982) have failed to find this association. Also no increased incidence of neonatal infection or low birth weight in babies born from sexually active and/or orgasmic women during pregnancy was found in these studies. Therefore, there is no confirmatory evidence for the data presented by Naeye (1981) that indicates an increased chance of the neonate dying from sepsis if the mother is sexually active. It is known, however, that coitus can indirectly result in fetal and neonatal morbidity and mortality through the spread of sexually transmitted diseases such as herpes, gonorrhea, and chlamydia. To date, no good studies have been done correlating these problems with the frequency of sexual relations, number of partners, socioeconomic group, and other factors. One would assume that in patients who are more likely to be exposed to these sexually transmitted diseases a high-risk subgroup could be identified. The evaluation of this problem awaits further study.

## Air Embolism

Air embolism due to aerocolpos is one complication of sexual activity during pregnancy with which no one disagrees as being associated with a higher incidence of morbidity in the mother and fetus. (Aronson and Nelson, 1967; Bray et al., 1983). Eleven cases have been described in the world literature, all of which have been associated with fetal demise and ten of which have resulted in maternal death. It is postulated that the vagina, being a distensible organ, can accomodate up to 1000 cc of air. When 500–600 ml of air is forceably blown into the vagina during pregnancy the patients may develop abdominal tightness, desire to urinate, pain, seizures, hypertension, cyanosis, and coma. It is postulated that the air dissects, via the cervical canal, to separate the amniotic membranes from the uterine wall. This air then enters a subplacental site that allows it to travel to the right atrium. The air then enters the arterial system via either a septal defect or patent ductus arteriosis. This then produces cerebral air embolism. The bubbles cause obstruction to the arterial blood flow and damage to the endothelial lining. Disseminated intravascular coagulation may then ensue. In the one case in which the mother survived she was treated with hyperbaric oxygen therapy. This therapy theoretically compresses the size of the bubbles and allows for a larger gradient for gas elimination. Because of the severe consequence of this problem, as well as the specific therapy required to treat it, it is suggested that if a patient presents *in extremis* during pregnancy one should actively ask about a history of air being blown into the vagina. If there is the possibility of aerocolpos determined from the history, hyperbaric oxygen therapy should be commenced as soon as possible (Bray et al., 1983).

## PERCEPTION OF SEXUALITY DURING PREGNANCY

When one considers the effects of pregnancy on human sexuality the perception of the participants of themselves and their mates at this time in their lives is an important consideration. Prochazka and Cernoch (1970) maintain that many women continued having intercourse during pregnancy only for the fear that their husbands would become unfaithful. Perkins (1982) found that 60 percent of men complained of their wives' sexuality during the pregnancy as compared to a 16 percent frequency of complaints prepregnancy. The complaints were over the frequency of sexual relations as well as their partners' decreased interest. He found that 52 percent of patients without problems prior to pregnancy developed sexual problems during this stage of their lives. Despite this, 15 percent of women enjoy the extra attention they receive from their partners during the pregnancy and about 6 percent felt closer to their husband and family at this time than prior to the pregnancy (Kenny, 1973). In Holtzman's (1976) study, it was found that 12 percent of women perceive themselves to be more attractive, 40 percent found no change in the level of attractiveness, and 24 percent found themselves less attractive, especially in the eighth and ninth month of pregnancy. Falicov (1973) found that in four out of 19 patients quickening introduced the feeling of a third person into the marital unit and this seemed to disturb the sexual intimacy of the couple, possibly inhibiting sexual activity and expression throughout the rest of pregnancy. Goodlin (1985) also has noted that when patients see the baby during an ultrasound examination the mother may tend to bond with the baby at that time. After this time, the couple may report a decreased interest in sexual activity.

Pregnancy is a time in which women question the fidelity of their husbands. Masters and Johnson (1966) found that 12 of the 79 men studied sought sexual release outside the home when they were denied the conjugal opportunity because of pregnancy. Six more of these men had extramarital affairs during the postpartum period. Three of these men had their first extramarital affair either during the pregnancy or immediately thereafter. Semmens (1971) found that 6 percent of men had extramarital affairs during their wives' pregnancy regardless of the presence of nausea and vomiting. Three times this number of men (18 percent) whose wives gained excessive amounts of weight during the first and second trimester had extramarital affairs.

When the question of male perception of sexual activity was looked into by Masters and Johnson (1966), they found that 31 of the 79 men who participated in the study of sexual response during pregnancy had withdrawn from active coital demands upon their wives by the beginning of the third trimester. Only 20 out of the 31 wives noticed this decrease. These men stated that there was a fear of injuring the fetus or the wife. Five of these men suggested that the physical appearance of their wife was so objectionable that they did not want to have coitus. Coleman and Coleman (1971) found that some men become impotent during pregnancy because pregnancy precipitates an identification with the feminine aspects of man's history and make-up. The Couvade syndrome has been identified. Here symptomatic emotional problems among husbands of pregnant women occur; these include nausea, vomiting, gastrointestinal upset, anxiety, unexplained fevers, and compulsions (Coleman and Coleman, 1971). White and Reamy (1982) identified factors that inhibit the male from participating in sexual activity during pregnancy. They describe fear of harming the woman or the fetus, the finding of the wife as being an asexual being when she is pregnant, being turned off by the pregnant body, an underlying belief that sex with the pregnant woman is immoral, and a feeling of inadequacy to meet the wife's needs. There is also the thought that the fetus is an observer to the sexual act and this inhibits sexual spontaneity. Some men also express a fear that damage to the fetus can occur during coitus. Therefore, pregnancy is a time that not only affects the pregnant woman, but the man whose mate is carrying a fetus. It can be a time when the father feels excluded, and he may turn to other sources in the home or outside the home for comfort and understanding (Zalor, 1976). Every effort should be made to minimize the detrimental effects of pregnancy on sexual behavior so that the marital unit may be maintained during this difficult period.

## PHYSICIAN INPUT INTO SEXUALITY DURING PREGNANCY

To fully understand sexual activity during pregnancy we must evaluate what instructions are given to those pregnant patients. As we have seen, pregnancy presents a stress on any marriage and when sexual intercourse is restricted the relationship is tested. When physicians tell the patient to abstain, an added stress may be placed on the marriage. Furthermore, failure to follow those instructions may result in increased guilt that could also have lasting detrimental effects. Battacchi (Battacchi et al., 1978) found that only 23 percent of obstetricians spontaneously discussed sexuality in pregnancy. Of those physicians who actually discussed sex approximately 20 percent just said to be more careful during the pregnancy, 19 percent said not to change anything, 15 percent advised abstaining during the last six weeks of pregnancy, 15 percent suggested abstaining throughout pregnancy, 3 percent told their patients not to have intercourse during the first trimester, 1.5 percent suggested changes in position, .5 percent suggested abstaining only during the third trimester. Eight percent offered no advice, and 15 percent offered questionable advice. In studies by Solberg (Solberg et al., 1973) and Falicov (1973) it appears that approximately 25 percent of patients are told to abstain from sexual relations at some point during pregnancy. Despite this advice only 8 percent of patients base their sexual behavior on physician recommendations. These investigators also found that only 10 percent of the patients were given advice on alternative positions during pregnancy, and only 2 percent were given recommendations concerning techniques of sexual stimulation other than coitus that could be used during pregnancy. Kumar (Kumar et al., 1981) found that 30 percent of patients would find sexual counseling beneficial at three months of gestation, but very few mention it to their physicians. Therefore, we can see that most physicians neglect the discussion of sexuality during pregnancy and when they do discuss it they do not often include alternative methods of stimulation and gratification, as well as suggestions that would improve comfort of sexual intercourse during pregnancy. This is an area that we as physicians must include in the counseling of the pregnant patient at the initial visit and throughout the pregnancy.

## CONCLUSION

Most studies suggest that the sexual desire in each couple before pregnancy may be the leading factor in determining the frequency of sexual intercourse and orgasmic response, the libido, and the incidence of total abstinence during pregnancy. Normal sexual activity does not seem to have any major adverse influence on the gestation. Herbst (1979), in reviewing all the data relating coitus and the fetus, states that "current data do not permit dogmatic statements about coitus and pregnancy outcome." He suggests that patients with obvious pregnancy complications, such as bleeding, rupture of membranes, premature dilatation of the cervix, threatened abortion, and threatened premature labor should abstain from coitus and orgasm, but the interdiction of coitus or any form of sexual activity during pregnancy for the large majority of perfectly healthy females without any intervening or previous obstetrical complication is unreasonable—in fact it may have such long lasting detrimental effects to the marital unit that any minor benefit gained from prohibiting sexual relations would be overwhelmingly negated. Therefore, Masters and Johnson's (1966) statement that "blanket medical interdiction of coital activity for arbitrarily established periods of time, both before and after delivery, has done far more harm than good" seems to be just as appropriate in 1985 as it was in 1966.

What we learn from all of these studies is that we, as physicians caring for pregnant women, need to be quite explicit with the instructions that we give these patients about sexuality during pregnancy. We should not make broad generalizations and we should tailor the instructions to the needs of the specific patient, her husband, and specific medical complications. In the patients without problems during the pregnancy we should inform them of the following seven points. (1) Sex during pregnancy is good; it provides a security and bonding of a marital relationship that is needed during a period of stress. (2) Normally sexual desire, frequency of intercourse, satisfaction with intercourse, and orgasmic response decrease to some extent, mostly during the third trimester. This decrease in sexuality should not be interpreted as a failure of one or the other of the sexual partners. (3) There are many physiological and anatomical changes occurring during pregnancy that account for this decrease in sexuality. These changes should be explained to the patients and alternatives to intercourse, including masturbation and orogenital sex, should be specifically ennunciated to the patient and her mate so they know that this type of behavior is considered normal. Alternatives to the male superior position during intercourse should also be explained to the patient to make her feel comfortable with what she may feel to be sexual practices that are not within the norm. (4) We must reassure the perfectly healthy gravid patient who had no previous pregnancy problems, such as habitual abortion or incompetent cervix, or a current problem, such as premature labor or antepartum hemorrhage, that sexual activity during pregnancy has not been found to be harmful to either the mother or the fetus. We should explain that sex or orgasm may initiate uterine contractions, but these will not place an undue stress on her baby or cause early delivery. (5) Specific instructions to avoid forceful blowing of air into the vagina should be told to every pregnant patient because this is the one sexual activity that is definitely known to be harmful to the gravid patient. (6) Both partners should be made aware of the sexual changes that occur during pregnancy. The physician should encourage open communication between the patient and her partner during the pregnancy to alleviate stresses that may result in seeking sexual gratification outside the family unit. (7) Finally, we must encourage patients to communicate openly with the physician at each visit if there are any sexual problems that occur so that these problems can be dealt with quickly and effectively. If this information is given to every normal pregnant patient, she and her mate can be made to feel more comfortable with their sexuality during pregnancy. Hopefully this will allow both of them to enjoy the pregnancy with minimal risk to the mother, the fetus, or the marital unit.

## REFERENCES

Aronson, M. E., and Nelson, P. K.: Fatal air embolism in pregnancy resulting from an unusual sexual act. *Obstet. Gynecol.,* 30:127, 1967.

Bartova, D.; Kolrova, O.; Uzel, R.; et al: Sex life during pregnancy. *Cesk. Gynekol.,* 34:560, 1969.

Battacchi, M.; Bottiglioni, F.; Codispoti, O.; DeAloysio, D.: Personality and stress factors in women's sexuality in pregnancy. *Proc. Serona Symposia,* 22, 1978.

Beach, F. A.: A review of physiological and psychological studies of sexual behavior in mammals. *Physiol. Rev.,* 27:240, 1947.

Bejar, R.; Curgello, V.; Davis, C.; and Gluck, L.: Premature labor. II Bacterial sources of phospholipase. *Obstet. Gynecol.*, 57:479, 1981.

Bray, P.; Myers, R. A. M.; and Cowley, R. A.: Orogenital sex as a cause of nonfatal air embolism in pregnancy. *Obstet. Gynecol.*, 61:653, 1983.

Cohn, S. D.: Sexuality in pregnancy. *Nurs. Clin. North. Am.* 17:91, 1982.

Coleman, A.; and Coleman, L.: In pregnancy. The psychological experience. *N.N., Herder and Herder,* 1971.

*Courier Post.* (Rochester). Title, December 13, 1983, 7B.

Cravitz, E., and Hayes, L.: A comparison of pregnant adolescents and non-pregnant sexually active peers. *J. Am. Med. Wom. Assoc.*, 34:179, 1979.

Dameron, G. W.: Helping couples cope with sexual changes pregnancy brings. *Contemp. Obstet. Gynecol.*, 21:23, 1983.

Driscoll, S. G.: The significance of acute chorioamnionitis. *Clin. Obstet. Gynecol.*, 22:339, 1979.

Elliott, J. P., and Flaherty, J. F.: The use of breast stimulation to ripen the cervix in term pregnancies. *Am. J. Obstet. Gynecol.*, 145:553, 1983.

Falicov, C. J.: Sexual adjustment during first pregnancy and postpartum. *Am. J. Obstet. Gynecol.*, 117:991, 1973.

Ford, C., and Beach, F.: Patterns of sexual behavior. *Perennial,* Harper and Row, New York, 1951.

Fox, C. A., and Knoggs, G. S.: Milk-ejection activity (oxytocin) in peripheral venous blood in man during lactation and in association with coitus. *J. Endocrinol.,* 45:145, 1969.

Fox, C. A.; Wolff, H. S.; and Baker, J. A.: Measurement of intravaginal and intrauterine pressures during human coitus by radio-telemetry. *J. Reprod. Fertil.*, 22:243, 1970.

Goodlin, R. C.: Orgasm and Premature Labor. *Lancet,* 2:646, 1969.

Goodlin, R. C.: Can sex in pregnancy harm the fetus. *Contemp. Obstet. Gynecol.,* 8:21, 1976.

Goodlin, R. C.; Keller, D. W.; and Raffin, M.: Orgasmic response during pregnancy: Its possible deleterious effects. *Obstet. Gynecol.,* 38:916, 1971.

Goodlin, R. C.; Schmidt, W.; and Creevy, D. C.: Uterine tension and fetal heart rate during maternal orgasm. *Obstet. Gynecol.,* 39:125, 1972.

Grudzinkas, J. G.; Watson, C.; and Chard, T.: Does sexual intercourse cause fetal distress. *Lancet,* 2:692, 1979.

Hallender, M. H., and McGehee, J. B.: The wish to be held during pregnancy. *J. Psychosom. Res.*, 18:193, 1974.

Herbst, A. L.: Coitus and the fetus. *N. Engl. J. Med.,* 301:1235, 1979.

Holtzman, L. C.: Sexual practices during pregnancy. *J. Nurse Midwife,* 21:29, 1976.

Javert, C. T.: The role of the patient's activities in the occurrence of spontaneous abortion. *Fertil. Steril.*, 11:550, 1960.

Kenny, J. A.: Sexuality of pregnant and breastfeeding women. *Arch. Sex. Behav.,* 2:215, 1973.

Kumar, R.; Brant, H. A.; and Robson, K. M.: Childbearing and maternal sexuality: A prospective survey of 119 primiparas. *J. Psychosom. Res.*, 25:373, 1981.

Kyndely, K.: The sexuality of women in pregnancy and postpartum—a review. *J. Obstet. Gynecol. Nurs.,* Jan/Feb:28, 1978.

Landes, J.; Thomas, P.; and Paffenberger, S.: *Am. Sociol. Rev.,* 15:766, 1950.

Limner, R.: *Sex and The Unborn Child.* Julian Press, New York, 1970.

Lumley, J.: Sexual feelings in pregnancy and after childbirth. *Aust. NZ J. Obstet. Gynecol.*, 18:114, 1978.

Masters, W. H., and Johnson, V. E.: *Human Sexual Response.* J. and A. Churchill Ltd., London, 1966.

Mills, J. L.; Harlap, S.; and Harley, E. E.: Should coitus late in pregnancy be discouraged? *Lancet,* 2:136, 1981.

Morris, N. M.: The frequency of sexual intercourse during pregnancy. *Arch. Sex. Behav.,* 4:501, 1975.

Naeye, R. L., and Peters, E. C.: Amniotic fluid infections with intact membranes leading to perinatal death. *Pediatrics,* 61:171, 1978.

Naeye, R. L.: Coitus and associated amniotic fluid infection. *N. Engl. J. Med.,* 301:1198, 1979.

Naeye, R. L.: Seasonal variation in coitus and other risk factors and the outcome of pregnancy. *Early Hum. Devl.,* 4:61, 1980.

Naeye, R. L.: Coitus and antepartum hemorrhage. *Br. J. Obstet. Gynaecol.,* 88:765, 1981.

Naeye, R. L., and Ross, S.: Coitus and chorioamnionitis. *Early Hum. Devl.,* 6:91, 1982.

Newton, N.: The role of oxytocin reflexes in three interpersonal reproductive acts: coitus, birth and breastfeeding. *Proc. of the Serona Symposia,* 22:411, 1978.

Nuckolls, K. B.; Cassel, J.; and Kaplan, B. H.: Psychosocial assets, life crises and the prognosis of pregnancy. *Am. J. Epidemiol.,* 95:431, 1972.

Ohry, A.; Peleg, D.; Goldman, J.; David A.; and Rozin, R.: Sexual function, pregnancy and delivery in spinal cord injured women. *Gynecol. Obstet. Invest.,* 9:281, 1978.

Perkins, R. P.: Sexual behavior and response in relation to complications of pregnancy. *Am. J. Obstet. Gynecol.,* 134:498, 1979.

Perkins, R. P.: Sexuality in pregnancy—What determines behavior. *Obstet. Gynecol.,* 59:189, 1982.

Pongthai, S.; Sakornratanakul, P.; and Chaturachinda, K.: Sexual behavior during pregnancy. *J. Med. Assoc. Thai,* 62:483, 1979.

Prochazka, J., and Cernoch, A.: Coitus in pregnancy. *Cesk. Gynekol.,* 35:282, 1970.

Pugh, W. E., and Fernandez, F. L.: Coitus in late pregnancy. *Obstet. Gynecol.,* 2:636, 1955.

Rabach, J.; Bartak, V.; and Nedoma, K.: Types of sexual activity in gynecological patients. *J. Sex. Res.,* 4:282, 1968.

Rayburn, W. F., and Wilson, E. A.: Coital activity and premature delivery. *Am. J. Obstet. Gynecol.,* 137:972, 1980.

Reamy, K.; White, S.; Daniell, W.; and LeVine, E.: Sexuality and pregnancy. *J. Reprod. Med.,* 27:321, 1982.

Semmens, J. P.: Female sexuality and life situations. *Obstet. Gynecol.,* 38:555, 1971.

Slate, W. G.: Coitus as a cause of abortion. *Med. Aspects Hum. Sex.,* 2:25, 1970.

Sloan, D., and Bing, E.: Sex in pregnancy. *The Female Patient,* 8:18, 1983.

Solberg, D. A.; Butler, J.; and Wagner, N. N.: Sexual

behavior in pregnancy. *N. Engl. J. Med.,* 288:1098, 1973.

Speroff, L., and Ramuiell, P. W.: Prostaglandins in reproductive physiology. *Am. J. Obstet. Gynecol.,* 107:1111, 1970.

Steege, J. F., and Jelovsek, F. R.: Sexual behavior during pregnancy. *Obstet. Gynecol.,* 60:163, 1982.

Swanson, J.: The marital sexual relationship during pregnancy. *J. Obstet. Gynecol. Nurs.,* 9:267, Sept./Oct., 1980.

Tolar, A., and DiGrazia, P. V.: Sexual attitudes and behavior patterns during and following pregnancy. *Arch. Sex. Behav.,* 5:539, 1976.

Wagner, N.; Butler, J.; and Sanders, J.: Prematurity and orgasmic coitus during pregnancy. Data on a small sample. *Fertil. Steril.,* 27:911, 1976.

White, S. E., and Reamy, K.: Sexuality and pregnancy: A review. *Arch. Sex. Behav.,* 11:429, 1982.

Zalor, M. K.: Sexual counseling for pregnant couples. *Am. J. Matern. Child Nurs.,* May/June:176, 1976.

Zlatnik, F. J., and Burmeister, L. F.: Reported sexual behavior in late pregnancy. *J. Reprod. Med.,* 27:627, 1982.

# CHAPTER 6  SEXUALITY AND THE MENOPAUSE

*John S. Rinehart, M.D., Ph.D., and Isaac Schiff, M.D.*

## INTRODUCTION

As the taboo surrounding the sexual behavior of the elderly falls away—perhaps the last of the sexual barriers to do so—both the anecdotal and the clinical evidence indicates that sexual activity, for both women and men, can continue until very late in life. Human sexuality derives from psychosocial factors, which include the changing cultural environment, and biological factors, which include the changing hormonal milieu. It is therefore the responsibility of the physician who treats a menopausal patient experiencing sexual dysfunction to try to assign a relative importance to all the various factors affecting the condition, and to prescribe a therapy accordingly. Thus, for example, estrogen therapy would not be a suitable treatment for a case of middle-age emotional distress; conversely, psychotherapy in any form would not really remedy an estrogen-deficiency problem. The purpose of this chapter is to list the main components of the sexuality of the menopausal patient. The chapter concludes with a discussion of the role of replacement therapy for the sexuality of the menopausal patient.

## SEXUALITY IN THE AGING MALE

Perhaps the most important "environmental" factor influencing sexual behavior of the menopausal patient is the sexual behavior of her partner. Gynecologists, who are accustomed to dealing with only one half, and always the same half, of the sexual equation, may at times find it difficult to keep an accurate perspective concerning the sexuality of the menopausal patient. Sexuality involves not only the menopausal patient but also her spouse or lack of spouse. Thus, for example, simply noting a woman's changing coital frequency can prove misleading, for that changing frequency may reflect more of her partner's situation than her own.

Kinsey studied the evolution of male sexuality as a function of age. The data show a gradual decline in frequency of marital coitus in first marriage, going from 4.1 per week among 16- to 20-year-old, white, college men to .96 among 61- to 65-year-old men, the oldest men examined (Gebhard and Johnson, 1979).

For their part, Masters and Johnson (1970) note four basic physiological changes in the male as he ages:

1. a longer time needed to achieve full penile engorgement
2. a decrease in expulsive pressure
3. a reduction in volume of seminal fluid ejaculated
4. an occasional loss or reduction in ejaculatory demand.

The aging male, the authors further note, may experience any combination of these four changes—at varying rates—or no change at all. Elsewhere, Pfeiffer and colleagues (1972) conducted a longitudinal study on 260 volunteers, male and female, over the age of 60. The data showed a general decline with age in sexual activity. From 40 to 65 percent between the ages of 60 and 71 engaged in intercourse, but once age 78 was achieved, the rate dropped to 10 to 20 percent. However, some individuals within the group actually noted a rise in sexual activity with age. Moreover, both men and women seemed to agree that when a couple ceased having intercourse, the man was the cause. In a follow-up study, the authors found that all the men in the 40–50 age group said they continued to be sexually active, but 24 percent of the men in the 66–71 age group said they no longer were (Pfeiffer et al., 1972). The decline with age in male sexual activity is concomitant with a gradual decline in testosterone levels that occurs after the age of 50. Vermeulen's study (Vermeulen et al., 1972) report average testosterone values of 616 to 640 ng/100 ml in 20- to 50-year-old males, which gradually decreases to 245 ng/100 ml in 80 to 90 year olds.

Sarrel (1982) reported on sexual dysfunction in 50 couples in which the woman was postmenopausal. Of the 50 men, 39 acknowledged that the dysfunction was theirs, and of these 38 said their problem was sustaining an erection. Twenty-eight of these men observed that their difficulties appeared either shortly before or within three years after their partner's menopause. Since secondary erectile difficulty occurs in many cases as the result of a change perceived in the sexual partner, the men were questioned on the subject. Twenty-two men reported feelings of rejection and anger during unsuccessful intercourse, brought on by one or more female reactions (or lack of), the most common being vaginal dryness, vaginismus, and not wanting to be touched. Twelve men feared that sex might physically injure their wives; five of them developed the fear after intercourse produced postcoital vaginal bleeding secondary to atrophic vaginitis. For ten men the increasing slowness of their spouse's response created erectile difficulty, exemplified in one case by a man whose efforts to bring his wife to orgasm brought on angina and, once during intercourse, actually a coronary thrombosis. Sarrel summarized the data by delineating three conditions creating difficulty in the male sexual response: (1) physical difficulties with penetration; (2) slowness of the female's sexual response; (3) any of a wide range of inhibiting emotions, such as fear of hurting and a feeling of rejection, inadequacy, or anger.

One ought also to mention here that, on the average, women live longer than men. Thus the sexuality of the menopausal woman is affected by the absence of a partner, by a general decline in male sexual drive, or by a partner whose own response is undercut by his spouse's menopause.

## SEXUALITY AND MENOPAUSE

The menopause describes the permanent cessation of menses, which is preceded by the gradual decline in ovarian function. The consideration of menopausal sexuality must take into account that two different processes affect the situation simultaneously—one related to the reproductive system and the other related to aging in general. Most investigators, Utian (1980) among them, maintain that only vasomotor flushes and vaginal atrophy are causally related to the cessation of the reproductive hormones. But since the matter has not been carefully studied, one might still ask whether there are not other sexual changes related only to the menopause, and if there are, whether therapy would help in cases of distressful change.

To answer the first question, one begins with general considerations. As in the case of the male, there appears to be a steady decline in the sexual activity of the aging female. For example, Kinsey noted an average frequency of intercourse for college females of 3.58 per week among 16- to 20-year-old, married, white, college females, decreasing to 1.34 per week among the 56- to 60-year-old women (Gebhard and Johnson, 1979). Kinsey also recorded a decline in the frequency of masturbation to orgasm among married women from once per week at 16 to 20 years to 0.34 at 56 to 60 years. Of the women who experienced natural menopause, 40 percent reported that their sexual response had decreased at the time of menopause. But overall the Kinsey data show essentially a decline only in female sexual activities that are dependent upon the male, and in some cases a decline related to women using menopause as an *excuse* to avoid sexual activity, but no decline due to aging *per se*. If there was any effect of aging upon sexual activity it was only experienced much later in life.

Newman and Nichols (1960) studied 250 women age 60 to 93. Of the 101 of these women who were either single, divorced, or, primarily, widowed, only 7 percent reported any sexual activity. Of the other 149 who were married and living with their spouses, 54 percent were sexually active. Frequency for the active group varied from three times weekly to once every other month. Among those women who were married, the frequency of sexual activity related to age did not markedly decrease until after the age of 75. The authors further noted, especially in the 75 and older age group, there was an increase in concomitant serious illness, and while there were still strong sexual feelings felt, the opportunities for actual sexual activity decreased.

As noted earlier, however, coital frequency is not an accurate indicator of female sexuality. The above figures, showing essentially no change as a function of age are at variance with other data which may more accurately reflect the changing state of the female libido with age. In Pfeiffer's study one variable measured was sexual interest (Pfeiffer *et al.*, 1972). In the 46 to 50 age group 7 percent reported no interest; 23 percent reported mild interest; 61 percent reported moderate; and 9 percent reported strong. In the 66 to 71 age group the percentages were 51 percent, no interest; 26 percent, mild; 22 percent, moderate; and 2 percent, strong. The dramatic shift occurred between ages 50 to 60 years, that is, the age of menopause. In another study, Hallstrom (1977) reports a study of 800 perimenopausal women. The figures show that between the ages of 38 and 54 years, there was a definite downward trend in sexual interest, capacity for orgasm, and coital frequency. Hallstrom concludes from the data that there was a real decline in female sexual activity after a certain age and that the decline was related to the postmenopausal state. It is perhaps appropriate to speculate here whether premenopausal sexual activity affects postmenopausal sexual activity. Clark and Wallin (1965) found that for marriages characterized as negative, a marked decrease in female sexual activity occurred in the later years of the marriage. Christenson and Gagnon (1965) divided women into three categories depending on whether the frequency of their early sexual experience was high, intermediate, or low. For women in the high frequency category, the frequency of marital coitus was higher than in the other categories.

A recent report by Consumers Union (Breecher, 1983) addresses some of the issues of aging and sexuality. They found that for both men and women the incidence of masturbation decreased with age (*e.g.*, 47 percent of women in 50s [N = 801] to 33 percent of women 70 and older [N = 324]). At each age a larger percentage of men masturbated than women. They also reported that the status of a person's health affected the sexual activity. For those women over age 50, 87 percent of those in excellent health were sexually active and for men in excellent health 93 percent were sexually active. These percentages dropped to 72 percent for women and 82 percent for men in fair or poor health. However, they emphasized that poor health was a minor contribution to the decline in the proportion of sexually active people. The authors state *two* major findings in their study of 4246 respondents: both male and female sexual function gradually declines from the 50s on. Broken down by decades, they report that the proportion of sexually active females was 93 percent in their 50s, 81 percent in their 60s, and 65 percent over 70; for males the percentages are 98 percent in their 50s, 91 percent in their 60s, and 79 percent over 70. Also relevant is their finding that the following four measures for women and five measures for men show an age dependent decade-by-decade decline; *women:* (1) orgasm when asleep or while waking up; (2) number of women who masturbate; (3) wives having sex with their husbands; (4) frequency of sex with their husbands—*men:* (1) orgasm when asleep or while waking up; (2) number of men who masturbate; (3) frequency of masturbation among men who masturbate; (4) husbands having sex with their wives; (5) frequency of sex with their wives. There was also a decade-by-decade decline in the interest of sex both at the time the question was asked and compared to interest at age 40.

Perhaps the best way to summarize these sometimes inconsistent data is to quote Masters and Johnson (1966). "It has become increasingly evident that the psyche plays a part at least equal to, if not greater than, that of an unbalanced endocrine system in determining the sex-drive of women during the postmenopausal period of their lives" (p. 242). Most probably older women possess the potential for an active sexual life, but whether this potential is realized depends upon other, nonbiological, contingencies.

There are a number of ways to assess endocrine influence versus other influences upon sexual activity. For one, if the sexual activity of a particular woman is mainly affected by her hormonal status, a very definite cyclical pattern to sexual arousal should be found. For another, surgical menopause should allow us to study the endocrine consequences of menopause independent of the aging process. Moreover, if the sexual activity is endocrine related, then replacement therapy should prove of some benefit. Lastly, cross-cultural studies might elucidate any sociological influence.

## The Menstrual Cycle and Sexuality

Although the evidence is often conflicting, a relationship between the menstrual cycle and sexual activity, at least for the periovulatory peak, does not appear to exist. Perhaps much of the controversy would be eliminated if one could accurately describe which phase of the menstrual cycle a woman was in. Udry and Morris (1977) studied the sexual behavior of 85 married women in relation to their menstrual cycle. The authors report that while certain techniques of aggregation produced similar results, by and large, different techniques produced widely differing frequency curves. Adams and coworkers (1978) studied female-initiated sexual activity, to eliminate the male factor as much as possible, in 35 white, married females. These authors found a statistically significant increase in both autosexual and female-initiated heterosexual activity periovulatory as determined by being 13 to 15 days premenstrual. The increases, however, were not in evidence for oral contraceptive users. But the study was severely criticized on methodological grounds by Kolodny and Bauman (1979) and may not truly be accurate. Persky's study (Persky *et al.,* 1976) divided the menstrual cycle into three phases, administered the Moos Menstrual Distress Questionnaire, and measured reproductive hormones in a group of 30 women. Sexual activity as determined by frequency of sexual intercourse was found to be related to testosterone at ovulation and progesterone during the luteal phase. In another study, Abplanalp and colleagues surveyed 33 women by means of a variety of psychological tests and found no relationship between cycle phase and mood or enjoyment of activities (Abplanalp *et al.,* 1974). It does seem, though, that there exists a subset of women within the general population who suffer from premenstrual syndrome (PMS) and who experience a cyclical variation in sexual arousal (Sanders and Bancroft, 1982). Sanders and Bancroft (1982) found that a recent study reviewing 32 studies looking at peak sexual activity at the periovulatory period showed 17 women with a sexual peak premenstrually, 18 with a peak postmenstrually, 4 with peak during the menses, and 8 at time of ovulation. Such inconsistency leads one to question the validity of the argument for a periovulatory peak in sexual activity. The authors note, however, that discrepancies may be accounted for by failure to relate activities to time of cycle accurately and by the inclusion in the studies of PMS patients, who do show a cyclic variation in their sexual arousal.

SOCIOLOGICAL VARIABLES

As is often the case with many kinds of behavior, it is possible that responses to menopause may be learned responses. If that is indeed the case, then cross-cultural studies should shed some light on the matter. Flint (1975) observed that Indian women, for whom menopause resulted in cultural gains, experienced fewer menopausal symptoms than did women in most other societies. Winn and Newton (1982) studied 106 different cultures and found that in 20 of the 28 societies for which the relevant data was available, males demonstrated continued sexual activity into old age. In the 26 cultures for which the relevant data was available, women demonstrated continued sexual activity into old age in 22 of them. Consistent with previously mentioned data on our own culture, in any comparisons made between men and women, it is women who appear to retain sexual interest until an older age. The authors conclude that: "The continuance of sexuality in some societies during aging and the limitation of sexuality in other societies suggest that cultural as well as biologic factors may be key determinants in sexual behavior in the later part of life" (Winn and Newton, 1982, p. 283).

One biological role that ceases at menopause is that of procreant. The new situation eventually leads to children moving away from home, producing what some researchers have called the "empty nest syndrome." Evidence for the syndrome was found by Crawford and Hooper (1973), who studied 106 women and reported that at menopause a child, particularly a daughter, leaving home was felt to be more stressful than grandparenthood. (Of these women, 63 were about to become grandparents and 43 were about to become postparental.) VanKeep and Kellerhals (1974) studied 418 women and found that direct climacteric complaints and subjective difficulty in adaptation to daily life were more severe in lower social classes than in upper, but that if children were still home the adverse effects occurred less frequently. A recent study, however, has cast doubt upon the theory of the empty nest syndrome: Krystal and Chiriboga (1979) reported a positive rather than a negative response to the empty nest. They did note, though, that a period of readjustment was required by some women following the moving away of children. In another study, Schneider and Brotherton (1979) were not able to single out the loss of reproductive capability as distinguishing depressed versus nondepressed patients, thus calling into question whether a postmenopausal woman becomes depressed because of loss of reproductive function. However, of the 20 women studied, seven of the ten depressed patients suffered a disturbed childhood. These studies thus suggest that premenopausal functioning and personality are important factors affecting a woman's ability to cope with menopause. Consistent with the findings of Masters and Johnson, the sociology of menopause plays a rather important role in sexual functioning.

## THE EFFECT OF HYSTERECTOMY ON SEXUAL FUNCTIONING

Most studies agree that hysterectomy has a negative effect on the sexual functioning of some women, but not on the majority of women. Huffman (1950) studied a number of private patients who had undergone either total hysterectomy with removal of ovaries, total hysterectomy, or simple removal of the uterus. The majority of patients (approximately 90 percent), whatever category they fell in, reported no change in their postoperative sexual activity. Dodds and coworkers (1961) studied the marital relationship of 108 women about to undergo total hysterectomy and oophorectomy of whom 50 percent reported unsatisfactory marital relations preoperative. After the operation 38 percent reported improved marital relations; 47 percent noted no change; and 15 percent (half of whom had previously unsatisfactory marital relations) noted a worsening of relations. Patterson and Craig (1963) found that only 18 percent of the patients in their study of hysterectomy patients noted a decreased erotic drive postoperative; 20 percent noted an increase; and 62 percent reported no change. Of the 18 percent who experienced decreased erotic drive, 5 percent admitted severe domestic stress. On the other hand, Utian (1975) noted a high incidence of decreased libido after hysterectomy, reporting 37 percent of 18 cases showing decreased sexual response respectively. Thus removal of the ovaries contributed little to the decreased sexual functioning. In a study of 49 randomly selected women undergoing noncancer hysterectomy, Martin and colleagues (1980) found no evidence of so-called posthysterectomy syndrome. In general preoperative psychological problems persisted postoperative. The predominant presurgical psychological diagnosis was hysteria; 27 percent of the sample admitted no diagnosis.

Dennerstein and colleagues (1977) retrospectively studied 809 women who had undergone hysterectomy with oophorectomy. The authors reported deteriorated sexual relations in 37 percent of cases, but improved relations in 34 percent of cases. No relationship was found between postoperative estrogen replacement therapy and sexual dysfunction. Preoperative anxiety about loss of sexual function secondary to the operation was positively associated with a postoperative deterioration of sexual relations. Women with a frequency of sexual relations less than once per week experienced a worse outcome than women with a frequency of greater than once per week. The authors concluded that reduced postoperative sexual functioning was primarily related to psychological factors. Gath (Gath et al., 1982a; 1982b) studied 156 women, both preoperatively and postoperatively, and found that psychiatric morbidity was actually higher preoperatively than postoperatively (58 percent preoperatively versus 29 percent at the 18 month follow-up). Thus it would seem that at most 15 to 20 percent of women undergoing hysterectomy with oophorectomy actually experience decreased sexual functioning. Most of the reported decrease seems to be related to the preoperative psychologic state of the patient. If ovarian removal were the significant factor, it would be expected that the majority of women undergoing oophorectomy would experience sexual impairment.

## REPLACEMENT THERAPY AND SEXUAL RELATIONSHIP

When considering recommendation of estrogen replacement therapy, the key question is what symptoms are estrogen related. Only if these symptoms are related to sexual function will estrogen be efficacious. Estrogen deficiency has been cited as causing vaginal atrophy and concomitant structural changes in the pelvis, hot flashes, and osteoporosis. For practical purposes osteoporosis need not be considered here although one could argue that a broken hip secondary to osteoporosis would certainly inhibit sexual activity. Hot flashes can affect a woman's life quite severely secondary to sleep loss. This would certainly have an effect upon sexual activity. Utian (1975) studied the effects of estradiol upon libido in a placebo-controlled study. The results indicated no beneficial effect upon libido.

However, estrogen does appear to improve vaginal lubrication and to restore some structural changes. Masters and Johnson (1966) note certain physiological changes that occur with aging. One of the first in response to sexual stimulation is vaginal lubrication, which can take as long as 5 minutes in the 50- to 70-year-old woman compared to 15 to 30 seconds in her 20- to 40 year old counterpart. Associated with this atrophic change is a delay in expansion of the vaginal barrel. Other changes noted were a loss of involuntary uterine elevation, a loss of labial skin color changes, and a slight loss in clitoral size and fat pad thickness near the mons. The orgasmic phase for the 50 to 70 year old is shortened with only 4 to 5 contractions as compared to 8 to 12 for the younger woman. A postmenopausal woman may actually experience a uterine spasm lasting up to one minute, which can be quite painful. All of these changes are due to a decrease in estrogen. Masters and Johnson (1966) note that of 54 women over the age of 60, three responded sexually as if they were younger and these three women were the only ones who had remained sexually active. Leiblum and colleagues (1983) studied 52 postmenopausal women to determine the effects of sexual activity upon the vagina. They found less vaginal atrophy was apparent in the sexually active women.

Campbell (1976) in a controlled study notes a diminution in vaginal dryness and heightening in coital satisfactions with PREMARIN, but no increase in frequency of masturbation, orgasm or coital frequency. Dennerstein and coworkers (1980) used a double-blind cross-over protocol to assess the effect of estrogen or levonorgestrel upon sexual desire, sexual enjoyment, and amount of spontaneous vaginal lubrication. After three months of therapy with estrogen, this resulted in heightened sexual desire and enjoyment. It would seem, therefore, that estrogen replacement may work more through its effect on vaginal lubrication than on libido. The lack of effect of estrogen on arousal is consistent with a report by Persky (Persky et al., 1978) that failed to show any relationship between sexual activity and serum estradiol levels.

The final choice whether to begin estrogen replacement therapy remains with the informed patient. For a patient not at risk from estrogen therapy, the combined benefit upon sexual function and osteoporosis may tip the scales in favor of treatment. Present studies suggest that combined estrogen–progestogen is the therapeutic regimen of choice. But, as any perceptive observer would have foreseen, the mystery of sexual fulfillment remains intractable to simple chemical or biologic manipulations.

## REFERENCES

Abplanalp, J. M.; Donnelly, A. F.; and Rose, R. M.: Psychoendocrinology of the menstrual cycle. I. Enjoyments of daily activities and moods. *Psychosom. Med.,* 41:587, 1974.

Adams, D. B.; Gold, A. R.; and Burt, A. D.: Rise on female-initiated sexual activity at ovulation and its suppression by oral contraceptives. *N. Engl. J. Med.,* 299:1145, 1978.

Breecher E. M.: *Love, Sex and Aging: A Consumers Union Report.* Little, Brown, Boston, 1985.

Campbell, S.: (ed.): Double-blind psychometric studies on the effects of natural estrogens on postmenopausal women. In *Management of the Menopause and Postmenopausal Years.* MTP Press, Lancaster, 1976, 148–158.

Christenson, C. V., and Gagon, J. H.: Sexual behavior in a group of older women. *J. Gerontol.* 20:351, 1965.

Clark A. L., and Wallin, P.: Women's sexual responsiveness and the duration and quality of their marriages. *Am. J. Sociol.,* 71:187, 1965.

Crawford, M. P., and Hooper, D.: Menopause, aging and family. *Soc. Sci. Med.,* 7:469, 1973.

Dennerstein, L.; Burrows, G. D.; Wood, C.; and Wyman, G.: Hormones and sexuality: effect of oestrogen and progestogen. *Obstet. Gynecol.,* 56:316, 1980.

Dennerstein, L.; Wood, C.; and Burrows, G. D.: Sexual response following hysterectomy and oophorectomy. *Obstet. Gynecol.,* 49:92, 1977.

Dodds, D. O.; Potgieter, C. R.; Turner, P. J.; Schupers, G. A. F.: The physical and emotional results of hysterectomy: A review of 162 cases. *S. Afr. Med. J.,* 1 53, 1961.

Flint, M.: The menopause: Reward or punishment? *Psychosomatics,* 16:161, 1975.

Gath, D.; Cooper, P.; and Day, A.: Hysterectomy and psychiatric disorder. I. Levels of psychiatric morbidity before and after hysterectomy. *Br. J. Psychiatr.,* 140:335, 1982a.

Gath, D.; Cooper, P.; Bond, A.; and Edmonds, G.: II. Demographic psychiatric and physical factors in relation to psychiatric outcome. *Br. J. Psychiatr.,* 140:343, 1982b.

Gebhard, P. M., and Johnson, A. B.: *The Kinsey Data: Marginal tabulations of the 1938–1963 interviews conducted by the Institute for Sex Research.* Saunders, Philadelphia, 1979.

Hallstrom, T.: Sexuality of the climacteric. *Clin. Obstet. Gynecol.,* 4:227, 1977.

Huffman, J. W.: The effect of gynecologic surgery on sexual reactions. *Am. J. Obstet. Gynecol.,* 59:915, 1950.

Kolodny, R. C., and Bauman, J. E.: To the editor. *N. Engl. J. Med.,* 300:626, 1979.

Krystal, S., and Chiriboga, D. A.: The empty nest process in mid-life men and women. *Maturitas,* 1:2 5, 1979.

Leiblum, S.; Bachmann, G.; Kemmann, E.; and Colburn, D.: Vaginal atrophy with postmenopausal women: The importance of sexual activity and hormones. *JAMA,* 249:2195, 1983.

Martin, R. L.; Roberts, W. V.; and Clayton, P. J.: Psychic status after hysterectomy: a one-year prospective follow-up. *JAMA,* 244:350, 1980.

Masters, W. H., and Johnson, V. E.: *Human Sexual Response.* Little, Brown, Boston, 1966.

Masters, W. H., and Johnson, V. E.: *Human Sexual Inadequacy.* Little, Brown, Boston, 1970.

Newman, G., and Nichols, C. R.: Sexual activities and

attitudes in older persons. *JAMA,* 1973:33, 1960.

Patterson, R. M., and Craig, J. B.: Misconceptions concerning the psychological effects of hysterectomy. *Am. J. Obstet. Gynecol.,* 85:104, 1963.

Persky, H.; O'Brien, C. P.; and Khan, M. A.: Reproductive hormone levels, sexual activity and moods during the menstrual cycle. *Psychosom. Med.,* 38:63, 1976.

Persky, M.; Charney, N.; Lief, M. I.; O'Brien, C. P.; Mellis, W. R.; and Strauss, D.: The relationship of plasma estradiol level to sexual behavior in young women. *Psychosom. Med.,* 40:523, 1978.

Pfeiffer, E.; Verwoerdt, A.; and Wang, H.: Sexual behavior in aged men and women. 1. Observation on 254 community volunteers. *Arch. Gen. Psychiatr.,* 19:753, 1968.

Pfeiffer, E.; Verwoerdt, A.; and Davis, A. C.: Sexual behavior in middle life. *Am. J. Psychiatr.,* 128:82, 1972.

Sanders, D., and Bancroft, J.: Hormones and the sexuality of women—the menstrual cycle. *Clin. Endocrinol. Metab.,* 11:639, 1982.

Sarrel, P. M.: Six problems after menopause: A study of fifty married couples treated in a sex counseling programme. *Maturitas,* 4:231, 1982.

Schneider, M., and Brotherton, P.: Physiological, psychological and situational stresses in depression during the climacteris. *Maturitas,* 1:153, 1979.

Udry, J. R., and Morris, N. M.: The distribution of events in the human menstrual cycle. *J. Reprod. Fertil.,* 51:419, 1977.

Utian, W. H.: Effect of hysterectomy, ooporectomy and estrogen therapy on libido. *Int. J. Gynaecol. Obstet.,* 13:97, 1975.

Utian, W. H.: *Menopause in Modern Perspective: A Guide to Clinical Practice.* Appleton–Century Crofts, New York, 1980.

Van Keep, P. A., and Kellerhals, J. M.: The impact of sociocultural factors on symptom formations. *Psychother. Psychosom. Med. Psychol.,* 23:251, 1974.

Vermeulen, A.; Rubes, R.; and Verdonck, L.: Testosterone secretion and metabolism in male seniscence. *J. Clin. Endocrinol. Metab.,* 37:730, 1972.

Winn, R. L., and Newton, N.: Sexuality in aging: a study of 106 cultures. *Arch. Sex. Behav.,* 11:283, 1982.

# UNIT II PATHOPHYSIOLOGY OF HUMAN SEXUALITY IN OBSTETRICAL AND GYNECOLOGIC DISEASE

CHAPTER **7.** EXTERNAL GENITAL AMBIGUITY

*Bertrand L. New, M.D., and Maria I. New, M.D.*

## INTRODUCTION

The perpetuation of the human species has depended upon the ontogenic differentiation of individuals into male or female, establishment of reciprocal mating and copulatory behavior, and fertilization of the female egg by a male sperm. Reproductive sexual activity first becomes possible after the completion of puberty. However, gender differentiation in all of its complex aspects begins well before then.

## BIOLOGICAL COMPONENTS

Early sexual identification can be divided into several aspects, which appear in chronological order in Figure 7-1. It can be noted that the nursery room sex, which is the key to the child's later gender role, depends on the external genitalia, generally evaluated by an obstetrician's examination in the delivery room. When all aspects of sexual identification are the same (isosexual), then the nursery room sex assignment is correct. However, in situations in which all aspects of sexual identification are not homologous, the external body sex may be misleading.

Ambiguous sex in the newborn infant is a medical emergency. The decision as to sex assignment at birth has obvious long-term implications. A rational approach permits a careful assessment of the problem and choice of sex assignment.

Male pseudohermaphroditism is the condition of incomplete male differentiation of the external genitalia in an individual with a Y chromosome. The gonads of the male pseudohermaphrodite, when present, are either streak gonads or testes. The term "male pseudohermaphroditism" encompasses a wide range of disorders and phenotypic presentations. The disorders resulting in male pseudohermaphroditism may be classified into three groups on the basis of pathophysiology:

1. disorders of testosterone biosynthesis: gonadal dysgenesis and deficiencies of any of the steroidogenic enzymes necessary for testosterone synthesis
2. disorders of testosterone metabolism: deficiency of 5α-reductase, an enzyme necessary for the conversion of testosterone to dihydrotestosterone
3. disorders of androgen receptors: complete or incomplete forms of testicular feminization.

Female pseudohermaphroditism is the condition of virilized genitalia in an individual with an XX karyotype. By far the most common cause of female pseudohermaphroditism is congenital adrenal hyperplasia due to 21-hydroxylase deficiency. Female pseudohermaphroditism may also occur due to exposure to excess maternal androgens, either exogenous or due to an androgen-producing tumor, or may be idiopathic.

The management of the patient who pres-

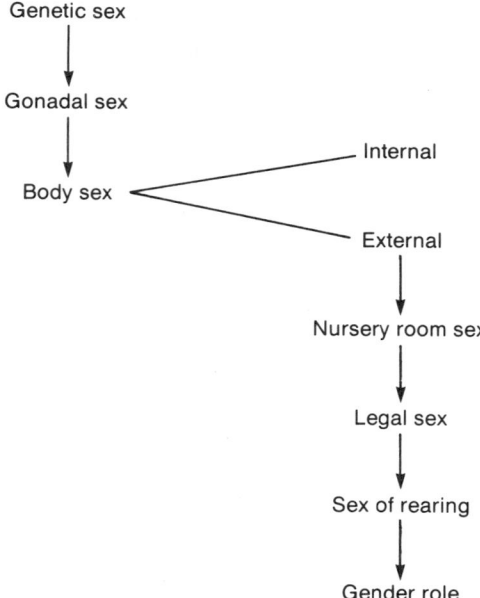

**FIGURE 7-1.** Aspects of sexual identification. (Reprinted with permission from New, M. I., and Levine, L. S.: Congenital adrenal hyperplasia. In Harris, H., and Hirschhorn (eds.): *Advances in Human Genetics.* Vol. 4. Plenum, New York, 1973, pp. 251-326.

ents with ambiguous genitalia is, in part, dependent upon the age of presentation. It is recommended that a neonate with ambiguous genitalia be referred to a major medical center, where resources necessary for performing sophisticated diagnostic studies and medical personnel with expertise in dealing with the problem of genital ambiguity are available.

When examining a newborn with ambiguous genitalia, it is usually not possible to distinguish between male and female pseudohermaphroditism on the basis of the appearance of the external genitalia (Figure 7-2). However, gonads that have descended to labial, scrotal, or inguinal regions are almost always testes. In addition, an evaluation of the internal organs will be helpful to delineate the diagnosis. A rectal examination should be performed in an attempt to palpate a uterine cervix. It should be noted that the presence of Mullerian derivatives in an infant with ambiguous genitalia excludes most forms of male pseudohermaphroditism, except for the cyto-

genetic forms resulting in gonadal dysgenesis. Hence, the presence of a cervix indicates that the infant probably has a form of female pseudohermaphroditism, true hermaphroditism, or gonadal dysgenesis. A careful search for the presence of other somatic anomalies is of great importance in the examination of the neonate. The presence of somatic anomalies associated with Ullrich–Turner's syndrome, occurring in conjunction with genital ambiguity, strongly suggests 45X/46XY mosaicism.

In the newborn period the physician must bear in mind that the patient may be at risk for the development of an adrenal crisis until the diagnosis of one of the forms of adrenal hyperplasia, associated with the impairment of glucocorticoid and mineralocorticoid production and ambiguous genitalia, is ruled out. Hence, the most common form of congenital adrenal hyperplasia, 21-hydroxylase deficiency, either of the salt-losing or simple virilizing form, should be considered in an infant presenting with ambiguous genitalia. Deficiency of 21-hydroxylase is associated with female pseudohermaphroditism. Deficiency of 11$\beta$-hydroxylase, which is much less common than 21-hydroxylase deficiency, is also associated with female pseudohermaphroditism. Male neonates with 11$\beta$-hydroxylase or 21-hydroxylase deficiency have normal genitalia. Hypertension may be present in 11$\beta$-hydroxylase deficiency and is attributed to elevation of deoxycorticosterone resulting from accumulation of precursors proximal to the enzymatic block. Deficiency of 3$\beta$-hydroxysteroid dehydrogenase is another form of congenital adrenal hyperplasia, which may present with virilization of the female neonate and undervirilization of the male neonate. Depending on the degree of enzymatic impairment, frank salt wasting and hypocortisolemia may occur in the newborn period.

Other less common forms of congenital adrenal hyperplasia, that is, congenital lipoid adrenal hyperplasia and 17$\alpha$-hydroxylase deficiency, should also be considered in the differential diagnosis of a neonate with genital ambiguity, as these disorders also are associated with adrenal insufficiency. Serial serum

7 EXTERNAL GENITAL AMBIGUITY    89

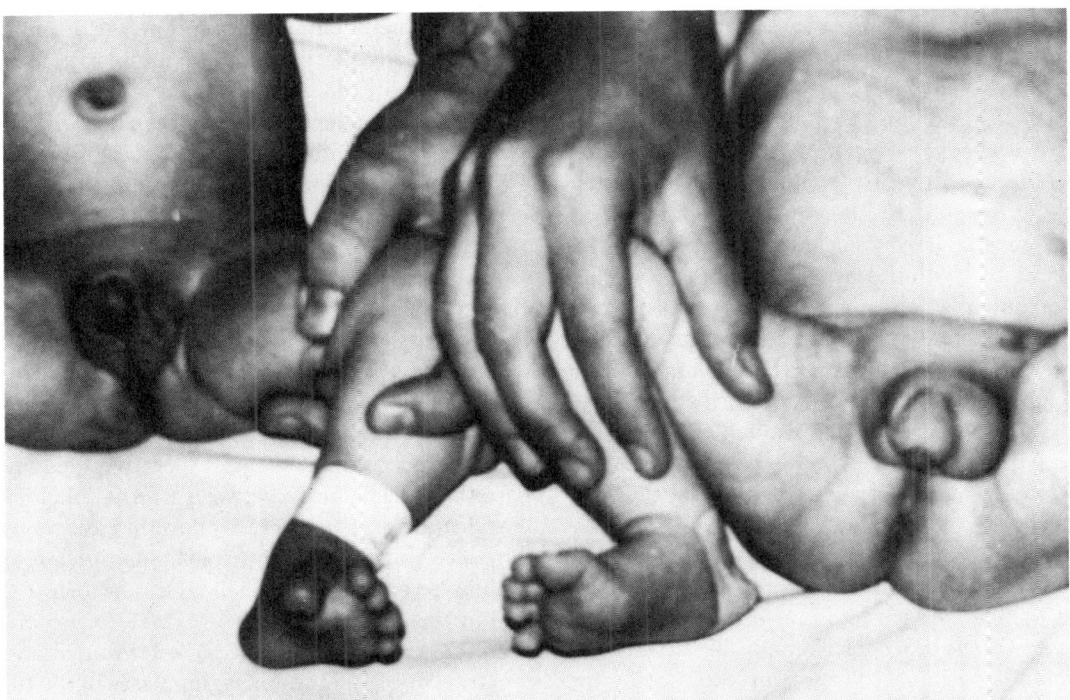

FIGURE 7-2. Marked similarity of genitalia of two infants pictured emphasizes fact that it is usually not possible to distinguish between a male and female pseudohermaphrodite on basis of external genitalia alone. Neonate on left has unclassifiable form of male pseudohermaphroditism (normal 46,XY chromosomal complement, normal adrenal and testicular steroidogenesis, positive nitrogen retention in response to exogenous testosterone treatment) and very undervirilized genitalia. Infant on right is female pseudohermaphrodite whose condition was diagnosed as a salt-wasting form of congenital adrenal hyperplasia due to 21-hydroxylase deficiency. (Reprinted with permission from Levy, D. J.; Levine, L. S.; and New, M. J.: *Male pseudohermaphroditism Pediatrics in Review.* 3:273–283, 1982.

and urinary electrolytes should be followed in all neonates with genital ambiguity in the event that a salt-wasting form of congenital adrenal hyperplasia exists. Careful attention to the general medical status of the neonate is imperative. Appropriate hormonal tests to assess adrenal as well as gonadal function will be useful for diagnosing congenital adrenal hyperplasia and detecting other causes of impaired testosterone biosynthesis, should they exist. These tests include baseline serum and urine androgens, mineralocorticoids, and glucocorticoids, as well as serum 17-hydroxyprogesterone levels. Determination of urinary 17-ketosteroids, 17-hydroxycorticosteroids, pregnanetriol, and aldosterone levels should also be performed. Measurement of serum 17-hydroxyprogesterone is recommended, as this hormone is elevated in 21-hydroxylase deficiency. An adrenocorticotropic hormone (ACTH) stimulation test may also be performed to further assess adrenal function. A human chorionic gonadotropin (hCG) stimulation test to assess gonadal function more carefully is necessary in most cases of male pseudohermaphroditism in order to define the etiology of the genital ambiguity.

While closely observing the neonate with ambiguous genitalia and pursuing hormonal studies, the issue of gender assignment must be addressed. This issue is of a critical nature, and sensitivity to the concerns of the patient's relatives is imperative. It is prudent to delay gender assignment until sufficient data are available to allow for the determination of the optimal sex assignment. However, too long a delay may be harmful. The results of the buccal smear can be obtained within 24 hours, but a chromosome study should be initiated at the same time in all patients with ambiguous genitalia. The results of many of the critical diagnostic hormonal tests discussed can be available within a week. Radiologic studies, including genitourograms and ultrasonography, can be employed in some cases to define the internal genitalia in the neonatal period. Once the critical data required for making an accurate diagnosis are available, a panel of experts should determine the sex of rearing. Consideration as to whether puberty will conform to the sex of assignment and as to the patient's potential for normal sexual functioning and fertility is critical in the determination of gender assignment. If reconstructive surgery of the external genitalia is necessary, it should be initiated sometime before the age of 2½ years.

A male sex assignment to a female pseudohermaphrodite with congenital adrenal hyperplasia due to 21-hydroxylase deficiency is particularly tragic, since with proper treatment, the infant could become a reproductive female, capable of normal sexual function and childbearing. The error can be avoided by a systematic approach to the problems of ambiguous genitalia in the newborn. With the ascertainment of female genetic sex by means of buccal smear or karyotype, the diagnosis of female pseudohermaphroditism is established and the previously discussed laboratory tests define the etiology and treatment.

Appropriate surgical measures may be taken to repair the ambiguous genitalia once a sex assignment has been made based on a reliable diagnosis of the underlying enzyme disorder. The aim of surgical repair should be to remove the redundant erectile tissue, preserve the sexually sensitive glans clitoris, and provide a normal vaginal orifice that will function adequately for menstruation and intromission. Because of the normal internal genitalia in these patients, normal puberty, fertility, and childbearing are possible when there is early therapeutic intervention. Additional reconstructive surgery (i.e., vaginoplasty) may be required in later years.

Rarely, female infants have been so virilized as to have a penile urethra. In these infants, surgical correction of the external genitalia to conform to the female sex presents a much greater challenge to the skill and experience of the surgeon. Before undertaking corrective surgery, several questions must be raised and answered. (1) What is the radiographic and endoscopic appearance of the proximal urethra and its spatial relationship to the vaginal "diverticulum"? In order to have a functioning and competent postoperative female urethra, the distance between internal bladder neck and point of juncture of urethra and vaginal diverticulum (the future vaginal introitus) must be at least 2.0 cm in the newborn. (2) How well developed is the vaginal "diverticulum"? A shallow vaginal pocket will demand extensive augmentation vaginoplasty in the future, thereby presenting a potential hazard to continence should the urethra and bladder base have to be undermined extensively during such a surgical procedure. Should there be serious doubt as to the eventual outcome of corrective surgery as far as urinary continence is concerned, based upon the above considerations and the ready availability of surgical expertise, then due consideration should be given to a male sex assignment in such a newborn with a prominent phallus and a completely formed male-type urethra. Of course, fertility would be sacrificed in the female given the male sex assignment, for a complete hysterectomy and oophorectomy would have to be done to complete such a sex reversal.

In congenital adrenal hyperplasia, treatment with hydrocortisone is necessary in both sex assignments for growth and prevention of early epiphyseal fusion, while treatment with testosterone is necessary after puberty to induce male secondary sex characteristics in the castrated genetic female raised as a male. In the case of female sex assignment, the surgery for phallic correction must be carried out in early infancy, while in the case of male sex assignment, hysterectomy and oophorectomy, relatively simple procedures, can be delayed until prepuberty. The hysterectomy and oopherectomy are necessary in genetic females raised as males in order to avoid menstrual flow at puberty, which may present as cyclical hematuria. The function of the urethra is not compromised in the male assignment, while it may be in the female. The certain loss of fertility in the case of male sex assignment to a 46XX individual must be balanced against possible urological complications in the potentially difficult surgical correction when the baby is assigned to the female sex. A rational and judicious choice of sex assignment is a critical aspect of treatment, since the sex assignment has life-long implications.

Gonadectomy prior to adolescence may be indicated to avoid pubertal virilization in certain cases of male pseudohermaphroditism in which a female gender assignment has been made (*e.g.,* incomplete testicular feminization). In those forms of male pseudohermaphroditism associated with an increased risk of testicular neoplasm (*i.e.,* both forms of testicular feminization and all forms of gonadal dysgenesis associated with the presence of Y chromosomal material), gonadectomy is also indicated.

These recommendations for evaluation of the newborn with ambiguous genitalia are summarized in Figure 7–3. Patients with ambiguous genitalia presenting after early infancy, or those who present in adolescence with pubertal failure, also require prompt medical attention and evaluation in a manner similar to that outlined for the neonate. A severe form of adrenal insufficiency, however, is virtually ruled out by later presentation, although milder forms must still be considered and investigation of adrenal function, along with gonadal function, is warranted.

## PSYCHOLOGICAL COMPONENTS

A bisexual potential exists within each individual, both biologically and psychologically. Gender dimorphism, or the divergent paths of individuals toward maleness or femaleness, begins with the physical and hormonal aspects and then proceeds to the more complicated psychological and social behavioral aspects. Courting, gender role, and gender-specific behavior are significantly modified by prevailing cultural values.

The psychological aspects of human sexuality are complex, multiply determined, and extensively varied. Data are difficult to establish

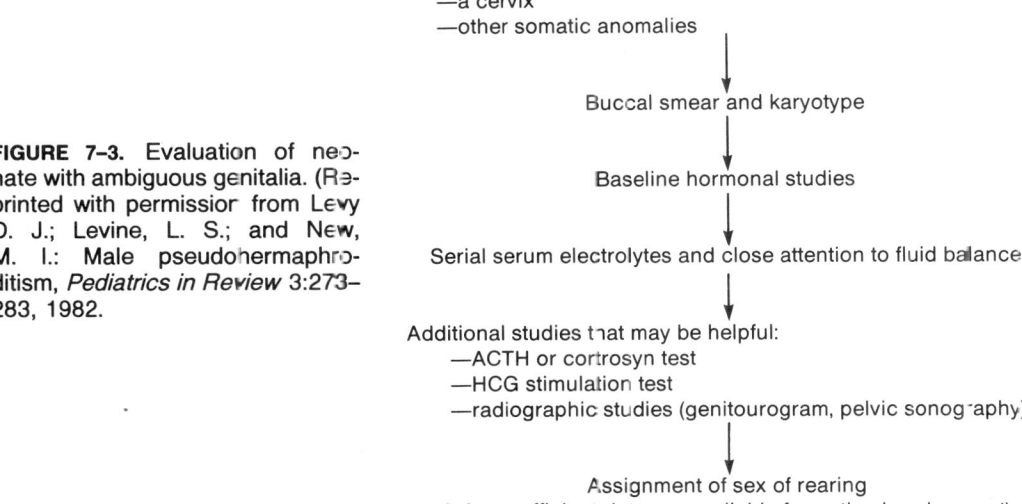

**FIGURE 7–3.** Evaluation of neonate with ambiguous genitalia. (Reprinted with permission from Levy D. J.; Levine, L. S.; and New, M. I.: Male pseudohermaphroditism, *Pediatrics in Review* 3:273–283, 1982.

because it is almost impossible to separate out simple cause and effect relationships in this highly complex system. For the sake of clarity one can divide psychosexual development into three components: gender identity, gender role, and sexual behavior.

Gender identity is the personal experience and persistence of one's individuality as a male or female. Gender role is the public expression and perception of one's gender identity (Money and Ehrhardt, 1972). Sexual behavior consists of internally or externally directed acts for the purpose of erotic gratification.

In addition to these aspects, recent interest has been directed to the question of whether male and female brains are organized differently in nonsexual areas, beginning perhaps as early as the third or fourth month of gestation in response to the impact of early gonadal hormones (Gorski and Jacobson, 1981; Witelson, 1976). Preliminary data suggest that boys develop a greater right hemispheric specialization at an earlier age and that girls may therefore retain a greater plasticity for the development of cognitive functions and thus be more resistant to unilateral defects. This finding might account for the fact that impairment of cognitive functions is found about five times as frequently in school-aged boys as in school-aged girls.

Sexual behavior, gender role practices, and gender identity are generally isosexual but can be relatively independent of each other. So, for example, a male practicing homosexual behavior might have a largely male identity and carry out male roles. Prior to the onset of puberty, sexual behavior is usually frowned upon and often punished by adults. However, observation of children demonstrates that male infants, even prior to birth, have erections. Casual autoerotic genital play is almost universal in male infants and common in female infants. The self-stimulation precedes gender identity and seems predicated on repeating pleasurable experiences discovered by accident. It is not clear whether the increased incidence in boys is based upon easier access to genital manipulation or hormonal differences. Gradually, at some stage in development, probably after the first few years of life, masturbatory play becomes associated with sexual fantasies. Since we have no methods of observing or measuring these fantasies, one must rely upon the individual to communicate them, either directly or indirectly by psychological tests or questionnaires (Higham, 1981).

However, observable sexual behavior in children, even autoerotic play, is often limited because of societal prohibitions against such behavior. This behavior is usually detected when adults surprise children in autoerotic, heterosexual, or homosexual play. Freud has directed us to the normal "polymorphous" nature of childhood sexuality (Freud, 1953). Occasional homosexual and masturbatory activity can be found in normal children of both sexes and does not necessarily predict adult sexual preference or orientation. It is important to note that children are vulnerable to seduction by same sex or opposite sex adults. These seductions can affect the individual child, but in unpredictable ways which may set up inhibition of all sexual gratification, resistance to specific types of sexual partners, or a predilection towards specific sexual partners or specific forms of sexual behavior.

Ford and Beach (1951), in their comprehensive study of patterns of sexual behavior, have illustrated the wide variety of sexual practices sanctioned by or prohibited by diverse human cultures. These include courtship, foreplay, sexual positions, and heterosexual, bisexual, and homosexual partner choice. Although prepubertal children are seldom participants, they are educated in socially acceptable sexual behavior by the parenting adults. The cultural prohibition that appears to remain most constant over a variety of human cultures is sexual activity with animals. However, even this is practiced by occasional individuals, especially in the prepubertal and pubertal years when animals are more accessible than other humans.

Gender role, or the culturally accepted gender-specific activities for males and females, begins at birth when hospital staff, parents, and families, on the basis of the external genitalia, designate the newborn as male, female or, rarely, as being of ambiguous gender. Designation of the majority of infants as male or female is done routinely by the delivery room physician and communicated to the parents who, in turn, raise the child as a boy or girl. This begins with the selection of a boy's or a girl's name, followed by selection of gender dimorphic clothing, colors, and early playthings. If there is a question about the gender or ambiguity of the genitalia, the normal happy birth announcements must be delayed. This constitutes a medical emergency, as long-delayed designation of the infant as boy or girl may lead to the family's perception of the child as somehow defective or damaged and may modify the family's wholehearted acceptance of the baby.

One may wonder whether individuals who have undergone corrective genital surgery can function successfully in sexual behavior, gender role, and gender identity. In one such group of genetic females who had been virilized by prenatal progestins, Money and Ehrhardt (1972) found that nine out of ten described themselves as tomboys, but at a later follow-up none wanted to change sex. They all had adequate female genitalia, some naturally and some by surgery. All had been raised as females. Five out of six women available for later follow-up had found satisfactory and exclusively heterosexual relations and interests (Money and Mathews, 1982). The remaining woman reported no special interest in sexual activity. None became lesbians. Comparable studies on males are impaired by other complicating variables.

This leads to the question of whether tomboyishness without known hormonal factors leads to an increased incidence of lesbianism. (In this context, tomboyishness is defined as increased interest in physical athletic activity and decreased interest in self-adornment and in doll play.) Current information indicates that tomboys without genital or hormonal anomalies may not have a higher incidence of lesbianism than non-tomboy girls. However, they do become involved in heterosexual activity and interests at a later stage in puberty than socially and culturally comparable girls. Green and coworkers (1982) are engaged in a study of this question, but the follow-up has not yet been completed.

Boys who show some effeminate behaviors are a more mixed group and range from boys whose slim build and hair coloring lead peers to consider them effeminate, to boys who are frightened of physical sports, to boys who dress as girls. The latter group appears to be at highest risk for adult homosexual or bisexual orientation. Transvestitism, in which an individual, most often a male, dresses in some or all of the clothing of the opposite sex with accompanying sexual excitement, occurs in adults. In preadolescent boys, this behavior is sometimes associated with sexual excitement but is more often seen as a compliance with parental wishes and ambiguous messages about the child's gender. Transvestite behavior, which may be compatible with normal heterosexual choice of partner and reproduction, is not the same as transsexualism in which the gender identity is incongruent with the genetic, hormonal, and physical sexual development.

Gender identity, or one's personal inner sense of being either a male or a female, is the most difficult aspect of psychosexual development to document because it is by definition an exclusively mental phenomenon. It is postulated that, as biologic human gender dimorphism is derived from a bisexual potential, all humans carry a psychological bisexual potential. In fact, men's and women's capacities to meet each other's needs may derive from the capacity to identify with and understand opposite sex needs. However, most individuals have a core gender identity of one sex or the other. Much of the controversy in the literature is derived from whether gonadal hormones are the primary influence on gender identity or whether externally assigned gender role based upon the external genitalia of the newborn is the primary determinant. In addition, this controversy raises the important question of whether there is a "critical" period for the establishment of core gender identity. A critical period is a specific time span within the course of development during which an attribute or function must develop. If it fails to develop within that time span, then it is either difficult or impossible for the attribute to develop fully later. This might apply to such diverse factors as gonadal differentiation, speech development, and gender identity.

Most researchers and clinicans in this field (Baker, 1981; Ehrhardt and Meyer-Bahlburg, 1981; Money and Ehrhardt, 1972) recognize that hormonal factors can influence the characteristics of gender dimorphic behavior, but believe that in most cases sex of rearing exerts the most important influence. However, Imperato-McGinley has studied a Dominican Republic population of 18 patients with $5\alpha$-reductase deficiency and draws a different conclusion. These individuals were genetic males who had normal testosterone levels at the fetal, neonatal and pubertal periods. However, the enzyme deficiency led to reduced dihydrotestosterone levels *in utero* with consequent ambiguity of the genitalia. These 18 males were raised "unambiguously" as girls until puberty when the pubertal increases in circulating testosterone led to masculinization of body and genitals. Imperato-McGinley reports that 17 of the 18 who were raised as girls made a dramatic reversal of gender identity over the period of a few years to become unequivocally male. She postulates that fetal and pubertal hormone levels were more significant determinants of satisfactory adult male gender identity than sex of rearing (Imperato-McGinley *et al.*, 1979, 1981). Others have questioned her conclusions (Rubin *et al.*, 1981) on the grounds that data in regard to unambiguous female designation at birth and during rearing were not sufficient. In addition, five male infants with $5\alpha$-reductase deficiency in the United States who had average male testosterone levels *in utero* but were then raised as females apparently maintained a feminine gender identity despite pubertal virilization.

One of the more dramatic examples of the importance of sex of rearing is reported by Money and Ehrhardt (1972). In this case one of a set of male identical twins completely lost his penis through a surgical accident at seven months of age. The parents agonized their way to the decision to rear the twin who had lost his penis as a girl. From 17 months onward the parents reared the unaffected child as a boy and the identical twin as a girl with genital reconstitution and estrogen hormone replacement therapy. Parental observation and studies by Money and his coworkers indicated that these two children found gender identities of opposite sex despite having started life as identical twins.

## CONCLUSION

It can be said that most humans grow up with a clear genetic, hormonal, physical, and gender identity as either male or female. Unambiguous biological givens lead to designation as either male or female by professionals and parents. The parents, in turn, raise the child to be a boy or a girl. Ambiguity of genitalia or of parental perceptions may confuse a clear, unequivocal gender identity. A confused or changing gender identity may lead to gender dysphoria. An occasional episode of cross-gender toileting behavior, that is, standing versus sitting during urination, and occasional heterosexual, homosexual, or autoerotic play in the child from infancy to preadolescence, does not necessarily indicate pathology. However, prolonged repetitive cross-dressing or deviant sexual play may set a pattern for adult sexuality or gender dysphoria, and a child is especially vulnerable to influence by adults who may use children for their own sexual purposes. Sex assignment and sex of rearing are major contributors to gender identity and should be made as early as possible in the infant's life, since gender identity begins before age one. The earlier that a sex assignment can be made, the less chance there is of subsequent confusion by the child and the family. The determinants of adult sexual orientation and behavior are multiple and at this point major deviations are seldom predictable.

# REFERENCES

Baker, S.: Psychological management of intersex children. In Josso, N.: (ed.): *The Intersex Child*. S. Karger AG, Basel/New York, 1981.

Ehrhardt, A. A.; and Meyer-Bahlburg, H. F. L.: Effects of prenatal sex hormones on gender-related behavior. *Science*, 211:1312–1318, 1981.

Ford, C. S., and Beach, F. A.: *Patterns of Sexual Behavior*. Harper and Brothers, 1951.

Freud, S.: Three essays on the theory of sexuality. In *The Complete Psychological Works of Sigmund Freud*, Vol. VII. Hogarth Press, London, 1953.

Gorski, R. A., and Jacobson, C. D.: Sexual differentiation of the brain. In Kogan, S. J.; Hafez, E. S. E.: (eds.): *Pediatric Andrology*, Martinus Nijhoff. The Hague, Boston/London, 1981, p. 109.

Green, R.; Williams, K.; and Goodman, M.: Ninety-nine "tomboys" and non-tomboys. Behavioral contrasts and demographic similarities. *Arch. Sex. Behav.*, 11:247–266, 1982.

Higham, E.: Gender identity/role (G-I/R) in male hermaphroditism. In Kogan, S. J.; Havez, E. S. E.: (eds.): *Pediatric Andrology*, Martinus Nijhoff. The Hague, Boston, London, 1981, p. 135.

Imperato-McGinley, J.; Peterson, R. E.; Gautier, T.; and Sturla, E.: Androgens and the evolution of male-gender identity among male pseudohermaphrodites with 5α-reductase deficiency. *N. Engl. J. Med.*, 300:1233, 1979.

Imperato-McGinley, J.; Peterson, R. E.; Gautier, T.; and Sturla, E.: The impact of androgens on the evolution of male gender identity. In Kogan, S. J.; Hafez, E. S. E.: (eds.): *Pediatric Andrology*, Martinus Nijhoff. The Hague, Boston, London, 1981, p. 99.

Money, J.: In regard to sex rearing and sexual orientation (Comments). *J Sex. Res.*, 12:152–157, 1976.

Money, J., and Ehrhardt, A. A.: *Man and Woman, Boy and Girl*. Johns Hopkins University Press, Baltimore and London, 1972.

Money, J., and Mathews, D.: Prenatal exposure to virilizing progestins: An adult follow up study of twelve women. *Arch. Sex. Behav.*, 11:73–84, 1982.

New, M. I., and Levine, L. S.: Congenital adrenal hyperplasia. In Harris, H., and Hirschhorn, K.: (eds.): *Advances in Human Genetics*, Vol. 4. Plenum Press, London, pp. 251–326.

Rafoch, J., and Horejsi, J.: Sexual life of women with the Küstner–Rokitansky syndrome. *Arch. Sex Behav.*, 11:215–220, 1982.

Resko, J. A., and Ellinwood, W. E.: Sexual differentiation of the brain of primates. In: Serio, M.; Zanisi, M.; Motta, M.; Martini, L.: (eds.): *Sexual Differentiaction: Basic and Clinical Aspects*. Raven Press, New York, 1984.

Rubin, R. T.; Reinish, J. M.; and Haskett, R. F. Postnatal gonadal steroid effects on human behavior. *Science*, 211:1318–1324, 1981.

Witelson, S. F.; Sex and the single hemisphere: specialization of the right hemisphere for spatial processing. *Science*, 193:425–427, 1976.

# CHAPTER 8  ANOMALOUS FEMALE GENITAL DUCT DEVELOPMENT

*Martin Farber, M.D., Joel Noumoff, M.D., and Martin Freedman, M.D.*

## INTRODUCTION

Human embryology is largely a descriptive, biological science. The early pioneering work of investigators, which documented the chronology and sequence of topographical changes in the development of the gonads and female urogenital ducts, still serves as the basis for our understanding of the embryogenesis of the kidneys, ureters, ovaries, fallopian tubes, uterus, cervix, and vagina (Gruenwald, 1941; Hunter, 1930; Koff, 1933; Streeter, 1942; Witschi, 1963). At present those subcellular inductive factors responsible for organogenesis are only beginning to be elucidated.

Prerequisite to an accurate understanding and a subsequent intelligent clinical management of patients with congenital anomalies of the paramesonephric ducts is not only a thorough working knowledge of urogenital duct and ovarian embryology, but an equally important thorough working knowledge of prepubertal and pubertal psychosexual development (Chapter 2). In this way the clinician will be able to correlate those symptoms produced by anomalous genital duct development with the existent anatomic abnormality, and chart a therapeutic course in the best psychosexual and physical interests of the patient.

## EMBRYOLOGY

### OVARIES

In the fourth week of embryonic life the germ cells are first recognized in the epithelium of the dorsal wall of the yolk sac above the allantoic stalk. They migrate dorsally in the wall of the hindgut and then through the mesentery to reach the genital ridge by the end of the fifth week. The genital ridge is an area of thickening on the ventro-medial surface of the mesonephros which becomes demarcated by lateral and medial grooves by the sixth week and then elongates. Cells from the germinal epithelium covering the developing gonad grow down into the mesenchyme and form the medullary or primary sex cords. In the seventh week there is sexual divergence in the further development of the gonads marked by the commencement of regression of the sex cords in the female, and their persistence in the male to give rise to the seminiferous tubules (Gray and Skandalakis, 1972; Streeter, 1942). The germ cells (oogania) continue to rapidly proliferate until the fifteenth week of fetal life when their number is estimated to be five to six million. Transformation of the oogania into primary oocytes when they enter prophase of their first maturation division commences in the tenth week and is completed by the twentieth week. Granulosa cells derived from the germinal epithelium surround the primary oocytes from the twentieth to the thirty-eighth week to form increasing numbers of primary follicles. Flattened mesenclymal cells form the thecal tunic peripheral to the layer of granulosa cells. Follicular atresia commences at 38 weeks in the ovary filled with primary follicles, and progression of the process mainly in the medulla leads to cortical dominance by puberty.

## UTERUS, FALLOPIAN TUBES, CERVIX, VAGINA

The paramesonephric ducts, the progenitors of the fallopian tubes, uterus, cervix, and a portion of the vagina, appear at six weeks as invaginations of the coelomic epithelium at the level of the third thoraccic somite lateral and cephalic to the mesonephros. Solid plugs of cells comprise their leading (caudal) tips which lie within the basement membranes of their ipsilateral mesonephric ducts. A proliferation of cells then appears between the openings of the mesonephric ducts in the dorsal wall of the urogenital sinus in the seventh week. Further caudal growth, simultaneous canalization, and ultimately deviation medially of the paramesonephric ducts results in their union at the sinusal tubercle by the eighth week. Continued fusion of their medial walls and concomitant resorption of the resultant intervening median septum in a craniad direction results in a single utero-vaginal canal by 10½ weeks.

The sinuvaginal bulbs, bilateral evaginations from the dorsal wall of the urogenital sinus, obliterate the sinusal tubercle and fuse with the solid tips of the paramesonephric ducts in the 11th week. Continued proliferation results in a solid mass of cells, the vaginal plate, which completely occludes the vaginal canal and grows caudally to reach the vestibule. Cavitation of the vaginal plate results in a fully canalized vagina by the twentieth week (O'Rahilly, 1973, 1977).

Although it has been claimed that the upper four-fifths of the vagina is formed from the caudally migrating vaginal plate derived from the paramesonephric ducts, and the lower one-fifth from the sinuvaginal bulbs, (presumably derived from the urogenital sinus) which precede the vaginal plate to reach the vestibule, there is controverting data to suggest that the mesonephric ducts also participate in formation of the vaginal plate. There is a general consensus that the hymen marks the point of junction of the sinuvaginal bulbs with the sinusal tubercle after caudal migration of the vaginal plate.

By week 20 the uterine corpus is half the length of the cervix, but well demarcated from it. The muscular layer of the uterus is almost completely differentiated by 23 weeks and at 25 weeks the V-shaped notch that had marked the craniad point of union of the paramesonephric ducts is obliterated by muscular growth.

In the rodent, gonadal ablation and transplantation experiments suggest bipotentiality for the sexual development of the embryonic genital ducts. In the male, the paramesonephric ducts involute due to an inhibitor secreted by the fetal testicle, while an androgenic steriod (presumably testosterone) is necessary for mesonephric ductal persistence and development. The anomalous genital duct development present in genetic males with the testicular feminization syndrome suggest a similar mechanism to be operative in the human Castration in the fetal rodent (whatever the genetic sex) leads to feminine genital duct development and mesonephric duct involution suggesting the female fetal gonad does not play an important role in feminine genital duct development. Most humans (regardless of their chromosomal sex) with gonadal dysgenesis develop female genital ducts (Jost, 1970).

## SYMPTOMATIC CLASSIFICATION OF PARAMESONEPHRIC DUCT ANOMALIES

The complicated and only partially elucidated embryogenesis of the female genital ducts suggests the potential for a myriad of congenital malformations. Although this is theoretically true, clinical experience reveals that a limited number of anomalies present, and they can be symptomatically categorized (Table 8–1). The patient with anomalous genital duct development who presents with failure of menses to be established at the proper time subsequent to thelarche will be found to have absence of the uterus, cervix, and vagina (Rokitansky–Kuster–Hauser syndrome). Complete obstruction to the egress of the menstruum presents with cyclic, intractible pelvic pain due to cryptomenorrhea and is due to imperforate hymen, transverse vaginal septum, partial vaginal agenesis, or congenital atresia of the uterine cervix. Cyclic pelvic pain due to cryptomenorrhea together with concomitant egress of the menstruum per vagina is due to duplication of the genital ducts with unilateral obstruction, such as duplication of the uterus, cervix, and vagina with unilateral vaginal or cervical blockage, and also menstrual retention in a functioning, noncommunicating uterine horn. Pregnancy wastage may occur when there is complete or partial duplication of the uterus of the bicornuate (externally divided) or septate (internally divided and externally united) variety, or unilateral paramesonephric ductal failure (unicornuate uterus). Very uncommonly the fallopian tubes are anomalous, almost always coexist with an anomalous uterus, and present no symptoms (Farber and Mitchell, 1977).

## Amenorrhea

**Congenital Vaginal Agenesis.** Eponymously designated the Rokitansky–Kuster–Hauser syndrome, congenital vaginal agenesis

TABLE 8–1 **Symptomatic Classification of Congenital Anomalies of the Paramesonphric Ducts**

| Symptom(s) | Anomalies |
|---|---|
| Amenorrhea | Congenital vaginal agenesis (Rokitansky–Kuster–Hauser syndrome) |
| Amenorrhea and cryptomenorrhea | Imperforate Hymen |
| | Transverse vaginal septum |
| | Partial vaginal agenesis with functional uterus |
| | Cervical atresia with normal vagina and functional uterus |
| | Cervical atresia with absent vagina and functional uterus |
| Cryptomenorrhea and menstrual egress per vagina | Double uterus and double cervix with unilaterally imperforate vagina |
| | Double uterus and double cervix with unilaterally imperforate cervix |
| | Double uterus and single cervix with rudimentary, noncommunicating uterine horn |
| Reproductive failure | Bicornuate uterus (partial or complete) |
| | Septate uterus (partial or complete) |
| Asymptomatic | Complete duplication of the fallopian tube |
| | Small accessory fallopian tube |
| | Segmental atresia of the fallopian tube |
| | Ectopic location of the fallopian tube |

Source: Farber, M.; Noumoff, J.; Freedman, M.; and Oberkotter, L.: Understanding and correcting genital anomalies. *Contemporary OB/GYN,* 24:113–129, 1984.

is a very unusual malformation of the paramesonephric ducts, and has been estimated to occur in 1 in 4,000 to 1 in 20,000 women (Evans et al., 1981). After gonadal dysgenesis, it is the second most common cause of primary amenorrhea (Willemsen, 1982B) and is generally discovered at a mean age of 17.5 years (Rock et al., 1983). Pubertal events are normal in their chronology and sequence in these phenotypically normal women. Their histologically normal ovaries, which reflect their almost invariably normal karyotype, secrete normal quantities of steriod hormones in response to normal stimuli from the hypothalamic-pituitary axis (Fraser et al., 1973). Internally the fallopian tubes are normally formed and terminate in noncanalized, functionless muscle nubbins located in the lateral pelvis bilaterally, which are joined by a broad fold of visceral peritoneum containing the bladder (Figures 8-1 and 8-2). The uterus is totally absent, and the vagina is represented by a small pouch one to two cm in depth (Hauser et al., 1961).

The etiology of the syndrome is unknown. A recent report of eight women with the syndrome found to have paternal relatives with the identical disorder suggested it is inherited as a female-limited autosomal dominant trait transmitted by males with a mutant gene (Shokeir, 1978). A report describing three karyotypically normal sisters with the syndrome suggests the malformation may be due to variable expression of a recessive trait (Jones and Mermut, 1972). Contraindicating a genetic etiology is the existence of three sets of monozygotic twins discordant for congenital vaginal agenesis. A teratogen present at the sixth to the eighth week of embryonic life and causing the syndrome has not been found.

Associated malformations most commonly involve the urinary system in up to 50 percent of cases, and 15 percent of these women have unilateral renal agenesis (Garcia et al, 1979). The frequent concomitant involvement of the urinary tract is explained by the chronologic and anatomic proximity of the two organ systems in the developing embryo. Experimentally, unilateral paramesonephric ductal failure results following interruption of the ipsilateral mesonephric duct in the chick embryo (Gruenwald, 1941). Interestingly, in all

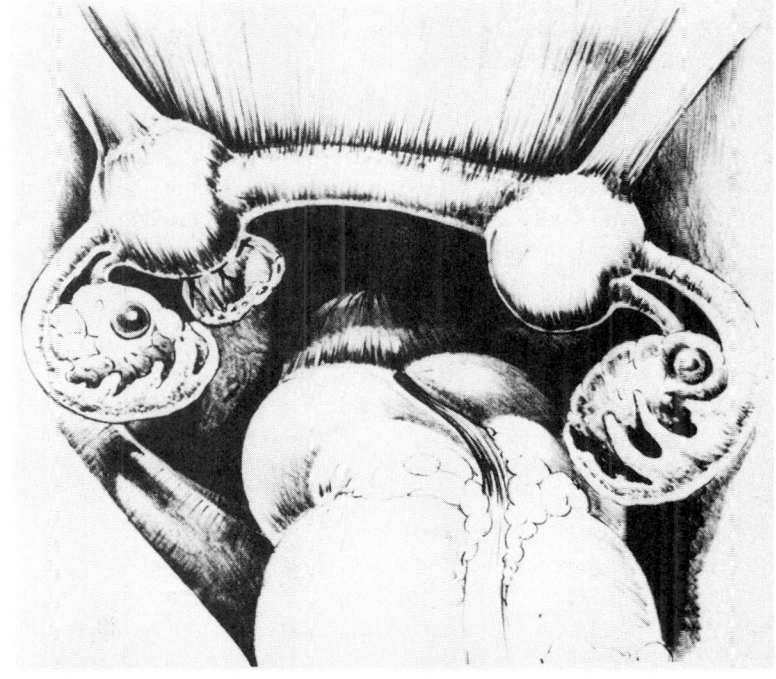

**FIGURE 8-1.** Internal genitalia of a patient with Rokitansky Kuster Hauser Syndrome. Normally formed fallopian tubes (A) terminate in functionless muscle nubbins (B) joined by a fold of peritoneum which contains the bladder. A leiomyoma has been resected from the right muscle nubbin. The uterus is absent and the ovaries (C) are in the normal position bilaterally.

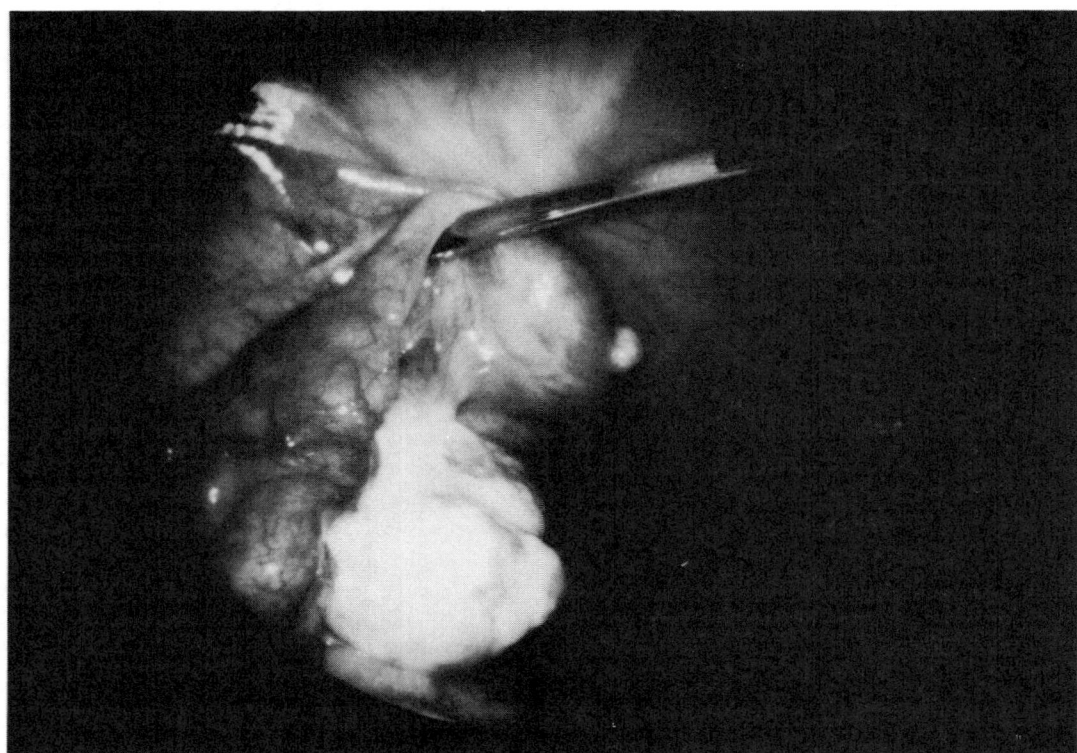

FIGURE 8-2. Laparoscopic photograph of the internal genitalia of a patient with Rokitansky Kuster Hauser Syndrome. The left fallopian tube (A) terminates in a muscle nubbin (B) and the left ovary (C) is normally situated.

three female fetuses described by Potter (1946) with congenital bilateral renal agenesis together with the typical facies, which is the hallmark of Potter's syndrome, there was associated vaginal and uterine agenesis. The skeletal system is involved in up to 25 percent of cases; most commonly a malformation of the vertebral column due to scoliosis. Fourteen cases of Klippel–Feil syndrome (short neck, low hairline, and limited neck movements due to variable degrees of fusion of the cervical vertebrae) have been reported to coexist with the syndrome (Willemsen, 1982A). In rare cases, congenital heart disease, femoral and inguinal herniae, deafness, cleft palate, situs inversus (Vasquez, 1982), and hypothalamic hypogonadism are also found (Check et al., 1983). Despite the relatively independent embryogenesis of the ovaries from the paramesonephric ducts, recently the Rokitansky–Kuster–Hauser syndrome has been found in a patient with Turner's syndrome and another with pure gonadal dysgenesis (Phansey et al., 1981).

Although these women are irreversibly sterile, the creation of a vagina by surgical or nonsurgical means permits them to function coitally. A fully functional neovagina can be created by intercourse for a variable period of time in a couple usually unaware of the diagnosis (D'Alberton and Santi, 1972). Alternatively numerous case reports document fully satisfactory uretheral (Figure 8–3) or anal intercourse in sexual partners prior to revelation of the congenital anomaly (Shukla and Tripathi, 1982). Frank's (1938) nonoperative technique involves the insertion of a series of dilators graduated in size into in the small existent vaginal pouch, and with persistence results in a vaginal tube of adequate length in a significant number of determined women (Wabrek et al., 1971). Segments of small

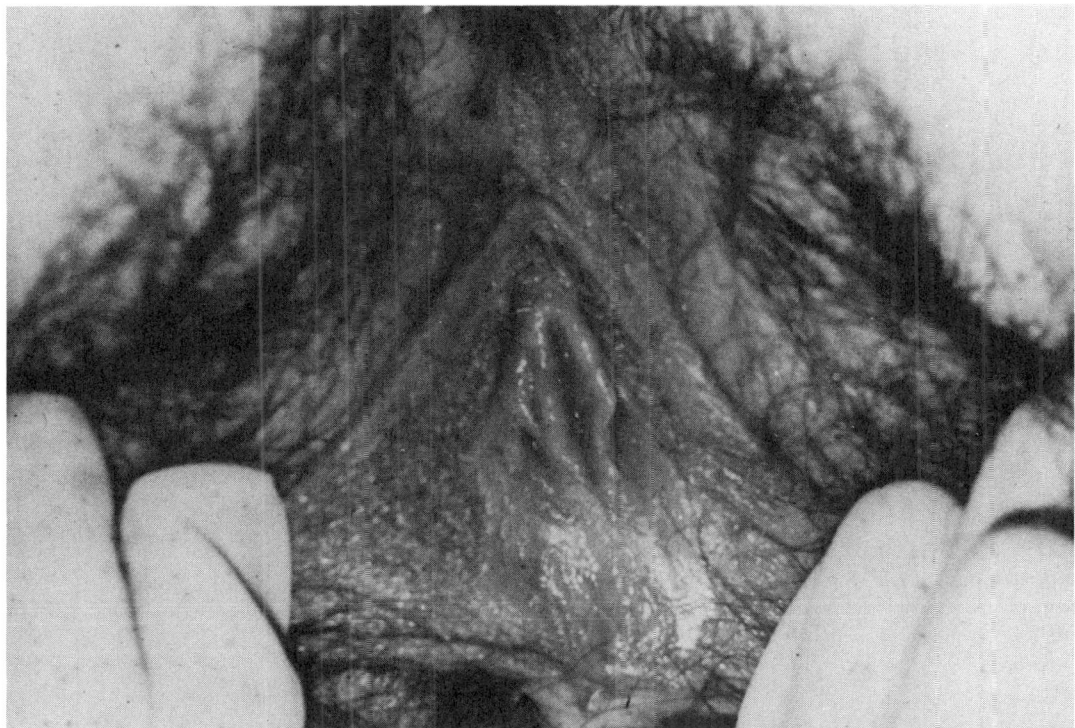

**FIGURE 8–3.** Widely dilated urethra (A) of a patient who engaged in urethral intercourse and was unaware of her vaginal agenesis.

(Baldwin, 1907) and large intestine (Pratt, 1966) have been utilized to create a neovagina, but their significant incidences of postoperative morbidity and occasional mortality obviate the modern applicability of these methods. The dissection of a space between the bladder and rectum to the level of the peritoneal reflection with the placement intraoperatively of a suitable stent to maintain patency of the neovaginal tube may be followed by epithelialization of the newly created tract (Wharton, 1938), presumably from the vestibular mucosa and squamous metaplasia of paramesonephric glandular epithelium present in the rectovesical space (Herman et al., 1982). Alternatively, a tube formed by pedicle grafts taken from the labia majora and labia minora and inverted over iodoform gauze to line the neovaginal space has recently been reported to yield excellent postoperative results (Song et al., 1982). A semilunar incision may be made in the medial aspects of the labia majora, the contralateral medial skin edges sutured in apposition, covered by subcutaneous tissue, and then covered by apposing the skin of the lateral aspects of the semilunar incision. The axis of the newly created pouch, which is perpendicular to the floor, is redirected by the use of dilators (Capraro and Gallego, 1976).

Counsellor's modification (Counsellor and Flor, 1957) of MacIndoe's procedure (1950) is most commonly used for the creation of a vagina in the Rokitansky-Kuster-Hauser syndrome. Subsequent to blunt and sharp dissection of a space between the bladder and rectum to the level of the peritoneal reflection, a mold is fashioned of foam rubber made to conform to the dimensions of the neovaginal space. Split thickness skin grafts taken from the buttocks or medial aspects of the thighs are sutured everted around the mold (Figure 8–4) which is then placed in the neovagina and sutured in place to the labia majora to be removed in one week. The incidence of major

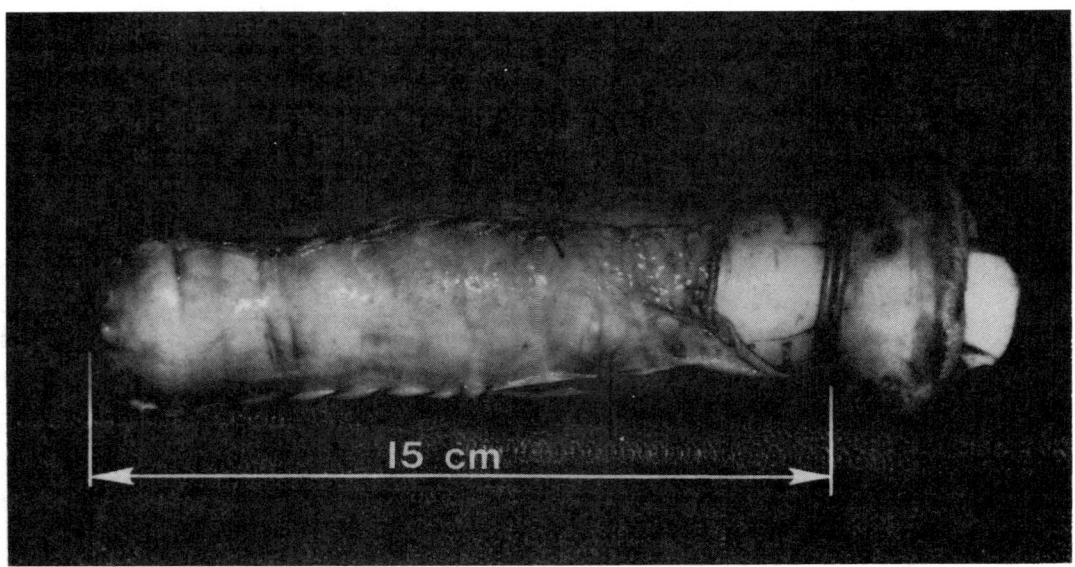

**FIGURE 8–4.** The split thickness skin grafts are sutured everted about a mold fashioned of foam rubber to conform to the space created between the bladder and rectum.

intraoperative and postoperative complications such as hemorrhage and infection, and the formation of urethrovaginal, vesicovaginal, and rectovaginal fistulae have been remarkably reduced by infiltration of the operative site with a dilute neosynephrine solution, the application of topical thrombin to the newly dissected endopelvic fascial space, the utilization of prophylactic antibiotics, and the placement of a urinary catheter suprapubically obviating the necessity for transurethral urinary drainage (Evans, 1981).

With all of these operative and nonoperative techniques for the creation of a vagina, it is mandatory for the patient to insert a mold into the neovagina at least twice a day and keep it in place for at least 15 minutes to maintain patency of the newly created space (Farber and Mitchell, 1978). Realization of the potential for self-imposed fatigue of the fingers and hands, the necessity for assuming the lithotomy or squatting position for an acceptably long period of time, and the inability of the patient to concomitantly perform other activities, a recent investigator fashioned a bicycle seat stool on which the girdled patient is instructed to sit and then lean forward to cause the stent to stretch the neovagina (Ingram, 1981).

Despite the excellent anatomic results (assessed in terms of the dimensions of the neovagina) and the excellent functional results (measured in terms of satisfactory sexual intercourse) ranging from 75 to 100 percent in most large series, it has been observed that these parameters of success are commonly disparate in a given patient (Cali and Pratt, 1968).

Patients with satisfactory postoperative coital function have been intensively studied and the anatomic reactions of the neovagina to sexual excitation are analogous to other women without the malformation. Bartholin's glands are normally situated and function normally. In the excitation phase lubricating droplets appear on the walls of the neovagina in 20–30 seconds of the initiation of stimulation, but in less than average quantity. After the first several penile thrusts, the droplets are quantitatively sufficient for satisfactory coition and are probably derived from the engorged venous plexus surrounding the neovaginal barrel. The neovaginal tube lengthens and distends, although its elasticity is less than the naturally formed organ. In the plateau phase there is marked congestion of the blood vessels surrounding the vaginal barrel and the labia minora which accounts for their assumption of a scarlet red color. Constriction of the levator ani muscles leads to the formation of a platform at the lower third of the vagina which undergoes rhythmic contractions in the orgasmic phase. A reversal of these phenomena occurs in the resolution phase of sexual stimulation (Masters and Johnson, 1961).

The observation that anatomic results may be disparate from functional results in a significant number of posttreatment patients has lead to retrospective psychological studies of patients with Rokitansky–Kuster–Hauser Syndrome (Raboch, 1982). Reactions such as denial, anger, guilt, and extreme depression on the part of the patient as well as her parents have led to the realization that the optimal age to initiate counseling of the patient and her parents is during puberty prior to the anticipated age of menarche and at a time judged optimum by a sensitive and well-informed health care provider (Hecker and McGuire, 1977; Kaplan, 1968). To accomplish this an adequate assessment of vaginal patency should be made in every female neonate. The feminine sexual identity of the patient must be firmly established by emphasizing that her gender is unequivocally, biologically female. Retrospectively it has been noted that although vaginoplasty may strengthen the patient's concept of her own feminine body image, the operation will not completely abolish the persistent psychological doubts over sexual identity (Kaplan, 1974). Feelings of sexual inadequacy (causing these women to seek out inferior consorts with ambivalent sexual identities) may be obviated by introducing techniques to "open" the vagina as opposed to "creating" a neovagina (Harkins et al., 1981). The invariable sterility must be countered by the potential to adopt children (David et al., 1975). Marriage and normal coital function should be stressed, and the observation that postoperatively the consorts of these women were unaware of the pre-existent malformation should be stressed.

The vagina should be "opened" only after the patient has reached full somatic growth, and when she wants the procedure (operative or nonoperative) initiated. Unquestionably the postoperative anatomic success rate will depend on her willingness to repetitively insert a vaginal mold until her coital frequency is adequate to maintain patency of the neovagina. Reports to indicate that these women develop gonadal neoplasms, myometrial neoplasms (Farber, Stein, and Adashi, 1978), pelvic endometriosis (Rosenfeld and Lecher, 1981), hematometra in a noncommunicating functional uterine horn (Rock et al., 1980) and squamous cell carcinoma (Rotmensch et al., 1983) or adenocarcinoma in the neovagina, suggest these women be followed by a qualified gynecologist for the rest of their lives.

## Amenorrhea and Cryptomenorrhea

**Imperforate Hymen.** This malformation is reported to occur in 1 in 1000 women. Most commonly it is discovered prepubertally when a bulge in the hymeneal membrane is caused by hydromucocolpos, and it is simply treated by cruciate incisions to permit egress of the obstructed secretions. Recent reports of the spontaneous formation (within the first year of life) of openings in the hymeneal membrane found to be imperforate upon a neonatal examination suggest that watchful waiting (in the absence of hydromucocolpos) without surgical intervention is acceptable for the infant (Kahn et al., 1975). In the postmenarchial girl, complete imperforate hymen presents with amenorrhea and cyclic pelvic pain due to cryptomenorrhea. The purpuric distended hymeneal membrane obstructs the egress of blood which commonly results in the formation of an abdominal-pelvic mass. After the administration of a broad spectrum antibiotic the hymen should be excised, the obstructed menstruum permitted to drain freely (not forcefully expressed), and the resultant epithelial edges sutured with interrupted sutures of polyglycolic acid. Adenosis of the craniad surface of the excised membrane together with varying degrees of adenosis of the vagina will spontaneously regress due to squamous metaplasia (Amortequi et al., 1979; Hansen et al., 1975). A variation of this theme is the well-described clinical entity microperforate hymen, which presents with cyclic hypomenorrhea and dysmenorrhea, recurrent vulvogainitis, and urinary tract infection. A pinpoint opening in the hymen, typically just suburethrally at 12 o'clock, permits the cyclic expression of a small quantity of menstrual blood, but the relative hymeneal obstruction accounts for the remainder of the symptoms. The lesion is treated identically to complete imperforate hymen (Capraro et al., 1974).

Preoperatively a full explanation of the nature of the lesion must be explained to the pubertal girl and her parents, and it is often helpful to demonstrate the obstructing membrane to the patient with a mirror held by an assistant. Both the patient and her parents should be advised of the excellent postoperative anatomic results together with the fact that retrospective clinical data has shown that fertility is normal postoperatively (Rock et al., 1982). Subsequent yearly gynecological office visits are sufficient to insure that vaginal outlet synechiae (very uncommon) have not formed and to retain a healthy rapport with the patient as she reaches adulthood.

**Transverse Vaginal Septum.** Among the most unusual anomalies of the paramesonephric ducts, the incidence of transverse vaginal septum has been estimated as 1 in 80,000 (Beyth and Kopolovic, 1982). Symptoms such as amenorrhea, dyspareunia, cyclic pelvic pain, urinary tract obstruction, painful defecation, hypomenorrhea, and dysmenorrhea will present depending on the presence (most commonly) of small perforations in the septum centrally or at 3 and 9 o'clock, or their absence leading to complete obstruction to menstrual egress (Suidan and Azoury, 1979; Wenof et al., 1979). On examination an abdominal-pelvic mass is invariably present and the obstructing vaginal septum easily identified. Most commonly it is situated at the junction of the middle and upper third of the vagina, but it has been reported at virtually any location along the vaginal tube (Deppisch, 1972). The mean fertility of a group of patients with the lesion was retrospectively found to be significantly reduced (47 percent of the patients conceived), and the fertility of individual patients varied inversely with the craniad location of the septum. In several instances, the septum was discovered at parturition when it obstructed descent of the presenting fetal part (Rock et al., 1982).

The transverse vaginal septum is excised subsequent to the prophylactic administration of intravenous antibiotics utilizing a cold knife or electrocautery, and the vaginal mucosal edges reapproximated utilizing fine interrupted sutures of polyglycolic acid. When the septum is very thick it might be necessary

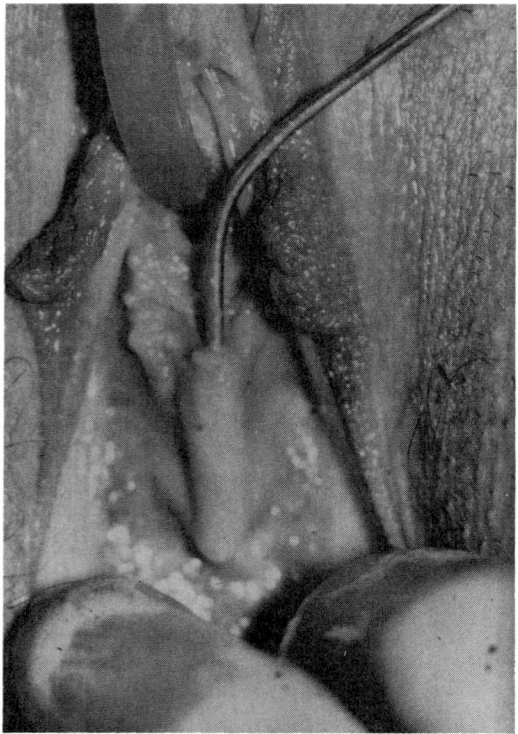

**FIGURE 8–5.** A fine probe is placed in the microperforate hymen suburethrally.

to place a hollow mold for up to six months in the vagina over which epithelialization will ultimately unite the separated mucosal edges.

The inverse relationship that exists between the craniad location of the septum and postoperative fertility rates suggests a negative effect from the reflux of menstrual blood into the pelvis. The triad of cyclic pelvic pain (due to cryptomenorrhea), hypomenorrhea or amenorrhea, and an abdominal pelvic mass with hematocolpos should alert the attending physician to the correct diagnosis and the necessity for an aggressive therapeutic course. Knowledge of genital duct embryology and the limited number of anatomic abnormalities described with this presentation would suggest a primary vaginal approach to remedy the problem and obviate unnecessary abdominal extirpative surgery in these young women and the inevitably devastating postoperative psychosexual effects.

**Partial Vaginal Agenesis.** In very unusual cases (6 to 20 percent) of ostensible vaginal agenesis a functional uterus is present, and egress of the menstruum is obstructed at a level about 3 cm caudal to the external cervical os. Amenorrhea, cyclic pelvic pain due to cryptomenorrhea, and partial urinary tract obstruction, together with an ostensibly absent vagina and a palpation of high hematocolpos communicating with an abdominal-pelvic mass should suggest the diagnosis. Dissection in the endopelvic fascia between the bladder and rectum to the apical canalized vaginal segment, and mobilization of the apical vagina for its anastomosis to the edges of the shallow inferior vaginal dimple yields the best postoperative results (Jeffcoate, 1969). When this is not technically feasible, skin grafts over a stent may be placed in the newly dissected space, but this commonly results in an hour glass deformity of the neovagina. All of these patients should have their internal genitalia assessed laparoscopically as there is a reported high incidence of concomitant anomalous development of the internal genitalia. An unusual variant of this theme (13 reported cases) is partial vaginal agenesis with a urinary (urethral or vesical) vaginal fistula. The vaginal abnormality is the same, and the fistula results in cyclic hematuria. The surgical approach is similar, but includes resection of the fistulous communication between the urinary tract and the apical vaginal segment (Figure 8–6).

The preoperative psychosexual counseling of these patients and their parents should em-

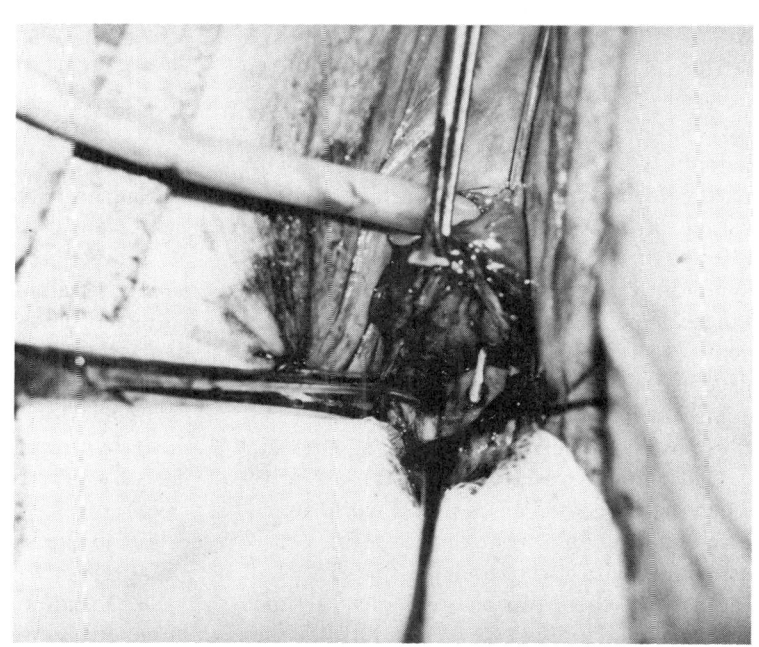

FIGURE 8–6. Partial vaginal agenesis with a urethrovaginal fistula. The apical vaginal pouch (A) has been entered. The transurethral probe (B) has negotiated the urethrovaginal fistula and terminates in the apical vaginal pouch.

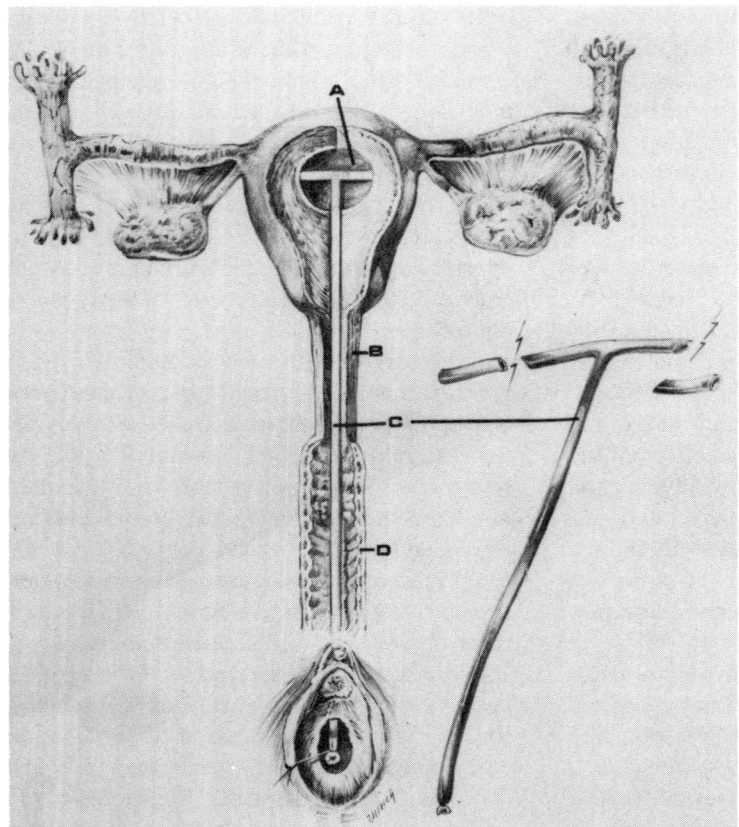

FIGURE 8-7. The uterine corpus and atretic cervix are incised and a rubber T-tube is extended the entire length of the incision, to be sutured to the labia minora. A, Endometrial cavity, B, atretic cervix; C, rubber T-tube; D, vagina.

phasize the anticipated favorable postoperative results in terms of coital function and fertility. Laparotomy is not necessary as the internal genitalia may be adequately assessed by laparoscopy. Interestingly, three of the four patients who presented postpubertally with partial vaginal agenesis and a urinary vaginal fistula did so at a later than anticipated age (18 to 21 years) suggesting their denial of the symptom (cyclic hematuria) or naive acceptance of the symptom as the norm. In a recently reported case pre- and postoperative psychosexual counseling greatly aided the achievement of fully satisfactory coital function postoperatively. (Genest et al., 1981).

**Congenital Atresia of the Uterine Cervix.** There have been 35 cases in the world literature of congenital atresia of the uterine cervix associated with a functional uterus. In 14 of the patients there was also complete absence of the vagina and in 7 of them multiple other genital duct anomalies, such as complete or partial uterine duplication and complete or partial fallopian tubal atresia were found. All of the patients, whose ages ranged from 11 to 31 years, presented with primary amenorrhea and cyclic, recurrent pelvic pain due to entrapment of the menstruum. Ten of the patients were initially treated by the performance of a hysterectomy when their genital duct anomaly was judged uncorrectible either pre- or intraoperatively. In the remaining 25 patients, there was an initial attempt to establish a communication between the endometrial cavity and the vagina, either by direct attachment (bypassing the atretic cervix) or by utilizing the atretic cervix as a conduit for a surgically created fistula from the endometrial cavity to the vaginal apex (Farber and Marchant, 1975, 1976; Figure 8-7).

Of the latter group of patients, there were numerous subsequent surgical procedures to maintain patency of the endometrial-vaginal communication, and nine of them ultimately came to hysterectomy. Although two of the group died postoperatively from sepsis, another two of these patients conceived and were delivered of viable fetuses at term by cesarean section five and eight years respectively after their primary surgery (Singh and Lakshmi, 1983; Zarou et al., 1973).

At present, controversy rages over the appropriate therapy for this very unusual anomaly, that is, primary hysterectomy versus an attempt at endometrial-vaginal communication. The fact that there is a very small experience with this anomaly reported in the world literature, that the presence of other associated genital duct anomalies makes this a heterogeneous group, that numerous surgical techniques have been utilized in subgroups of these patients to establish an endometrial-vaginal communication, and that the postoperative results have varied from death of the patient to the delivery of a fetus at term, suggests that no broad generalization can be made concerning the appropriate mode of therapy in a given patient. In that the incidence of depression manifested by a deterioration in self-image and then sexual function together with a persistent wish for children is significant following hysterectomy (Kaltreider et al., 1979) and inversely related to the age at which the operation is performed (Ananth, 1978) suggests a full psychological, and psychosexual assessment be accomplished preoperatively. High-risk factors for posthysterectomy depression would include a poor gender identity, previous adverse reactions to stress, a family history of mental illness, and an expressed desire for children, and the like (Roeske, 1979). The ultimate therapeutic decision must be made by a well-informed patient and her gynecologic surgeon after all factors that bear on the quality of life are considered.

## Cryptomenorrhea and Menstrual Egress per Vagina

Severe cyclic dysmenorrhea, which increases in severity from the onset of menarche, strongly suggests the possibility of persistent duplication of the paramensonephric ducts with unilateral obstruction to menstrual egress and cryptomenorrhea. While dysmenorrhea is a common complaint of adolescent women, the symptom usually appears several months to several years after the menarche when ovulatory cycles are regularly established. Despite the chronology, all of these young women should have a thorough history and a physical examination performed including a pelvic examination to rule out an anatomic cause of pelvic pain. The inability of the patient to relax her levator ani muscles to permit a complete pelvic assessment should not lead to admonishments from medical personnel or her parents, or persistence on the part of the examining physician, but to the liberal use of general anesthesia for a thorough pelvic examination including diagnostic laparoscopy if indicated. In this way a developmental abnormality will be accurately diagnosed at the incipiency of cryptomenorrhea to obviate the devastating effects of menstrual entrapment on the pelvic viscera.

**Complete Duplication of the Uterus and Cervix with a Unilaterally Imperforate Vagina.** To date 56 cases of complete duplication of the uterus and cervix with a unilaterally imperforate vagina have been reported (Figure 8–8). All of the patients presented with severe and progressive dysmenorrhea since menarche (except for the 14 patients in whom a small communication existed in the endocervical septum), and a unilateral abdominal-pelvic mass which terminated in a large purpuric bulge in the lateral vaginal wall. In the 38 patients for whom an intravenous pyelogram was performed there was renal agenesis ipsilateral to the imperforate vagina (Eisenberg et al., 1982). Recently pelvic sonography has been utilized to define the nature of the large abdominal-pelvic mass and its separation from the urinary bladder (Rosenberg et al., 1982; Stangl et al., 1983). Other accompanying symptoms included dysparuenia, rectal pressure, back pain, urinary retention, and vaginal discharge (Venter and Theron, 1981).

Prompt recognition of the lesion should be followed by an explanation of the abnormality

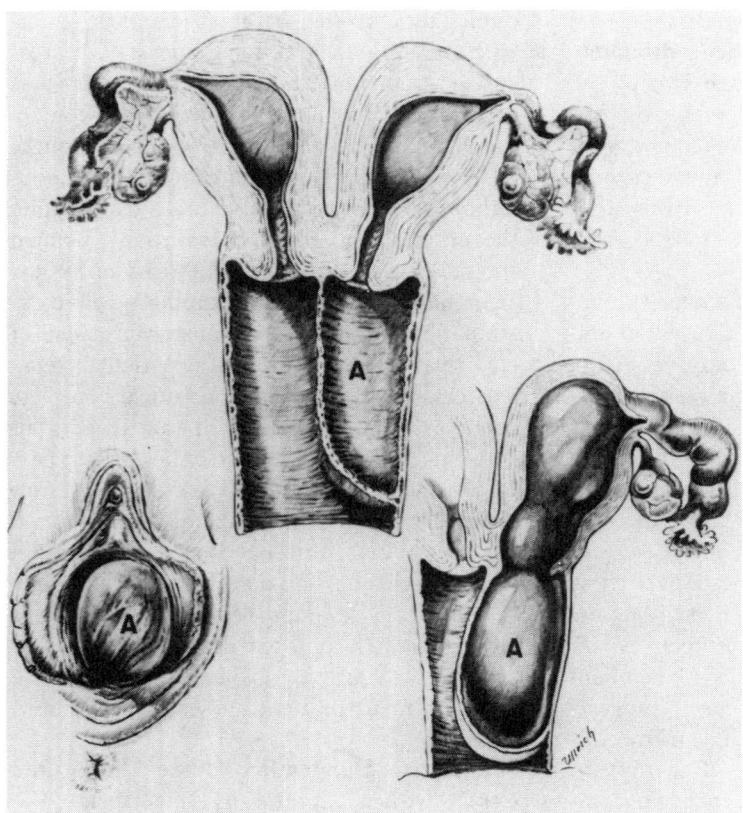

FIGURE 8–8. Double uterus and double cervix with unilaterally imperforate vagina (A). Insert at right demonstrates hematocolpos, hematotrachelos, hematometra, and hematosalpinx. Insert at left demonstrates hematocolpos that almost totally obscures the contralateral vagina at the time of pelvic examination.

to the patient and her parents including the overwhelmingly favorable prognosis for satisfactory coital function and future fertility. The septum should be widely incised after the intravenous administration of a broad septum antibiotic to release the trapped menstrual blood. Several months later, when the widely dilated cervix has resumed a normal appearance, the septum should be excised. Unfortunately, failure to accurately and promptly diagnose the lesion has led to a large number of inappropriate surgical procedures on these patients and severely compromised the fertility of the group.

**Complete Duplication of the Uterus and Cervix with a Unilaterally Imperforate External Cervical Os.** Several cases of unilateral obstruction to menstrual egress due to failure of canalization of the external cervical os in a completely duplicated uterus have been reported. The diagnosis was made at laparotomy and resulted in hysterectomy in one young woman who developed a pelvic abscess subsequent to curettage of the uterine horn from which a pregnancy had been aborted, and inadvertent perforation of the endocervical septum resulting in innoculation of the obstructed contralateral uterine horn (Farber and Mitchell, 1977).

**Complete Duplication of the Uterus with a Noncommunicating Uterine Horn.** Complete duplication of the uterus of the bicornuate variety with a noncommunicating, functioning uterine horn will be accurately and promptly diagnosed when hysterosalpingography (if necessary under general anesthesia) reveals a unicornuate uterus contralateral to a rubbery pelvic mass in a young woman with intractable and increasing dysmenorrhea (McRae and Kim, 1979). The noncommunicating uterine horn and its associated fallopian tube should be resected (Farber, 1973). Failure to define the lesion has led to its diagnosis most frequently at the time of catastrophic rupture of the pregnant noncommunicating horn (Wahlen, 1972). Recently a woman with the lesion was delivered of a viable fetus by cesarean section of the noncommunicating horn (Jarrell et al., 1977). A dead fetus was found at term in the peritoneal cavity of another woman whose noncommunicating uterine horn was presumed to have ruptured six weeks preoperatively (Cohn and Goldenberg, 1976).

## Reproductive Failure

**Complete or Partial Duplication of the Uterus.** Complete or partial duplication of the uterus of the bicornuate or septate variety may be completely asymptomatic or may be causally related to recurrent midtrimester abortion, preterm delivery of a low birth weight infant, or fetal malpresentation in successive pregnancies. The psychosexual effects of these high-risk pregnancies are discussed in Chapter 17. There are conflicting data suggesting either type of uterine configuration (septate or bicornuate) confers a greater likelihood on the gravida of pregnancy loss, but there is a consensus that subsequent to the exclusion of other causes of fetal wastage a unification metroplasty results in increased fetal salvage (Heinonen et al., 1982; Jones and Wheeless, 1969). The bicornuate uterus may be united by the Strassman technique which involves the transverse incision of the entire length of the uterine fundus, the identification of both endometrial cavities, and the unification of both endometrial cavities by vertically joining their incised opposite walls (Strassman, 1966). The septum of a septate uterus may be excised (Jones and Jones, 1953) or hysteroscopically incised (Daly et al., 1983). Transperitoneal vertical incision of the septum for its entire length followed by the bisection of each half of the septum to permit its incorporation in a uterine unification procedure has also been described (Tompkins, 1962). In all these metroplasty procedures, myometrial hemostasis should be accomplished by utilization of figure of eight sutures, but the most superficial myometrium should be reapproximated by the subserosal placement of fine polyglycolic acid sutures to minimize postoperative adhesions and a decrease in fertility.

**Unicornuate Uterus.** Small case series of patients with a unicornuate uterus suggest an increased chance of a poor obstetrical outcome, that is, abortion, malpresentation, intrauterine growth retardation, and preterm delivery of a low birth weight infant (Andrews and Jones, 1982).

## Asymptomatic

**Anomalous Fallopian Tubal Development.** Very rarely an anomalous development of the fallopian tube occurs. It is usually asymptomatic and found in conjunction with a major maldevelopment of the uterus. Unilateral duplication of the tube (Daw, 1973) and unilateral tubal ectopia (Dabby and Nardone, 1977) have each been reported once. Unilateral atresia of the isthmic segment and part of the ampullary portion of the fallopian tube has been reported in seven cases (Farber and Mitchell, 1979) (Figure 8–9). Unilateral midsegmental fallopian tubal atresia resulting in ectopic pregnancy in the isolated ampullary tubal segment has recently been described (Szlachter and Weiss, 1979). Small accessory tubes recently demonstrated in up to 5 percent of women have been suggested to result in infertility and should be carefully resected when discovered at laparotomy (Beyth and Mor-Yosef, 1982). Great caution should be exercised when performing adnexal surgery (especially extirpative surgery) in women with anomalous genital duct formation, and the contralateral adnexa should always be meticulously inspected.

## Conclusion

An accurate and timely diagnosis of anomalous female genital duct development will be

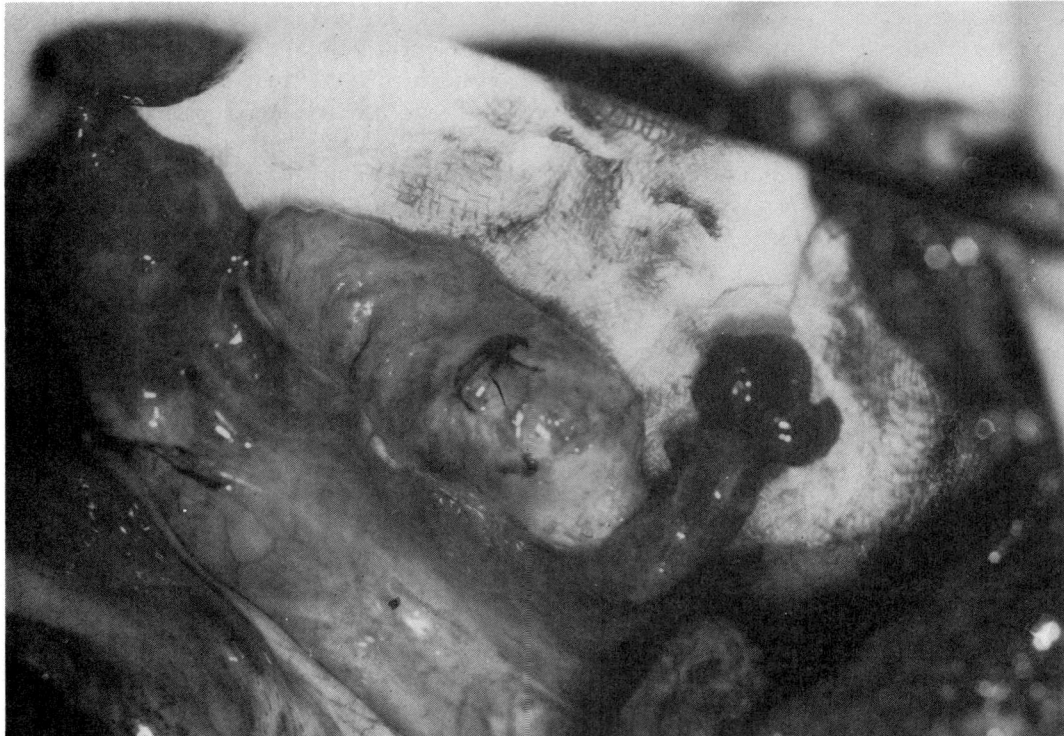

FIGURE 8-9. Partial fallopian tubal atresia. The ovary (A) is interposed between the 1½ cm segment of left fallopian tube (B) which merges imperceptibly with the broad ligament (C) lateral to the rudimentary left uterine horn (D).

made by a clinician with an appropriate index of suspicion resultant from a thorough working knowledge of the embryology of the paramesonephric ducts. Therapeutic interventions will succeed only when the psychosexual effects of the anomaly are fully considered by the health care team.

## REFERENCES

Amortequi, A. J.; Kanbour, A. I.; and Silverstein, A.: Diffuse vaginal adenosis associated with imperforate hymen. *Obstet. Gynecol.,* 53:760–762, 1979.

Ananth, J.: Hysterectomy and depression. *Obstet. Gynecol.* 52:724–730, 1978.

Andrews, M. C., and Jones, H. W.: Impaired reproductive performance of unicornuate uterus. Intrauterine growth retardation, infertility, and recurrent abortion in five cases. *Am. J. Obstet. Gynecol.,* 144:173–176, 1982.

Baldwin, J. F.: Formation of an artificial vagina by the intestinal transplantation. *Am. J. Obstet.* (NY), 36:636–640, 1907.

Beyth, Y., and Kopolovic, J.: Accessory tubes: A possible contributing factor in infertility. *Fertil. Steril.,* 38:382–383, 1982.

Beyth, Y., and Mor-Yosef, S.: Combined medical and surgical treatment for transverse vaginal septum associated with anovulation. *Fertil. Steril.,* 37:704–706, 1982.

Cali, R. W., and Pratt, J. H.: Congenital absence of the vagina: Long-term results of vaginal reconstruction in 175 cases. *Am. J. Obstet. Gynecol.,* 100:752–763, 1968.

Capraro, V. J., and Gallego, M. B.: Vaginal agenesis. *Am. J. Obstet. Gynecol.,* 124:98–107, 1976.

Capraro, V. J.; Dillon, W. P.; and Gallego, M. B.: Microperforate hymen: A distinct clinical entity. *Obstet. Gynecol.,* 44:903–905, 1974.

Check, J. H.; Weisberg, M.; and Laeger, J.: Sexual infantilism accompanied by congenital absence of the uterus and vagina: Case report. *Am. J. Obstet. Gynecol.,* 145:633–634, 1983.

Cohn, F. L., and Goldenberg, R. L.: Term pregnancy in an unattached rudimentary uterine horn. *Obstet. Gynecol.,* 48:234–236, 1976.

Counsellor, V. S., and Flor, F. S.: Congenital absence of the vagina: further results of treatment and a new technique. *Surg. Clin. N. Am.,* 37:1107–1118, 1957.

D'Alberton, A., and Santi, F.: Formation of a neovagina by coitus. *Obstet. Gynecol.,* 40:763, 1972.

Dabby, V., and Nardone, R.: Ruptured ectopic pregnancy

in an ectopic tube: First case report. *J. Fla. Med. Assoc.,* 64:809–810, 1977.

Daly, D. C.; Walters, C. A.; and Soto-Albors, C. E.: Hysteroscopic metroplasty: Surgical technique and obstetric outcome. *Fertil. Steril.,* 39:623–628, 1983.

David, A.; Carmil, D.; Bar-David, E.; et al: Congenital absence of the vagina: Clinical and psychological aspects. *Obstet. Gynecol.,* 46:407–409, 1975.

Daw, E.: Duplication of the Uterine tube. *Obstet. Gynecol.,* 42:137–138, 1973.

Deppisch, L. M.: Transverse vaginal septum: Histologic and embryologic considerations. *Obstet. Gynecol.,* 39:193–198, 1972.

Eisenberg, E.; Farber, M.; Mitchell, G W.; et al: Complete duplication of the uterus and cervix with a unilaterally imperforate vagina. *Obstet. Gynecol.,* 60:259–262, 1982.

Evans, T. N.; Poland, M. L.; and Boving, R. L.: Vaginal malformations. *Am. J. Obstet. Gynecol.,* 141:910–920, 1981.

Farber, M.: Uterus bicornis unicollis with a noncommunicating rudimentary uterine horn: An unusual cause of dysmenorrhea. *Int. J. Gynaecol. Obstet.,* 11:190–194, 1973.

Farber, M., and Marchant, D. J.: Congenital absence of the uterine cervix. *Am. J. Obstet. Gynecol.,* 121:414–417, 1975.

Farber, M., and Marchant, D. J.: Reconstructive surgery for congenital atresia of the uterine cervix. *Fertil. Steril.,* 11:1277–1282, 1976.

Farber, M., and Mitchell, G. W.: Surgery for congenital anomalies of Mullerian ducts. *Contemp. OB/GYN,* 9:63–69, 1977.

Farber, M., and Mitchell, G. W.: Surgery for congenital absence of the vagina. *Obstet. Gynecol.,* 51:364–367, 1978.

Farber, M., and Mitchell, G. W.: Bicornuate uterus and partial atresia of the fallopian tube. *Am. J. Obstet. Gynecol.,* 134:881–884, 1979.

Farber, M.; Stein, A.; and Adashi, E.: Rokitansky-Kuster-Hauser Syndrome and leiomyoma uteri. *Obstet. Gynecol.,* 51:70S–73S, 1978.

Frank, R. T.: The formation of an artificial vagina without operation. *Am. J. Obstet. Gynecol.,* 35:1053–1055, 1938.

Fraser, I. S.; Baird, D. T.; Hobson, B. M.; et al: Cyclical ovarian function in women with congenital absence of the uterus and vagina. *J. Clin. Endocrinol. Metab.,* 36:634–637, 1973.

Garcia, J., and Jones, H. W., Jr.: The split thickness graft technique for vaginal agenesis. *Obstet. Gynecol.,* 49:328–332, 1977.

Genest, D.; Farber, M.; and Mitchell, G W., Jr.; et al: Partial vaginal agenesis with a urinary–vaginal fistula. *Obstet. Gynecol.,* 58:130–134, 1981.

Gray, S. W., and Skandalakis, J. E.: The ovary and testis, *Embryology for Surgeons.* In Gray, S. W., and Skandalakis, J. E. (eds.): *The Embryological Basis for the Treatment of Congenital Defects,* 1st ed., Saunders, Philadelphia, 1972, pp. 563–593.

Gruenwald, P.: The relation of the growing Mullerian duct to the Wolffian duct and its importance for the genesis of malformations. *Anat. Rec.,* 81:1–19, 1941.

Hansen, K., and Egholm, M.: Diffuse vaginal adenosis.

Three cases combined with imperforate hymen and haematocolpos. *Acta Obstet. Gynec. Scand.,* 54:287–292, 1975.

Harkins, J. L.; Gysler, M.; and Cowell, C. A.: Anatomical amenorrhea: The problems of congenital vaginal agenesis and its surgical correction. *Pediatr. Clin. N. Am.,* 28:345–354, 1981.

Hauser, Von G. A., and Schreiner, W. E.: Das Mayer-Rokitansky-Kuster-Syndrome: Uterus Bipartis Solidus Rudimentarius Cum Vagina Solida. *Schweiz. Med. Wochenschr.* 91:381–384, 1961.

Hecker, E. R., and McGuire, L. S.: Psychosocial function in women treated for vaginal agenesis. *Am. J. Obstet. Gynecol.,* 129:543–547, 1977.

Heinonen. P. K.; Saarikoski, S.; and Pystynen, P.: Reproductive performance of women with uterine anomalies: An evaluation of 182 cases. *Acta Obstet. Gynecol. Scand.,* 61:157–162, 1982.

Herman, C. J.; Erp, V. A.; Willemsen, W. N. P., et al: Artificial vaginas: Possible sources of epithelialization. *Hum. Pathol.,* 13:1100–1105, 1982.

Hunter, R. H.: Observations on the development of the human female genital tract. *Contrib. Embryol. Carnegie Inst.,* 22:91–108, 1930.

Ingram, J M.: The Bicycle Seat Stool in the treatment of vaginal agenesis and stenosis: A preliminary report. *Am. J. Obstet. Gynecol.,* 140:867–873, 1981.

Jarrell, J.; Effer, S. B.; and Mohide, P. T.: Pregnancy in a rudimentary horn with fetal salvage *Am. J. Obstet. Gynecol.,* 127:676–677, 1977.

Jeffcoate, T. N. A.: Advancement of the upper vagina in the treatment of haematocolpos and haematometia caused by vaginal aplasia. Pregnancy following the construction of an artificial vagina. *Br. J Obstet. Gynaecol.,* 76:961–968, 1969.

Jones, H. W., Jr., and Jones, G. E. S.: Double uterus as an etiological factor of repeated abortion, indication for surgical repair. *Am. J. Obstet. Gynecol.,* 65:325–339, 1953.

Jones, H. W. Jr., and Mermut, S.: Familial occurrent of congenital absence of the vagina. *Am. J Obstet. Gynecol.,* 114:1100–1101, 1972.

Jones, H. W., and Wheeless, C. R.: Salvage of the reproductive potential of women with anomalous development of the Müllerian ducts: 1868–1968–2068. *Am. J. Obstet. Gynecol.,* 104:348–364, 1969.

Jost, A.: Hormonal factors in the sex differentiation of the mammalian foetus. *Philos. Trans. R. Soc. Lond.,* B259: 19–130, 1970.

Kahn, R.; Duncan, B.; and Bowes, W.: Spontaneous opening of imperforate hymen. *J. Pediatr,* 87:768–770, 1975.

Kaltreider, N. B.; Wallace, A.; and Horowitz, M.: A field study of the stress response syndrome: Young women after hysterectomy. *JAMA,* 242:1499–1503, 1979.

Kaplan E. H.: Congenital absence of vagina: Psychiatric aspects of diagnosis and management. *NY State J. Med.,* 68:1937–1941, 1968.

Kaplan, E. H.: Congenital absence of the vagina. *Psychoanal. Q.,* 39:52–70, 1974.

Koff, A. K.: Development of the vagina in the human fetus. *Contrib. Embryol. Carnegie Inst.,* 24:59–90, 1933.

Lischke J. H.; Curtis, C.; and Lamb, E. Discordance

of the vaginal agenesis in monozygotic twins. *Obstet. Gynecol.,* 41:920–924, 1973.
Masters, W. H., and Johnson, V. E.: The artificial vagina: Anatomic, physiologic, psychosexual function. *West. J. Surg. Obstet. Gynecol.,* 69:192–213, 1961.
McIndoe, A.: The treatment of congenital absence and obliterative conditions of the vagina. *Br. J. Plast. Surg.,* 2:254–267, 1950.
McRae, M. A., and Kim, M. H.: Dysmenorrhea in uterus unicornis with rudimentary uterine cavity. *Obstet. Gynecol.,* 53:134–137, 1979.
O'Rahilly, R.: The embryology and anatomy of the uterus. In Norris, H. J.; Hertig, At.; Abell, M. R.: (eds.): *The Uterus by 23 Authors,* 1st ed. Williams and Wilkins, Baltimore, 1973, pp. 17–39.
O'Rahilly, R.: The development of the vagina in the human. *Birth Defects,* 13:123–136, 1977.
Phansey, S. A.; Tsai, C. C.; and Williamson, H. O.: Vaginal agenesis in association with gonadal dysgenesis. *Obstet. Gynecol.,* 57:565–575, 1981.
Potter, E. L.: Bilateral renal agenesis. *J. Pediatr.,* 29:68–76, 1946.
Pratt, J. H., and Smith, G. R.: Vaginal reconstruction with a sigmoid loop. *Am. J. Obstet. Gynecol.,* 96:31–40, 1966.
Raboch, J., and Horejsi, J.: Sexual life of women with the Kustner–Rokitansky syndrome. *Arch. Sex. Behav.,* 2:215–220, 1982.
Rock, J. A.; Baramki, T. A.; Parmley, T. H. et al: A unilateral functioning uterine anlage with Müllerian duct agenesis. *Int. J. Gynaecol. Obstet.,* 18:99–101, 1980.
Rock, J. A.; Zacur, H. A.; Dlugi, A. M. et al: Pregnancy success following surgical correction of imperforate and complete transverse vaginal septum. *Obstet. Gynecol.,* 59:448–451, 1982.
Rock, J. A.; Reeves, L. A.; Retto, H. et al: Success following vaginal creation for Müllerian agenesis. *Fertil. Steril.,* 39:809–813, 1983.
Roeske, N. C. A.: Hysterectomy and the quality of a woman's life. *Arch. Intern. Med.,* 139:146–147, 1979.
Rosenberg, H. K.; Udassin, R.; Howell, C. et al: Duplication of the uterus and vagina unilateral hydrometrocolpos, and ipsilateral renal agenesis: Sonographic aid to diagnosis. *J. Ultrasound Med.,* 1:289–291, 1982.
Rosenfeld, D. L., and Lecher, B. D.: Endometriosis in a patient with Rokitansky–Kuster–Hauser syndrome. *Am. J. Obstet. Gynecol.,* 139:105–107, 1981.
Rotmensch, J.; Rosenshein, N.; Dillon, M. et al: Carcinoma arising in the neovagina: Case report and review of the literature *Obstet. Gynecol.,* 61:534–536, 1983.
Shokeir, M. H. K.: Aplasia of the Müllerian ducts: Evidence for probable sex-limited autosomal dominant inheritance. *Birth Defects,* 14:147–165, 1978.
Shukla, V. K., and Tripathi, V. N. P.: Urethral coitus. *Urology,* 19:542–543, 1982.
Singh, J., and Lakshmi, Y.: Pregnancy following surgical correction of nonfused Müllerian bulbs and absent vagina. *Obstet. Gynecol.,* 61:267–269, 1983.
Song, R.; Wang, X.; and Zhou, G.: Reconstruction of the vagina with sensory function. *Clin. Plast. Surg.,* 9:105–108, 1982.
Stangl, W.; Frank, R. C.; and Frank, W. et al: Sonographic findings in a case of uterine and vaginal duplication (didelphys) with unilateral hematocolpometra salpinx. *JCU,* 11:40–41, 1983.
Strassman, E. O.: Fertility and unification of double uterus. *Fertil. Steril.,* 17:165–176, 1966.
Streeter, G. L.: Developmental horizons in human embryos. Description of the age group XI, 13 to 20 Somites, and age group XII, 21 to 29 Somites. *Contrib. Embryol Carnegie Inst.,* 30:211–245, 1942.
Suidan, F. G., and Azoury, R. S.: The transverse vaginal septum a clinicopathologic evaluation. *Obstet. Gynecol.,* 54:278–283, 1979.
Szlachter, N., and Weiss, G.: Distal tubal pregnancy in a patient with a bicornuate uterus and segmental absence of the fallopian tube. *Fertil. Steril.,* 32:602–603, 1979.
Tompkins, P.: Comments on the bicornuate uterus and twinning. *Surg. Clin. North Am.,* 42:1049–1061, 1962.
Vasquez, S. B.: Müllerian duct agenesis and other congenital anomalies. *J. Adolesc. Health Care,* 2:289–290, 1982.
Venter, P. F., and Theron, M. S.: Double uterus with a unilateral blind vagina. *S. Afr. Med. J.,* 59:838–840, 1981.
Wabrek, A. J.; Millard, P. R.; Wilson, W. B. et al: Creation of a neovagina by the Frank nonoperative method. *Obstet. Gynecol.,* 37:408–413, 1971.
Wahlen, T.: Pregnancy in non-communicating rudimentary uterine horn. *Acta Obstet. Gynecol. Scand.,* 51:155–160, 1972.
Wenof, N.; Reyniak, J. V.; Novend-Stern, J. et al: Transverse vaginal septum. *Obstet. Gynecol.,* 54:60–64, 1979.
Wharton, L. R.: A simple method of constructing a vagina. Report of four cases. *Ann. Surg.,* 107:842–854, 1938.
Willemsen, W. N. P.: Combination of the Mayer–Rokitansky–Kuster and Klippel–Feil Syndrome—A case report and literature review. *Eur. J. Obstet. Gynec.,* 13:229–235, 1982a.
Willemsen, W. N. P.: Renal–Skeletal–Ear-and Facial anomalies in combination with the Mayer–Rokitansky–Kuster (MRK) Syndrome. *Eur. J. Obstet. Gynec. Reprod. Biol.,* 14:121–130, 1982b.
Witschi, E.: Embryology of the ovary. In Grady, H. G., Smith, D. E.: (eds.): *The Ovary.* 1st ed. Williams and Wilkins Company, Baltimore, 1963, pp. 1–10.
Zarou, G. S.; Esposito, J. M.; and Zarou, D. M.: Pregnancy following the surgical correction of congenital atresia of the cervix. *Int. J. Gynaecol. Obstet.,* 11:143–146, 1973.

# CHAPTER 9  ENDOCRINE CORRELATES AND ONTOGENY OF FEMININE SEXUAL BEHAVIOR: BASIC AND CLINICAL CONSIDERATIONS

*Eli Y. Adashi, M.D., and Bruce Parsons, Ph.D.*

## INTRODUCTION

Although the role of feminine sexual behavior in the preservation of the species is undisputed, its relative contribution to human reproduction remains uncertain. Although multiple mammalian species heavily rely on hormonally triggered feminine sexual behavior, the human species and subhuman primates appear to have modified this pattern. The existence of such interspecies differences becomes immediately apparent when one considers that in the human, feminine sexual behavior is not merely channeled toward procreation, but that recreational considerations may also be at play. It is the intent of this chapter to discuss basic and clinical considerations as they pertain to the feminine sexual behavior of the mammalian female, including the human.

## BASIC CONSIDERATIONS

During the rat estrous cycle, estradiol ($E_2$) and progesterone (P) synergize to activate and terminate feminine reproductive behavior and to induce ovulation. A 36–48 h rise in plasma $E_2$ levels is followed by a surge in both plasma P and luteinizing hormone (LH) (Smith et al., 1975), which occurs several hours prior to the appearance of reproductive behavior on the evening of proestrus. During the initial phase of P action, P activates proceptive behaviors, such as soliciting and ear wiggling, and facilitates sexual receptivity, as measured by the frequency and quality of the lordosis posture (Ball, 1937; Beach, 1942; Hardy, 1972; Hardy and DeBold, 1977; Kuehn and Beach, 1963). Ovulation occurs during the early morning hours of estrus, and reproductive behavior disappears several hours later.

The sequential application of estrogen and progesterone to ovariectomized rodents restores feminine reproductive behavior. The manipulation of exogenous $E_2$ and P has permitted a more precise characterization of the $E_2$–P synergism which underlies the activation of proceptivity and receptivity in the rat. In this chapter, we will describe some of the key neuroendocrine and neurochemical events that underlie the activation by estradiol and progesterone of feminine reproductive behavior in the rat. In addition, we will review that literature which suggests that other hormones or neuropeptides may contribute to the expression of feminine reproductive behavior in this species. These include the leutinizing hormone-releasing hormone (LHRH), prolactin, vasopressin, and opioid peptides.

ACTIVATION OF FEMININE SEXUAL BEHAVIOR BY ESTROGEN AND PROGESTERONE

**Estradiol: Spatial Correlations.** Autoradiographic studies of the neuroanatomy of estrogen-concentrating neurons have identified precise areas of $E_2$ action and have facilitated correlations with estrogen function. In the female rat, a system of limbic, medial preoptic and medial hypothalamic cells show the highest concentration of estrogen receptors in the central nervous system (Pfaff, 1968, 1973; Stumpf, 1968). Recent physiochemical studies utilizing microdissection of rat brain nuclei have provided quantitative measurements of estrogen receptors in specific areas of concentration (Rainbow et al., 1982b). The greatest number of estrogen receptors (20–35 fm/mg protein) in the rat brain are located within the periventricular preoptic area, the medial preoptic area, and the periventricular hypothalamus, particularly the rostral portion. High numbers of $E_2$ receptors (10–20 fm/mg protein) are found within the arcuate nucleus; the ventromedial nucleus, particularly the lateral portion; and the bed nucleus of the stria terminalis. Fewer estradiol receptors (5–10 fm/mg protein) are located within the medial amygdala, the paraventricular nucleus, the ventral premammillary nucleus, and the dorsomedial nucleus.

Many of these areas have been implicated in the control of feminine reproductive behavior, as well as in aggression and gonadotropin secretion. Two basic types of studies have provided such information: (1) those based on lesions of specific brain areas (for reviews, see Barfield and Chen, 1977; Malsbury et al., 1977; McEwen et al., 1979; Modianos et al., 1975; Morrell et al., 1975); and (2) those based on localized implantation of $E_2$ onto specific brain regions. Lesion studies have demonstrated that regions within the hypothalamus and preoptic area contribute differentially to the control of various neuroendocrine endpoints. For example, lesions in and in close proximity to the ventromedial nucleus abolish the expression of feminine reproductive behavior in the rat (see Malsbury et al., 1977); whereas lesions in the anterior hypothalamus-preoptic area abolish masculine sexual behavior (see McEwen et al., 1979). However, lesions within the ventromedial nucleus-arcuate region also alter normal food intake, gonadotropin secretion and aggressive behavior (see Martin et al., 1970; Moyer, 1976). Thus, it is conceivable that a specific $E_2$-concentrating region, or even a single steroid-concentrating cell, may participate in the multiple control of neuroendocrine endpoints.

Because brain lesions can produce a deficit in neuroendocrine function by disrupting fibers of passage or ablating nonsteroid-concentrating cells, more direct evidence regarding specific sites of estrogen action has been provided by studies utilizing stereotaxic application of hormone. Two recent studies that have employed refined techniques of $E_2$ implantation to minimize steroid diffusion have indicated that the primary site of estrogen action in the activation of the lordosis reflex is the ventromedial nucleus (Davis et al., 1979; Rubin and Barfield, 1980). A similar type of implantation study has demonstrated that the primary site of estrogen action governing positive feedback is the medial preoptic area (Goodman, 1978). Thus, the principal sites of estrogen action regulating feminine reproductive behavior and gonadotropin secretion in the rat appear to be, at least partially, anatomically distinct.

**Estradiol: Temporal Correlations.** Green, Luttge, and Whalen (1970) demonstrated that a single intravenous injection of a large dose of $E_2$ (100 g) can activate progesterone-facilitated reproductive behavior in the female rat. Green and coworkers reported that no activation of feminine reproductive behavior was seen within 16h of $E_2$ administration; but thereafter, an almost linear increase in receptivity was observed until maximal receptivity was attained at 24h. Parsons and coworkers (1980) reported that implantation of Silastic capsules, which produced physiological concentrations of $E_2$ in plasma, increased progesterone-facilitated receptivity as early as 18h after capsule insertion. Such latent periods between $E_2$ initiation and expression of receptivity are consistent with the hypothesis that $E_2$ activates reproductive behavior, at least in part, by altering protein synthesis in hypothalamic neurons.

If $E_2$ can activate feminine reproductive behavior within 18–24h of administration, then any change in hypothalamic biosynthesis which is causally related to that activation must also occur within 18–24h of $E_2$ treatment. However, relatively few biosynthetic events in the hypothalamus of the female rat have been shown to respond to estrogen treatment within 24h. Kelner, Miller, and Peck (1980) observed an increase in the activity of RNA polymerase II, which occurred *in vivo* within 8h of $E_2$ administration. An increase in hypothalamic levels of cystine aminopeptidase was noted 18h after an injection of $E_2$ (Heil et al., 1971). Luine and McEwen *1977) found that estradiol benzoate produces an increase in the *in vivo* levels of choline acetylase in the preoptic area within 24h of administration. Rainbow and colleagues (1980) report that $E_2$ elicits an increase in muscarinic receptors in the ventromedial nucleus of female rats within 24h of administration.

Perhaps the best example of a biosynthetic event in the hypothalamus of the female rat, which can be temporally correlated with the appearance of feminine reproductive behavior, is the induction of the progestin receptor by $E_2$. Parsons and coworkers (1980) report that progesterone-facilitated mating behavior and hypothalamic progestin receptors increased monotonically when Silastic capsules containing $E_2$ were implanted and decreased monotonically when these capsules were removed. Several aspects of these data merit emphasis:

1. A significant increase in progesterone-facilitated mating behavior was first observed 18h after capsule insertion; at this time, estrogen-inducible progestin receptors in the mediobasal hypothalamus (MBH) and preoptic area (POA) have increased to 26 percent of their maximal level.
2. After 48h of $E_2$ treatment, progestin receptors in the MBH–POA were maximal, and progesterone-facilitated receptivity was approaching maximal levels.
3. After removal of Silastic capsules, progesterone-facilitated sexual receptivity was last observed at 36h, when inducible progestin receptors in the MBH–POA had declined to 34 percent of the maximal levels.
4. Within 48h after capsule removal, inducible progestin receptors in the MBH–POA were approaching unstimulated levels, and sexual receptivity was not observed.

Based on these observations, Parsons and coworkers (1980) suggest that a "threshold level" (25 to 35 percent maximal induction) of estrogen-inducible progestin receptors in the MBH–POA is associated with the appearance and disappearance of progesterone-facilitated sexual receptivity in the female rat.

Many investigators have attempted to describe the minimal length of time that estradiol need be retained by hypothalamic cell nuclei in order to activate feminine reproductive behavior. Such knowledge would permit a characterization of the temporal pattern of nuclear estrogen receptors in the MBH–POA, associated with the activation of lordosis. One could also begin to select those cellular events implicated in the control of sexual receptivity by their response to this regimen of $E_2$ treatment. Some reports have suggested that $E_2$ levels in the hypothalamus must be elevated significantly at the time of mating for the full expression of lordosis (Blaustein et al., 1979; Johnson and Davidson, 1979), while others have indicated that $E_2$ need not be present in hypothalamic nuclear acceptor sites during the time of induced sexual receptivity (McEwen et al., 1975; Soderstein et al., 1981). A recent series of studies (Parsons et al., 1981b, 1982a, 1982c) has demonstrated that receptivity comparable to 24h of continuous $E_2$ treatment was seen in female rats which received only two 1-hour periods of $E_2$ (administered via Silastic capsules), provided that the second treatment began not less than 4h nor more than 13h after the end of the first period (*Sufficient treatment*). If animals received only 2 ½h exposures to $E_2$ during these times, receptivity was not observed (*Insufficient treatment*). *Sufficient treatment* elicited an essentially discontinuous pattern of estrogen receptors in MBH–POA cell nuclei, whereby two "peaks" representing 60 percent of receptor capacity were separated by a "valley" representing no more than 4 percent of receptor capacity. Thus, there appears to be an essentially discontinuous requirement in the brain for $E_2$ to activate progesterone-facilitated reproductive behavior. In addition, *Sufficient treatment* elevated estrogen-inducible progestin receptors in the MBH–POA to threshold levels (25 to 35 percent maximal), whereas *Insufficient treatment* did not. These findings are consistent with the hypothesis that the induction of cytosol progestin receptors in the MBH–POA is one of the neurochemical events mediated by $E_2$ that accompanies the activation of sexual receptivity in the female rat.

**Estradiol: Functional Correlations.** The genomic origin of the lordosis reflex has been implicated by the work of several investigators. Terkel, Shryne, and Gorski (1973) demonstrated that stereotaxic application of actinomycin D into the preoptic area was effective in depressing sexual receptivity if applied before, or within 6h of, the initiation of $E_2$ treatment. Quadagno and Ho (1975) observed that stereotaxic application of cycloheximide into the preoptic area was effective in depressing feminine reproductive behavior if given before, or within 12h of, the initiation of estrogen treatment. Application of cycloheximide to the ventromedial nucleus produced an inhibition of receptivity comparable to that observed when cycloheximide was applied to the preoptic area (Meinkoth et al., 1979). However, the interpretation of these studies is complicated by the fact that the extent of cycloheximide diffusion from the sites of implantation was not assessed.

More recent studies have employed the protein synthesis inhibitor, anisomycin (ANI), in order to provide additional correlates of $E_2$ action. In one such study, ANI significantly decreased the lordosis quotient score at 24h, when applied bilaterally to the ventromedial nucleus 6h after the initiation of estrogen treatment (Rainbow et al., 1981, 1982a). Moreover, at 4h after ANI application, protein synthesis (as estimated by [$^3$H]-leucine incorporation into soluble protein) in the mediobasal hypothalamus was inhibited by 70 percent, but no inhibition was observed in the preoptic area, corticomedial amygdala, or pituitary. Thus, the activation of feminine reproductive behavior can be blocked by inhibiting protein synthesis in a discrete region of the hypothalamus, consisting primarily of the ventromedial nucleus.

Anisomycin has also been used to elucidate the time course of the changes in protein synthesis following *sufficient treatment* with $E_2$ which are essential for the activation of the lordosis reflex in the female rat. If ANI is applied 15 minutes prior to the first, 15 minutes prior to the second, or between the two 1-hour segments of $E_2$ treatment, little or no sexual receptivity is observed at 24h (Parsons et al., 1981b, 1982c). However, if ANI is delayed until 2h or 6h after the end of the second period of $E_2$ treatment, no significant decrease in receptivity is observed at 24h. Thus, at least a large portion of the protein synthesis essential for the activation of lordosis is completed within 2h after the termination of *sufficient treatment*. In addition, experiments which employed different doses of ANI revealed that inhibition of protein synthesis by 60 percent in the MBH–POA for the 1h duration of either segment of $E_2$ treatment is adequate to decrease significantly, but not abolish, sexual receptivity at 24h. To abolish sexual receptivity at 24h, protein synthesis had to be inhibited by 40 to 80 percent in the MBH–POA for two consecutive hours, both during and one hour after the termination of either segment of $E_2$ treatment.

**Progesterone: Spatial Correlations.** The availability of a high-affinity synthetic progestin, [$^3$H]-R5020, facilitated the physiochemical identification of specific saturable cytosol progestin binding molecules in both ovariectomized and estrogen-primed rodents (Kato and Onouchi, 1977; MacLusky and McEwen, 1980; Moguilewsky and Raynaud, 1979; Warembourg, 1978). One major feature of progestin receptors isolated from the rat brain is the presence of two classes of receptors, one of which is induced by $E_2$, the other of which is not (MacLusky and McEwen, 1978). Although the physiological significance of the noninduced progestin receptor is unclear, it is important to note that $E_2$ induces progestin receptors in those areas of the brain implicated in the control of feminine reproductive behavior and gonadotropin secretion, in the MBH, and in the POA (Blaustein and Feder, 1979; MacLusky and McEwen, 1978; Parsons et al., 1981a).

Autoradiographic studies of the neuroanatomy of progestin-concentrating neurons which employed [$^3$H]-progesterone as a radioligand often resulted in negative results. One exception was the autoradiographic study by Sar and Stumpf (1973), which identified some progestin-concentrating cells in the basal hypothalamus and pituitary of the estrogen-primed guinea pig. Using [$^3$H]-R5020 as a radioligand, Warembourg (1978) examined the neuroanatomical distribution of estrogen-inducible progestin receptors in the female rat brain with autoradiography. Few labeled cells were observed outside of the preoptic area and mediobasal hypothalamus (Warembourg, 1978). Recently, physiochemical analyses employing microdissection of rat brain nuclei have permitted quantification of both estrogen-inducible and noninducible progestin receptors in specific areas of concentration (Parsons et al., 1982b). The greatest number of estrogen-inducible progestin receptors (20–45 fm/mg protein) in the female rat brain are located in the periventricular preoptic area, the medial preoptic area, the suprachiasmatic preoptic area, the periventricular anterior hypothalamus, the arcuate-median eminence and the ventromedial nucleus. Areas which show a lesser, although significant, induction of progestin receptors (3–10 fm/mg protein) are the anterior hypothalamus, the cingulate cortex, the lateral preoptic area, the medial nucleus of the amygdala, and the CA1 hippocampal subfield. Significant concentrations of noninducible receptors were observed in many, but not all, of the above regions that contained inducible receptors, as well as in regions that did not contain inducible receptors, such as the parietal cortex and the olfactory tubercle.

Direct evidence regarding sites of progesterone action in the activation of feminine reproductive behavior has been provided by Rubin and Barfield (1983). These workers found that the stereotaxic application of P to the ventromedial nucleus, but not to other brain areas, facilitated reproductive behavior in estrogen-primed rats. Ineffective sites of P application included the preoptic area, the mesencephalic reticular formation, the central grey, and the hippocampus. Thus, the ventromedial nucleus of the hypothalamus appears to be the principal, but not exclusive, site of gonadal steroid action in the activation of feminine reproductive behavior.

**Progesterone: Temporal Correlations.** The overall effects of progesterone on a target tissue are partially determined by that target tissue's endocrine environment. Specifically, pretreatment with an estrogen appears to be prerequisite for most target tissues to respond optimally to progesterone. In such tissues, the role of estrogen is primarily that of inducing progesterone-sensitive target cells by inducing receptors specific for progestins.

Pretreatment with estrogen appears to be a major requirement for optimal progestational responses in the nervous system. Unfortunately, very few events in the hypothalamus of the estrogen-primed rodent have been characterized with respect to their time of induction by progesterone. In the $E_2$-treated rat, the administration of intravenous P can increase both the frequency and quality of the lordosis posture within 30–60 minutes (Kubli-Garfias and Whalen, 1977; Lisk, 1960; McGinness et al., 1981; Meyerson, 1972; Tennet et al., 1980). In addition to facilitating sexual receptivity, progesterone can activate components of sexual proceptivity, such as hopping, darting and ear wiggling, within 30–60 minutes of intravenous administration (McGinnis et al., 1981). If the progesterone dose is sufficiently large, a refractory period follows at 18–24h postinjection, during which time animals are less sensitive to additional P (Blaustein and Feder, 1980; Blaustein and Wade, 1977; Powers and Moreines, 1976; Zucker, 1966). This refractory period has been termed "sequential inhibition" by progesterone (Powers and Moreines, 1976). The minimal length of time that progesterone must be retained by hypothalamic or pituitary cell nuclei in order to promote the above changes in feminine reproductive behavior or gonadotropin secretion has not been characterized. One recent study by McGinnis and colleagues (1981) has demonstrated that the rapid behavioral effects of intravenous P administration in $E_2$-primed rats are preceded by rapid progestin receptor translocation to MBH–POA cell nuclei. Furthermore, the facilitation of feminine reproductive behavior by P continues to be observed several hours after nuclear progestin receptor in the MBH–POA have returned to control levels (McGinnis et al., 1981). These findings are consistent with the hypothesis that P-induced effects on feminine reproductive behavior involve genomic activation and subsequent protein synthesis.

**Progesterone: Functional Correlations.** The antibiotic, ANI has been shown to be effective in blocking protein synthesis in the central nervous system when administered systemically. Rainbow, McGinnis, Davis, and McEwen (1982a) found that ANI, when given 15 minutes prior to the administration of P, blocked the activation of proceptivity and the facilitation of receptivity in ovariectomized rats primed with estrogen. More recently, Rainbow and coworkers (1982a) have demonstrated that stereotaxic application of ANI to the ventromedial nucleus also blocks the facilitation of feminine reproductive behavior seen 4–6h after subcutaneous P administration. Four hours after intracranial ANI application, protein synthesis in the MBH was inhibited by 70 percent, but no inhibition was observed in the preoptic area, corticomedial amygdala, or pituitary. These findings are consistent with, but not proof of, the hypothesis that progesterone's activation of proceptivity and facilitation of receptivity in the female rat is a result of altered genomic expression and protein synthesis in the ventromedial nucleus.

In addition to facilitating sexual receptivity acutely, P also may play a role in the subsequent termination of reproductive behavior. As mentioned above, animals, which receive P initially, are less sensitive to additional P 24h later than animals which did not receive initial P ("sequential inhibition"). A study by Parsons and McEwen (1981) demonstrated that administration of ANI, 15 minutes prior to and again 3h after initial P treatment, can block the "sequential inhibition" of reproductive behavior. According to the time course of effective ANI application, the presumed protein synthesis responsible for the inhibition of sexual receptivity occurs between 3h and 13h after the administration of P (Parsons and McEwen, 1981). The identification of the proteins associated with the sequential inhibition of receptivity, as well as those associated with the facilitation of reproductive behavior by P, remains an area for future investigation.

## MODULATION OF FEMININE SEXUAL BEHAVIOR BY THE LEUTINIZING HORMONE-RELEASING HORMONE

During the rat estrous cycle, a surge of LH from the pituitary precedes the appearance of ovulation and reproductive behavior by several hours. The release of LH from the pituitary has been shown to be regulated by the hypothalamic decapeptide, LHRH, which has been isolated, sequenced, and synthesized (Amoss et al., 1971; Burges et al., 1972; Matsuo et al., 1971a, 1971b). Initial experiments by Pfaff (1973), and Moss and McCann (1973, 1975) demonstrated that systemic administration of LHRH to ovariectomized rats primed with estrogen or estrone facilitated behavioral receptivity. Because the animals which received estrogen were also hypophysectomized, the observed increase in behavioral receptivity could not have been produced by an increase in pituitary LH or follicle-stimulating hormone (FSH) release.

The behavioral efficacy of systemically administered LHRH in hypophysectomized animals suggests that some hypothalamic LHRH-producing neurons may project to other brain regions involved in the regulation of feminine reproductive behavior. One region implicated in the control of receptivity, the central grey or the midbrain, has been shown by immunohistochemical techniques to contain axons that stain with LHRH antiserum (Liposits and Setalo, 1980). Both Riskind and Moss (1979) and Sakuma and Pfaff (1980) have reported that microinfusion of LHRH into the midbrain central grey rapidly facilitates the lordosis reflex in estrogen-primed female rats. In addition, Sakuma and Pfaff (1983) demonstrated that microinfusion of an LHRH antiserum into the dorsal portion of the central grey completely abolishes the expression of the receptivity for as long as 7h after infusion. A tentative conclusion that emerges from these studies is that LHRH-containing neurons, which project from the hypothalamus to the midbrain central grey, may be important for the regulation of lordosis in the female rat.

Recent studies of Shivers and coworkers (1983a, 1983b, 1983c) also suggest, but do not prove, that LHRH may modulate the expression of feminine reproductive behavior in the rat. These investigators have reported that there are marked effects of gonadal manipulation on the LHRH content of two hypothalamic terminal fields, as determined by immunocytochemical procedures. An important question that emerges from this study is whether estrogen modulates hypothalamic LHRH content by acting directly on LHRH-containing cell bodies, or by acting secondarily on neurons which project to LHRH cell bodies. Shivers and coworkers have elegantly demonstrated that a second hypothalamic cell type must mediate the genomic actions of estradiol on LHRH synthesis and/or release. Out of more than 400 LHRH cell bodies localized in rat brain sections processed for autoradiography, only one LHRH cell body concentrated estradiol (Shivers et al., 1983b). However, the location of many LHRH neurons was only a few micrometers from estrogen-concentrating cells, suggesting that LHRH neurons may receive monosynaptic projections from cells containing estrogen receptors.

## Modulation of Feminine Sexual Behavior by Opiate Peptides

Several lines of evidence have indicated that endogenous opiate peptides may participate in the regulation of masculine reproductive behavior in the rat (McIntosh et al., 1980; Meller et al., 1980; Meyerson and Terenius, 1977; Myers and Baum, 1979, 1980). In addition, two recent studies suggest that endogenous opiates may be implicated in the regulation of feminine reproductive behavior. Sirinathsinghji and coworkers (1983) report that the infusion of naloxone into the midbrain central grey produced a prompt facilitation of the lordosis response in estrogen-primed rats, occurring within 5 minutes and persisting for 90 minutes. To test whether this facilitation was produced by naloxone-induced LHRH release, these investigators pretreated the central grey with a LHRH antiserum or a LHRH antagonist prior to naloxone infusion. Pretreatment of the midbrain central grey with a LHRH antiserum diminished the naloxone-induced increase in lordosis, while pretreatment with a LHRH antagonist abolished lordosis.

Sirinathsinghji and colleagues also sought to determine which of the endogenous opiate receptor ligands might be involved in the modulation of LHRH release and the regulation of feminine reproductive behavior. The infusion of met-enkephalin into the midbrain central grey had no inhibitory effects on lordosis quotient scores in estrogen-primed female rats. By contrast, infusion of β-endorphin completely abolished the expression of receptivity within 2h of infusion. This suppressive effect of β-endorphin could be overcome not only by pretreatment with systemic naloxone, but also by the prior application of LHRH to the central grey. Taken together, these results suggest that endogenous opiates, specifically β-endorphin in the midbrain central grey, may contribute to the expression of sexual receptivity by modulating the release of LHRH.

A recent report by Allen, Renner, and Luine (in press) also indicates that opioid peptides may modulate the expression of receptivity in the female rat. Systemic administration of naltrexone facilitated lordosis quotient scores in estrogen-primed females, with significant increases observed 3h and 4h after administration. Interestingly, the facilitative effects of naltrexone were not blocked by the concurrent administration of the protein synthesis inhibitor, ANI. These experiments indicate that the modulation of receptivity by opioid peptides does not require macromolecular synthesis; a conclusion consistent with the provisional hypothesis that endogenous opiates inhibit receptivity by modulating LHRH release.

## Modulation of Feminine Sexual Behavior by Vasopressin

Although the antidiuretic hormone vasopressin has been implicated in the maintenance of learned avoidance behaviors and in memory consolidation (Bohus *et al.*, 1978; deWied, 1976; LeMoal *et al.*, 1981; Walter *et al.*, 1978), its possible role in the regulation of reproductive behavior has received scant attention. However, a recent study by Sodersten and colleagues (1983) suggests that vasopressin may inhibit the expression of feminine reproductive behavior in the rat. These workers observed that the intracerebroventricular (i.c.v.) injection of arg-vasopressin (AVP) decreased lordosis quotient scores in females primed with estrogen and progesterone within 15 minutes of application. This inhibition was blocked by the prior i.c.v. injection of an AVP antiserum, and could not be overridden by increasing the priming dose of estrogen. Thus, if vasopressin is found to play a physiological role in the regulation of feminine reproductive behavior, it is likely that it may regulate neurochemical events which are different from those regulated by the steroid hormones. Sodersten and coworkers tentatively suggest that the suprachiasmatic nucleus may release vasopressin rhythmically, and that such release may contribute to the inhibition of reproductive behavior in the female rat.

## Modulation of Feminine Sexual Behavior by Prolactin

Unlike estradiol, progesterone, and LHRH, prolactin has not been implicated in the control of sexual receptivity until quite recently. Studies by Toubeau and coworkers (1979) have demonstrated that a prolactin-like substance is present in cell bodies of the mediobasal hypothalamus, as well as in the midbrain central grey. Harlan, Shivers, and Pfaff (1983) report that microinfusion of prolactin into the midbrain central grey facilitates lordosis in a dose-dependent manner in female rats primed with estrogen. In addition, these workers have established that infusion of a prolactin antiserum into the dorsal midbrain significantly decreases the lordosis quotient scores of estrogen-primed females for as long as 2h after infusion. These findings are consistent with the postulate that hypothalamic cells may partially facilitate lordosis by releasing a prolactin-like substance in the midbrain.

Shivers, Harlan, and Pfaff (1983a) have extended their investigations to include a detailed neuroanatomical description of immunoreactive prolactin fibers. Using immunocytochemical procedures, these workers have estimated that there are approximately 2000–3000 immunoreactive prolactin-containing cell bodies within the mediobasal hypothalamus. These cell bodies are localized exclusively within the arcuate nucleus and in a band extending ventral and lateral to the ventromedial nucleus. Immunoreactive prolactin fibers appear to take both medial and lateral pathways from the hypothalamus to the central grey, a finding consistent with the neural circuitry controlling lordosis. In addition, high concentrations of immunoreactive prolactin-containing fibers are observed in and adjacent to the midbrain central grey. Taken collectively, these findings provisionally suggest that prolactin, transported from the hypothalamus to the midbrain central grey, may facilitate lordosis in the female rat.

## CLINICAL CONSIDERATIONS

### ONTOGENETIC TRACING

The evolution of sex steroids by the reproductive axis constitutes the primary means of regulating sexual behavior. Sexual behavior is strictly governed by sex steroids in lower mammals, but this regulation is of somewhat lesser importance in primates and least of all in man. The hormonal effects on feminine sexual behavior are of two kinds:

1. differentiation of the somatic and central nervous systems
2. expression of feminine sexual behavior in the sexually mature woman.

In the first case, it is understood that sex steroids are capable of exerting an organizing effect on the developing central nervous system acting at key developmental milestones. The continued expression of feminine sexual behavior, on the other hand, is a function of the elaboration of sex steroids in the adult as a reflection of reproductive competence. The differentiating and the activating roles of sex steroids in the regulation of sexual behavior are closely interrelated—the organizing effects of a hormone may set the stage for subsequent responsiveness of key tissues as they relate to sexual behavior phenomena. It is the objective of this section to trace in an ontogenetic manner physiologic and pathophysiologic considerations of sexual behavior in the human, as they may be encountered by the practicing obstetrician or gynecologist.

### PRENATAL PERIOD

In certain subhuman primates, prenatal androgenic exposure of genetic females may lead to higher prevalence of male-oriented behavior. A similar phenomenon in the human has not been convincingly demonstrated, a fact which may be attributed to the complexity of human sexual behavior as compared with that of subhuman primates, further stressing the complicating effect of social reinforcement of sex-role stereotypes. This difference between human and subhuman sexual behavior also serves to underscore the point that whatever the prenatal programming of the central nervous system, additional subsequent programming by social environment inevitably takes place. According to Money and Higham (1979) "most of the masculinity, femininity, or bisexuality of a person's gender identity and behavior is a product of his or her postnatal biography." Indeed, the prenatal component of differentiating gender identity and role as either masculine or feminine would not predetermine or preordain the postnatal factor (Money and Higham, 1979).

**Turner's Syndrome.** Turner's syndrome represents a state of gonadal insufficiency and a consequent total lack of gonadal estrogen biosynthesis (Turner, 1938). Most commonly attributed to a 45X chromosomal constitution, Turner's syndrome is characterized clinically by primitive gonadal streaks, sexual infantilism, short stature, and multiple congenital abnormalities of varying expression and severity (McDonough and Byrd, 1977). Due to the failure of ovarian development, the embryo differentiates along female lines, developing the external features of a normal female. Such individuals are usually assigned a female gender at birth with subsequent differentiation to a typical feminine gender identity except for inevitable infertility.

According to some authorities (Money and Higham, 1979), girls afflicted by Turner's syndrome do dream of romance, marriage, and maternalism, display a substantial interest in doll play and baby care, but limited, if any, interest in athletics and fighting (attack and dominance assertion) behavior. They also suggest that subsequent realization of the inevitable infertility and the handicap of short stature characteristic of this syndrome do not generally alter the urge for marriage and motherhood. After the achievement of pubertal maturation by the administration of exogenous sex steroids, individuals afflicted by Turner's syndrome appear to look their age even though short in stature. It remains uncertain whether current regimens of estrogen replacement therapy are compatible with optimal erotic function.

**Congenital Virilizing Adrenal Hyperplasia.** Prenatal androgenization due to androgen excess is best exemplified by a group of autosomally recessive inherited entities collectively referred to as congenital virilizing adrenal hyperplasia or the adrenogenital syndrome (Amrhein et al., 1976). In this situation, a steroidogenic block is congenitally present resulting in the accumulation of adrenal androgenic precursors present in excess prenatally and persisting postnatally unless recognized and treated. A related disorder of an iatrogenic nature has been known to occur rarely as a result of exogenous hormone administration during pregnancy. Indeed, female hermaphroditism could be inadvertently induced by the prenatal administration of synthetic progestins with androgenic potential. Such steroids have been sporadically used with the intent of prevention of spontaneous miscarriage.

Prior to the introduction of cortisol by Lawson Wilkins for the treatment of congenital virilizing adrenal hyperplasia, abnormal androgen production as characteristic of this syndrome resulted in progressive masculinization. With the initiation of treatment, additional postnatal masculinization can now be controlled, but abnormally differentiated genitalia still require surgical correction. To date, infants born with the adrenogenital variant of female hermaphroditism are invariably assigned a female gender at birth given their genetic female constitution and the presence of internal female ductal structures (Jones and Verkauf, 1971; Klingensmith, et al., 1977).

Based on the thorough studies of Money (Money and Higham, 1979), it is currently thought that treated individuals afflicted by congenital virilizing adrenal hyperplasia "differentiate a feminine gender identity although with tomboy traits. In fact, it has been stated that such individuals proudly describe themselves as tomboys." These patients are said to engage in strenuous physical activity such as competitive sport, often in the company of boys. However, "fighting" patterns are quite uncommon. It is generally felt that in individuals afflicted by the adrenogenital syndrome, the "threshold for the emergence of parental behavior, as for romantic response, is elevated but not insuperable" (Money and Higham, 1979).

Although relatively little information is available with respect to women with inordinately high androgen levels leading to substantial masculinization, pretherapy eroticism consisted of "moderate frequency of homosexual and bisexual imagery, rare frequency of actual lesbian encounters and absence of transsexual desire for sex reassignment" (Money and Higham, 1979).

According to Lev-Ran (1974), most women afflicted by congenital virilizing adrenal hyperplasia did not display homosexual tendencies though a slightly increased tendency to bisexuality may be operative. These findings suggest that the role of androgens in congenital virilizing adrenal hyperplasia may be to alter libido as opposed to sexual preferences.

In summary, there is limited evidence to suggest that prenatal hormonal exposure affects gender role behavior and identity. However, one cannot exclude the possibility that these postnatal endpoints may in fact be social consequences resultant from anatomical variation.

The maintenance of menstrual cyclicity in the adult human female heavily relies on the presence of intact positive feedback mechanisms responsible for the generation of the midcycle LH and FSH ovulatory surge. Consequently, one prevalent and legitimate past concern regarding individuals afflicted by congenital virilizing adrenal hyperplasia, was the possible adverse effect of prenatal androgenization on the ability to develop positive feedback mechanisms. It has been envisioned that prenatal exposure to excess androgen levels may lead to irreversible androgenization of those portions of the central nervous system responsible for the control of the cyclic mode of gonadotropin release. Stated differently, prenatal androgenization might lead to chronic anovulation and the permanent absence of cyclic gonadotropin release. However, it is now generally held that primates appear to be insensitive to the early effect of androgenization. In marmosets, both sexes possess positive feedback capabilities. Moreover, female rhesus monkeys subjected to androgenization *in utero*, as human females afflicted with congenital virilizing adrenal hyperplasia are exposed *in utero* to virilizing steroids, do usually ovulate displaying intact positive feedback mechanisms (Klingensmith, *et al.,* 1976; Reiter, *et al.,* 1975). These observations have generally been taken to mean that positive feedback capabilities in the human cannot be employed as marker of earlier sexual differentiation of the brain. For further discussion see Chapter 7.

**Androgen Insensitivity Syndromes.** Individuals with a 46XY chromosomal complement afflicted by the X-linked recessive trait of androgen insensitivity, represent a spectrum of entities characterized by quantitative and qualitative abnormalities of androgen receptor tissue proteins. In the complete form characterized by total androgen insensitivity, also referred to as testicular feminization (Morris, 1953), afflicted individuals differentiate along female lines to display a typical phenotypic female gender with the exception of a small or absent vagina and the absence of any pubic or axillary hair. Although the external genitalia are indistinguishable from those of the normal female, internal female genitalia are absent due to testicular secretion of the so-called Mullerian inhibiting factor.

Given that sex of assignment and rearing is universally female and that the phenotypic expression is along female lines, gender identity is feminine as well. It is, therefore, apparent that neither chromosomal nor gonadal sex *per se* necessarily regulate the expression of gender identity and role. Indeed, according to Money and Higham (1979) childhood rehearsal play of girls afflicted by testicular feminization is characterized by a high preference for marriage and raising a family. Moreover, the adult posture is one of satisfaction with the feminine role, with eroticism and sexuality manifesting characteristic heterosexual feminine orientation.

Since, for the most part, information relating to their chromosomal and gonadal sex has been withheld from individuals with testicular feminization, it is difficult to predict the effect of this later realization of the limitations set up by karyotype and gonadal sex (*e.g.,* infertility, need for vaginoplasty). It has generally been assumed that such realization would be detrimental to the psychological well being of individuals afflicted by testicular feminization. However, little or no evidence supports this concern or supports the practice of withholding information on karyotype and gonadal sex from such patients. There may be, in fact, some room for the re-evaluation of the advisability of withholding such information from the patient given that such information may ultimately surface in connection with future litigation.

PERIPUBERTAL PERIOD

Relatively little is known about hormonal–behavioral relationships in the peripubertal period. This, according to Money and Higham (1979), may be accounted for, at least in part, by the "relative similarity of physical and mental growth in both sexes during childhood and the Freudian conception of childhood as a latency period." A detailed account of peripubertal events is provided in Chapter 2.

REPRODUCTIVE PERIOD

Steroid hormones assume an important role in the animal kingdom with respect to the expression of sexual behavior. At least in nonprimates, female heat, characterized by sexual receptivity and attractivity to the male, is clearly hormone dependent. In fact, little or no sexual activity occurs at any other time. In contrast, the role of hormones in sexual behavior of primates remains uncertain. Some studies suggest that there appears to be no correlation between sexual activity and specific hormonal patterns (Bancroft, 1980; 1981; Persky, et al., 1978; Spitz, et al., 1975). In contrast, studies in gorillas and orangutans suggest midcycle peaking of feminine sexual behavior. Similar uncertainties exist as regards human sexual behavior.

The pattern of sexual behavior throughout the human menstrual cycle is unpredictable. Some studies, however, suggest peaks of sexuality prior to or following menstruation. The issue may be further complicated by the cyclic mood alterations throughout the cycle. The reasons underlying the perimenstrual peaks of feminine sexual behavior remain uncertain. Possibly, androgens, the putative libidinal agents, may be at play during the perimenstrual period. However, testosterone and androstenedione peak at midcycle (Frohlich, et al., 1976; Judd and Yen, 1973; Vermeulen and Verdonck, 1976). Women afflicted with the polycystic ovary syndrome and its associated hyperandrogenism are found to be more sexually assertive than controls (Gorzynski and Katz, 1977).

Perhaps the most recent and definitive study on this issue is one performed by Adams and colleagues (1978). This study was designed to test the hypothesis that women exhibit peaks of sexual activity at ovulation as might be predicted from estrous effects in animals. According to this study, married women using contraceptive devices other than combination oral contraceptives, experience a significant increase in sexual behavior at the time of ovulation. It has also been suggested that previous failures to find an ovulatory peak may have been due to the use of measures of sexual behavior that are primarily determined by initiation by the male partner. Significantly, women using combination oral contraceptives did not show a rise in female-initiated sexual activity at the time corresponding to midcycle, presumably due to suppression of the preovulatory hormonal alterations.

## CLIMACTERIC PERIOD

"Active sexuality in the geriatric years has often been viewed negatively as a concomitant of senility and of the failure of suitable impulse repression rather than as the expression of desire for erotic and affectionate relationship continued throughout life" (Money and Higham, 1979). This misconception and the current outlook on climacteric feminine sexual behavior is covered at length in Chapter 6.

## CONCLUSION

We attempted to summarize the current views of the differentiation of feminine sexual behavior. To this end, use was made of experimental information derived from animal models as well as clinical observations made in several pathophysiologic conditions. Although subprimate studies may not be immediately applicable to the human, such an approach nevertheless outlines the direction of future research in this area. Given the dynamic nature of this area of research, novel observations are clearly to be expected in the relatively near future.

## REFERENCES

Adams, D. B.; Gold, A. R.; and Burt, A. D.: Rise in female-initiated sexual activity at ovulation and its suppression by oral contraceptives. *N. Engl. J. Med.*, 299:1145–1150, 1978.

Allen, D.; Renner, K.; and Luine, V. N.: Naltrexone facilitation of lordosis in the female rat. *Horm. Behav.*, in press.

Amoss, M.; Burges, R.; Blackwell, R.; Vale, W.; Fellows, R.; and Guillemin, R.: Purification, amino acid composition and n-terminus of the hypothalamic luteinizing hormone releasing factor (LRF) of ovine origin. *Biochem. Biophys. Res. Commun.*, 44:205–210, 1971.

Amrhein, J. A.; Meyer, W. J. III; Jones, H. W. Jr.; and Migeon, C. J.: Androgen insensitivity in men: Evidence for genetic heterogeneitity. *Proc. Natl. Acad. Sci. USA*, 73:891–894, 1976.

Ball, J.: A test for measuring sexual excitability in the female rat. *Comp. Psychol. Mon.*, 14:1–37, 1937.

Bancroft, J.: Endocrinology of sexual function. *Clin. Obstet. Gynaecol.*, 7:253–281, 1980.

Bancroft, J.: Hormones and human sexual behavior. *Br. Med. Bull.*, 37:153–158, 1981.

Barfield, R. J., and Chen, J. J.: Activation of estrous behavior in ovariectomized rats by intracerebral implants of estradiol benzoate. *Endocrinology*, 101:1716–1725, 1977.

Beach, F. A.: Importance of progesterone to induction of sexual receptivity in spayed female rats. *Proc. Soc. Exp. Biol. Med.*, 51:369–371, 1942.

Blaustein, J. D., and Feder, H. H.: Cytoplasmic progestin receptors in the female guinea pig brain and their relationship to refractoriness in expression of female sexual behavior. *Brain Res.*, 177:489–498, 1979.

Blaustein, J. D., and Feder, H. H.: Nuclear progestin receptors in guinea pig brain measured by an in vitro exchange assay after hormonal treatments that affect lordosis. *Endocrinology*, 106:1061–1069, 1980.

Blaustein, J. D., and Wade, G. N.: Sequential inhibition of sexual behavior by progesterone in female rats: comparison with a synthetic antiestrogen. *J. Comp. Physiol. Psychol.*, 91:752–760, 1977.

Blaustein, J. D.; Dudley, S. D.; Grey, J. M.; Roy, E. J.; and Wade, G. N.: Long-term retention of estradiol by brain cell nuclei and female rat sexual behavior. *Brain Res.*, 173:355–359, 1979.

Bohus, B.; Urban, J.; van Greidanaus, T. B.; and deWied, D.: Opposite effects of oxytocin and vasopressin on avoidance behavior and hippocampal theta rhythm in the rat. *Neuropharmacology*, 17:239–247, 1978.

Burges, R.; Butcher, M.; Amoss, M.; Ling, N.; Fellows, R.; Blackwell, R.; Vale, W.; and Guillemin, R.: Primary structure of the ovine hypothalamic luteinizing hormone releasing-factor (LRF). *Proc. Natl. Acad. Sci. USA*, 69:278–282, 1972.

Davis, P. G.; McEwen, B. S.; and Pfaff, D. W.: Localized behavioral effects of tritiated estradiol implants in the ventromedial hypothalamus of female rats. *Endocrinology*, 104:893–903, 1979.

deWied, D.: Behavioral effects of intraventricularly administered vasopressin and vasopressin fragments. *Life Sci.*, 19:685–690, 1976.

Frohlich, M.; Brand, E. C.; and Van Hall, E. V.: Serum levels of unconjugated aetiocholanolone, androstenedione, testosterone, dehydroepiandrosterone, aldosterone, progesterone and oestrogen during the normal menstrual cycle. *Acta Endocrinol.*, 81:548–562, 1976.

Goodman, R. L.: The site of positive feedback action of estradiol in the rat. *Endocrinology*, 102:151–159, 1978.

Gorzynski, G., and Katz, J. L.: The polycystic ovary syndrome: psychosexual correlates. *Arch. Sex. Behav.*, 6:215–222, 1977.

Green, R.; Luttge, W. G.; and Whalen, R. E.: Induction of receptivity in ovariectomized female rats by a single intravenous injection of estradiol-17. *Physiol. Behav.*, 5:137–141, 1970.

Hardy, D. F.: Sexual behavior in continuously cycling rats. *Behavior*, 41:288–297, 1972.

Hardy, D. F., and DeBold, J. F.: The relationship between levels of exogenous hormones and the display of lordosis by the female rat. *Horm. Behav.*, 9:380–386, 1977.

Harlan, R. E.; Shivers, B. D.; and Pfaff, D. W.: Midbrain microinfusions of prolactin increase the estrogen-dependent behavior, lordosis. *Science*, 219:1451–1453, 1983.

Heil, H.; Meltzer, V.; Kuhil, H.; Abraham, R.; and Taubert, H. D.: Stimulation of L-cystine-aminopeptidase activity by hormonal steroids and steroid-analogs in the hypothalamus and other tissues of the female rat. *Fertil. Steril.*, 22:181–187, 1971.

Johnson, P. G., and Davidson, J. M.: Priming action of estrogen: minimum duration of exposure for feedback and behavioral effects. *Neuroendocrinology*, 28:155–159, 1979.

Jones, H. W. Jr., and Verkauf, B. S.: Congenital adrenal hyperplasia: age at menarche and related events at puberty. *Am. J. Obstet. Gynecol.*, 109:292–299, 1971.

Judd, H. L., and Yen, S. S. C.: Serum androstenedione and testosterone levels during the menstrual cycle. *J. Clin. Endocrinol. Metab.*, 36:475–481, 1973.

Kato, J., and Onouchi, T.: Specific progesterone receptors in the hypothalamus and anterior hypophysis of the rat. *Endocrinology*, 101:912–928, 1977.

Kelner, K. L.; Miller, A. L.; and Peck, E. J.: Estrogens and the hypothalamus: nuclear receptor and RWA polymerase activation. *J. Recept. Res.*, 1 215–227, 1980.

Klingensmith, G. J.; Garcia, S. C.; Jones, H. W. Jr.; Migeon, C. G.; and Blizzard, R. M.: Glucocorticoid treatment of girls with congenital adrenal hyperplasia: effects on height, sexual maturation, and fertility. *J. Pediatr.*, 90:996–1004, 1977.

Klingensmith, G. J.; Wentz, A. C.; Meyer, W. J. III; and Migeon, C. G.: Gonadotropin output in congenital adrenal hyperplasia before and after adrenal suppression. *J. Clin. Endocrinol. Metab.*, 43:933–938, 1976.

Kubli-Garfias, C., and Whalen, R. E.: Induction of lordosis behavior in female rats by intravenous administration of progestins. *Horm. Behav.*, 9:380–386, 1977.

Kuehn, R. F. and Beach, F. A.: Quantitative measurement of sexual receptivity in female rats. *Behaviour*, 21:282–299, 1963.

LeMoal, M.; Koob, G. F.; Kooda, L. Y.; Bloom, F. E.; Manning, M.; Sawyer, W. H.; and River, J.: Vasopressor receptor antagonist prevents behavioral effects of vasopressin. *Nature*, 291:491–493, 1981.

Lev-Ran, A.: Sexuality and educational level of women with the late-treated adrenogenital syndrome. *Arch. Sex. Behav.*, 3:27–32, 1974.

Liposits, Z., and Setalo, G.: Descending luteinizing hormone-releasing hormone (LHRH) nerve fibers to the midbrain of the rat. *Neurosci. Lett.*, 20:1–4, 1980.

Lisk, R. D.: A comparison of the effectiveness of intravenous, as opposed to subcutaneous, injections of progesterone for the induction of estrous behavior in the rat. *Canad. J. Biochem. Physiol.*, 38:1331–1383, 1960.

Luine, V. N., and McEwen, B. S.: Effects of an estrogen antagonist on enzyme activities and H-estradiol nuclear binding in uterus, pituitary and brain. *Endocrinology*, 100:903–910, 1977.

MacLusky, N. J., and McEwen, B. S.: Oestrogen modulates progestin receptor concentration in some brain regions but not in others. *Nature*, 274:276–277, 1978.

MacLusky, N. J., and McEwen, B. S.: Progestin receptors in rat brain: distribution and properties of cytoplasmic progestin binding sites. *Endocrinology* 106:192–202, 1980.

Malsbury, C.; Kow, L. M.; and Pfaff, D. W.: Effects of sexual receptivity in the hormone-primed female hamster by electrical stimulation of the medial preoptic area. *Physiol. Behav.,* 19:223–237, 1977.

Martin, L.; Molla, M.; and Fraschini, F.: *The Hypothalamus.* Academic Press, New York, 1970.

Matsuo, H.; Arimura, A.; Nair, R. M. G.; and Schally, A. V.: Synthesis of the porcine LH- and FSH-releasing hormone by the solid-phase method. *Biochem. Biophys. Res. Commun.,* 45:822–827, 1971.

Matsuo, H.; Baba, Y.; Nair, R. M. G.; Arimura, A.; and Schally, A. V.: Structure of the porcine LH and FSH-releasing hormone. I. The proposed amino acid sequence. *Biochem. Biophys. Res. Commun.,* 43:1334–1339, 1971b.

McDonough, P. G., and Byrd, J. R.: Gonadal dysgenesis. *Clin. Obstet. Gynecol.,* 20:565–579, 1977.

McEwen, B. S.; Davis, P. G.; Parsons, B.; and Pfaff, D. W.: The brain as a target for steroid hormone action. *Annu. Rev. Neurosci.,* 2:65–112, 1979.

McEwen, B. S.; Pfaff, D. W.; Chaptal, C.; and Luine, V. N.: Brain cell nuclear retention of H-estradiol doses able to promost lordosis: temporal and regional aspects. *Brain Res.,* 86:155–161, 1975.

McGinnis, M. V.; Parsons, B.; Rainbow, T. C.; Krey, L. C.; and McEwen, B. S.: Temporal relationship between cell nuclear progestin receptor levels and sexual receptivity following intravenous progesterone administration. *Brain Res.,* 218:365–371, 1981.

McIntosh, T. K.; Vallano, M. L.; and Barfield, R. J.: Effects of morphine, β-endorphin and naloxone on catecholamine levels and sexual behavior in the male rat. *Pharmacol. Biochem. Behav.,* 13:435–441, 1980.

Meinkoth, J.; Quadagno, D.; and Bast, J. P.: Depression of steroid induced sex behavior in the ovariectomized rat by intracranial injection of cycloheximide: Preoptic area compared to the ventromedial hypothalamus. *Horm. Behav.,* 12:199–204, 1979.

Meller, R. E.; Keverne, E. B.; and Herbert, J.: Behavioral and endocrine effects of naltrexone in male talapoin monkeys. *Pharmacol. Biochem. Behav.,* 13:663–672, 1980.

Meyerson, B.: Latency between intravenous injection of progestins and the appearance of estrous behavior in estrogen-treated ovariectomized rats. *Horm. Behav.,* 3:1–9, 1972.

Meyerson, B. J., and Terenius, L.: β-endorphin and male sexual behavior. *Eur. J. Pharmacol.,* 42:191–192, 1977.

Modianos, D.; Hitt, J. C.; and Popolow, H. B.: Habenular lesions and feminine sexual behavior of ovariectomized rats: Diminished responsiveness to the synergistic effects of estrogen and progesterone. *J. Comp. Physiol. Psychol.,* 89:231–237, 1975.

Moguilewsky, M., and Raynaud, J.-P.: The relevance of hypothalamic and hypophyseal progestin receptor regulation in the induction and inhibition of sexual behavior in the female rat. *Endocrinology,* 105:516–522, 1979.

Money, J., and Higham, E.: Sexual behavior and endocrinology (normal and abnormal). In DeGroot, L. J.; Cahill, G. F. Jr.; Martini, L.; Nelson, D. H.; Odell, W. D.; Potts, J. T. Jr.; Steinberger, E.; and Winegrad, A. I.: (eds.): *Endocrinology,* 1st ed. Grune and Stratton, New York, 1979.

Morrell, J.; Kelley, D.; and Pfaff, D. W.: Sex steroid binding in the brains of vertebrates: Studies with light microscopic autoradiography. In Knigge, K.; Scott, D.; Kobayashi, H.; and Ishii, S.: (eds.): *Brain-Endocrine Interaction,* Vol. 2. Karger, Basel, 1975, pp. 230–256.

Morris, J. M.: The syndrome of testicular feminization in male pseudohermaphrodites. *Am. J. Obstet. Gynecol.,* 65:1192–1211, 1953.

Moss, R. L., and McCann, S. M.: Induction of mating behavior in rats by luteinizing hormone-releasing factor. *Science,* 181:177–179, 1973.

Moss, R. L., and McCann, S. M.: Action of luteinizing hormone-releasing factor (LRF) in the initiation of lordosis behavior in the estrone-primed ovariectomized rat. *Neuroendocrinology,* 17:309–318, 1975.

Moyer, K. E.: *The Psychobiology of Agression.* Harper and Row, New York, 1976.

Myers, B. M., and Baum, M. J.: Facilitation by opiate antagonists of sexual performance in the male rat. *Pharmacol. Biochem. Behav.,* 10:615–618, 1979.

Myers, B. M., and Baum, M. J.: Facilitation of copulatory performance in male rats by naloxone: effects of hypophysectomy, 17-estradiol, and luteinizing hormone releasing hormone. *Pharmacol. Biochem. Behav.,* 12:365–370, 1980.

Parsons, B.; MacLusky, N. J.; Krey, L. C.; Pfaff, D. W.; and McEwen, B. S.: The temporal relationship between estrogen-inducible progestin receptors in the female rat brain and the time course of estrogen activation of mating behavior. *Endocrinology,* 107:774–779, 1980.

Parsons, B., and McEwen, B. S.: Sequential inhibition of sexual receptivity by progesterone is prevented by a protein synthesis inhibitor and is not causally related to decreased levels of hypothalamic progestin receptors in the female rat. *J. Neurosci.,* 1:527–531, 1981.

Parsons, B.; McEwen, B. S.; and Pfaff, D. W.: A discontinuous schedule of estradiol treatment is sufficient to activate progesterone-facilitated feminine reproductive behavior and to increase cytosol progestin receptor levels in the hypothalamus of the rat. *Endocrinology,* 110:613–619, 1982a.

Parsons, B.; McGinnis, M. V.; and McEwen, B. S.: Sequential inhibition by progesterone: effects on sexual receptivity and associated changes in brain cytosol progestin binding in the female rat. *Brain Res.,* 221:149–160, 1981a.

Parsons, B.; Rainbow, T. C.; MacLusky, N. J.; and McEwen, B. S.: Progestin receptor levels in rat hypothalamic and limbic nuclei. *J. Neurosci.,* 2:1446–1452, 1982b.

Parsons, B.; Rainbow, T. C.; Pfaff, D. W.; and McEwen, B. S.: Oestradiol, sexual receptivity and cytosol progestin receptors in the hypothalamus. *Nature,* 292:58–59, 1981b.

Parsons, B.; Rainbow, T. C.; Pfaff, D. W.; and McEwen, B. S.: Hypothalamic protein synthesis essential for the activation of the lordosis reflex in the female rat. *Endocrinology,* 110:620–624, 1982c.

Persky, H.; Charney, N.; Lief, H. I.; O'Brien, C. P.; Miller, W. R.; and Strauss, D.: The relationship of plasma estradiol level to sexual behavior in young women. *Psychosom. Med.,* 40:523–535, 1978.

Pfaff, D. W.: Uptake of estradiol-17-H in the female rat brain. An auto-radiographic study. *Endocrinology,* 82:1149–1145, 1968.

Pfaff, D. W.: Luteinizing hormone-releasing factor potentiates lordosis behavior in hypophysectomized ovariectomized female rats. *Science,* 182:1148–1149, 1973.

Pfaff, D. W., and Keiner, M.: Atlas of estradiol-concentrating cells in the central nervous system of the female rat. *J. Comp. Neurol.,* 151:121–158, 1973.

Powers, J. B., and Moreines, J.: Progesterone: examination of its postulated inhibitory actions on lordosis during the rat estrus cycle. *Physiol. Behav.,* 17:492–498, 1976.

Quandagno, D. M., and Ho, G. K.: The reversible inhibition of steroid-induced sexual behavior by intracranial cycloheximide. *Horm. Behav.,* 6:19–26, 1975.

Rainbow, T. C.; Davis, P. G.; and McEwen, B. S.: Anisomycin inhibits the activation of sexual behavior by estradiol and progesterone. *Brain Res.,* 194:548–555, 1981.

Rainbow, T. C.; DeBroff, V.; Luine, V. N.; and McEwen, B. S.: Estradiol-17 increases the number of muscarinic receptors in hypothalamic nuclei. *Brain Res.,* 198:239–243, 1980.

Rainbow, T. C.; McGinnis, M. V.; Davis, P. G.; and McEwen, B. S.: Application of anisomycin to the lateral ventromedial nucleus of the hypothalamus inhibits the activation of sexual behavior by estradiol and progesterone. *Brain Res.,* 233 417–423, 1982a.

Rainbow, T. C.; Parsons, B.; MacLusky, N. J.; and McEwen, B. S.: Estradiol receptor levels in rat hypothalamic and limbic nuclei. *J. Neurosci.,* 2:1439–1445, 1982b.

Reiter, E. O.; Grumbach, M. M.; Caplan, S. L.; and Conte, F. A.: The response of pituitary gonadotrophs to synthetic LRF in children with glucocorticoid-treated congenital adrenal hyperplasia: lack of effect of intrauterine and neonatal androgen excess. *J. Clin. Endocrinol. Metab.,* 40:318–325, 1975.

Riskind, P., and Moss, R. L.: Midbrain central grey: LHRH infusion enhances lordotic behavior in estrogen-primed ovariectomized rats. *Brain Res. Bull.,* 4:203–205, 1979.

Rubin, B. S., and Barfield, R. J.: Priming of estrous responsiveness by implants of 17-estradiol in the ventromedial hypothalamic nucleus of female rats. *Endocrinology,* 106:504–509, 1980.

Rubin, B. S., and Barfield, R. J.: Progesterone in the ventromedial hypothalamus facilitates estrous behavior in ovariectomized, estrogen-primed rats. *Endocrinology,* 113:797–805, 1983.

Sakuma, Y., and Pfaff, D. W.: Effects of LHRH and antibody to LHRH infused in central grey on lordosis behavior in female rats. *Nature,* 283:566–567, 1980.

Sakuma, Y., and Pfaff, D. W.: Modulation of the lordosis reflex of female rats by LHRH, its antiserum and analogs in the mesencephalic central grey. *Neuroendocrinoly,* 36:218–224, 1983.

Sar, M., and Stumpf, W. E.: Neurons of the hypothalamus concentrate H-progesterone or its metabolites. *Science,* 182:1266–1268, 1973.

Shivers, B. D.; Harlan, R. E.; and Pfaff, D. W.: Immunocytochemical mapping of immunoreactive prolactin in female rat brain. *Abstracts, Soc. Neurosci.,* 9:1018, 1983a.

Shivers, B. D.; Harlan, R. E.; Morrell, J. I.; and Pfaff, D. W.: Absence of oestradiol concentration in cell nuclei of LHRH-immunoreactive neurons. *Nature,* 304:345–347, 1983b.

Shivers, B. D.; Harlan, R. E.; Morrell, J. I.; and Pfaff, D. W.: Immunocytochemical localization of luteinizing hormone-releasing hormone in male and female rat brain: quantitative studies on the effect of gonadal steroids. *Neuroendocrinoly,* 36:1–12, 1983c.

Sirinathsinghji, D. J. S.; Whittington, P. E.; Audsley, A.; and Fraser, H. M.: $\beta$-endorphin regulates lordosis in female rats by modulating LHRH release. *Nature,* 301:62–64, 1983.

Smith, M. S.; Freeman, M. E.; and Neill, J D.: The control of progestin secretion during the estrous cycle and early pseudopregnancy in the rat: prolactin gonadotropin and steroid levels associated with resue of the corpus luteum of pseudopregnancy *Endocrinology,* 96:219–226, 1975.

Sodersten, P.; Eneroth, P.; and Hansen, S.: Induction of sexual receptivity in ovariectomized rats by pulse administration of oestradiol-17. *J. Endocrol.,* 89:55–62, 1981.

Sodersten, P.; Henning, M.; Melin, P.; and Ludin, S.: Vasopressin alters female sexual behavior by acting on the brain independently of alterations in blood pressure. *Nature,* 301:608–610, 1983.

Spitz, C. J.; Gold, A. R.; and Adams, D. B.: Cognitive and hormonal factors affecting coital frequency. *Arch. Sex. Behav.,* 4:249–264, 1975.

Stumpf, W. E.: Estradiol-concentrating neurons topography in the hypothalamus by dry mount autoradiography. *Science,* 162:1001–1003, 1968.

Tennet, B. J.; Smith, E. R.; and Davidson, J. M.: The effects of estrogen and progesterone on female rat proceptive behavior. *Horm. Behav.,* 14:65–75, 1980.

Terkel, A. S.; Shryne, J.; and Gorski, R. A.: Inhibition of estrogen facilitation of sexual behavior by the intracerebral influence of actinomycin D. *Horm. Behav.,* 4:377–386, 1973.

Toubeau, G.; Desclin, J.; Parmentier, M.; and Pasteels, J. L.: Cellular localization of a prolactin-like antigen in the rat brain. *J. Endocrinol.,* 83:261–266, 1979.

Turner, H. H.: A syndrome of infantilism, congenital webbed neck, and cubitus valgus. *Endocrinology,* 23:566, 1938.

Vermeulen, A., and Verdonck, L.: Plasma androgen levels during the menstrual cycle. *Am. J. Obstet. Gynecol.,* 125:491–494, 1976.

Walter, R.; van Ree, J. M.; and deWied, D.: Modification of conditioned behavior of rats by neurohypophyseal hormones and analogues. *Proc. Natl. Acad. Sci., USA,* 5:2493–2496, 1978.

Warembourg, M.: Uptake of H-labeled synthetic progestin by rat brain and pituitary. A radiographic study. *Neurosci. Lett.,* 7:1–8, 1978.

Ydstebo, R., and Sodersten, P.: Induction of sexual receptivity in ovariectomized female rats by subcutaneous implants of estradiol-17. *Horm. Behav.,* 9:130–140, 1977.

Zucker, I.: Facilitatory and inhibitory effects of progesterone on sexual responses of spayed guinea pigs. *J. Comp. Physiol. Psychol.,* 62:376–381, 1966.

# CHAPTER 10  CONTRACEPTION AND PSYCHOSEXUAL FUNCTION

*Roger C. Toffle, M.D., and George E. Tagatz, M.D.*

## INTRODUCTION

Unwanted pregnancy and sexually transmitted diseases are only two of many deterrents to the uninhibited pursuit of sexual gratification. Pregnancy can be prevented with variable success by utilizing contraception, but the decision to use contraception and the choice of contraceptive method present a dilemma for many women. The apparently simple decision to interfere with the biological processes required to achieve pregnancy is affected by many of the same variables that affect the decision to engage in sexual activity: cultural heritage, religious commitment, educational experience, and emotional status. In turn, the utilization of contraception has the potential of altering one's sexual expression and behavior within society. We intend to explore the evidence linking hormonal events, sociocultural experience, and psychological circumstances with contraception and the expression of human sexuality.

## SEXUAL EXPRESSION

### HORMONAL INFLUENCES ON ANIMAL SEXUAL BEHAVIOR

In contrast to observed human conduct, animal behavior is characterized by periodic sexual activity. Changes in the concentration of sexual hormones have been implicated as the stimuli primarily responsible for this periodicity. Sexual behavior has been analysed in relation to attractivity (perceived value), proceptivity (appetite for sexual contact), and receptivity (consummation of sexual encounter) (Beach, 1976). Rats and mice demonstrate heightened sexual receptivity at estrus; as a result of similar observations in other non-human mammals, attempts have been made to elucidate the relationship of specific hormones to sexual behavior (Ford and Beach, 1951).

**Estrogen.** As anticipated from the association of increased concentration of estrogen with estrus, the administration of exogenous estrogen to female rhesus monkeys increased proceptive and receptive behavior (Beach, 1976). Replacement of estrogen deficiency induced by ovariectomy also restored attractivity in female rhesus monkeys (Michael and Keverne, 1968).

**Progesterone.** Rhesus monkeys exhibited no change in attractivity (frequency of mounting) in relation to changes in the phase of the menstrual cycle, but the mean number of ejaculations was decreased during the luteal phase (Michael and Zumpe, 1970). After estrogen therapy restored attractivity in ovariectomized monkeys, the administration of exogenous progesterone diminished this response (Baum *et al.*, 1976; Michael and Keverne, 1968).

**Androgens.** Baum observed that androgens modified proceptivity and receptivity in female primates (Baum et al., 1977). Androgens may affect sexuality indirectly since androgens are transformed into estrogens by aromatization at peripheral sites. Beyer and coworkers (1970) found that only those androgens which could be converted into estrogens were capable of inducing estrus and increased sexual activity in female rabbits.

**Pheromones.** The observation that male rhesus monkeys rendered anosmic failed to initiate sexual activity until olfaction was restored suggests that pheromones might influence sexual behavior in primates (Michael and Keverne, 1968).

## HORMONAL INFLUENCES ON HUMAN SEXUAL BEHAVIOR

In the ovulating human female, the concentrations of hormones associated with reproduction exhibit predictable changes. During the perimenstrual (early follicular) phase, the estrogen (estradiol and estrone) and progesterone concentrations are low and the androgen (testosterone and androstenedione) concentrations are baseline. In the periovulatory phase at midcycle, estradiol, and to a lesser extent, estrone rise to peak concentrations, androgens exhibit a slight increase, and progesterone begins to be secreted. The luteal phase, which follows, is characterized by high levels of both estrogens and progesterone and concentrations of androgens which are not significantly different from those present during the first half of the cycle (Speroff et al., 1983).

**Estrogen, Progesterone, and Androgens.** Numerous studies have attempted to correlate altered human sexual behavior with changes in the concentrations of reproductive hormones. Many studies have purportedly observed increased human sexual activity at one or more phases of the menstrual cycle (Adams et al., 1978; Cavanagh, 1969; Davis, 1926; Hart, 1960; Hite, 1977; McCance et al., 1937; Spitz et al., 1975; Udry and Morris, 1968). These studies have been criticized for defects in study design which included errors of patient selection, failure to utilize rigorous definitions of behavior, inadequate data collection, indirect measurements of hormone concentrations as inferred from cycle phase, failure to recognize the role of the sexual partner, and errors of statistical analysis (Adams et al., 1978; James, 1971; Kolodny and Bauman, 1979; Persky et al., 1979; Schreiner-Engel, 1980; Schreiner-Engel et al., 1981).

The sources of bias in study design and interpretation are illustrated by the following examples. The lack of validity of retrospective studies was shown by Englander-Golden and colleagues (1980), who found that retrospective recall of sexual activity did not correlate with the patterns of behavior noted in daily logs.

Studies utilizing subjective reports are prejudiced by anticipating expected events and inappropriate interpretation of physiological responses. Ruble (1977) altered women's perception of their cycle phase by deluding them into believing that the onset of the next menses could be predicted by a—simulated—EEG. Although all were in the same phase of the menstrual cycle, those women who believed that menses was imminent reported a higher incidence of premenstrual symptoms than those who perceived the onset of menses as being remote.

Apparently objective studies employing vaginal plethysmography utilize recordings of vaginal pulse pressure and blood volumes as the sign of physiological response to psychosexual arousal. However, this monitored response is dissociated from conscious awareness of arousal (defined by reports of subjective feelings) in some subjects (Heiman, 1975). Other studies utilizing plethysmographic recordings have demonstrated changes consistent with sexual arousal in 95 percent of REM sleep cycles (Fisher et al., 1983). Studies reporting subjective awareness of dream content did not suggest that sexual themes were so commonly encountered during sleep (Lewis and Burns, 1975; Swanson and Foulkes, 1968). In addition to the previous demonstration of dissociation between the physiological state and intellectual perception, an additional study demonstrated the dissociation of perception and reporting (Wincze et al., 1977). Wincze observed women's responses to a series of erotic scenes in which some of the pictures depicted behavior expected to be socioculturally taboo. With regard to these scenes, subjective reports of arousal and measurements of vaginal blood flow were often discordant. Schreiner-Engel and coworkers (1981) found that objective plethysmographic changes and subjective reports of arousal has no observable correlation with changes in the serum concentrations of estrogens, progesterone, and testosterone obtained by direct measurement. In addition to the apparent difficulties posed for the validation of subjective reports of arousal, it is possible that the physiological standard, changes in vaginal blood flow, may result from multiple and diverse stimuli, not all of which are sexual.

The majority of human studies show no correlation between fluctuations in the serum concentrations of estrogen and progesterone and sexual behavior, as long as these hormone concentrations remain in the ranges observed in the ovulatory female. Although several studies suggest that increased concentrations of testosterone in the female are associated with increased sexual activity, this is not a consistent finding (Ablanalp et al., 1979; Carney et al., 1978; Daniels, 1943; McCauley and Ehrhardt, 1976; Persky et al., 1976, 1978a, 1978b, 1982; Schreiner-Engel et al., 1981). It is not unexpected that significant deficiencies of estrogen and androgen are associated with decreased sexual activity in the female and that appropriate hormonal replacement restores sexual interest (Davidson et al., 1979; Dennerstein et al., 1980; Perloff, 1949; Salamies et al., 1982; Waxenberg et al., 1959).

**Pheromones.** Several findings suggest that pheromones and olfaction figure significantly in human sexual activity. Humans are capable of distinguishing the odors of specific steroids (Kloeck, 1961) and women demonstrate cyclic changes in their ability to detect synthetic musk-like odors (Vierling and Rock, 1967). In a study of sexual response to testosterone replacement, the wives' reports of sexual desire correlated directly with the husbands' serum concentrations of testosterone (Persky et al., 1978a). Cyclic changes have also been observed in the content of volatile fatty acids in the human vagina (Michael et al., 1974). A group of couples increased the frequency of coitus when vaginal secretions rather than control substances were applied to the wife's chest (Morris and Udry, 1975).

### INFLUENCE OF SEXUAL BEHAVIOR ON HORMONES

The possibility that human sexual activity may directly influence hormonal levels is not compelling. Specific attempts have been made to correlate a preovulatory surge of the luteinizing hormone (LH) with coitus as is found in those animals which exhibit reflex ovulation. Morris and coworkers (1977) found that sexual intercourse did not influence the concentrations of LH in married couples. Clark and Zarrow (1971) cited investigators who have shown that conception can occur after rape during all phases of the menstrual cycle. Others have noted that women with regular sexual contact are more likely to have regular menstrual cycles and that sporadic sexual contact is associated with menstrual irregularity (Cutler et al., 1979, 1980). However, this observation fails to delineate cause and effect.

### NONHORMONAL INFLUENCES ON SEXUAL BEHAVIOR

Since hormonal changes do not alter sexual activity, it follows that nonhormonal factors are of primary importance.

**Age.** The age of initial coitus has steadily decreased; by age 19 over 50 percent of females have engaged in sexual intercourse (Freeman, et al., 1980; Zelnik and Kantner, 1976).

**Social Encounters.** Women's reports of sexual arousal were related to the type of heterosexual encounter experienced that day (Spitz et al., 1975).

**Socioeconomic Status.** Although in 1953 Kinsey found that socioeconomic status correlated directly with the occurrence of premarital coitus, studies of the contemporary population have blurred this distinction (Zelnik and Kantner, 1977).

**Religion.** In 1953 Kinsey could and in 1973 Kantner and Zelnick could correlate religious denomination, degree of fundamentalism, and the frequency of church attendance with the frequency of coital activity. Barrett (1980) found that religious variables had a more predictable effect on sexual behavior in 1968 than ten years later in 1978.

**Sexual Education.** Family relationships are the primary influence affecting the socialization and sexual expression of the individual. In families which disapprove of premarital coitus, it is found that identification with the parental value system coupled with open communication with the parents served as the principal deterrent to engaging in sexual activity (Kantner and Zelnick, 1973; Miller, 1976). Children of parents who support or encourage sexual activity are much more likely to have premarital intercourse (Davis, 1974).

**Psychosocial Factors.** Self-image, like physical attractiveness, is not a reliable predictor of sexual involvement. It appears that self-expression, self-fulfillment, and self-control, as well as control and commitment within a sexual relationship are interdependent variables which defy meaningful analysis (Campbell and Barnlund, 1977; Strahle, 1983).

**Educational Career.** Aspirations for a competitive career requiring extensive education discourage sexual involvement. Contrarily, women who perceive the establishment of a family as a primary goal are more likely to engage in sexual intercourse (Strahle, 1983).

## INFLUENCES AFFECTING CONTRACEPTIVE CHOICE AND USE

### HORMONAL INFLUENCES

Since hormonal influences are not the primary stimulus-controlling sexual interest, they would not be expected to affect the decision to utilize contraception. However, hormonal status and regularity of ovulation may be the most significant factors in the selection of method. As examples, the woman with regular ovulatory cycles is more likely to choose and be successful with symptothermic methods, and the anovulatory or irregularly ovulatory woman with androgen excess is a prime candidate for oral contraception.

### NONHORMONAL INFLUENCES AFFECTING USE

**Socioeconomic Status, Academic Achievement, Geographical Location.** The use of contraception is directly related to increasing socioeconomic status, particularly when status is associated with higher levels of parental education (Kantner and Zelnick, 1973). A college education and aspirations for a successful career also have been associated with a higher likelihood of using contraception (Strahle, 1983). Although the level of education is more important than the location of residence, women with a rural background are less likely to use contraception (Kantner and Zelnick, 1973).

**Religion.** In one recent study, contraception was elected more frequently by women of Catholic and Jewish faiths than by members of a fundamentalist Protestant religion (Mosher, 1981). Regular church attendance is associated with increased use of contraception by blacks, but decreased use of contraception by whites (Kantner and Zelnick, 1973).

**Education and Psychology.** Miller (1976) found that women were more likely to elect and to use contraceptives effectively when their mother provided the initial useful contraceptive counseling. Women who believe that pregnancy is not very likely to result from infrequent sexual intercourse, and those who believe that contraception will interfere with sexual pleasure, rarely use contraceptive techniques. Miller explored the relationship of awareness of the objective risk of pregnancy and the perceived anxiety concerning the risk to the utilization of contraception. High objective risk assessment coupled with moderate anxiety were associated with frequent contraceptive use. Women who perceived the risk of pregnancy to be minimal and who experienced little anxiety were unlikely to use contraception. Paradoxically, women with very high levels of anxiety rarely used contraception because of a "sense of powerlessness."

Other psychometric characteristics appear to be associated with the use of contraception. Effective contraceptors have good ego strength, a high degree of self-esteem, good problem-solving ability, and they are oriented to future accomplishments. Poor contraceptors tend to idealize but are less effective in interpersonal relationships, are often impulsive, and frequently have negative expectations of future events (Campbell and Barnlund, 1977; Harvey, 1976; Herold et al., 1979; Joe et al., 1979; Keller and Sack, 1982; Miller, 1976; Mindick et al., 1977; Steinlauf, 1979).

PARTNER INFLUENCES

Although males often initiate sexual intercourse at a younger age than females (Finkel and Finkel, 1975), young males are less likely to recognize the associated risk of pregnancy. It has been found that males are less knowledgeable about contraception than their female classmates, despite exposure to similar programs of sexual instruction in school. The lack of awareness among young males has been attributed to the rarity of primary or reinforcing education from family members (Freeman et al., 1980). One can surmise that a relationship requiring the male to make contraceptive decisions is more likely to result in unprotected intercourse.

NONHORMONAL INFLUENCES AFFECTING CHOICE OF CONTRACEPTIVE METHOD

In addition to the factors which influence the decision to utilize contraception, the choice of method is also influenced by age, socioeconomic status, health condition, and lifestyle of the woman. Developing sexual relationships are characterized by evolving contraceptive choices and the contraceptive regimen chosen within mature relationships is influenced by family size. The selection and availability of a method may require the interposition of a physician or other healthcare provider. Communications media also have affected contraceptive choice.

**Maturity of Relationship.** Miller (1976) observed an evolving sequence of contraceptive behavior in sexual relationships: Complete or partial abstinence and withdrawal were commonly used in new relationships. Subsequently, more effective nonprescription methods such as foam and condoms were employed. Finally the couples used the most effective prescription methods, such as oral contraceptives and intrauterine devices. This progression of contraceptive sophistication was associated with an enhancement of the relationship as subjectively perceived by the participants.

**Socioeconomic Status, Race, Education.** Mosher (1981) observed that white women of high socioeconomic status and black women of low socioeconomic status were more likely than others to use effective contraception. Among those women choosing effective contraceptive methods, black women consistently selected oral contraceptives more frequently than did white women (Mosher, 1981).

Postcoital contraception was requested most frequently by nulligravid, highly educated, affluent white women at a Philadelphia family planning clinic during the 1970s (Rosenfeld et al., 1976).

**Religion.** Although of decreasing significance, religious affiliation continues to play an important role in the choice of contraceptive method. During 1976, Catholics used the rhythm method twice as frequently as did Protestants, although this ratio was seven to one in 1965. Sterilization or permanent contraception is elected more frequently by Protestants than Catholics (Mosher, 1981).

**Life style.** Despite the popularity of oral contraceptives among most women, female runners rarely choose this method (Jarrett and Spellacy, 1983).

**Age.** Women entering the fourth decade of life elect the more efficient methods of contraception. These women are generally better informed about increasing medical risks associated with pregnancy and perceive an increased potential for personal inconvenience as a result of an unplanned pregnancy. In 1976, sterilization was the most common method of contraception selected by women between the ages of 30 and 44 (Mosher, 1981).

**Family Size.** Although marked individual differences exist in personal preferences for family size, sterilization was elected seven times more frequently by couples with four or more children than those with one or two children (Gavin, 1979).

**Health Care Provider.** The health care provider ideally assumes the roles of evaluator, educator, and advisor prior to recommending a specific method. To the multiple factors which will affect personal choice, the physician is obliged to add those conditions of medical health which will affect this choice. The interposition of a third party also introduces the religious, social, and psychological attitudes of the health care provider. Since the most effective contraceptives must be prescribed or implemented by a physician, this requirement limits the availability of these methods (Gavin, 1979). Miller (1976) found that many women did not consider effective forms of contraception because of fears associated with the required medical examination.

**Communications Media.** The decrease in the use of oral contraceptives after 1976 was clearly related to the widespread dissemination of adverse publicity at that time. Gavin (1979) notes that those patients least able to cope with problems were most likely to respond to sensational news reports, and, therefore, were most likely to discontinue the use of oral contraceptives.

## CONTRACEPTIVE METHODS

Contraceptive methods have been classified as coital-dependent, coital-independent, and postcoital. Withdrawal, rhythm with or without symptothermic charting, and physical and chemical barriers are coital-dependent. Coital-independent methods include intrauterine devices (IUD), hormonal regimens, and surgical procedures for male and female sterilization. Hormonal regimens and the IUD are used as postcoital contraceptives.

### COITAL-DEPENDENT METHODS

Coital-dependent contraception focuses on the act of intercourse. The methods include the elimination of exposure during the fertile phase of the cycle or the prevention of sperm entry into the vagina or cervix.

**Abstinence.** Abstinence has been classified as absolute, partial, and periodic. Only the latter categories are applicable to the couple having coitus. Withdrawal, or partial abstinence, involves removal of the penis from the vagina immediately prior to ejaculation. The presence of sperm within pre-ejaculatory secretions and difficulty in timing effective withdrawal, together with inhibition of psychological gratification result in as high as a 25 percent failure rate with this method (Hatcher et al., 1980).

Periodic abstinence, or the rhythm method, requires the couple to avoid intercourse during the fertile phase of the menstrual cycle. Specific methods include: (1) the sole use of a calculated safe interval determined from the duration of preceding cycles and the assumption that ovulation precedes a 14-day luteal phase; and (2) the symptothermal methods, which employ evaluation of the cervix and cervical mucus together with the changes in the basal body temperature to modify the equation, arriving at the time of predicted ovulation. Avoidance or rhythm methods are most effective when the couple has intercourse only during the luteal phase, beginning a few days after apparent ovulation and ceasing with the onset of menses. As the result of significant differences in knowledge and motivation, the success of rhythm methods ranges from failure rates of one to 25 percent (Hatcher et al., 1980; The Couple to Couple League, 1981).

Adverse medical complications have not resulted from the use of abstinence methods. The commitment and motivation of both participants are required to achieve pregnancy prevention and emotional satisfaction.

**Barrier Methods.** Barrier methods include physical and chemical barriers designed to deny access of the spermatozoa to the site of fertilization in the upper reproductive tract of the female or to destroy the reproductive potential of the spermatozoa. Physical barriers include the condom, diaphragm, cervical cap, and contraceptive sponge. Chemical spermicides are marketed as creams and jellies. Physical and chemical barriers are commonly used in combination and are most effective when used together. The sponge, condom, and spermicides may be obtained without prescription, but the diaphragm and cervical cap require a physician's prescription.

Theoretical failure rates have been calculated to be less than 3 percent, but failure rates have been as high as 25 percent (Hatcher et al., 1980). As with partial abstinence, the effective use of barriers requires education and motivation on the users' parts.

Barrier methods have much to recommend their use. They are relatively easy to use and are associated with a decreased incidence of sexually transmitted diseases (Berberian et al., 1959; Berger et al., 1975; Postic et al., 1978). Untoward reactions are essentially limited to occasional chemical vaginitis. The mortality rates attributed to barrier methods are the lowest observed for any active method of contraception, even when the method-failure complications of elective abortions and pregnancy related conditions are considered (Tietze, 1976).

## Noncoital Dependent Methods

Noncoital dependent methods are the most effective mode of contraception and permit sexual spontaneity by dissociating the contraceptive regimen from the isolated act of coitus. Hormonal regimens and the use of the IUD are temporary noncoital dependent methods; male and female sterilization procedures are considered to be permanent since they may not be reversible.

**IUD.** Intrauterine devices have been marketed with several design configurations, and one type has copper added to enhance its effectiveness. The IUD is placed into the endometrial cavity and prevents implantation of the pre-embryo by altering tubal motility and endometrial physiology (Hatcher et al., 1980). Use–failure rates of the IUD are approximately 5 percent (Hatcher et al., 1980; Keith et al., 1982). Users of IUD's experience a low mortality rate but serious morbidity consists of uterine perforation and an increased likelihood of ectopic pregnancy, pelvic inflammatory disease, and septic abortion. Menorrhagia, intermenstrual spotting, and dysmenorrhea may be of enough significance to prompt removal of the IUD (Nagel, 1983).

**Hormonal Contraceptives.** Hormonal regimens provide the greatest degree of contraceptive protection. Only the oral contraceptives and injectable progestins utilized by women are of practical significance.

Oral contraceptives are currently marketed in combined estrogen–progestin and progestin-only preparations. The primary contraceptive effect of combination oral contraceptives is the inhibition of ovulation resulting from suppression of the secretion of pituitary gonadotropins (Bronson, 1981; Goldzieher et al., 1970; Spellacy et al., 1980). Periodic injections of medroxyprogesterone acetate also inhibit ovulation by the same mechanism. Oral preparations containing only progestins in low doses have a variable effect on ovulation and are less effective than the combination types. Progestin-only regimens change the composition and amount of cervical mucus and alter the histology and function of the endometrium and fallopian tubes.

Combination oral contraceptive regimens have a theoretical use–failure rate of about one percent and study subjects can achieve similar rates of use-effectiveness, but failure of compliance among routinely motivated populations accounts for use–failure rates in the range 4 to 10 percent (Hatcher et al., 1980). The regimen utilizing the injection of depo-medroxyprogesterone acetate (DMPA) at 90-day intervals has a use–failure rate similar to the theoretical failure rate of one percent. Oral administration of low dosage progestin-only preparations is associated with a use–failure rate of about 5 percent, which is similar to that of the IUD (Hatcher et al., 1980).

Combination oral contraceptives have many beneficial effects. Withdrawal bleeding is predictable and regular, and the amount of withdrawal flow is reduced so that users are less likely to develop iron-deficiency anemia. Oral contraceptive users have a decreased likelihood of having an ectopic pregnancy or developing pelvic inflammatory disease. The incidence of malignancies of the endometrium and ovary is reduced in oral contraceptive users. The relationship to breast cancer and cervical dysplasia remains unsettled. However, benign ovarian and breast diseases are less likely to occur in oral contraceptive users (Center for Disease Control Cancer and Steroid Hormone Study, 1983; Pike et al., 1983; *Population Reports*, 1982; Rosenfield, 1983; Swan and Brown, 1981; Vessey et al., 1983b).

The incidence of adverse reactions associated with the use of oral contraceptives is extremely low, but the serious complications are devastating. It appears that most of the vascular complications occur in smokers or other high-risk groups with pre-existing medical conditions such as hypertension, diabetes mellitus, hyperlipidemia, and advancing age. Serious complications include cerebrovascular accidents (strokes), myocardial infarctions, and venous thromboembolism. The development of gallbladder disease, hypertension, and hepatocellular adenomas has been associated with the duration of use (Rosenfield, 1983).

As of this writing, possible relationship between injectable DMPA and breast cancer has not been definitively excluded and is the reason that DMPA has not been sanctioned for use as a contraceptive by the U.S. Federal Drug Administration (Liang et al., 1983).

As for male contraceptives, hormonal regimens designed to inhibit spermatogenesis have the untoward effect of concomitantly inhibiting testosterone production with consequent suppression of libido and potency. More subtle efforts to inhibit epididymal functions and alter spermatozoal functions have not been acceptable for clinical application (Bremner and Dekrester, 1976; Darney, 1982).

**Male and Female Sterilization.** Vasectomy in the male and tubal ligation in the female are surgical procedures that prevent the delivery of the sperm or ovum and are equally effective, but permanent, forms of contraception.

Both procedures have use–failure rates of about .5 percent (Hatcher et al., 1980). The surgical procedures are occasionally complicated by infection and bleeding and, on rare occasion, surgical mortality. Premature atherosclerosis has been observed after vasectomy in monkeys, but the complication has not been documented in human males (Alexander and Clarkson, 1978; Alexander and Anderson, 1979; Goldacre et al., 1978; Walker et al., 1981; Wallace et al., 1981). Although Donnez and Jackson noted that some groups of women have an increased incidence of menstrual dysfunction after tubal ligation (Donnez et al., 1981; Jackson and Lander, 1980), such an increase was not observed in two studies of large populations (Destefano et al., 1983; Vessey et al., 1983a).

Surgical procedures are required to reverse the consequences of prior sterilization, and the success rate is variable. The development of antispermatozoal antibodies may affect the outcome despite successful surgical reversal of vasectomy.

**Postcoital Methods.** Hormonal regimens utilizing high doses of estrogens alone or in combination with progestin and intrauterine devices have been used as postcoital contraceptives. Since the goal is to prevent implantation after fertilization has occurred, therapy must be instituted within a few days after the coital event. Hormonal regimens are expected to be effective if instituted within 3 days (72h) after coital exposure and IUD's may be effective if instituted as late as 7 days after coitus (Chez and Yuzpe, 1982). Yuzpe (1979) studied 152 patients who were treated with hormonal regimens after midcycle coitus and observed only one pregnancy, although 12 to 30 pregnancies were expected to occur without treatment. The high doses of estrogen and progestin commonly induce nausea and vomiting. Although the IUD may induce any of the complications previously noted, the usual problem of short-term use is limited to abnormal bleeding.

To assess the effectiveness of postcoital contraception a physician may monitor women with serial assays of human chorionic gonadotropin (HCG) and offer menstrual extraction if pregnancy occurs.

## EFFECTS OF CONTRACEPTION ON PSYCHOSEXUAL FUNCTION

It is generally agreed that the use of any of the currently available contraceptive methods does not significantly alter libido. Advocates of natural family planning methods state that the method used has the added advantage of improving the marital relationship because of increased mutual respect and communication, peace of conscience, relief from sexual satiation or boredom, freedom from worry about complications associated with other contraceptive methods, and the necessity of developing nongenital methods for expressing love and affection (Couple to Couple League, 1981).

### COITAL-RELATED CONTRACEPTION AND THE IUD

Coital activity must be avoided during the periovulatory interval for rhythm methods to be effective. Women using coital-related techniques and the IUD have been observed to increase their sexual activity during the periovulatory phase; to the contrary their male partners are less likely to initiate sexual activity at midcycle (Adams et al., 1978). In addition, Adams and colleagues (1978) found that women using the IUD exhibited an increase in the frequency of masturbation and sexual fantasies during the periovulatory phase.

### NONCOITAL DEPENDENT METHODS

**Hormonal Regimens.** Gambrell and colleagues (1976) observed an improvement of libido but no change in orgasmic potential or enjoyment among single women using oral contraceptives (Morris and Udry, 1971). Despite the suspicion lingering from experiments among animals, Cullberg (1972) could relate no change in libido to increasing doses of progestins in oral contraceptives. Although a causal relationship has not been demonstrated, a few women develop psychological depression while taking oral contraceptives; in these women a loss of libido is a concomitant of the depression (Herzberg et al., 1971; Mathew and Weinman, 1982).

Coital activity is probably not significantly affected by the use of oral contraceptives. Studies by Morris and Udry (1971) and the Adams group (1978) report no change in the frequency of coitus; Westoff and coworkers (1969) observed an increase, and Gambrell's study (1976) found that sexual activity increased or decreased according to the specific population studied. Gambrell and colleagues observed that sexual activity increased more frequently than it decreased among single users, but married users were equally likely to increase or decrease coital frequency.

In the male, loss of libido and potency are the principal reasons for the failure to develop an acceptable method of hormonal contraception (Bremner and DeKretser, 1976).

**Male and Female Sterilization.** Studies by Vessey and Jackson found that for women tubal ligation resulted in no significant change in sexual activity (Jackson and Lander, 1980; Vessey et al., 1983a).

Men who have had vasectomies exhibit no change in coital frequency, sexual dysfunction, extramarital affairs, or divorce, although Ziegler and coworkers (1966) suggested that vasectomy has an adverse effect upon marital satisfaction and adjustment (Dias, 1983; Rodgers and Ziegler, 1968).

### POSTCOITAL CONTRACEPTION

A study of 120 women presenting for postcoital contraception were found to suffer transiently from anxiety, guilt, and depression. These symptoms were markedly diminished when they returned two weeks later for follow-up (Huggins et al., 1979). Unfortunately, they were not re-evaluated at a later date to determine lasting effects on libido and sexual activity.

## CONCLUSION

Three major findings emerging from this study are: (1) Nonhormonal cues are the predominant determinants of human sexual behavior during the reproductive years. (2) The decision to utilize contraception and the choice of method are also primarily conditioned by cultural, social, educational, and psychological factors. Hormonal dysfunctions and other medical diseases are important considerations in the selection of contraceptive method. (3) Currently available contraceptive methods do not appreciably alter human psychosexual function, with the exception of the rhythm method which requires periodic abstinence to be effective.

## REFERENCES

Ablanalp, J. M.; Rose, R. M.; Donnelly, A. F.; and Livingston-Vaughn, L.: Psychoendocrinology of the menstrual cycle: The relationship between enjoyment of activities moods, and reproductive hormones. *Psychosom. Med.*, 41:605–614, 1979.

Adams, D. B.; Gold, A. R.; and Burt, A. D.: Rise in female initiated sexual activity at ovulation and its suppression by oral contraceptives. *N. Engl. J. Med.*, 299:1145–1150, 1978.

Alexander, N. J. Anderson, D. J.: Vasectomy: Consequences of autoimmunity to sperm antigens. *Fertil. Steril.*, 32:253–260, 1979.

Alexander, N. J. and Clarkson, T. B.: Vasectomy increases the severity of diet-induced atherosclerosis in Macaca fasicularis. *Science*, 201:538–541, 1978.

Barrett, F. M.: Sexual experience, birth control usage, and sex education of unmarried canadian university students: Changes between 1968 and 1978. *Arch. Sex. Behav.*, 9:367–390, 1980.

Baum, M. J.; Everitt, B. J.; Herbert, J.; and Keverne, E. B.: Suppression of sexual interaction in rhesus monkeys by intravaginal administration of progesterone to the female. *Nature*, 263:606–608, 1976.

Baum, M. J.; Everitt, B. J.; Herbert, J.; and Keverne, E. B.: Hormonal basis of proceptivity and receptivity in female primates. *Arch. Sex. Behav.*, 6:173–192, 1977.

Beach, F. A.: Sexual attractivity, proceptivity, and receptivity in female mammals. *Horm. Behav.*, 7:105–138, 1976.

Berberian, D. A.; Coulston, F.; and Slighter, R. G.: Laboratory evaluation of a new contraceptive gel with trichomonadicidal and moniliastatic properties. *Toxicol. Appl. Pharmacol.*, 1:366–376, 1959.

Berger, G. S.; Keith, L.; and Moss, W.: Prevalence of gonorrhea among women using various methods of contraception. *Br. J. Vener. Dis.*, 51 307–309, 1975.

Beyer, C.; Vidal, N.; and Mijares, A.: Probable role of aromatization in the induction of estrus behavior by androgens in the ovariectomized rabbit. *Endocrinology*, 87:1386–1389, 1970.

Bremner, W. J., and De Kretser, D. M.: The prospects for new, reversible male contraceptives. *N. Engl. J. Med.*, 295:1111–1117, 1976.

Bronson, R. A.: Oral contraception: Mechanism of action. *Clin. Obstet. Gynecol.*, 24:869–877, 1981.

Campbell, B. K., and Barnlund, D. C.: Communication style: A clue to unplanned pregnancy. *Med. Care*, 15:181–186, 1977.

Carney, A.; Bancroft, J.; and Mathews, A : Combination of hormonal and psychological treatment for female sexual unresponsiveness: A comparative study. *Brit. J. Psychiatr.* 132:339–346, 1978.

Cavanagh, J. R.: Rhythm of sexual desire in women. *Med. Aspects Hum. Sex.*, 3:29–39, 1969.

Chez, R. A., and Yuzpe, A. A.: Postcoital contraception for unprotected intercourse. *Contemp. OB/GYN*, 20:79–84, 1982.

Clark, J. H., and Zarrow, M. X.: Influence of copulation on time of ovulation in women. *Am. J. Obstet. Gynecol.*, 109:1083–1085, 1971.

Cullberg, J.: Mood changes and menstrual symptoms with different gestagen/estrogen combinations. *Acta Psychiat. Scand.* (Suppl), 236:1–84, 1972

Cutler, W. B.; Garcia, C. R.; and Krieger, A. M. Sexual behavior frequency and menstrual cycle length in mature premenopausal women. *Neuroendocrinology*, 4:297–309, 1979.

Cutler, W. B.; Garcia, C. R.; and Kreiger, A. M.: Sporadic sexual behavior and menstrual cycle length in women. *Horm. Behav.*, 14:163–172, 1980.

Daniels, G. E.: An approach to psychological control studies of urinary sex hormones. *Am. J. Psychiatr.* 100:231–239, 1943.

Darney, P. D.: What's new in contraceptives? *Contemp. OB/GYN*, 19:81–91, 1982.

Davidson, J. M.; Camargo, C. A.; and Smith, E. R.: Effects of androgen in sexual behavior in hypogonadal men. *J. Clin. Endocrinol. Metab.*, 48:955–958, 1979.

Davis, K. B.: Periodicity of sex desire. *Am. J. Obstet. Gynecol.*, 12:824–838, 1926.

Davis, P.: Contextual sex-saliency and sexual activity: The relative effects of family and peer group in the sexual socialization process. *J. Marriage Fam*, 36:196–202, 1974.

Dennerstein, L.; Burrows, G. D.; Wood, C.; and Hyman, G.: Hormones and sexuality: Effect of estrogen and progestogen. *Obstet. Gynecol.*, 56:316–322, 1980.

Destefano, F.; Huezo, C. M.; Peterson, H. B.; Rubin, G. L.; Layde, P. M.; and Ory, H. W.: Menstrual changes after tubal sterilization. *Obstet. Gynecol.*, 62:673–681, 1983.

Dias, P. L. R.: The long-term effects of vasectomy on sexual behaviour. *Acta Psychiatr. Scand.,* 67:333–338, 1983.

Donnez, J.; Wauters, M.; and Thomas, K.: Luteal function after tubal sterilization. *Obstet. Gynecol.,* 57:65–68, 1981.

Englander-Golden, P.; Chang, H. S.; Whitmore, M. R.; and Dienstbier, R. A.: Female sexual arousal and the menstrual cycle. *J. Human Stress,* 6:42–48, 1980.

Finkel, M. L., and Finkel, D. J.: Sexual and contraceptive knowledge, attitudes and behavior of male adolescents. *Fam. Plann. Perspect.,* 7:256–260, 1975.

Fisher, C.; Cohen, H. D.; Schiavi, R. C.; Davis, D.; Furman, B.; Ward, K.; Edwards, A.; and Cunningham, J.: Patterns of female sexual arousal during sleep and waking: Vaginal thermo-conductance studies. *Arch. Sex. Behav.,* 12:97–122, 1983.

Ford, C. S., and Beach, F. A.: *Patterns of Sexual Behavior.* Harper and Row, New York, 1951.

Freeman, E. W.; Rickels, K.; Huggins, G. R.; Mudd, E. H.; Garcia, C. R.; and Dicken, H. O.: Adolescent contraceptive behavior use: Comparisons of male and female attitudes and information. *Am. J. Public Health,* 70:790–799, 1980.

Gambrell, R. D. Jr.; Bernard, D. M.; Sanders, B. I.; Vanderburg, N.; and Buxton, S. J.: Changes in sexual drives of patients on oral contraceptives. *J. Reprod. Med.,* 17:165–171, 1976.

Gavin, J.: Selecting the optimum method of contraception for each patient. *Int. J. Gynaecol. Obstet.,* 16:542–546, 1979.

Glick, B. B.; Baughman, W. L.; Jensen, J. N.; and Phoenix, C. H.: Endogenous opiate systems and primate reproduction: Inability of nalaxone to induce sexual activity in rhesus males. *Arch. Sex. Behav.,* 11:267–275, 1982.

Goldacre, M. J.; Clarke, J. A.; and Heasman, M. A.: Follow-up of vasectomy using medical record linkage. *Am. J. Epidemiol.,* 108:176–180, 1978.

Goldzieher, J. W.; Kleber, J. W.; Moses, L. E.; and Rathmacher, R. P.: A cross-sectional study of plasma FSH and LH levels in women using sequential, combination or injectable steroid contraceptives over long periods of time. *Contraception,* 2:225–248, 1970.

Hart, R. D.: Monthly rhythm of libido in married women. *Br. Med. J.,* 1:1023–1024, 1960.

Harvey, A. L.: Risky and safe contraceptors: Some personality factors. *J. Psychol.,* 92:109–112, 1976.

Hatcher, R. A.; Stewart, G. K.; Stewart, F.; Guest, F.; Schwartz, D. W.; and Jones, S. A.: *Contraceptive Technology,* 1980–1981, 10th ed. Irvington Publishers, New York, 1980.

Heiman, J.: Women's sexual arousal. The physiology of erotica. *Psychology Today,* April:90–94, 1975.

Herold, E. S.; Goodwin, M. S.; and Lero, D. S.: Self-esteem, locus of control, and adolescent contraception. *J. Psychol.,* 101:83–88, 1979.

Herzberg, B. H.; Draper, K. C.; Johnson, A. A.; and Nichol, G. C.: Oral contraceptives, depression and libido. *Br. Med. J.,* 3:495–500, 1971.

Hite S: *The Hite Report.* Macmillan Publishing Co., New York, 1977.

Huggins, G. R.; Rosenfeld, D. L.; Rickels, L.; Garcia, D. R.; and Fischer, E. L.: Emotional distress in morning-after pill patients. *Acta Obstet. Gynecol. Scand.,* 58:65–68, 1979.

Jackson, P., and Lander, J. L.: Female sterilization: A five-year follow-up in Auckland. *N. Z. Med. J.,* 91:140–143, 1980.

James, W. H.: Coital rates and the pill. *Nature,* 234:555–556, 1971.

Jarrett, J. C., and Spellacy, W. N.: Contraceptive practice of female runners. *Fertil. Steril.,* 39:374–375, 1983.

Joe, V. C.; Jones, R. N.; Noel, A. S.; and Roberts, B.: Birth control practices and conservatism. *J. Pers. Assess.,* 43:536–540, 1979.

Kantner, J. F., and Zelnik, M.: Contraception and pregnancy: Experience of young unmarried women in the United States. *Fam. Plann. Perspect.,* 5:21–35, 1973.

Keith, L.; Berger, G. S.; and Jackson, M.: Vaginal contraception. *Curr. Probl. Obstet. Gynecol.,* 8:3–47, 1982.

Keller, J. F., and Sack A. R.: Sex guilt and the use of contraception among unmarried women. *Contraception* 25:387–393, 1982.

Kinsey, A. C.; Pomeroy, W. B.; Martin, C. E.; and Gebhard, P. H.: *Sexual Behavior in the Human Female.* Saunders, Philadelphia, 1953.

Kloeck, J.: The smell of some steroid sex-hormones and their metabolites. Reflections and experiments concerning the significance of smell for the mutual relation of the sexes. *Psychiatria, Neurologia, Neurochirurgia,* 64:309–344, 1961.

Kolodny, R. C. and Bauman, J. E.: To the Editor. *N. Engl. J. Med.,* 300:626, 1979.

Lewis, S. A., and Burns, M.: Manifest dream content: Changes with the menstrual cycle. *Br. J. Med. Psychol.,* 48:375–377, 1975.

Liang, A. P.; Levenson, A. G.; Layde, P. M.; Shelton, J. D.; Hatcher, R. A.; Potts, M.; and Michelson, M. J.: Risk of breast, uterine corpus, and ovarian cancer in women receiving medroxyprogesterone injections. *JAMA,* 249:2909–2912, 1983.

Mathew, R. J., and Weinman, M. L.: Sexual dysfunctions in depression. *Arch. Sex. Behav.,* 11:323–328, 1982.

McCance, R. A.; Luff, M. C.; and Widdowson, E. E.: Physical and emotional periodicity in women. *J. Hyg.,* 37:571–611, 1937.

McCauley, E., and Ehrhardt, A. A.: Female sexual response. *Primary Care,* 3(3):455–476, 1976.

Michael, R. P., and Keverne, E. B.: Pheromones in the communication of sexual status in primates. *Nature,* 218:746–749, 1968.

Michael, R. P., and Zumpe, D.: Rhythmic changes in the copulatory frequency of rhesus monkeys (*Macaca Mullata*) in relation to the menstrual cycle and a comparison with the human cycle. *J. Reprod. Fert.,* 21:199–201, 1970.

Michael, R. P.; Bonsall, R. W.; and Warner, P.: Human vaginal secretions: volatile fatty acid content. *Science,* 186:1217–1219, 1974.

Miller, W. B.: Sexual and contraceptive behavior in young unmarried women. *Primary Care,* 3:427–453, 1976.

Mindick, B.; Oskamp, S.; and Berger, D. E.: Prediction of success or failure in birth planning: An approach to prevention of individual and family stress. *Am. J. Commun. Psychol.,* 5:447–459, 1977.

Morris, N. M., and Udry, J. R.: Sexual frequency and contraceptive pills. *Soc. Biol.,* 18:40–45, 1971.

Morris, N. M., and Udry, J. R.: An experimental search for pheromonal influences on human sexual behavior. (Abstract) *Eastern Conference on Reproductive Behavior.* Nags Head, North Carolina, May, 1975.

Morris, N. M.; Udry, J. R.; and Underwood, L. E.: A study of the relationship between coitus and the luteinizing hormone surge. *Fertil. Steril.,* 28:440–442, 1977.

Mosher, W. D.: Methods in contraceptive practice. *Vital Health Stat.,* 23:1–58, 1981.

Nagel, T. C.: Intrauterine contraceptive devices. Complications associated with their use. *Postgrad. Med.,* 73:155–164, 1983.

Perloff, W. H.: Role of the hormones in human sexuality. *Psychosom. Med.,* 11:133–139, 1949.

Persky, H.; Obrien, C.; and Khan, M. A.: Reproductive hormone levels, sexual activity and moods during the menstrual cycle. *Psychosom. Med.,* 38:62, 1976.

Persky, H. P.; Charney, N.; Leif, H. I.; O'Brien, C. P.; Miller, W. R.; and Strauss, D.: The relationship of plasma estradiol level to sexual behavior in young women. *Psychosom. Med.,* 40:523–535, 1978a.

Persky, H.; Lief, H. I.; Strauss, D.; Miller, W. R.; and O'Brien, C. P.: Plasma testosterone level and sexual behavior of couples. *Arch. Sex. Behav.,* 7:157–173, 1978b.

Persky, H.; O'Brien, C. P.; Lief, H. I.; Strauss, D.; and Miller, W. R.: To the Editor. *N. Engl. J. Med.,* 300:626, 1979.

Persky, H.; Driesbach, L.; Miller, W. R.; O'Brien, C. P.; Khan, M. A.; Lief H. I.; Charney, N.; Strauss, D.: The relation of plasma androgen to sexual behaviors and attitudes of women. *Psychosom. Med.,* 44:305–319, 1982.

Pike, M. C.; Henderson, B. E.; Krailo, M. D.; Duke, A.; and Roy, S.: Breast Cancer in young women and use of oral contraceptives: Possible modifying effect of formulation and age at use. *Lancet,* 8356:926–929, 1983.

Population Reports: Oral contraceptives in the 1980's. Series A, Number 6:A191–A222, 1982.

Postic, B.; Singh, B.; Squeglia, N. L.; and Guevarra, L. O.: Inactivation of clinical isolates of herpesvirus hominis, types 1 and 2 by chemical contraceptives. *Sex. Transm. Dis.,* 5:22–24, 1978.

Rodgers, D. A., and Ziegler, F. J.: Changes in sexual behavior consequent to use of noncoital procedures of contraception. *Psychosom. Med.,* 30:495–505, 1968.

Rosenfeld, D. L.; Huggins, G. R.; Jusczyk, A. M.; Garcia, Rickels, K.: Medical, psychologic, and social factors in morning-after pill utilization. *Advances in Planned Parenthood* 11:19–23, 1976.

Rosenfield, A.: The pill's many concontraceptive benefits. *Contemp OB/GYN,* 22:136–154, 1983.

Ruble, D. N.: Premenstrual symptoms: A reinterpretation. *Science,* 197:291–292, 1977.

Salmimies, P.; Kockott, G.; Pirke, K. M.; Vogt, H. J.; and Schill, W. B.: Effects of testosterone replacement on sexual behavior in hypogonadal men. *Arch. Sex. Behav.,* 11:345–353, 1982.

Schreiner-Engel, P.: Female sexual arousability: The relation to gonadal hormones and the menstrual cycle. *Dissertations and Abstracts International,* 41(2):80–17, 527, 1980.

Schreiner-Engel, P.; Schiavi, R. C.; Smith, H.; and White, D.: Sexual arousal and the menstrual cycle. *Psychosom. Med.,* 43:199–214, 1981.

Spellacy, W. N.; Kalra, P. S.; Buhi, W. R.; and Birk, S A.: Pituitary and ovarian responsiveness to a graded gonadotropin releasing factor stimulation test in women using a low estrogen or a regular type of oral contraceptive. *Am. J. Obstet. Gynecol.,* 137:109–115, 1980.

Speroff, L.; Glass, R. H.; and Kase, N. G.: *Clinical Gynecologic Endocrinology.* Williams and Wilkins, Baltimore, 1983.

Spitz, C. J.; Gold, A. R.; and Adams, D. B.: Cognitive and hormonal factors affecting coital frequency. *Arch. Sex. Behav.,* 4:249–262, 1975.

Steinlauf, B.: Problem solving skills, locus of control, and the contraceptive effectiveness of young women. *Child. Dev.,* 50:268–271, 1979.

Strahle, W. M.: A model of premarital coitus and contraceptive behavior among female adolescents. *Arch. Sex. Behav.,* 12:67–94, 1983.

Swan, S. H., and Brown, W. L.: Oral contraceptive use, sexual activity, and cervical carcinoma. *Am. J. Obstet. Gynecol.,* 139:52–57, 1981.

Swanson, E. M., and Foulkes, D.: Dream content and the menstrual cycle. *J. Nerv. Ment. Dis.,* 145:358–363, 1968.

Tessman, I.: To the Editor. *N. Engl. J. Med.,* 300:626, 1979.

The Centers for Disease Control Cancer and Steroid Hormone Study: Long-term oral contraceptive use and the risk of breast cancer. *JAMA,* 249:1591–1595, 1983.

The Couple to Couple League: *A Physician's Reference to Natural Family Planning.* The Couple to Couple League International, Inc., Cincinnati, 1981.

Tietze, C.; Bongaarts, J.; and Schearer, B.: Mortality associated with the control of fertility. *Fam. Plann. Perspect.,* 8:6–14, 1976.

Udry, J. R., and Morris, N. M.: Distribution of coitus in the menstrual cycle. *Nature,* 220:593–596, 1968.

Vessey, M.; Huggins, G.; Lawless, M.; McPherson, K.; and Yeates, D.: Tubal sterilization: Findings in a large prospective study. *Br. J. Obstet. Gynaecol.,* 90:203–209, 1983a.

Vessey, M. P.; Lawless, M.; McPherson, K.; and Yeates, D.: Neoplasia of the cervix uteri and contraception: A possible adverse effect of the pill. *Lancet,* 8356:930–933, 1983b.

Vierling, S. C., and Rock, J.: Variations in olfactory sensitivity to exaltolide during the menstrual cycle. *J. Appl. Physiol.,* 22:311–315, 1967.

Walker, A. M.; Jick, H.; Hunter, J. R.; Danford, A.; Watkins, R. N.; Alhadeff, L.; and Rothman K. J.: Vasectomy and nonfatal myocardial infarction. *Lancet,* 1:13–15, 1981.

Wallace, R.; Lee, J.; Gerber, W. L.; Clarke, W. R.; and Lauer, R. M.: Vasectomy and coronary disease in men under 50: Absence of correlation. *J. Urol.,* 126:182–184, 1981.

Waxenberg, S. E.; Drellich, M. G.; and Sutherland, A. M.: The role of hormones in human behavior. I. Changes in female sexuality after adrenalectomy. *J. Clin. Endocrinol. Metab.,* 19:193–202, 1959.

Westoff, C. F.; Bumpass, L.; and Ryder, N. B.: Oral contraceptives, coital frequency, and the time required to conceive. *Soc. Biol.,* 16:1–10, 1969.

Wincze, J. P.; Hoon, P.; and Hoon, E. F.: Sexual arousal in women: A comparison of cognitive and physiological responses by continuous measurement. *Arch. Sex. Behav.,* 6:121–133, 1977.

Yuzpe, A. A.: Postcoital contraception. *Int. J. Gynaecol. Obstet.,* 16:497–501, 1978–79.

Ziegler, F. J.; Rodgers, D. A.; and Kriegsman, S. A.: Effect of vasectomy on psychological functioning. *Psychosom. Med.,* 28:50–63, 1966.

Zelnik, M., and Kantner, J. F.: Sexual and contraceptive experience of young unmarried women in the United States, 1976 and 1971. *Fam. Plann. Perspect.,* 9:55–71, 1977.

# CHAPTER 11 PSYCHOSEXUAL DYSFUNCTION AND INFERTILITY

Jay S. Schinfeld, M.D.

## INTRODUCTION

Couples facing infertility frequently experience a sense of desperation and loss of sexuality in a society where childbearing appears to complete the individual's or couple's growth and development. People used to achieving success by hard work, initiative, and expenditure of finances and time are extremely frustrated and threatened by the discovery that potentially there is something wrong that is beyond their control. These individuals, who are considered "normal" by our society in most ways, become "abnormal" simply by being unable to procreate. Furthermore, this sense of abnormality may distort their relationship with other individuals and other aspects of their world.

Infertility is a difficult issue for many to discuss even with friends, not only because of its relationship to personal sexual issues, but also because of the many superstitions and myths surrounding it. Open discussion often evokes uninvited advice and lay psychological counseling, exposing the couple to speculation about sexual and marital difficulties or inadequacies. Infertility becomes a psychosexual, conjugal problem. A great deal of guilt comes into the relationship; partners hope to spare each other from being the one "at fault," while simultaneously hoping that the problem is not theirs. The projection of anger on to the other partner, family members, or the health care specialist is especially common (McGuire, 1975).

Despite the option that individuals or couples can lead a mature and satisfied adult life without children, conflicts and fears remain. However, the major psychosexual problem in an infertile couple seems related to the fact that their essential maleness and femaleness appears to be open to public ridicule (Kaufman, 1969). The infertility investigation probes the private lives of individuals in a manner that can make them helpless and dependent.

Can psychosexual dysfunction and related stress be a *cause* of male or female infertility? Is this stress a necessary and natural reaction to infertility, and can the long-term effects of this problem be overcome with the establishment of normal sexuality and self-esteem? This chapter will discuss these and other critical questions.

## IDENTIFICATION

Almost 50 percent of individuals who present with infertility will be found to have some identifiable psychosexual dysfunction during the work-up (Moghissi and Wallach, 1983).

Frequently, however, the health professional is unable to decide when the psychosexual dysfunction began, and its direct relationship to the problem at hand. Most studies have suggested that there is no increase in psychosis or neurosis in couples suffering from infertility (Mandelbrote and Monro, 1964). Eisner (1963) has suggested that there are certain personality differences between members of fertile and infertile couples—especially among the women. In the past, it was felt that these personality differences emanated from problems and concerns about the individual's sexual role, feelings about parenthood, sexual identity, and sexual relationships. However, no long-term prospective study in newly married couples with a normal past history (including psychiatric history) has been performed evaluating them during the time they attempt conception, which notes changes that occur subsequent to failure to conceive. Therefore, it remains hard to assess which couples and individuals truly have an "infertile personality type" (Benedek et al., 1953; Seward et al., 1963).

Mai, Mundy, and Rump (1972) suggest that although in general there are no more neuroses or psychoses in infertile couples than in normals, the women tend to be "more hysterical and aggressive" with an increased ambivalence about parenthood and sexuality. Eisner (1963), trying to find psychological differences between fertile and infertile women, suggests that there was indeed emotional disturbance to some degree in infertile women. Again conflicts concerned primarily the female role and sexuality. In an excellent psychiatric study by Platt and colleagues (1973), personality traits and self ideals were again found related to infertility, but no etiologic mechanism or definite causal relationship was demonstrated. Singh and Nicki (1982) used the Eysenck personality inventory and Ryle's marital patterns test with a separate inventory for depressive illness. No significant differences in genetic and nongenetic forms of infertility were found. Finally, in a psychoanalytic study, 32 women were seen and 15 studied completely; emotional dynamics characteristic of functional infertility were found in 10 (Ford et al., 1953). However, in this study and most of the papers previously mentioned, coexisting organic abnormalities sufficient to explain a barren marriage were either ignored or not evaluated completely.

Proving that psychosexual dysfunction is the cause of infertility is difficult. "Normal infertile couples" or patients with "unexplained infertility," have previously been described to have a 48 percent incidence of psychologically caused male or female infertility (Heiman, 1959). However, many of the articles demonstrating this are from the 1940s. Subsequently, immunologic infertility, endometriosis, and several degrees of oligoasthenospermia have been identified. Therefore, where psychological infertility was once considered obvious, organic problems would now be identified.

Seward and coworkers (1963), in a study of infertility in 50 couples, suggests that psychological evaluation immediately after any gynecological visit for infertility revealed no deep-rooted problems with sexual function or sexual feelings, and no deep-rooted psychiatric problems. They identified the existence of an "infertility personality disorder" caused by a developmental defect or pathological trends in the personality structure. These couples experienced minimal subjective anxiety and little or no sense of distress, although they tended to be under more stress shortly following the menstrual period.

Subsequently, in a study of frigidity and sterility Labandibar and Benzecry (1959), found no correlation between the woman's physical and orgasmic reaction and the conception rate. In women capable of regular orgasm and those considered anorgasmic or preorgasmic, conception rates were approximately the same. However, due to increased sexual exposure in responsive women, the chances for conception per cycle were increased (Kostic and Mladenovic, 1960). Therefore, little evidence suggests that orgasm is required to speed the sperm to the fallopian tubes or to dip the cervix into the vaginal pool of seminal fluid.

## INCIDENCE

Psychosexual dysfunction is identified by at least one member of the health care team in as many as 50 percent of couples (Dorfman, 1969). Previous studies suggest that 10 to 25 percent of couples with no other obvious causes of infertility have a primary psychogenic etiology for infertility (Moghissi and Wallach, 1983). This study includes the fact that 4 to 5 percent of marriages appear never to be consummated (Dawkins and Taylor, 1961), and that studies by Amelar, Dubin, and Walsh (1977) suggest that 10 percent of all infertility is due to overt male sexual dysfunction. The actual percentage of dysfunction in normal fertile couples, and the significance of the problem in infertile couples, remains undefined.

## ETIOLOGIES AND MECHANISMS

Many possible causes of infertility in a couple exist. By dividing these into the possible female and male factors, one can discuss in detail the evidence of possible causal relationships between psychosexual stress and infertility. Much of the data from the past are anecdotal and theoretical, but in certain situations both an etiology and possible mechanism for infertility can be stated (Morris and Sturgis, 1959).

### Female Factors

In the female, psychological stress can indeed result in anovulation, shown by the fact that 25 percent of women, who have had a previously normal work-up, may become anovulatory or amenorrheic when donor insemination begins. When the complete responsibility for pregnancy is placed on her shoulders, a woman's stress level apparently interferes with normal hypothalamic-pituitary-ovarian function. It has recently been suggested that this is mediated through endorphins, nature's own narcotics. These endogenous opioid peptides have been related to many behavioral patterns, such as schizophrenia, response to hypnosis, acupuncture, or the ability to undergo natural childbirth. Endorphins inhibit the release of luteinizing hormone-releasing hormone (LHRH), which results in a loss of the secretion of luteinizing hormone (LH) and follicle-stimulating hormone (FSH) from the pituitary, which may result in an hypoestrogenic state, or simply preclude the midcycle LH surge with its accompanying ovulation.

Quigley and colleagues (1980), in eight women with hypothalamic hypogonadotropic amenorrhea, found evidence of increased hypothalamic, dopaminergic and opioid activity. Using the dopamine receptor antagonist metoclopramide, four of eight patients had increased LH response and a slight increase in prolactin compared to the great increase in the normal controls. Naloxone, a narcotic antagonist with no agonistic actions, increased LH pulses in four of eight patients. A dramatic increase in prolactin was noted if there was no change in LH in these patients. If gonadotropins were very low, LH changes were rarely noted. Since psychosexual dysfunction and stress could alter dopamine or endorphin release, a subtle mechanism might lead to poor corpus luteum function.

Other factors, such as catechol estrogens, weak estradiol metabolites, may be somewhat antiestrogenic or interfere with catecholamine turnover. These catecholestrogens are primary substrates for catechol-o-methyl transferase, resulting in increased concentrations of dopamine and norepinephrine, both of which have been noted to have a role in LHRH release, as well as psychosexual function and dysfunction (Schinfeld et al., 1980).

Other pituitary hormones may also be involved in this same anovulatory process. Adrenocorticotrophic hormone (ACTH) or adrenal androgen-stimulating hormone accompanying the release of endorphins may result in an increase in adrenal androgens. These adrenal androgens, including dehydroepiandrosterone sulphate and androstenedione, may cause further anovulation either through aromatization in adipose tissue and other peripheral tissues or by direct negative effects on follicular development in the ovary. Similarly, prolactin, a stress-released hormone, can interfere with LH and FSH release. Prolactin may also have a luteolytic effect on luteinized granulosa cells in the ovarian corpus luteum. Thus, stress can either interfere with gonadotropin release or ovarian function.

Thyroid dysfunction as part of psychological difficulties may be demonstrated on occasion by abnormal results on thyrotrophin-releasing hormone (TRH) testing. In depressed patients, TRH tests and dexamethasone suppression tests may demonstrate abnormalities. These abnormal results in thyroid economy directly result in anovulation, affect general metabolism, and may reflect abnormalities in catecholamine metabolism, especially dopamine.

Therefore, it appears that etiologic associations and mechanisms do exist that can cause ovulatory dysfunction, psychogenic amenorrhea, and infertility generally mediated through hypothalamic-pituitary-ovarian axis disruption. These dysfunctions can be objectively identified and successfully treated medically. However, the possibility of polycystic ovarian disease, luteal phase defects, and anovulation—more subtle dysfunctions, not as well-documented—does exist.

It is unknown whether the "unruptured follicle syndrome," a mechanism currently thought to account for infertility with apparent ovulation, documented by basal body temperature charts, progesterone assays, or endometrial biopsy, exists at a higher frequency in normal infertile couples compared to those with other ovulatory dysfunction or organic fertility problems. In addition, no proof that stress causes the local entrapment of the eggs is available (Kerin et al, 1983). Likewise an antinidatory factor at the uterine level related to a woman's intense desire not to become pregnant has never been demonstrated.

In the normal ovulating woman, investigators (Noyes and Chapnick, 1964; Greenhill, 1956) suggest that there are alternate mechanisms which can result in infertility even though the woman is menstruating regularly. The concept of fallopian tubal spasm as a cause for infertility has been related in many anecdotal reports. The spasm, as noticed at the time of a hysterosalpingogram, may prevent sperm passage or result in rejection of the egg at the fimbriated end. Few earlier studies and reports can document that such a continued and prolonged painless tubal spasm capable of midcycle tubal blockage exists (Greenhill, 1956).

## Male Factors

In the male, sexual dysfunction accompanying infertility and its concomitant physical work-up is also common. Failure to maintain an erection, premature ejaculation, avoidance of intercourse, and poor orgasmic strength have been discussed in the past (Kaufman, 1969). Recently the concept of retrograde or anejaculation in the face of orgasm has been suggested as an alternative mechanism to explain poor semen samples or postcoital tests. The incidence in infertile couples of male psychosexual factors or dysfunctions, as causative, is not known. However, failure to produce a masturbated specimen for semen analysis or the inability to participate in any timed postcoital test does not necessarily seem to correlate with other sexual or psychological dysfunction in male partners in our experience. The threat of these tests can cause impotence in otherwise normal individuals. The physician should work with the male to establish alternative reliable testing methods.

Suggestions that oligospermia and azoospermia may be due to psychological problems have been discussed by Palti (1969). There is little evidence that psychological mechanisms influence the mobility or morphology of spermatozoa. The male hypothalamic-pituitary-testicular axis is thought to be less easily disturbed due to its tonic mode. Any long-term stress that affects this axis should be accompanied by obvious changes in testosterone metabolism, libido, and potency.

Recently Gagnon and colleagues (1982) demonstrated an enzyme defect accompanying poor motility or azoospermia and oligospermia that resolves when the semen analysis returns to normal. The use of the human sperm–hamster egg penetration test can also show apparent defects in the sperm that prevent them from fertilizing or, at least, penetrating the zona pellucida or vitelline membrane of the hamster egg, and, presumably, the human egg as well. No information has been obtained to suggest that such abnormalities in enzymes or sperm function can be caused by psychological stress, but such subtle defects could be the mechanisms for stress-related infertility. It is interesting to note that 10 percent of men who discontinued infertility work-ups had an immediate improvement in their semen analyses. Palti (1969) showed that sex by the clock or the calendar resulted in both periodic impotence and retrograde or anejaculation in infertile male partners.

## Psychosocial Factors Influencing Infertility

Psychosexual dysfunction, resulting in infertility in the female, is quite obvious. If repeatedly placed in stressful situations when dealing with family and friends who question her lack of fertility, the woman's self-doubts, or those suggested or suspected by her partner, and her own concern of an inate defect in her body or femininity can result in infertility. The mechanisms for infertility in these patients could, of course, be similar to those previously discussed: Ovulatory dysfunction is quite common, with low or absent progesterone levels and frequent abnormalities in adrenal and ovarian androgens and estrogen secretion. Also, infertile women frequently experience definite changes in their libido. They no longer care whether their partner is enjoying the sexual experience, but become anorgasmic and solely concerned with simply getting the sperm where they belong. These women often become extremely depressed at the time of their menstruation (Chamberlain et al, 1984).

For the infertile couple, the menstrual cycle becomes a repetitive cycle of stresses. Menses represents the obvious losing of the struggle.

This loss is then followed by a short period of frustrating abstinence during which the couple prepares for a heightened frequency of sexual intercourse that may be totally foreign to their normal sexual desires. The fertile period becomes an automated attempt to engage in coitus frequently enough to achieve the desired result. While the male frequently feels like a "sperm machine" with little or no apparent caring or response from his partner, the wife is powerless and dependent on his performance. After the midcycle stress, the man and woman frequently shy away from each other, unable to communicate or share the deep hurt and frustration, as well as the physical and psychological fatigue that are all too commonly overlooked. The time of the next menstrual period initiates the anger, sadness, and feelings of guilt that represent the couple's reaction to their failure to achieve a pregnancy.

It is not infrequent, therefore, that many infertile women develop an aversion or avoidance reaction to sex. Especially if the male partner is the initiator of the desire for parenthood, frigidity, vaginismus, and dyspareunia can become major complaints in the female. Women may complain of an inability to lubricate and deeply resent their husband's impatience or disinterest in their orgasm. The incidence of chronic pelvic pain, dysmenorrhea, and unusual illnesses is unknown, but these difficulties may represent mechanism's meant to displace the anxiety and tension from conception.

Many social factors contribute to stress and the frequency with which it interferes with fertility. Keye and coworkers (1983) tried to predict a woman's emotional response to infertility. A Utah Infertility Reaction Scale was developed and used for determination of the response to infertility based on type and duration. This 127 item questionnaire measured changes in body image, self-esteem, sense of loss, helplessness, and sexual satisfaction. For the 214 infertile women who completed the questionnaire, feelings of inadequacy and hopelessness increased with the duration of infertility, although older infertile women suffered somewhat less emotional distress than younger ones.

This study noted a relationship between the underlying causes of infertility and the nature of the emotional distress. Women with anovulatory infertility typically felt inadequate with a poor body image and reduced self-esteem. Women with tubal disease or pelvic adhesions often felt guilty; they thought they had caused their infertility and therefore were being punished. Women with endometriosis felt helpless, while women whose infertility was attributed to the male partner frequently were dissatisfied with their sexual relationship.

In infertility practice we frequently find evidence of psychosexual problems. These difficulties require discussion or even regular counseling, but rarely is there firm evidence that these problems caused the infertility. The intensity of psychological disturbances appears to be the same in couples with and without confirmed organic pathology.

One of the most common reactions to infertility is guilt. Patients try to attribute a direct cause and effect relationship between past actions and current problems in conceiving. Couples commonly blame a previous abortion, use of birth control, or premarital sex. Others, especially the very religious, may relate their infertility to a general sense of unworthiness or unholiness. The degree of stress and desperation felt by a couple can eventually result in destructive behavior. Divorce and spouse abuse are more frequent in childless couples (Walker, 1978), and it has been said that suicide is approximately twice as frequent in infertile couples as in fertile couples (Stallworthy, 1948).

Couples who had normal and fulfilling sexual function prior to infertility problems may develop temporary or permanent decreases in their ability to achieve coitus. Coital infrequency and orgasmic dysfunction are common according to Moghissi and Wallach (1983), and they may provide secondary gain by presenting an obvious cause for the barren marriage.

Dyspareunia and vaginismus may result in temporary or permanent inability to conceive due to lack of vaginal intercourse. However, couples who have at least a spoken desire for conception can achieve a pregnancy without normal vaginal penetration. In recent years two such couples conceived: one by ejaculation on the inner thigh on a repeated basis and the second by homologous artificial insemination performed by the husband using a small syringe.

In approximately 25 percent of consecutive infertility study cases (67 out of 268), there was an "apparent significant stress induced factor" in the infertile couples (Sandler, 1959). After counseling, there was a 48 percent pregnancy rate in this group versus a 32 percent pregnancy rate in couples with obvious organic factors and less evidence of psychosexual stress. Menning (1980) states that "infertile people frequently relate stories of feeling like perpetual adolescents until they achieve parenthood by some means." A couple that does not conceive loses some sense of purpose especially in a traditional marriage where having children may be one of the most important functions of the relationship.

## THE PHYSICIAN AND THE INFERTILITY WORK-UP: CAUSING OR PREVENTING STRESS

Prevention of psychosexual dysfunction related to infertility, or treatment of established difficulties can begin the first time the physician meets with the couple. The physician's attitude, explanations, and sense of timing can make the difference between eliminating or dramatically increasing stress.

On the initial visit it is best to schedule at least 30 minutes to spend with the couple. The physician should relate that he or she understands the frustrations and the sense of desperation the couple may have. Also, the physician can discuss the frequency of psychosexual dysfunction as a result of the stress of infertility. In a general discussion concerning the causes of infertility and the explanation for tests, care must be taken to protect the couple's privacy whenever possible. It is probably inappropriate to get more than a general sexual history on the initial visit. Timing and frequency of intercourse is generally sufficient. Later in the work-up, especially after the results of the postcoital tests and semen analysis are known, specific instructions concerning positions and techniques may be more appropriate. The physician must be comfortable with and concerned about psychological and sexual issues, as well as prepared and available to discuss these topics.

For the male patient, after a general history and physical examination, separate questioning concerning the effects of the infertility on his sexuality followed by questions concerning a previous history of venereal disease, are all germane. He should be asked whether he has fathered a child with a previous sexual partner. An advance explanation of the semen analysis, stating the necessity and reason for producing a masturbated specimen, is especially useful. It should be explained to the man that sperm counts, motility, and morphology frequently fluctuate. The effects of stress, alcohol, diet, medications, and previous illnesses on a semen analysis should be mentioned to prepare the patient for the possibility of repeated specimen collection. A special discussion of the postcoital test is also indicated. In my experience failure at a postcoital test is frequently related to the onset of midcycle impotence and followed by discontinuation of the infertility work-up.

Although couples must be told when and sometimes how to have intercourse, enjoyment and preservation of sexuality is very important. Therefore, if the scheduled postcoital test results in sexual dysfunction or discord, the physician should simply be notified. It may be rescheduled when the couple feels confident that previous problems have been resolved. Careful counseling prior to ordering postcoital tests is far more successful in avoiding psychosexual dysfunction, especially in the male, than attempts at treatment following failure to perform or a poor result.

Similarly, in discussing various tests with the female partner, the physician must take care to use words which do not convey a sense of guilt or failure to the patient. Words like luteal phase "inadequacy" and "insufficiency" are especially burdensome to women, as is the term "hostile mucous" (mucous of poor quality or suspected of harboring antibodies). When describing to the patient the presence or absence of pathology at the time of laparoscopy, one must consider psychosexual dynamics. The woman is being searched, and her genitals poked and plotted. Physicians without the proper training or those who lack proper sensitivity to participate in the infertility work-up, should refer infertile patients for psychological counseling and diagnostic evaluation whenever possible.

Lack of information and confusion causes stress and frustration in these couples. Allowing the couple to ask questions reduces anxiety, and an immediate discussion of the test results is useful. Separately asking each partner intrusive questions may not only yield useful information, but also reveal the degree of stress in the relationship. History-taking is the first attempt at diagnosis, and questionnaires and brochures can be less effective and potentially harmful in establishing the proper physician–couple relationship.

While infertility can cause depression, some deeply troubled patients may present with the complaint of infertility (Ellenberg and Koren, 1982). If one of the spouses is clinically depressed or even psychotic or if both partners show significant psychiatric disturbance, it is suggested that this problem be treated prior to continuing the infertility work-up. Patients who do well with psychotherapy or on psychomimetic medication may be candidates for continued infertility evaluation.

Physicians should remember that the basal body temperature chart can be a potentially important factor causing sexual dysfunction. This piece of paper is the first thing a couple sees in the morning. The wife may never forget that she is infertile since as soon as she awakens she is forced to take her temperature—she may not brush her teeth, kiss her husband, or get up and check on the other children. Couples can view the temperature chart with a magic all its own and maintaining the proper charting can become a compulsion. One can advise the couple to discontinue charting the basal body temperature after several months.

In a time when television and printed media frequently discuss infertility, one would suspect that taking the inability to conceive "out of the closet" would be viewed as positive by infertile patients. On the contrary, many couples are not relieved to learn that they are not alone, and they only feel more stressed to be part of this unfortunate, involuntary minority. Therefore, reassurance during the first visit is extremely important. Allowing the couple to relax by openly discussing problems can result in avoiding common stress reactions.

Furthermore, some couples are ambivalent about parenthood and are unprepared for success. When pregnancy occurs early in the course of an evaluation, these couples may release a great deal of anger and rethink whether or not they really want to become parents. In other words, once they have proven their fertility, the man and woman—the couple—are faced with the reality that their lifestyle will be changed by the myriad challenges and responsibilities of parenthood.

## THE PHYSICIAN AND THERAPY FOR INFERTILITY: CAUSING OR PREVENTING STRESS

### Artificial Insemination

The establishment that the problem is irreversible male infertility requiring donor artificial insemination (AID) presents significant problems for a couple. The male must accept the fact that he will not be the biological father of the child. Furthermore, his ability to pass on his genes, and to an extent his perceived sexuality, must be acknowledged as impaired. The woman is then presented with the entire responsibility for pregnancy success as she will be given sperm from a "proven fertile man." Glezerman and Insler (1981) show that this situation presents a critical identity crisis in the male with accompanying guilt and anger. In addition to self-doubts, the male may experience jealousy directed toward the female partner, who can still prove her sexuality and femininity and pass on her biological make-up.

The female partner, presented with what may be overt resentment from her partner along with the total responsibility for fertility or infertility, frequently ceases to ovulate regularly. This reaction can happen in women who have never missed a menstrual period since menarche. Glezerman and Insler (1981) suggested that 67 percent of artificially inseminated women develop evidence of disturbed luteal function. It is not infrequent for patients who previously had 28-day regular cycles to change their menstrual pattern from 21 to 46 days. When frozen sperm is used, changes in ovulation timing or supervening anovulation can essentially negate the possibility of success in that cycle. When fresh donors are involved, they are frequently put on call while cervical mucous evaluations or ultrasounds to note ovarian follicular size are employed. In my practice clomiphene citrate must be employed in 25 percent of patients to obtain a more regular cycle.

Some authors note that the presence of the husband accompanying the patient for appointments is of critical importance (Glezerman and Insler, 1981). If there is evidence of resistance toward artificial insemination by either partner, Glezerman and Insler (1981) observed a pregnancy rate of only 28.6 percent versus 93.6 percent in couples where the husband was present and supportive. They also noted increased miscarriage rates and more discontinuation of insemination in the group of women who were apparently pursuing artificial insemination with little support from their spouses. In our practice psychiatric and psychological support services are available for these patients when needed, and their effectiveness does not appear to be impaired by the lack of an initial psychological screening visit. The implementation of these services is frequently followed by a spontaneous return of regular menstrual cycles, as well as an apparent increase in interest on the part of the male partner.

We have encouraged the participation of

the infertile male in the insemination process depending on the couple's desire. Often husbands are in the examining room and, in selected cases, may actually perform the final step in artificial insemination themselves. During the 10 or 15 minutes (postinsemination) while the patient remains in the room, complete privacy is given. The response to these amenities has been overwhelmingly positive. The husbands who have noticed cyclic impotence and anger during previous artificial inseminations feel that they are now present at the moment of conception. Husbands who have participated in repeated courses of AID have stated that they have felt closer to the resulting child since they were present at its conception.

Psychosexual problems occurring in couples involved in programs such as *in vitro* fertilization, surrogate motherhood, homologous artificial insemination, and amniocentesis for chromosomal or genetic problems can be expected to be similar to those in couples in artificial insemination programs.

## ADOPTION

It is common among the general population to believe that once stress has been relieved by stopping an infertility investigation, by taking long vacations such as ocean cruises, or by adopting a baby, the chance for conception is dramatically increased. These myths are almost totally spurious and not well-supported by any scientific study. Andrews (1970) studied 60 couples who conceived after making application to adopt or after adopting a child. Only 37 couples in the group had documented infertility. Fourteen of the 37 couples conceived during the application process, 16 conceived within a few days to 18 months of adopting child, and three of the couples conceived after application for their second adopted child. Four additional couples conceived within a few months of receiving their second adopted child. The report concluded that these pregnancies supported a clinical "hunch" that adoption can be a powerful method for a couple to overcome its infertility.

Couples who applied for adoption and who did not conceive were not used as controls.

The previous study of Hanson and Rock (1950) shows completely conflicting results. Through the aid of adoption agencies, 202 couples who adopted over a 10-year period were contacted by means of a questionnaire to determine whether or not they had biological children following adoption and other pertinent information. Pregnancies were reported in only 15 cases. Of these 15 couples, 11 were studied to find the cause of the presumed infertility. Most couples (prior to the conception) had poorly documented causes for their infertility. Following adoption, 19 of the women in this study reported changes in their menstrual cycles including duration of the cycle, duration of the menstrual flow, and decreased intensity of dysmenorrhea. It is interesting to note that 26.2 percent of the women in the study reported improvement in their sexuality following adoption. The 8 percent postadoption conception rate was not judged to be significant compared to the random, infertile population. Subsequent studies have confirmed these conclusions. Tyler, Bonapart, and Gent (1960) found that 4 percent of the couples established a pregnancy within two years of adoption. Similarly, Aaronson and Glienke (1963) found that only 2.9 percent of the 188 couples who responded to a questionnaire had a pregnancy for the first time after adoption. Therefore, there is little to support the hypothesis that adoption increases the possibility of conception. However, this does not deny the fact that the reduction of stress in any manner might result in eventual fertility.

## HABITUAL ABORTION

Some investigators have suggested that recurrent spontaneous abortions might be psychologically induced (Kaij *et al.,* 1969). Tupper and Weil (1982) evaluated the results of psychotherapy in habitual aborters. Aware that approximately 67 percent of habitual aborters carry to term regardless of the therapy employed, they conclude that the patient's capacity to continue to term and achieve a successful pregnancy was related to her psychological state and attitude toward motherhood. After a thorough evaluation by an obstetrician, a psychiatric interview was obtained. Certain personality types were more common in women with multiple abortions. They divided their patients into two types; basically immature women who could not accept responsibility and mature women who were independent and frustrated in a male dominated world. The overall results show that supportive psychotherapy throughout the pregnancy resulted in an 84 percent full-term live birth rate in 19 cases, with two miscarriages and one premature delivery. There was only a 26 percent full-term pregnancy rate in the untreated controls who were only interviewed a maximum of two times. The data suggest supportive psychotherapy could prevent pregnancy losses.

Tupper and Weil (1982) also conclude that while it was not certain that recurrent abortions were triggered by emotional factors, there were specific identifiable psychosexual problems in these patients. Pregnancy, in fact, represented a threat to their psychological equilibrium. The investigators did not establish in relation to recurrent abortion whether these psychosexual problems were cause or effect (Weil and Tupper, 1960).

Grimm (1962) notes that there seem to be personality discriminators for habitual aborters. Women with and without a known organic basis for their miscarriages were studied. These patients, with an average number of four previous spontaneous abortions, had a successful pregnancy rate of 80 percent following use of psychotherapy alone. Using Wechsler–Bellevue, Rorschach and TAT testing, the patients were analyzed and separated into different comparison groups. The Rorschach test, in particular, showed that they lack control of emotions and had a tendency to act out conflicts. These women had very good reality testing on the whole, but appeared geared to excessive conformity and social adaptability. They also had problems and concerns dealing with hostile feelings, but could not in any sense be described as markedly, overtly, or covertly hostile. These results were paralleled by those from TAT testing. Their conclusions were that abortion-prone women had an impairment of the ability to plan and anticipate, poor emotional control, great tension about their hostile affect, and strong feelings of dependency. When 18 "successful" habitual aborters were retested at the 35th week of pregnancy, 4–7 indicators previously found to discriminate for habitual abortion had changed. The changes were in the direction of greater emotional control, less build-up of tension, correction of hostile feelings, and less guilt. These data suggest that many of their problems were effects of the stresses and dissatisfactions with the previously poor pregnancy outcomes.

Seibel and Graves (1980) found that women who had spontaneous miscarriages describe themselves as unhappy, depressed, hostile, and anxious. Approximately 25 percent admitted having a psychiatric problem. A fourth of the total number of patients had previous threatened abortions, 17.3 percent had previous miscarriages, and 25 percent felt that they were personally responsible for the miscarriage.

At present it is not possible to state whether or not psychosexual dysfunction results in recurrent pregnancy wastage (James, 1963). No prospective controlled data are available, but it appears that once a live birth has been accomplished, the incidence of recurrent miscarriage is decreased. Problems in corpus luteum function, placental blood supply, and immunologic mechanisms might result from a psychological rejection of the pregnancy. More overt acts including use of drugs, alcohol, overwork, poor nutrition, and other potential pregnancy-threatening processes can also be identified in some recurrent aborters.

## THERAPEUTIC MODALITIES FOR ESTABLISHED PSYCHOSEXUAL DYSFUNCTION IN INFERTILE COUPLES

If the initial interview has been sensitively conducted, psychosexual problems are usually diagnosed relatively early in the infertility evaluation. Simple reassurance, answering questions directly, and correcting misinformation from friends, relatives, and the media, will allow a decrease in anxiety and occasionally will result in an early pregnancy. Specific questions about sexual behavior to be asked during the initial interview include the number of times the couple engages in sexual intercourse per week, whether intravaginal ejaculation occurs, and whether a lubricating jelly is necessary. General questions about sexual dysfunction and sexual satisfaction then follow. Frequently, at this time the couple will reveal clues about possibly important, unresolved psychosexual difficulties even if complete revelation does not take place.

It is important to remember that sometimes bizarre sexual behavior on the part of one or both members of the couple occurs during an infertility evaluation. The male may feel compelled to prove himself by impregnating another woman, while the female, now doubting her femininity, may become indiscriminately seductive.

Once specific psychosexual problems are identified, treatment can be instituted (Marbach and Schinfeld, 1953). No firm conclusion can be drawn concerning the efficacy of a formal psychodynamic approach in an infertile population because of the absence of control studies. Noyes and Chapnick (1964) allude to suggestions in the literature that psychotherapy may indeed be helpful in some couples with particular personality disorders.

Harrison and colleagues (1981) used transcendental meditation (TM) as therapy for primary or secondary psychosexual dysfunction in infertile couples. Ten couples with longterm infertility and six control couples were evaluated in a preliminary study. They found an increased anxiety level in infertile couples that was dramatically decreased after TM in most of them. However, seven of the ten couples did not complete the course of therapy, and the only pregnancy that occurred was in a patient with secondary infertility after only one TM session. The authors felt that this pregnancy was probably coincidental. Hypnosis has also been used to treat amenorrhea and infertility. Reports of this technique are uncontrolled, and thus it is unclear whether hypnosis is superior to reassurance, specific instructions, and time.

When a particular sexual or a psychological problem is identified it must be concomitantly treated, as discontinuing the infertility treatment may increase the patients' frustration and is rarely necessary. A thorough discussion of the psychosexual problems and therapeutic options should ensue, and frequently only superficial therapy or education is needed. Support groups that can direct energy and thoughts in a positive manner are useful.

## Secondary Infertility

The emotional response of couples who have previously conceived and now face either recurrent pregnancy losses or the inability to conceive again is especially complex. If the couple had prior pregnancies with different partners, the new relationship becomes suspect, causing anxiety and guilt. The physician must explain that frequently one member of the couple is subfertile and that a previous partner might have compensated for a particular relative defect. Alternatively, the new couple's problems may be due to newly acquired infertility factors. Individuals that have accomplished pregnancies with multiple other partners are probably quite fertile and should be reassured.

It is very difficult for couples who have conceived easily the first time to deal with secondary infertility (deWatteville, 1957). They must recognize that factors such as age, postabortal or postpartum endometritis, endometriosis, immunologic factors, and changes in weight, and levels of stress may have affected their infertility. Mentally the couples examine themselves with a great deal of anxiety looking for missing or supervening factor(s). In secondary infertility a physician must look for marital discord and avoidance of properly timed sex as possible etiologic factors. Many times one member of the partnership may not want more children, while the other member, eager for additional children to recapture youth or marital harmony, pursues an infertility investigation. Avoidance of stress and reestablishment of rapport with the couple may be constructive while looking for potential organic problems.

### Support Groups

The advent of support groups for infertile couples has had a dramatically positive effect on psychosexual dysfunction in infertility. Groups like RESOLVE, frequently founded by infertile couples with the help of infertility specialists, educate patients to find available services and let them contact other couples with similar problems. These organizations promote the sharing of ideas, grief, and anger, and they disseminate information concerning adoption. Couples are encouraged to channel their energies into positive ways of dealing with this threat to their sexuality and are directed to obtain both medical and psychological help from qualified health care providers.

## EFFECT OF SUCCESS OR FAILURE ON PSYCHOSEXUAL DYNAMICS

While psychosexual factors are intimately involved in the diagnostic evaluation and therapy for infertility, success in achieving and maintaining a pregnancy can further reveal deep basic difficulties in the marriage or sexual interaction. Men and women who have previously been able to blame all psychosexual problems on their inability to produce a conceptus lose their thin protective veneer.

They may feel fatigue, sadness, and anger. Without the prescribed schedule of coital activity they may lack the initiative to have sexual intercourse for pleasure alone. Some couples fear that coitus may injure the fetus (see Chapter 5).

Menning (1980) maintains that the acceptance of terminating an infertility evaluation is crucial to the eventual resolution of feelings of anger and guilt. She states that depression "is a natural part of moving from anger and rage to the acceptance that a loss has occurred and that grief is imminent. When infertility is marked by an end-point, such as the final knowledge that pregnancy will never occur, depression gives way to grief" (pp. 317). Shock and disbelief must subside to allow the sense of loss felt by an individual to be truly experienced and discussed. The couple, successful in their grief reaction and admitting their feelings of object loss, can make new plans and strengthen their relationship. Problems arise when individuals experience a block in this process, manifested by fatigue, sadness, somatic complaints, and expressions of hopelessness.

## CONCLUSION

Clearly a need exists for long-term, prospective, controlled studies designed specifically to determine the relationship between infertility and psychosexual dysfunction. It is important to not presume psychosexual dysfunction as a cause for infertility until all other mechanisms have been excluded and this diagnosis confirmed by a multidisciplinary team of health care providers including gynecologists, psychologists and/or psychiatrists. Subsequently the couple must be guided toward psychosexual adjustment that, hopefully, results in achieving pregnancy.

## REFERENCES

Aaronson, H. G., and Glienke, C. F.: A study of the incidence of pregnancy following adoption. *Fertil. Steril.*, 14:547, 1963.

Amelar, R. D.; Dubin L.; and Walsh, P. C.: *Male Infertility*. Saunders, Philadelphia 1977, pp. 202–203.

Andrews, R. G.: Adoption and the resolution of infertility. *Fertil. Steril.*, 21:73–77, 1970.

Benedek, T.; Ham, G. C.; Robbins, F.; and Rubenstein, B.: Some emotional factors in infertility. *Psychosom. Med.*, 15:485–498, 1953.

Chamberlain, B.; Daugherty, D.; and Schinfeld, J. S.: Cyclic changes in mood during infertility work-ups. (Submitted to *Psychosomatics,* 1984.)

Dawkins, S., and Taylor R.: Non-consummation of marriage. *Lancet,* 2, 1029–1033, 1961.

De Watteville, H.: Psychologic factors in the treatment of sterility. *Fertil. Steril.*, 8:12–24, 1957.

Dorfman, W.: Psychosomatics, psychopharmacology, psychotherapy and sterility. *J. Reprod. Med.,* 34:39–41, 1969.

Eisner, B. G.: Some psychological differences between fertile and infertile women. *J. Clin. Psychol.,* 19:391–395, 1963.

Ellenberg, J. J., and Koren, Z.: Infertility and depression. *Int. J. Fertil.,* 27:219–223, 1982.

Ford, E. S. C.; Forman, I.; Willson, J. R.; Char, W.; Mixon, W. T.; and Scholz, C.: A psychodynamic approach to the study of infertility. *Fertil. Steril.,* 4:456–463, 1953.

Gagnon, C.; Sherins, R. J.; Phillips, D. M.; and Bardin, C. W.: Deficiency of protein-carboxyl methylase in immotile spermatozoa of infertile men. *N. Engl. J. Med.,* 306:821–825, 1982.

Glezerman, M., and Insler, V.: Some factors affecting successes of artificial donor insemination: Survey of 253 couples. In Insler, V. Bettendorf, G.: (eds.): *Advances in Diagnosis and Treatment of Infertility.* Elsevier/North Holland, New York, 1981.

Greenhill, J. P.: Emotional factors in female infertility. *Obstet. Gynecol.,* 7:602–607, 1956.

Grimm, E. R.: Psychological investigation of habitual abortion. *Psychosom. Med.,* 24:369–378, 1962.

Hanson, F. M., and Rock, J.: The effect of adoption on fertility and other reproductive functions. *Am. J. Obstet. Gynecol.,* 59:311–320, 1950.

Harrison, R. F.; O'Moore, A. M.; O'Moore, R. R.; and McSweeney, J. R.: Stress profiles in normal infertile couples: Pharmacological and psychological approaches to therapy. In Insler, V.; Bettendorf, F. G.: (eds.): *Advances in Diagnosis and Treatment of Infertility.,* Elsevier/North Holland, New York, 1981.

Heiman, M.: Toward a psychosomatic concept in infertility. *Int. J. Fertil.,* 4:247–252, 1959.

James, W. H.: Control data for evaluating the efficacy of psychotherapy habitual spontaneous abortion. *Br. J. Psychiatry,* 109:81–83, 1963.

Kaij, L.; Malmquist, A.; and Nilsson, A.: Psychiatric aspects of spontaneous abortion-II. Importance of bereavement, attachment, and neurosis in early life. *J. Psychosom. Res.,* 13:53–59, 1969.

Kaufman, S. A.: Impact of infertility on the marital and sexual relationship. *Fertil. Steril.,* 20:380–383, 1969.

Kerin, J. F.; Kirby, C.; Morris, D.; McEvoy, M.; Ward, B.; and Cox, L. W.: Incidence of the luteinized unruptured follicle phenomenon in cycling women. *Fertil. Steril.,* 40:620–626, 1983.

Keye, W. R. Jr.; Deneris, A.; Butell, S.; Wilson, T.; and Sullivan, J.: Predicting women's emotional response to infertility. Abstract from the *Am. Fertil. Soc. Suppl.,* In *Fertil. Steril.,* 39:417, 1983.

Kostic, T., and Mladenovic, D.: Influence of frigidity on sterility. *Int. J. Fertil.,* 5:417–420, 1960.

Labandibar, B., and Benzecry, L. V.: Frigidity and sterility. *Int. J. Fertil.,* 4:66–69, 1959.

Mai, F. M.; Munday, R. N.; and Rump, E. E.: Psychiatric interview comparisons between infertile and fertile couples. *Psychosom. Med.,* 34:431–440, 1972.

Mandelbrote, B. M., and Monro, M.: Neurotic illness as a factor in reproduction. *Acta Psychiatr. Scand.,* 40:419–426, 1964.

Marbach, A. H., and Schinfeld, L. H.: Psychosomatic aspects of infertility. *Obstet. Gynecol.,* 2:433–441, 1953.

McGuire, L. S.: Psychologic management of infertile women. *Postgrad. Med.,* 57:173–176, 1975.

Menning, B. E.: The emotional needs of infertile couples. *Fertil Steril.,* 34:313–319, 1980.

Moghissi, K. S., and Wallach, E. E.: Unexplained infertility. *Fertil. Steril.,* 39:5–21, 1983.

Morris, T A., and Sturgis, S. H.: Practical aspects of psychosomatic sterility. *Clin. Obstet. Gynecol.,* 28:2890–2899, 1959.

Noyes, R. W., and Chapnick, E. M.: Literature on psychology and infertility. A critical analysis. *Fertil. Steril,* 15:543–558, 1964.

Palti, Z.: Psychogenic male infertility. *Psychosom. Med.,* 31:326–330, 1969.

Platt, J. J.; Ficher, I.; and Silver, M. J.: Infertile couples: Personality traits and self-ideal concept discrepancies. *Fertil. Steril.,* 24:972–976, 1973.

Quigley, M. E.; Sheehan, K. L.; Casper, R. F.; and Yen, S. S. C.: Evidence for increased dopaminergic and opioid activity in patients with hypothalamic hypogonadotropic amenorrhea. *J. Clin. Endocrinol. Metab.,* 50:949–954, 1980.

Sandler, B.: Emotional stress and infertility. *Br. J. Clin. Pract.,* 13:328–330, 1959.

Schinfeld, J.; Tulchinsky, D.; Schiff, I.; and Fishman, J.: Supression of prolactin and gonadotropin secretion in post-menopausal women by 2-hydroxyestrone. *J. Clin. Endocrinol. Metab.,* 50:408–419, 1980.

Seibel, M., and Graves, W. L.: The psychological implications of spontaneous abortions. *J. Reprod. Med.,* 25:161–165, 1980.

Seward, G. H.; Bloch, S. K.; and Heinrich, J. F.: The question of psychophysiologic infertility: some negative answers. *Psychosom. Med.,* 109:81–83, 1963.

Singh, J. R. and Nicki, J. S.: Psychogenic factors in some genetic and non-genetic forms of infertility. *Int. J. Obstet. Gynaecol.,* 20:119–123, 1982.

Stallworthy, J.: Facts and fantasy in the study of female infertility. *Br. J. Obstet. Gynaecol.,* 55:171–180, 1943.

Tupper, C., and Weil, R. J.: The problems with spontaneous abortion. IX, The treatment of habitual aborters by psychotherapy. *Am. J. Obstet. Gynecol.,* 83:421–424, 1982.

Tyler, E. T.; Bonapart, J.; and Gent, J.: The occurence of pregnancy following adoption. *Fertil. Steril.,* 11:581–589, 1960.

Walker, H. E.: Sexual problems and infertility. *Psychosomatics,* 19:477–484, 1978.

Weil, R. J., and Tupper, C.: Personality, life situation and communication: Study of habitual abortion. *Psychosom. Med.,* 22:448–455, 1960.

# CHAPTER 12 PELVIC RELAXATION

*George W. Mitchell, Jr., M.D.*

## INTRODUCTION

There is a remarkable dearth of data in the literature relating to coital function in women whose vaginal outlet is relaxed as a result of childbirth trauma, and the muscular atrophy that is associated with the aging process. Based on what we know of the anatomy and physiology of sexual intercourse, it would seem that such women suffer from a certain degree of disability, but this remains largely unrecorded. The probability is that most patients so afflicted are attended by medical practitioners who fail to ask the pertinent questions and who adopt a mechanistic approach to therapy, but it is also possible that this condition seldom causes significant sexual problems. This chapter is an attempt to assess the extent of current knowledge on the subject and to make a few conjectures.

## SUPPORT OF THE VAGINA

The vagina, like the bladder and rectum, is supported by a broad muscular hammock which descends from the brim of the pelvis and attaches to the sacrum and coccyx. Its two principal components are the pubococcygeus and iliococcygeus muscles. Considered by some anatomists to be a single entity and referred to as the levatores ani, these are somatic striated muscles innervated by branches of the pudendal plexus. The pubococcygeus muscles closely invest the lateral surfaces of the vagina and send interdigitating fibers that meet in the midline between the posterior vagina and the anterior rectal wall. Anterior to the vagina, there is a triangular gap where the twin muscular components of the pubococcygeus fail to meet between the superior vaginal wall and the pubis. This space is filled by the urogenital diaphragm, which is composed of the deep transverse perineal muscles sandwiched between an inferior and a superior layer of fascia. Whether or not the levator muscles contain a sensory element which can be stimulated during coitus to produce a more profound erotic reaction is controversial and the subject of continuing research, but the importance of their power to constrict the vagina remains unquestioned.

At the perineal level, the vagina is surrounded laterally by the bulbocavernosus muscles, which run very close to its walls, and further out by the ischiocavernosus muscles. Posteriorly lie the superficial transverse perineal muscles and the superior margin of the external anal sphincter, meeting in the central tendonous raphe of the perineum and forming the perineal body between vaginal fourchette and anus. Anteriorly is the external urethral sphincter, which, in the female, is anatomically insignificant and, physiologically, relatively so. These muscles are also striated and are innervated by the external pudendal nerve. All assist in narrowing the introitus and are the principal local factor in dysfunctional sexual conditions such as vaginismus. The gripping action of the different muscle groups is further enhanced by the intense paravaginal venous congestion which occurs in response to sexual excitement (Graber, 1982; Netter, 1974).

## OBSTETRICAL TRAUMA

Obstetric trauma to the muscles supporting the vagina is very common, and lacerations may extend in any direction. Such injuries are likely to occur during nulliparous births when the pelvis is small or the baby is large, and when instruments are used. During delivery, the increased pressure exerted on the vaginal supports is most often directed posteriorly toward the perineal body, tearing the superficial muscles and fascia and the upper margin of the external anal sphincter. Prophylactic episiotomies may be directed down the midline or mediolaterally. Since the latter operation involves cutting through the bulbocavernosus, the superficial perineal, and the edge of the levator muscles on one side, the resultant healing of the repair may give rise to future difficulties in sexual function.

Lacerations may also involve the interdigitating fibromuscular extensions of the pubococcygeus muscles higher in the birth canal, causing stretching and separation of the main lateral pillars. Anterior tears damage the urogenital diaphragm, weaken the supports of the bladder and sometimes directly involve that organ. Lack of expertise in the use of forceps may lead to inadvertent avulsion of portions of the pubococcygeus close to its origin at the pelvic brim. Even in the absence of demonstrable damage, a considerable amount of muscular stretching is inevitable, and postpartum, even after complete involution, the vagina remains relaxed relative to the nulliparous state.

## PELVIC RELAXATION

Depending upon the degree of injury sustained, the genetic quality of the individual's elastic tissue, and the adequacy of surgical repair, the vagina may or may not return to a reasonably normal caliber with adequate support. Adverse factors include the state of nutrition, increasing multiparity, aging, and activities which tend to increase intraabdominal pressure. It seems likely that exercises specifically designed to strengthen the deep and superficial muscle groups are beneficial in preventing loss of tone in the muscles. As the end result of any or a combination of the above factors, especially aging—which leads to muscular disuse—herniations may develop. Adjacent organs press in or down upon the vagina, and there is a progressive widening of the vaginal barrel, particularly at the introitus. The relative magnitude of the hernia of bladder or rectum depends to some extent on the original injuries, but usually cystocele and rectocele coexist. They are present to a degree in most parous women and are usually asymptomatic. There may be a concurrent prolapse of the uterus, often associated with enterocele, but this condition rarely exists independently. It is interesting that the severity of the symptoms ascribed to vaginal herniae and vaginal relaxation may bear little relation to the observed anatomic derangement.

The symptoms associated with the vaginal outlet are the presence of a vaginal mass, a dragging sensation in the back and pelvis and a feeling of bladder or rectal pressure. Stress urinary incontinence may be present if there is a loss of support at the urethrovesical junction which alters the delicate balance of pressures in the proximal urethra and bladder. Chronic symptoms of this kind cause fatigue and may eventually become a factor in the development of anxiety and depression, with a focus in the genital area. Whether the dyspareunia or anorgasmic coitus sometimes associated with vaginal relaxation is actually a function of the altered anatomy or of concomitant psychiatric problems is debatable, but it seems likely that each plays a role.

From a rational viewpoint, one might expect that large cystoceles with redundant folds of vaginal mucosa might cause urethral and bladder irritation during coitus, especially when there is residual urine in the bladder, and that postcoital urgency and dysuria might result. In fact, cystoceles seldom contain significant quantities of residual urine and postcoital urethrotrigonitis is more common among nulliparous women. Rectoceles and disruptions of the external anal sphincter cause little sexual difficulty unless attempts at repair have left a buildup of tender scar tissue. Coital pain has been thought by some to be due to abnormal mobility of the uterus, but lack of mobility has been held responsible by others. Since a totally prolapsed uterus not trapped by edema can be pushed high up into the pelvis, it seems unlikely that even deep penile thrusting against the overstretched supports would produce much discomfort. In the occasional case when edema fixes the uterus outside of the introitus or immobilizes it at a low level in the vagina, coitus, obviously, will be difficult or impossible.

One disadvantage of having a very relaxed vagina is that diaphragms may not fit properly and, therefore may not be as comfortable or as safe a means of contraception. Even large diaphragms in a relaxed vagina tend to be displaced more easily than when vaginal supports are satisfactory, and when this happens, dyspareunia and orgasmic failure may ensue.

The question of whether a vagina of very large caliber contributes to sexual dysfunction and orgasmic failure has not been fully answered. Physiologic reasons why this might be so seem plausible. Stimulation of the clitoris during coitus is thought to be in large part responsible for intracoital orgasm, and the mechanism is not so much direct contact with the penis as the indirect effect of traction on the labia minora exerted by penile thrusting, causing clitoral excursion and stimulation. A woman with a normal vagina can accommodate for a discrepancy in penile size by contracting the supporting muscles, thereby obtaining coaptation; however, with weakened muscular supports and a dilated introitus, there would presumably be less pull on the clitoris and, therefore, diminished sensation. To those who believe that there is a sensate focus in the vagina or in the inner margins of the pubococcygeus muscles themselves, leading to "deep" orgasm, it is clear that chronic overdistension of the vagina must, in many cases, lead inevitably to at least qualitative orgasmic failure. Defects and scars in the muscles immediately adjacent to the vagina are also thought by some to induce pain and reduce responsiveness when direct contact is made with the injured area. In addition, the perivaginal vasocongestion known to be caused by sexual excitement may not be as effective in preparing the vagina for intercourse in the absence of good muscle tone. It has also been alleged that overrelaxation of the vagina, especially with gaping, exposes the mucosa to the outside and to friction with clothing and causes dryness and subsequent failure of lubrication (Masters and Johnson, 1966, 1970).

These hypothetical problems were posed to six experienced gynecologists, none of whom could remember more than two or three patients who had actually complained of orgasmic dysfunction as a result of severe degrees of vaginal relaxation, but all of whom could remember at least five or six patients, with and without relaxation, whose husbands had complained about the relative absence of vaginal tonicity. Although this was an informal retrospective survey among a group of physicians who might not always have asked questions appropriate to clarification of the sexual issue, it suggests that, in clinical practice, sexual complaints based on anatomy alone are not common. Because of insufficient contact between penis and the vaginal walls, it is possible that, in some cases of vaginal relaxation, ejaculation may be long deferred or may not occur, but many other factors would have to be elucidated before the vaginal condition could be pinpointed as the direct cause of such a disability. It has also been said that the overrelaxed vagina may make it difficult for a man to realize the approach of his orgasm and that he, therefore, may feel less excitement or be unable to withdraw in time, but specific data on this are lacking. Conversely, a nulliparous woman may not be able to retain the penis without discomfort when she or her partner is in an overriding position, whereas the relaxed outlet, which permits downward thrusting under these circumstances, could accommodate better and produce direct clitoral stimulation.

The use of oral and intravaginal estrogen has long been recommended to improve paravaginal muscle tone and thicken the vaginal mucosa. Undoubtedly this offers relief in terms of alleviating vaginal dryness and preventing or curing atrophic vaginitis and urethrotrigonitis, but its role in increasing vaginal tonicity is doubtful.

Since the early 1950s, exercises designed to strengthen the pubococcygeus muscles and associated supporting structures have become a ritual advocated by physicians, sexologists, and a host of other therapists. These exercises consist of repetitive contractions of the entire pelvic diaphragm, since the individual muscle groups cannot be exercised separately, and the maintenance of these contractions for several seconds at least three times a day for 20 minutes or 20 times a day for three minutes, depending upon the individual therapist's viewpoint. Intensive instruction in the proper technique for conducting these exercises is given to the woman seeking help, who may be there because of stress urinary incontinence, frigidity, spouse's request, or simply to bring her sexual performance to the level the media have led her to believe is normal. Most qualified observers believe that better urinary continence can be achieved through compliance with one of these modalities, although the intracoital, inadvertent voiding that sometimes occurs during coitus, particularly at the time of orgasm, is probably a reflex act and that will not be altered (Kegel, 1952).

Many studies of the tone of the paravaginal muscles have been done in both orgasmic and anorgasmic women, with conflicting results. Most of these studies are of faulty design, and interpretations derived from them can be criticized; however, in general, they suggest that women who are anorgasmic have more atrophic and weaker muscles than do women who are orgasmic. There is also a qualitative, as well as a quantitative factor, involved. The determinations are usually made by clinical examination, the use of a perineometer to determine intravaginal pressure, electromyography, or some combination of these methods (Gillian and Brindley, 1979; Graber et al, 1981; Logan, 1975). Further confusion is added by the fact that some authors (Huey et al, 1982) believe that vaginal deliveries have no effect on the strength of the pubococcygeus muscles and that there is no difference in this type of power between nulliparous and parous women. The beneficial effects of exercises are difficult to determine because of variability in the degree of compliance and because the data are necessarily subjective. Although there is no consensus, there is some agreement that the exercises are probably helpful in improving vascularization, which, in turn, permits better vasocongestion. The edges of the pubococcygeus muscles are brought closer to the midline, thus allowing them to be stroked during coitus, an important feature of the act in the minds of some sex counselors. This concept seems to be another turnabout toward the "vaginal orgasm," described by Freud as separate and distinct from the more superficial and cutaneous clitoral reflex. The theory is that contact with the medial pubococcygeus precipitates a dynamic stretch reflex, the basis for which is unknown, but which some believe is of autonomic rather than somatic nerve derivation. The clonic contractions of the pelvic diaphragm, including the external anal sphincter, which have been noted during orgasm, are thought to be related to this mechanism. Since autonomic nerves have not been demonstrated anatomically in the appropriate areas, it seems more likely that these contractions are cortically mediated.

The time-honored definitive treatment for vaginal relaxation associated with cystocele, rectocele, and uterine prolapse has been plastic surgery. In the repair of vaginal herniae, the uterus is usually removed and the uterosacral ligaments brought together in the midline to prevent recurrent descensus, thus shortening the vagina. Repair of cystocele and rectocele often results in narrowing and further shortening of the vaginal barrel, sometimes with the production of annular constrictions. These procedures should be undertaken only for symptoms directly referable to the anatomy and to organ function, since the outcome can be functionally deleterious. Seldom should they be done for improvement of sexual function alone, and then only after both partners and the entire marital experience have been carefully evaluated by experts to rule out more likely interpersonal factors. Operations designed to raise the perineum in order to further buttress the repair may eventually cause difficulty with intromission as the vagina shrinks with old age and the introitus narrows. Scars resulting from mediolateral episiotomies can cause similar difficulties in younger people. Frequently, it is necessary to widen the introitus by lowering the perineum and everting the posterior vaginal mucosa in order to permit painless intromission.

## SUMMARY

We need more information regarding sexual activity and satisfaction in women with moderate to advanced degrees of cystocele, rectocele and other manifestations of prolapse of the pelvic floor. Undoubtedly other symptoms, such as pressure sensation in the pelvis and urinary retention or incontinence predominate over coital dysfunction in the minds of many such patients and their physicians, and the sexual history is sketchy or nonexistent. History taking should include questions regarding frequency of intercourse, reasons for possible abstinence, orgasmic response, both qualitative and quantitative, and intra and post coital pain or discomfort. When a disability exists, other causes such as vaginal infection or dryness due to lack of estrogen must be ruled out. Emotional factors and the relationship with the sexual partner should be probed and adequate counseling provided. Exercise designed to strengthen the perivaginal musculature are taught. As a final resort, applicable in few cases for this purpose, surgery may be attempted.

## REFERENCES

Gillan, P., and Brindley, G. S.: Vaginal and pelvic floor responses to sexual stimulation. *Psychophysiology* 16:471, 1979.

Graber, B., and Kline-Graber, G.: Female orgasm: Role of pubococcygeus muscle. *J. Clin. Psychiatry* 35:157, 1981.

Graber, B.: (Ed.): *Circumvaginal Musculature and Sexual Function.* S. Karger, New York, 1982.

Huey, C. J.; Graver, B.; Kline, G.; and Golden, C. J.: Studies of the circumvaginal musculature in a treatment population. In Graber, B.: (ed.): *Circumvaginal Musculature and Sexual Function.* Karger, New York, 1982.

Kegel, A. H.: Sexual functions of the pubococcygeus muscle. *West. J. Surg. Obstet. Gynecol.,* 60:521–524, 1952.

Logan, T. G.: The vaginal clasp: A method of comparing contractions across subjects. *J. Sex Res.* 11:353, 1975.

Masters, W. H., and Johnson, V. E.: *Human Sexual Response.* Little, Brown, Boston, 1966.

Masters, W. H., and Johnson, V. E.: *Human Sexual Inadequacy.* Little, Brown, Boston, 1970.

Netter, F. H.: Reproductive system. In Oppenheimer, E.: (Ed.): *The CIBA Collection of Medical Illustrations,* Vol. 2. CIBA Pharmaceutical Co., Summit, New Jersey, 1974.

# CHAPTER 13  PSYCHOSEXUAL PROBLEMS RELATED TO PELVIC PAIN

*David Charles, M.D., and Douglas D. Glover, M.D.*

## INTRODUCTION

Sexual compatibility may not be the foundation of a happy marriage, but incompatibility can certainly have a destructive effect on any union. Anything that causes sexual dissatisfaction will adversely affect the patient, the partner, and the couple as a unit.

Sexuality is an important aspect of the patient's life. Discussion with the physician while the history is being taken and during physical examination can help to at least elucidate problems and aid the patient. Normal findings should be emphasized by simple reassurance or by furnishing facts that may serve to alleviate unnecessary anxiety. The physician's responsibility is the recognition of sexual dysfunction and the provision of support. Inability to do so necessitates referral to a physician who has both experience and expertise in the management of psychosexual problems.

Although the most common origins of sexual dysfunction have psychogenic and cultural bases, physicians should be able to recognize and modify the organic causes whenever possible. Identification of any organic etiology may prevent prolonged therapy at undue expense and inconvenience to the patient.

## PELVIC PAIN

Dyspareunia is the most common complaint associated with the organic causes of female sexual dysfunction. Dyspareunia may be due to pelvic congestion, vaginismus, or other specific syndromes. Another frequent complaint is orgasmic dysfunction. Though it is not usually associated with organic causes, orgasmic difficulties may result from pelvic pathology. Sometimes both of these symptoms are interrelated and may represent different stages of sexual dysfunction. Each is, however, related to one or more etiological factors.

Most females with dyspareunia can pinpoint the site of their coital pain without difficulty. Dyspareunia in a woman who cannot locate the site of the discomfort is most likely to be psychogenic in origin. Interrogation, investigation, and management should be predicated on such a presumption. Evaluation of a patient's emotional and psychic state is part of the study of her coital difficulty. Direct questions are asked about her sexual life. Once reticence has been overcome, much useful information can be forthcoming which will help not only in establishing a diagnosis, but also in the institution of therapy. If the patient desires to be relieved of her problem its nature will be revealed. In a patient with relatively superficial dyspareunia, psychogenic factors may be relieved by explanation and reassurance or through a readjustment in her environment. A conference may be held with her partner. Patients who have deep-seated psychological blockades related to sexual matters should be referred for psychiatric evaluation and therapy.

Most instances of dyspareunia, however, are due to organic, anatomic, or inflammatory disorders. Psychogenic dyspareunia is relatively uncommon.

By nature of her biological responsibilities, a woman's reproductive function can be separated from her enjoyment of coitus. Nature can be served whether or not she achieves any satisfaction; even her consent is unnecessary. Though there is obviously both a physical element to sexual satisfaction and a rhythm of response associated with the ovarian hormonal cycle in some individuals, psychological factors are important in the majority of women. Circumstances, therefore, can determine the woman's response in a way they do not in the man. Psychogenic factors may certainly influence the reaction, particularly when failure to achieve orgasm is primary, as this may result from faulty education, traumatic early experience, fear of being hurt, fear of pregnancy, or an unwillingness to do something that the woman believes necessitates surrender of a part of her personality. This personality problem is characteristic of women who are poor at sustaining personal relationships and would, perhaps, be more commonly seen if it was not in itself often a barrier to marriage. Faulty education may include the imperceptible absorption of ideas from friends and relatives as well as from parents. One sometimes encounters a woman whose problem appears to stem from the way in which the facts of biological reproduction have been acquired.

It is well recognized that the patient who has had previous pelvic inflammatory disease without any residual pelvic pathology may exhibit guilt and this may be associated with an excessive desire to prove her fertility. The overextending of a woman's desire to conceive can cause dyspareunia and this may be associated with vaginismus. Vaginismus can certainly be a cause of superficial dyspareunia in some of these patients.

Physicians are all too ready to ascribe deep dyspareunia to demonstrable pathology, but this may not always be the case. A retroverted uterus, however, even when mobile, may be associated with deep dyspareunia because the ovaries can be trapped in the cul-de-sac and pressed against the sacrum at the time of coitus. In such circumstances, the dyspareunia may be intermittent, since it depends on the ovaries being located deep in the pelvis. In most instances, this form of painful intercourse in the absence of pelvic adhesive disease is relieved by coitus in the left lateral position. Lesions in the pelvis, however, such as previous sepsis or endometriosis may result in pain which can be reproduced on pelvic examination and elicitation of pain is extremely important. Also, appropriate treatment can usually bring relief. Finally, back lesions, such as a prolapsed intervetebral disc or sacroiliac strain, can give rise to pain after coitus which may be referred around to the abdomen. This pain characteristically lasts for a day or more after coitus.

At the same time, it is necessary to discuss pelvic congestion because many women's problems have been attributed to pelvic congestion associated with sexual frustration. This may be part of the problem in pelvic inflammatory disease where the patient is frustrated that she has not conceived. It is difficult to know how much weight, however, to attribute to such a fact as pelvic congestion when sexual frustration is so often a symptom of a poor relationship and general discontent. Masters and Johnson (1970) were able to show a gradually developing, but eventually intense pelvic vasocongestion with enlargement of the uterus, in a woman subjected to repeated pelvic examination and coital stimulation over a period of six hours. The congestion was rapidly relieved by orgasm. It would not be surprising if such congestion repeatedly induced by sexual stimulation but never relieved by satisfactory climax did ultimately produce such problems as low-grade pain and menstrual abnormalities. It is, however, impossible to ascertain how common such factors are although it is recognized that counseling both partners will usually provide an improvement in general health and mental outlook.

Vaginismus, refers to the partly voluntary, partly spontaneous contraction of the pelvic muscles that occurs when coitus is attempted and, as a result, it may make coitus painful or at times impossible. In the majority of instances, vaginismus is psychological. Rarely, there is a painful lesion of the vulva such as a scar or an infection which causes involuntary spasm as a protective reflex. Usually, however, a physical examination discloses nothing whatsoever but a reluctance to be examined. In these circumstances a reluctant attitude about sex generally based on poor education will often be discovered. However, vaginismus may also be a reflex as a result of psychogenic disturbances related to previous pelvic inflammatory disease, specifically gonococcal infection. The gynecologist has an enormous advantage over the psychiatrist when dealing with vaginismus. The patient attending the gynecological outpatient clinic or the physician's office expects a pelvic examination whereas the woman attending the psychiatric clinic would reasonably look askance at such a suggestion. In practice the vaginal examination has both diagnostic and therapeutic benefits.

It is important to stress that no woman should be labeled as having dyspareunia of a psychosomatic or functional etiology without a very thorough investigation by a gynecologist. The responsibility rests on the individual who labels dyspareunia functional to make sure that all organic causes have been ruled out. A sound knowledge of the anatomic relationships of the female genital tract is essential to elicit the cause of dyspareunia. In the case of previous pelvic inflammatory disease, it has been well-established that the diagnosis is commonly in doubt, and errors in diagnosis are frequent. In fact, with deep dyspareunia, the two common causes are endometriosis or pelvic inflammatory disease. Frequently, endometriosis can mimic upper genital tract infection and consequently laparoscopy is necessary in order to establish the diagnosis.

ORGANIC CAUSES OF PELVIC PAIN

**Pelvic Inflammatory Disease.** The incidence of acute pelvic inflammatory disease, commonly referred to as an acute salpingitis or PID, seems to be rising and consequently is one of the most frequently encountered gynecological disorders. It usually afflicts young women and its late sequelae are often severe and result in involuntary sterility, an increased risk of ectopic pregnancy, and chronic pain.

Obstruction of the fallopian tubes is the most commonly identifiable cause of female infertility. Tubal occlusion most often follows pelvic infection. Pelvic inflammatory disease must now be considered to have a multifactorial microbial etiology. In women under 25 years of age it most often is caused by microbial agents transmittable during sexual intercourse. As a consequence of the world-wide epidemic of sexually transmitted diseases, the incidence of salpingitis is increasing as is the incidence of postinfection infertility. An intrauterine pregnancy, however, is the only unequivocal proof that tubal function has been preserved after pelvic inflammatory disease.

The role of *Neisseria gonorrhoeae* as the leading cause of salpingitis is now being questioned. *Chlamydia trachomatis* as well as anaerobic organisms are now recognized as etiological agents for upper genital tract infections.

The physician attempting to diagnose and treat infections of the genital tract caused by *Chlamydia trachomatis* faces a dilemma. On the one hand, he or she knows that chlamydial infections are both common and important, but on the other hand, laboratory diagnostic techniques are not, at present, universally available. The only escape from this paradox appears to be the physician's sound knowledge of the various clinical syndromes which result from infection by this organism, as well as exclusion of other causes, and treatment with suitable antimicrobial agents.

The availability of laboratory tests for sexually transmitted diseases is variable, but most physicians have ready access to facilities whereby most microbiological studies can be performed. The introduction of transport media for suitable cultures has entirely altered the diagnostic capabilities of the physician who has to deal with pelvic infections.

An accurate diagnosis of pelvic inflammatory disease requires the use of diagnostic laparoscopy as the diagnosis can be verified in only 70 percent of patients suspected on clinical grounds.

Chlamydial infections are not associated with distinctive symptoms or signs that would enable a clinician to make an accurate diagnosis without recourse to laboratory help. As noted, access to a diagnostic facility capable of isolating *Chlamydia trachomatis* is not widely available, and in the absence of such a service, most clinicians now treat female contacts of men with nongonococcal urethritis with antibiotics active against Chlamydia trachomatis, especially as it has been shown that about one-third of such women harbour this organism in the cervix. Furthermore, a similar proportion of women who have gonococcal infections or who are contacts of men with gonorrhoea are Chlamydia positive, and it has been proposed that treatment regimens for the management of patients with proven or suspected gonorrhoea should incorporate antichlamydial agents.

The symptoms of inflammation of the fallopian tubes and ovary resemble those of pelvic peritonitis. Acute lesions may develop rapidly with grave symptoms indistinguishable from other forms of the acute abdomen, which may develop without localizing signs. More frequently, the onset is less severe and the two main symptoms are fever and pain. Vomiting is rare, an important clinical point in distinguishing acute salpingitis from inflammation associated with the appendix. The pyrexia can be quite severe, up to 103° F, and may be associated with chills and rigors. Subsequently, the temperature pursues an irregularly intermittent course similar to that of septicemia. One should, however, be cognizant of the fact that with patients with Chlamydal salpingitis, only one-third have fever.

Salpingitis is usually a polymicrobial infection. In some cases of polymicrobial infection, recurrences of pyrexia occur with intervals of abatement; this indicates that the inflammatory process involving the tubes has succeeded in passing the barrier and has invaded fresh regions of the peritoneum and that the suppurative process has extended. In the severe cases, the pulse rate is proportionately elevated to the temperature and when it is disproportionately rapid, septicemia should be suspected.

Abdominal pain and distention, initially limited to the hypogastrium or to one or the other side, are usually present and indicate localized peritonitis. Great tenderness can be elicited on abdominal pressure. Defecation and micturition may be painful.

The symptoms indicative of suppuration and pus formation are not always clear. Chills and rigors may be absent and the temperature is not invariably elevated. After a time the general condition deteriorates, the pulse quickens and sweating occurs. Diaphoresis occurs only with a fulminant polymicrobial infection.

Assistance in the diagnosis of pus formation may be obtained by means of a differential blood count, which should be repeated on one or more occasions, as a single estimation is frequently unreliable. A count of 20,000–25,000 leukocytes, of which 80 percent are polymorphonuclear cells, indicates the presence of pus. The sedimentation rate may become elevated in severe cases to about 60 ml within one hour. On the other hand, if Chlamydia trachomatis is the cause of the pelvic inflammatory process, the sedimentation rate rarely exceeds 20 ml in an hour, and a leukocytosis is only present in 30 percent, of such individuals (Westrom, 1980). The patient may have no pelvic complaints but may present with the Fitz–Hugh–Curtis syndrome where the symptoms of perihepatitis can stimulate cholecystitis and, on occasion, cholelithiasis.

In the great majority of cases of chronic tubo-ovarian inflammation, a prolonged history of pain and general ill health is obtained which can be traced to a previous episode of infection. An important clinical feature of chronic adnexitis is a history of intercurrent acute attacks or exacerbations at irregular intervals. These exacerbations produce the usual clinical features of acute pelvic inflammation and are usually attended by slight to moderate abdominal pain and fever. Frequently they are sufficiently severe to necessitate confinement to bed for several days, and the onset is often synchronous with menses. These acute episodes do not, of necessity, indicate the presence of suppuration, but they imply that the infective agent is still active in the inflammatory focus. In the course of time the relapses cease, as the virulence of the infected agent becomes exhausted after suitable antimicrobial therapy.

During the quiescent phases, chronic inflammatory lesions give rise to few symptoms. They are aggravated by exertion, so that the patient becomes disinclined to any exertional effort and commonly falls into a state of chronic invalidism. Hypermenorrhea and dysmenorrhea are nearly always present and probably arise, in part, from associated chronic infection of the endometrium. Dyspareunia and sterility are common, and sooner or later nervous symptoms may be superimposed, which may distract attention from the true cause of the illness. Occasionally gross pelvic lesions, such as pyosalpinx, are tolerated so well they cause little or no trouble.

Of all the varieties of pelvic inflammatory swelling, the tubo-ovarian is by far the most common. Chronic cellulitis is rare. The most common result of adnexitis is the formation of adhesions, leading subsequently to displacement and loss of mobility of the uterus and its appendages.

The swelling produced by salpingo-oophoritis almost invariably lies in the posterior compartment of the pelvic cavity. As a rule, it is not mesial but posterolateral in location and in about three quarters of the cases both sides are involved, either in the form of a single mass, or two distinct swellings. The lesion on one side may be appreciably larger than the other, which is now more apparent since greater attention has been paid to unilateral inflammatory masses associated with the use of the intrauterine contraceptive device. In other cases, a definite swelling is formed on one side, and only an ill-defined thickening of the other tube and ovary can be felt. The actual characteristics of the swelling vary and the outline of the affected tube and ovary is often obscured by the presence of surrounding exudative peritonitis. The latter results in the formation of a firm, fixed, tender adnexal mass, the nature of which can only be inferred. This is a further reason why one should consider laparoscopy in pelvic inflammatory disease. At times, more details can be recognized: a pedunculated attachment to the uterine horn, a curved structure representing the tube, or a globular or oval portion representing the ovary. Again, it is important to evaluate these patients with ultrasound because real-time ultrasound has done a great deal to aid in the elucidation of gynecologic pathology. A rectal examination should always be performed for it will indicate the relationship of the swelling to the anterior rectal wall. A finger in the rectum can reach the lower and posterior surfaces of a cul-de-sac mass while through the vagina only the anterior surface can be felt. Consequently, a rectal examination is of great value in elucidating the diagnosis of pelvic inflammatory disease.

On infrequent occasions the inflammatory swellings are sufficiently large to extend above the pelvic brim and to be palpable on abdominal examination. In every case of pelvic inflammatory swelling the possibility of an endometriotic cyst of the ovary, as well as diverticulitis, must be considered in the differential diagnosis. Careful attention to the clinical history and symptomatology is of prime importance in this regard.

The medical consequences of this entity are significant as at least 20 percent of those who acquire salpingitis become infertile. The incidence of ectopic pregnancy increases, six to tenfold in these individuals and chronic pain due to adhesions is present in at least 20 percent of the patients. In fact, a quarter of the patients who have acute salpingitis develop long-term sequelae.

Unquestionably, emotional and/or psychological disturbances may interfere with sexual activity, but the importance of anatomic abnormalities and organic pathologic lesions as causes of dyspareunia tend to be underestimated. At times the psychic and physical causes are intertwined, and the examiner must unravel their respective roles. Many women following pelvic inflammatory disease hesitate to mention sexual difficulties to their physician unless they are severe and intense, yet these problems may directly affect their well-being. Thus, it is often necessary for the physician to explore a patient's sexual activities and attitudes tactfully as part of an approach to management of a presumably sexually unrelated condition.

**Tubal Ligation.** Another matter which must be addressed is coital difficulties after tubal sterilization. The incidence of menstrual disorders following sterilization varies from study to study but no doubt remains: Whether the procedure be tubal ligation or fulguration, late morbidity in the coital sense may be considerable. The late morbidity may on occasion emanate from guilt feelings as a result of the patient's loss of her procreating role. A feeling of mutilation can result and, as there are several myths about the results of tubal ligation, it is important that factual information be given to such individuals.

Deep perineal pain secondary to surgical incisions or deep pain in the cul-de-sac after vaginal tubal ligation with adhesions when infection ensued, produces sensations that result in muscle spasm. The levator-ani spasm syndrome, resulting in pain in the sacrococcygeal area, rectum, and pelvic diaphragm, is caused by spastic tender muscles. This syndrome is confirmed by rectal examination which elicits pain in the area described.

**Uterine Retrodisplacement.** Bilateral chronic salpingitis is the most common form of pelvic inflammation associated with dyspareunia, and the widespread peritoneal adhesions which are usually present result in loss of mobility of the uterus and adnexa. Reposition of the uterus except by surgical measures is impossible. The mass of inflamed structures filling the posterior pelvic compartment in women so afflicted may be the cause of intense suffering and dyspareunia.

It must be emphasized that in the majority of cases of uterine displacement, such as retroversion which is uncomplicated by previous pelvic inflammatory disease, there are usually no symptoms and no treatment is required. However, retroversion of the uterus may be associated with a greater or lesser degree of pain in the lower abdomen and sacral region, irregular menstruation, menstrual pain, and leukorrhea. Some women, as mentioned, will complain of dyspareunia and sterility. It must be remembered that a similar symptom complex, due to other causes, may be noted when the position of the uterus is normal; accordingly, the dependence of the symptoms on malposition of the uterus cannot always be postulated with certainty in any given case.

Pain when present may be of a dull aching variety, and most commonly it takes the form of backache or dragging sensation in one or both iliac regions. Characteristically the backache associated with uncomplicated retroversion is relieved when the patient lies down and should not be present at night nor upon waking in the morning. However, in cases where the uterus is tethered by adhesions, the backache is very severe and not related to posture. Sterility is not a common symptom of retroversion *per se,* but occasionally is the only factor that can be elicited after several years of nonfertile marriage, and the correction of the retrodisplaced uterus may result in conception.

A further source of error lies as previously mentioned in the fact that retrodisplacement may be found in women who present with a complex of functional disturbances referable to the pelvic organs. Great difficulty is encountered in elucidating the role of the pelvic adhesions and malposition of the uterus as a cause for the patient's symptoms. No clinical problem taxes the patience and judgment of the conscientious physician more than this one. If the rule, apparently followed by some, is observed of correcting every case of backward displacement it may be said safely that only a small proportion of the patients so treated would derive any benefit.

**Intrauterine Device.** Individuals who use an intrauterine device for contraception may complain of intermenstrual bleeding and cramping abdominal pain. Submucosal microabscesses may form underneath the intrauterine device, and once endometritis is established, bacteria may ascend the lymphatics to the perimetrial tissues and broad ligaments resulting in salpingitis. It is important to remember that unilateral pelvic inflammatory disease is often associated with the use of an intrauterine contraceptive device (Kaufman, Shapiro, Rosenberg, et al, 1980; Lee, Rubin, Ory et al, 1983). With the increasing incidence of various sexually transmitted diseases it is difficult to attribute these tubal infections specifically to intrauterine devices. While the prevalence of lower tract gonorrhea does not appear altered when patients use the intrauterine device, there is some evidence that suggests an increase in the risk of upper genital tract disease (Faulkner and Ory, 1976). However, most patients, who have developed pelvic infection associated with an intrauterine device, have in the previous months exhibited milder symptoms such as pelvic pain, bleeding, and uterine tenderness upon examination. Thus, if a patient has significant discomfort with the device, it is recommended that it be removed in an attempt to prevent more serious complications.

**Genital Herpes.** Today, genital herpes is receiving a great deal of publicity and, in the case of the married couple, the sudden and unexpected outbreak of genital lesions in either the male or female may be followed by accusations of that partner's infidelity. The stigma surrounding genital herpes infections can be blamed for the psychological trauma that results from such encounters. It is conceivable that there has been no marital infidelity in some cases, but nonetheless consideration of the psychological trauma that the individual may suffer from the exposure of his or her unfaithfulness is a concern that cannot be neglected. The psychological problems associated with recurrent episodes of genital herpes in unmarried individuals who desire to have a marriage and children are enormous. This group of individuals has to cope with problems that appear very similar to those presented by individuals having far more serious diseases. Although *Chlamydia trachomatis* is the most common of the sexually transmitted disease agents, herpes is the most feared. The reason for this is more attributable to the media than the medical community. However, the fact that there is no known cure or vaccine for herpes obviously contributes to the excessive worries patients have. Many recognize that the sexual revolution and the change in sexual mores of the last decade undoubtedly has played a role in elevating the incidence of herpes genitalis to epidemic proportions. One point which must not be overlooked: The sexual revolution may have played a significant role in allowing an unmarried individual to become infected, and its impact on present-day lifestyles may also contribute significantly to the psychological cruelty of the disease.

**Miscellaneous Problems.** Other causes of pelvic pain, however, should be considered and these are those associated with the lower intestinal tract, the urinary tract, or skeletal system. Chronic pelvic congestion can be associated with pelvic varicosities and previous pelvic inflammatory disease.

## PSYCHOLOGICAL CAUSES OF PELVIC PAIN

Lamont (1980), in a review of 230 women who complained of pain during intercourse, found that only 68 had a primarily physical problem. He concluded that a minority of patients who presented with the chief complaint of dyspareunia have an identifiable physical source for their pain. Seventy percent of the cases he evaluated were found to have a psychosocial cause of their pain such as vaginismus, failure of vaginal lubrication, or vaginal barrel changes. Lamont concluded that although dyspareunia is an important gynecological complaint, careful physical assessment and evaluation of intrapsychic relationships are necessary to insure that the source of the problem is identified so that appropriate therapy can be instituted.

Lamont also indicated that there were five patients who could not be assigned to any specific diagnostic category. Although they presented with pelvic findings compatible with pelvic inflammatory disease, laparoscopic examination revealed no abnormality. In his group of patients, however, there was only one patient who was referred to as having had adhesions associated with dyspareunia. This finding is surprising because the sexual mores of the last decade have been associated with an increased incidence of pelvic inflammatory disease. In Lamont's group of patients, many complained of premenstrual tension, dysmenorrhea, or infertility, but these symptoms could only on rare occasions be ascribed to chronic pelvic inflammatory disease.

Patients at every educational level present with advanced stages of serious sexual disorders. Here mechanisms other than sexual ignorance—avoidance and denial—may be operational. This state of affairs is commonly encountered in patients who have had pelvic inflammatory disease; they believe that if their sexual difficulties are ignored they will go away. In other individuals, minimal lesions are given undue importance so that many of their daily activities are unfavorably influenced. Sometimes the presence of a small lesion is used as an excuse to avoid sex or the patient will be abstinent because she is afraid that she is going to infect her partner.

A careful and instructive examination, however, may alleviate anxieties and provide the patient with sexual education which may prove curative. The latter is not, however, easy when the patient has severe chronic salingitis. Again it is necessary to emphasize that laparoscopy should be performed in patients with pelvic pain when the etiology is not readily discernible. In one study (Pent, 1972) about 50 percent of the patients with a diagnosis of pelvic pain with clinically normal findings had pelvic pathology that could have accounted for their symptomatology. On the other hand, about one-third of the patients whom gynecologists considered to have abnormal pelvic findings were found to have no abnormality at laparoscopy.

Psychosomatic disorders are common in gynecological practice and the symptoms of such disorders may closely simulate organic pelvic disease. It is well known that intense emotion may evoke somatic accompaniments. Such emotion may be but a brief incident or may be due to prolonged resentment or insecurity. Different emotions will produce different somatic reactions. What is important clinically is that different impulses from the periphery may dominate the patient's consciousness and may be the predominant complaint to the exclusion of any spontaneous reference to the psychological factor that originally evoked them. This psychological component can only be established by obtaining a well-documented history and if such a biography reveals no intelligible reason for assuming the existence of evidence for a morbid emotional state, it is unwise to regard any symptoms the patient may have as functional even if these bear no immediate evidence of organic pathology. Such an observation is obviously of the utmost importance in clinical gynecology and emphasizes the necessity to inquire into a patient's emotional background closely, especially in women who complain of symptoms where clinical evidence of an organic cause cannot be substantiated.

Psychosomatic disorders may express themselves as menstrual abnormalities, such as polymenorrhea, hypermenorrhea, or various types of abdominopelvic pain. These are also common manifestations of chronic salpingitis. Furthermore, such pelvic symptoms, whether physiological or pathological, may occur at a time when the woman has experienced some emotional distress or difficulty. This is especially true, for example, if her relations with her husband should take the form of neglect. Then, she will be in need of affection and sympathy, and if this particular symptomatology is successful in restoring the husband's attentions, it is possible that a woman may subconsciously prolong the symptoms for an indefinite period, long after the original cause has ceased to operate.

There are two types of patients encountered by the gynecologist who are particularly prone to adverse psychological reactions. The first is the patient who has had numerous surgical procedures for abdominopelvic pain without any relief. The second is the patient with chronic pelvic pain who may or may not have pelvic organic disease. Such patients are usually individuals who are unhappy and lonely with a prolonged history of sexual unresponsiveness. These individuals have been significantly deprived of parental affection or interest as children. They have a history of many childhood illnesses for which they have achieved strong secondary gains. Many such patients have had to assume adult responsibility at an early age, marry in their teens, and relate a history of hard, unremitting, and unappreciated work. Psychosocial pathology during adolescence including rape, incest, or running away from home are found in about 25 percent of such individuals, and these patients tend to marry to escape their nuclear family.

Gynecologists are likely to meet with a significant number of women who gravitate to the gynecological clinic complaining of a multiplicity of symptoms for which no obvious organic cause can be found. Many of these patients are convinced there is an underlying pelvic condition responsible for their illness and if such a condition could only be diagnosed or removed they would be well. Certainly in some of these patients, there may be some minor organic condition present. Indeed, in most women who have had children it is usually so, but the gynecologist knows that such conditions are not, as a rule, associated with symptoms in normal-functioning women. It would appear that these women experience increased nervous irritability and have a marked decrease in their pain threshold. They appear to be conscious of even normal physiologic functions and minor pathologic conditions that usually cause no symptoms, or, in the extreme case, only minor discomfort is associated with intense pain. Backache, bearing down pains, pain in both iliac fossae—though more frequently to the left—and morbid pelvic sensations are commonly complained of, often in the most extravagant terms. Palpation in these regions during examination can cause intense discomfort in the absence of any clinical evidence of pelvic pathology. Therefore, the medical attendant is prompted to ascribe such symptoms to organic disease in the absence of any pathology. The appendix may be blamed, if it has not already been sacrificed, and if it has, then the symptoms are ascribed to postoperative adhesions. When the pain is located mainly in the left iliac fossa, a spastic colon may be thought responsible for the symptoms. If pelvic in location, the ovary is considered to be the source of the patient's pain and a diagnosis of inflammation or enlargement of the organ made, in spite of the fact that such a state is, in the absence of tubal infection, a rare occurrence.

It is possible that infertility may result from psychological disorders, as it is well recognized that sterility can be associated with anxiety due to failure to conceive (Chapter 11). Frigidity is another example of a psychosomatic disorder. It is important not only for the distress and unhappiness it causes but because of its far-reaching effects. A multitude of symptoms may unfold when one tries to evaluate dyspareunia or frigidity. Such symptoms as insomnia, weakness, loss of weight, and vague pains over a wide distribution may be noted by these patients and in fact what they are referring to is that they are in a chronic state of ill health. As few women will volunteer information about their sexual inadequacies, the physician, when confronted with such individuals, should ascertain whether such a state of affairs exists, and, if possible, correct it.

## CONCLUSION

Although there is nothing new about the idea that sexual compatibility can be an important factor in the success of a marriage, today, unlike previous years, premarital sex is often an important part of premarital behavior. Even though sexual behavior is becoming more conservative in light of the media exploitation of herpes infection, the impact of the sexual revolution lingers on. Many individuals feel entitled to learn more about private physical parts, libido, as well as sexual techniques and inhibitions before making any long-term commitments. Demands such as these could place enormous pressure on individuals with a past history of pelvic inflammatory disease.

Upon recognition of such complex diseases in the pursuit of partners, some individuals are driven by hopelessness, depression, and despair to abandon the idea of finding a lifelong companion temporarily. Society promotes the institution of marriage and the pursuit of it, a concept instilled in children at an early age. But, if the risk of acquiring sexually transmitted diseases continues to rise at the present rate, in the year 2000, estimates predict that one out of every two women under the age of 23 will have some form of pelvic inflammatory disease.

## REFERENCES

Cunanan, R. G. Jr.; Courey, N. G.; and Lippes, J.: Laparoscopic findings in patients with pelvic pain. *Am. J. Obstet. Gynecol.,* 146:589–591, 1983.

Faulkner, W. L. and Ory, H. W.: Intrauterine devices and acute pelvic inflammatory disease. *JAMA,* 235:1851–1853, 1976.

Kaufman, D. W.; Shapiro, S.; Rosenberg, L.; et al.: Intrauterine contraception device use and pelvic inflammatory disease. *Am. J. Obstet. Gynecol.,* 136:159–162, 1980.

Lamont, J. A.: Female dyspareunia. *Am. J. Obstet. Gynecol.,* 136:282–285, 1980.

Lee, N. C.; Rubin, G. L.; Ory, H. W.; et al.: Type of intrauterine device and the risk of pelvic inflammatory disease. *Obstet. Gynecol.,* 62:1–6, 1983.

Masters, W. H., and Johnson, V. E.: *Human Sexual Inadequacy.* Little, Brown, Boston, 1970.

Osser, S.; Liedholm, M. D.; and Sjoberg, N-O.: Risk of pelvic inflammatory disease among users of intrauterine devices. *Am. J. Obstet. Gynecol.,* 138:864–867, 1980.

Pent, D.: Laparoscopy: Its role in private practice. *Am. J. Obstet. Gynecol.* 113:459–468, 1972.

Westrom, L.: Incidence, prevalence, and trends of acute pelvic inflammatory disease and its consequences in industrialized countries. *Am. J. Obstet. Gynecol.,* 138:888–892, 1980.

Zetzel, L.: Fertility, pregnancy, and idiopathic inflammatory bowel disease. In Kirsner, J. B., and Shorter, R. G.: (eds.): *Inflammatory Bowel Disease,* 2nd ed. Lea and Febiger, Philadelphia, 1980, pp. 241–253.

# CHAPTER 14  HUMAN SEXUALITY AND BENIGN NEOPLASIA

*Alan H. DeCherney, M.D., Dorothy A. Greenfeld, M.S.W., and Mary Lake Polan, M.D., Ph.D.*

## INTRODUCTION

Benign neoplasia of the female pelvic organs is a frequent occurrence and ranges in severity from a small inocuous cervical polyp to a 20-week size myomatous uterus or a frozen pelvis riddled with endometriosis. Clearly the psychosexual sequelae of such disparate pathology will range from nil to severe. In this chapter we will concern ourselves with the benign gynecologic conditions of endometriosis, pelvic inflammatory disease (PID), fibroid uterus, endometrial polyps, and disease of the Bartholin's gland, and the implications they present for impairment of psychosexual function. The primary immediate problems related to these conditions are, of course, pelvic pain or vaginal bleeding. These clinical manifestations bring the woman to her physician where an assessment of the degree of pathology and the extent of physical and emotional dysfunction are made. Depending on age, parity, and education, various forms of medical or surgical therapy are initiated. However, since these are all progressive conditions, pathology or dysfunction of long duration and increasing severity is ultimately resolved by removal of the offending organs. Thus, no discussion of benign gynecologic neoplasia is complete without consideration of hysterectomy and its psychosexual ramifications.

## VAGINAL BLEEDING

A number of benign gynecological conditions result in prolonged, heavy, or irregular vaginal bleeding. Menorrhagia has been operationally defined as loss of more than 80 cc of blood during the menstrual period (Chimbira et al., 1979).

Initial therapy of significant vaginal bleeding, after malignancy has been ruled out, is usually medical. Hormonal manipulation with or without additional curettages of the uterus (dilation and curettage; D&Cs) is often successful in controlling menometrorrhagia associated with anovulation or perimenopausal hormonal changes. Heavy vaginal bleeding may also result from benign mass lesions such as fibroids and endometrial polyps and in these cases is frequently unresponsive to steroid therapy. Severe blood loss associated with such benign neoplasias may result in anemia requiring blood transfusion or surgical intervention.

As DeCherney and Polan (1983) report, a group of 14 women with severe intractable menometrorrhagia unrelated to hormonal causes underwent hysteroscopy and all were found to have benign intrauterine neoplasia—either myomata or polyps—which were excised hysteroscopically with return of normal cycles. Thus, submucous fibroids or benign endometrial polyps can result in severe blood loss necessitating surgical intervention. In the vast majority of cases, however, definitive surgery is performed with removal of the uterus and in certain cases the ovaries as well. A full discussion of the ramifications of extirpative surgery is deferred until later.

However, we must not overlook the emotional and functional implications of heavy or prolonged vaginal bleeding. Menstruation is commonly termed "the curse" suggesting that despite the symbolic representation of the uterus and its cyclic functions as "a source of strength, health and general effectiveness" (Turpin and Heath, 1979), there must also be some negative associations. These can be most easily divided into the categories of inconvenience and fear. In a society where more than half the women under age 50 work outside the home (Roeske, 1978), prolonged, heavy vaginal bleeding can interfere with professional functions. Leaving aside the potential decrease in function resulting from long-term, chronic anemia, the social inconvenience of prolonged or unexpected bleeding is real. Many women express a fear of embarrassment, leading them to curtail activities outside the home.

A more serious fear for personal safety is expressed by women with severe menorrhagia. Frequently flow is heavy enough to immobilize a woman and the inability to control blood loss produces severe anxiety. Many women express this monthly anticipatory fear to the gynecologist seeking reassurance that, in an emergency, the physician can control the blood loss. Although studies are not available, this fear for bodily safety engendered by menometrorrhagia must have an effect on sexual function. Anecdotal experience related to the authors suggests that sexual partners in such a situation and, frequently the women themselves, abstain from sexual relations during episodes of bleeding for fear of exacerbating blood loss. In particular, spouses and partners fear the responsibility for serious injury to a loved one. At the very least, an atmosphere of anxiety and fear about bodily safety is not conducive to relaxed, uninhibited sexual function.

A more structured situation where vaginal bleeding interferes with sexual function is for the Orthodox Jewish couple. For these women, intercourse is prohibited during menstruation (a minimum of five days) and during seven days after cessation of vaginal bleeding (Leviticus 20:18). After this, the woman immerses herself in a ritual bath, mikveh, and is then permitted to have intercourse (Sheinfeld, 1983). Although rabbinic exemption from the proscription of intercourse may sometimes be obtained for therapy of infertility (Rosner and Tendler, 1974), lovemaking is otherwise restricted. For women with prolonged or irregular vaginal bleeding, intercourse may become virtually impossible, with the attendant potential marital problems.

In most situations menometrorrhagia uncontrolled by medical hormonal therapy is due to conditions of benign neoplasia such as fibroids or endometrial polyps. As the pathology becomes more severe ensuing emotional and functional problems are resolved by definitive surgical treatment. The resultant hysterectomy is followed by its own special and unique set of problems as will be discussed.

## PELVIC PAIN

Chronic pain from any source, including the pelvis, is debilitating. Chronic pain may result from the pathologic conditions of endometriosis and adenomyosis, pelvic inflammatory disease or uterine myomata. In addition, chronic pain may be reported with documented normal anatomy leaving the physician with few valid therapeutic choices.

### Uterine Myomata

An enlarged bulky uterus of 14 to 16 weeks gestational size becomes a space-occupying lesion. As such it presses on other pelvic viscera—bowel and bladder—causing discomfort often manifested as urinary frequency, constipation, and a feeling of "heaviness" or "fullness." Sometimes backache or lower back pain is ascribed to myomata as well. Although women may complain of discomfort, unless there is degeneration and necrosis, large myomata do not usually cause acute, severe pain. In the absence of dysfunctional bleeding there also appears to be little disturbance of psychosexual function in these women. Neubardt (1982) states "even in the presence of large and even painful tumors, most women do not complain of interference with intercourse or orgasm . . . they notice no change in their sexual functioning."

## ENDOMETRIOSIS

Endometriosis is a common problem occurring in young women (Goldstein et al., 1980; Schifrin et al., 1973) as well as older women and results from retrograde menstruation and implantation of viable bits of endometrium on peritoneal surfaces (Sampson, 1940). It may result in tender nodules on the uterosacral ligaments, endometriomas of the ovary, retroversion of the uterus, and severe pelvic adhesions particularly of the ovary to the pelvic sidewall or posterior broad ligament. Concomitant complaints are infertility and pelvic pain. The most frequent symptoms are dysmenorrhea and dyspareunia; the former may be explained by elevated levels of prostaglandins found in the peritoneal fluid of endometriosis patients (Badawy et al., 1982; Drake et al., 1981) which are assumed to cause increased vasoconstriction and cramping at menses. The latter symptom, dyspareunia, is thought to occur as a result of tender endometriotic nodules in the cul-de-sac coupled with posteriorly adherent ovaries that are traumatized during intercourse. In some endometriosis patients pain is so severe that intercourse is avoided by both partners.

## PELVIC INFLAMMATORY DISEASE

The incidence of PID is increasing as a result of infection with not only gonococci, but also anerobic and chlamydial pathogens (Mardh et al., 1977) Sequelae are infertility in as many as 21 percent of affected women and chronic abdominal pain reported in 18 percent of women with documented PID resulting from the formation of adhesions distorting normal anatomy, as well as occluded fallopian tubes (Westrom, 1975). Psychosexual dysfunction is also reported in this group of women when intercourse becomes associated with pain rather than pleasure.

## PELVIC PAIN IN THE ABSENCE OF PATHOLOGY

Pelvic pain resulting from endometriosis or PID has a clear etiology in adhesions and the distortion of normal anatomical relationships. With the advent of diagnostic laparoscopy even mild cases, with unremarkable physical findings can be diagnosed and treated appropriately. There is, however, another group of women with disabling pelvic pain who have an anatomically normal pelvis with no adhesions or endometriosis and patent tubes at lapararscopy. There are no magic tests to distinguish an organic as opposed to psychological cause for such pain, although many have been used (DeVaul and Zisook, 1978). However, women with chronic pelvic pain in the absence of demonstrable pathology are commonly assumed to be under stress and often have difficulty with sexual relationships suggesting a basic internal conflict (Beard et al., 1977; Duncan and Taylor, 1952; Renaer et al., 1979). In one study, such women appeared to have been deprived of warmth and affection during childhood, often with loss of a parent before the age of 10 (Duncan and Taylor, 1952). This background resulted in depressive and psychosomatic symptoms such as chronic fatigue, anxiety, headache, and shortness of breath (Castelnuovo-Tedesco and Krout, 1970) and suggested that chronic pelvic pain is only one of many possible manifestations of basic psychological problems.

Treatment of these women is difficult and often unrewarding. Although psychotherapy has been reported to decrease the number of attacks of pain (Beard et al., 1977), others have found that a total rehabilitation program rather than therapy alone is necessary to treat chronic pelvic pain (DeVaul and Zisook, 1978). Because other symptoms associated with chronic pelvic pain are often depressive, trials of tricyclic antidepressants have been given and are reported to be successful (Weddington, 1982). Even when laparoscopy reveals minor pathology, and it is treated appropriately, relief from pain may not occur because "the finding of an organic lesion does not necessarily explain the patient's pain, since it is necessary to understand the context and meaning of the pain for the patient" (Nadelson et al., 1983, p. 873). The following case reports are of two women from our clinic who reported severe pelvic pain but laparoscopy revealed no pelvic disease.

CASE I.

M. K. is a 28-year-old divorced white female, gravida 0, with a history of pelvic pain and endometriosis. She had had many surgical procedures prior to her admission to our clinic. Laparoscopy revealed no organic pelvic disease, although the patient continued to suffer from pain and was treating herself with narcotics and sleeping pills. The patient requested a presacral neurectomy for relief of the pain. She was referred to a psychiatrist for evaluation. He found the patient to be depressed and recommended tricyclic antidepressants. However, the patient refused treatment and went to another hospital for the surgery.

CASE II.

Mrs. L is a 25-year-old married white female, gravida 0, with a history of pelvic pain since menses began at 11 years. The patient reports difficulty tolerating pain during menses and painful sexual intercourse. The patient came to our clinic after her own gynecologist suggested a hysterectomy to relieve the pain. Mrs. L has a history of a difficult childhood, early sexual abuse by her stepfather and a non-nurturing relationship with her alcholic mother. Laparoscopy revealed no organic pelvic disease and the patient was referred to a psychiatrist. His recommendation was intense psychotherapy and the patient currently is following that recommendation.

## SURGICAL TREATMENT OF PELVIC PAIN

### Presacral Neurectomy

Pain impulses from the cervix, uterus, and proximal portions of the fallopian tubes travel through the superior hypogastric plexus, "presacral nerve," to the spinal column. These nerves overlay the sacrum and are easily accessible at the sacral prometory through a retroperitoneal incision. Interruption of these nerves, presacral neurectomy, has been used to treat central pelvic pain resulting from endometriosis, dysmenorrhea, and dyspareunia. In this setting, pain relief is achieved in 72 to 97 percent of operated patients (Black, 1964; Nadelson et al., 1983) with pregnancy rates of 40 to 75 percent (Garcia and David, 1977; Sadigh et al., 1977; Spangler et al., 1971).

Chronic pain resulting from PID is most often adnexal in origin, and the innervation of the ovaries and distal fallopian tubes travels through the infundibulopelvic ligament with the vessels to the inferior mesenteric plexus. Thus, presacral neurectomy has not been recommended for pain secondary to PID. However, in a group of eight women with PID, presacral neurectomy resulted in pain relief for 75 percent of them; results that were comparable to a group of endometriosis patients and significantly better than a 26 percent incidence of pain relief in women with simple lysis of adhesions for PID (Polan and DeCherney, 1980). Thus, the suggestion has been made to perform presacral neurectomy in cases of PID as well as endometriosis.

Theoretically, a presacral neurectomy could be performed through the laparoscope by interrupting the uterosacral ligaments at their uterine insertion utilizing a $CO_2$ laser.

Primary dysmenorrhea in the absence of any other pelvic pathology has been suggested as another indication for presacral neurectomy. Black (1964) describes a group of 24 women with incapacitating pain for several days a month, 86 percent of whom experienced pain relief after surgery with a follow-up of 10 years. The condition of dysmenorrhea may well be one which is amenable to surgical therapy even in the absence of anatomic pathology since the painful uterine cramps initiated by prostaglandins at the time of menses could theoretically be abolished by division of efferent uterine pain fibers such as occurs with presacral neurectomy.

Pelvic pain unresponsive to either medical or conservative surgical therapy is often treated, as a last resort, by hysterectomy. In situations of true, severe pathology such as PID or endometriosis, ovaries and uterus are removed with institution of estrogen replacement therapy. In most of these women extirpation of diseased pelvic organs results in significant pain relief and a dramatic increase in level of function. Most of these are young women with concomitant infertility and although loss of the reproductive organs prior to childbearing may result in postoperative depression, in the authors' experience the long-term adjustment and level of function is good. However, in a study of "hysterectomy when the uterus is grossly normal," D'Esopo (1962) found about 2 percent of all hysterectomies were performed for pelvic pain with removal of a normal uterus. Although specific outcomes were not specified he stated that the "follow-up of these women in the 1937–38 group showed a poor result in the majority." The implication is that extirpative surgery performed for valid pathologic reasons has a better outcome reflected in patient function than does the same surgery when pain is not of documented organic origin.

## Hysterectomy

Hysterectomy is the most commonly performed major surgical operation of women of reproductive age in the United States (Dicker et al., 1982). A study by the National Center for Health Statistics on trends of hysterectomy between 1970 and 1978 found that in 1973 there were 690,000 hysterectomies performed in this country. The number appears to have remained stable since then (Nadelson et al., 1983). Questions have been raised about such large numbers of elective hysterectomies. Indeed, in Canada when questions were raised about the same issue, a review board was formed in Saskatchewan and the hysterectomy rate declined by 33 percent prior to the institution of surgical guidelines (Dyck et al., 1977). Hysterectomy either with or without removal of the ovaries is a major procedure invested with significant emotional and psychological implications.

## The Psychosexual Impact of Hysterectomy

The association of the uterus and the psyche has been assumed since antiquity. Women manifesting symptoms of *hysteria*—a psychiatric term derived from the Greek word for uterus, *hustera*—were thought to be suffering from a condition caused by the movement of the uterus pressing on other parts of the body (Mora, 1980). The psychological aspects of hysterectomy were first discussed in detail by Lindemann in 1941. Lindemann studied 40 women who had recently undergone hysterectomy and compared them to a group of women who had been subjected to surgery on the upper abdomen. He found that the symptoms of mild agitation, restlessness, insomnia, and preoccupation with depressive thought content occurred twice as often with the pelvic surgery group. In 1962, Melody concluded that depression had replaced hemorrhage, infection, and intestinal obstruction as the most common complication following hysterectomy.

In a more recent review of the literature on hysterectomy and depression, Turpin and Heath (1979) found authors evenly divided between those whose studies suggested a possible link between hysterectomy and psychological sequelae, that is, "the post-hysterectomy syndrome" and those who found no connection between hysterectomy and psychiatric problems. In those studies that suggest an association between the two, one or more of the following risk factors was usually present: (1) patients under the age of 40 or in the childbearing years; (2) patients with a previous history of depression, anxiety, and hysteria; and (3) patients manifesting no evidence of organic uterine pathology (Anath, 1978; Barker, 1968; Richards, 1973). Less common but important risk factors are marital breakdown and divorce (Polivy, 1974), patients with an apparent lack of preoperative anxiety, and patients who have misconceptions and fears about the effects of surgery (D'Esopo, 1962; Drellich and Bieber, 1958).

When there are psychiatric sequelae for women following hysterectomy—and many researchers suggest that the morbidity was present prior to surgery—the diagnoses are most often primary depression and hysteria (Briquet's somatization syndrome). Richards (1973) found that women who had hysterectomies were "four times more likely to become depressed within three years of the operation than women who had not had hysterectomies" (p. 432). On the question of premorbid psychopathology, Martin and colleagues (1977) looked at 49 women before hysterectomy and found 57 percent to be psychiatrically ill. Twenty-seven percent had a diagnosis of Briquet's somatization syndrome and 18 percent had a diagnosis of primary depression. In a later study the same authors (Martin et al., 1980) looked at 44 women after hysterectomy and found, for the most part, that they lacked psychiatric symptoms. Those who did manifest psychological morbidity postoperatively had manifested the same symptoms before surgery—in particular the diagnosis of hysteria. The authors suggested that patients presenting with the symptoms of Briquet's somatization syndrome should be considered at-risk psychiatrically rather than gynecologically. The syndrome has symptoms that mimic "the posthysterectomy syndrome"—recurrent pains, nervousness, depression, and sexual and marital discord. They further suggested that it is not unusual to find such a diagnosis in the gynecology clinic given the fact that hysterics are prime utilizers of the medical system overall (Martin et al., 1977).

Not all evidence points to poor emotional outcome after hysterectomy. Meikle, Brody, and Pysh (1977) compared mood disorders after hysterectomy and found "no evidence . . . that the special psychological significance of the uterus results in greater post-surgery mood disturbance than occurs with a control procedure such as cholecystectomy" (p. 36). In addition, a comparison of sterilization by tubal ligation or hysterectomy revealed no difference in psychological impact (Meikle et al., 1977). Roeske (1978) in a small study of 21 middle- and upper-middle-class women, found that professional involvement positively affected posthysterectomy psychological outcome and quoted expressions of "better than ever" and "glad to get it over with." A British study of 60 premenopausal women undergoing hysterectomy reported an improved postoperative mood and unimpaired sexual enjoyment compared to preoperative baseline studies (Coppen et al., 1981).

It appears that the psychological impact of hysterectomy varies greatly among women. The ability to cope with the loss of the uterus and to recover emotionally from hysterectomy seem to be associated with the significance of the uterus in each woman's life. Historically, woman's sense of feminity and self-esteem was derived from her ability to bear children. Changes in society and attitudinal patterns have helped women to obtain gratification in other areas. Nevertheless, for many women the uterus remains an important symbol of femininity. Indeed, some women view the uterus as a literal source of strength and fear a loss of stability and personal independence after hysterectomy (Polivy, 1974).

In interviews with 23 women before hysterectomy, Drellich and Bieber (1958) found that women feared, in addition to the loss of the ability to bear children, the loss of ability to menstruate. Some women may be relieved at no longer having menses, but many mourn the loss nevertheless. A common fear of women who are having hysterectomies, is the loss of attractiveness and the fear of premature aging. Many women fear that following hysterectomy their partner will no longer find them sexually desirable. Certainly the positive reaction of a sexual partner can offer an important component to successful recovery (Melody, 1962; Roeske, 1978).

## VARIOUS SURGICAL TECHNIQUES OF HYSTERECTOMY

Surgically, there are several different techniques of performing a hysterectomy. Clearly removal of the ovaries in a premenopausal woman with estrogen deprivation and the onset of menopausal symptoms might affect postoperative psychosexual function. Indeed, comparison of 24 women undergoing bilateral oophorectomy as well as hysterectomy revealed a correlation between fatigue, headaches, and posthysterectomy syndrome with loss of ovarian function (Martin et al., 1980). When estrogen was not replaced in these women, fatigue was exacerbated but there was no correlation with posthysterectomy syndrome. In a prospective study of simple hysterectomy patients Coppen and coworkers (1981) found no evidence of impaired ovarian function as measured by serum estrogen level, suggesting that the surgical techniques involved in removal of the uterus do not damage ovarian blood supply or function. In addition, comparison of baseline and follow-up studies showed a beneficial psychological effect for hysterectomy (Coppen et al., 1981). In another study of women undergoing hysterectomy and oophorectomy, although 37 percent reported a poorer sexual relationship, this was not generally affected by estrogen replacement even though dyspareunia decreased (Dennerstein et al., 1977). Thus, psychosexual functional disturbances posthysterectomy can not be directly correlated with the removal or conservation of the ovaries and in the absence of ovarian function, estrogen replacement does not reverse any dysfunction experienced (Dennerstein et al., 1977; Kilkku et al., 1983).

The question of specific changes was addressed by the Kilkku study (1983) in a comparison of total hysterectomy with the now infrequently performed supracervical hysterectomy. Waning libido was clearly associated with an age of 45 or more but not with type of hysterectomy, parity, marital status, removal of the ovaries, or characteristic symptoms. A very interesting observation was the decreased frequency of orgasmic intercourse, with unchanged libido, in women undergoing total hysterectomy. Supracervical hysterectomy appeared to result in a maintenance of orgasmic ability which was partially lost by removal of the cervix. Whether this one report justifies performing a procedure which leaves a potential cancer-bearing organ in place is moot, and further studies comparing factors affecting libido versus orgasmic response are awaited.

## CONCLUSION

In essence, the association between sexual dysfunction and benign neoplasia seems vague. Sexual problems seem to be related more to symptoms than to a specific disease process. Effective therapy is difficult to evaluate because of the multifactorial causes and effects that are associated. Sarrel and colleagues' (1983) work on occlusion of Bartholin's gland duct illustrates in a tangible fashion how benign gynecologic neoplasia can cause demonstrable sexual dysfunction that can be precisely diagnosed and appropriately treated. What these authors illustrate is that by occlusion of the greater vestibular glands, secretions build up in this area during the plateau stage of sexual response. These entrapped secretions cause intense pelvic pain. "The pain is specific in location and is elicited regardless of mode of sexual stimulation" (Sarrel et al., 1983, p. 261). Sexual stimulation always causes the pain. Extripation of the gland in three cases and marsupialization in the fourth resulted in complete cure in these patients, as well as a return of sexual satisfaction, thus demonstrating how sexual dysfunction can directly be related to benign gynecologic disease.

Although disturbance of psychosexual function is rare in women with a fibroid uterus, menometrorrhagia resulting from polyps or submucus myomata may affect function through anxiety and fear. Benign neoplasia such as endometriosis, adenomyosis, and PID associated with pain most certainly inhibits sexual response. All of these pathologic states are progressive in that they usually do not resolve spontaneously. Appropriate therapeutic intervention, whether medical or with a hysteroscopic resection or laparotomy, may arrest or reverse symptoms associated with the disease process. However, in many instances pathology either recurs or is not amenable to available therapies. In such cases extirpative surgery is a final resort.

Despite the fact that some studies report no significant changes in sexual functioning following hysterectomy—Patterson, Craig, and Dinitz (1960) in fact found an improvement in the quality of sexual functioning for many women following hysterectomy—many women and men view the uterus as the organ of sexual responsiveness and fear its loss will cause cessation of sexual activity and desire. Indeed, for many women loss of the uterus is an event charged with meaning that evokes considerable anxiety and emotional turmoil. Caution should be exercised by physicians when patients considering hysterectomy present with symptoms of depression; have a history of psychosomatic complaints and exhaustion; are under 40 years of age or of childbearing potential; or when there is no obvious uterine pathology present. It seems clear that patients and their partners should be well-informed before hysterectomy about the surgery and its aftereffects. Other factors that suggest a good psychic outcome following surgery include a stable marital relationship; independent sources of self-esteem; (Roeske, 1978); a realistic preoperative understanding of the surgery; and a completion of childbearing.

## REFERENCES

Anath, J.: Hysterectomy and depression. *Obstet. Gynecol.*, 52:724–730, 1978.

Badawy, S. Z. A.; Marshall, L.; Gabal, A. A.; and Nusbaum, M. L.: The concentration of 13, 14-dihydro-15-keto prostaglandin $F_2$ and prostaglandin $E_2$ in peritoneal fluid of infertile patients with and without endometriosis. *Fertil. Steril.*, 38:166, 1982.

Barker, M.: Psychiatic illness after hysterectomy. *Brit. Med. J.*, 2:91–95, 1968.

Beard, R. W.; Belsey, E. M.; Lieberman, B. A.; and Wilkinson, J. C. M.: Pelvic pain in women. *Am. J. Obstet. Gynecol.*, 128:566–570, 1977.

Black, W. T. Jr.: Use of presacral sympathectomy in the treatment of dysmenorrhea. *Am. J. Obstet. Gynecol.*, 89:16–22, 1964.

Buttram, V. C. Jr.: Conservative surgery for endometriosis in the infertile female: a study of 206 patients with implications for both medical and surgical therapy. *Fertil. Steril.*, 31:117, 1969.

Castelnuovo-Tedesco, P., and Krout, B. M.: Psychosomatic aspects of chronic pelvic pain. *Psychiatr. Med.*, 1:109–126, 1970.

Chimbira, T.; Cope, E.; Anderson, A.; and Bolton, F.: The effect of Danazol on menorrhagia, coagulation mechanisms, naemotological indices and body weight. *Br. J. Obstet. Gynaecol.*, 86:46–50, 1979.

Coppen, A.; Bishop, M.; Beard, R. J.; Barnard, G. J. R.; and Collins W. P.: Hysterectomy, hormones and behaviour. *Lancet*, 126–128, 1981.

DeCherney, A., and Polan, M. L.: Hysteroscopic management of intrauterine lesions and intractable uterine bleeding. *Obstet. Gynecol.*, 61:392–397, 1983.

D'Esopo, D. A.: Hysterectomy when the uterus is grossly normal. *Am. J. Obstet. Gynecol.*, 83:113–121, 1962.

DeVaul, R. A., and Zisook, S.: Chronic pain: The psychiatrist's role. *Psychosom. Med.*, 19:417–421, 1978.

Dennerstein, L.; Wood, C.; and Burrows, G. D.: Sexual response following hysterectomy and oophorectomy. *Obstet. Gynecol.*, 49:92–96, 1977.

Dicker, R.; Scally, M.; Greenspan, J.; Layde, P.; Ory, H.; Maze, J.; and Smith, J.: Hysterectomy among women of reproductive age: Trends in the United States, 1970–1978. *JAMA*, 248:323–327, 1982.

Drake, T.; O'Brien, W. F.; Ramwell, P. W.; and Metz, S. A.: Peritoneal fluid thromboxane $B_2$ and 6-keto-prostaglandin $F_1$ endometriosis. *Am. J. Obstet. Gynecol.*, 140:401, 1981.

Drellich, M., and Bieber, I: The psychologic importance of the uterus and its functions. *J. Nerv. Ment. Dis.*, 126:322, 1958.

Duncan, C. H., and Taylor, H. C., Jr.: A psychosomatic study of pelvic congestion. *Am. J. Obstet. Gynecol.*, 64:1–12, 1952.

Dyck, F.; Murphy, F.; Murphy, J.; Road, D.; Boyd, M.; Osborne, E.; DeVlieger, D.; Korchinski, B.; Ripley, C.; Bromley, A.; Innes, P.: Effects of surveillance on the number of hysterectomies in the province of Saskatchewan. *N. Engl. J. Med.*, 296:1326–1328, 1977.

Garcia, C. R., and David, S. S.: Pelvic endometriosis: Infertility and pelvic pain. *Am. J. Obstet. Gynecol.*, 129:740, 1977.

Goldstein, D. P.; deCholnoky, C.; Emans, S. J.; and Leventhal, J. M.: Laparosocpy in the diagnosis and management of pelvic pain in adolescents. *J. Reprod. Med.*, 24:251, 1980.

Kilkku, P.; Gronroos, M.; Hirvonen, T.; and Rauramo,

L.: Supravaginal uterine amputation vs. hysterectomy: Effects on libido and orgasm. *Acta Obstet. Gynecol. Scand.,* 62:147, 1983.

Lindemann, E.: Observations of psychiatric sequelae to surgical operations in women. *Am. J. Psychiatry,* 98:132–139, 1941.

Mardh, P. A.; Ripa, K. T.; Svensson, L.; and Westrom, L.: *Chylamydia trachomatis* infections in patients with salpingitis. *N. Engl. J. Med.,* 296:1377, 1977.

Martin, R. L.; Roberts, M. V.; Clayton, P. J.; and Wetzel, R.: Psychiatric illness and non-cancer hysterectomy. *Dis. Nerv. Syst.,* 38:974–980, 1977

Martin, R. L.; Roberts, W. V.; and Clayton, P. J.: Psychiatric status after hysterectomy. *JAMA,* 244:350–353, 1980.

Meikle, S.; Brody, H.; and Pysh, F.: An investigation into the psychological effects of hysterectomy. *J. Nerv. Ment. Dis.,* 164:36–41, 1977.

Melody, G. F.: Depressive reactions following hysterectomy. *Am. J. Obstet. Gynecol.* 83:410–413, 1962.

Mora, G: Historical and Theoretical trends in psychiatry. In Kaplan, H. I.; Freedman, A. M.; and Sadock, G. J.: (eds.): *Comprehensive Textbook of Psychiatry Vol. III,* 3rd ed. Williams and Wilkins, Baltimore, 1980.

Nadelson, C. C.; Notman, M. T.; and Ellis, E. A.: Psychosomatic aspects of obstetrics and gynecology. *Psychosom. Med.,* 24:871–884, 1983.

Neubardt, S.: Fibroids and sexual function. *Med. Aspects of Hum. Sex.,* 16:42I–42J, 1982.

Patterson, R. M.; Craig, J. B.; Dinitz, S.: Social and medical characteristics of hysterectomized and nonhysterectomized psychiatric patients. *Obstet. Gynecol.,* 15:209, 1960.

Polan, M. L., and DeCherney, A.: Presacral neurectomy for pelvic pain in infertility. *Fertil. Steril.,* 34:557–560, 1980.

Polivy, J.: Psychological reactions to hysterectomy: A critical review. *Am. J. Obstet. Gynecol.,* 118:417–426, 1974.

Ranaer, M.; Vertommen, H.; Nijs, P.; et al: Psychological aspects of chronic pelvic pain in women. *Am. J. Obstet. Gynecol.,* 134:75–80, 1979.

Richards, D.: Depression after hysterectomy. *Lancet,* 2:430–432, 1973.

Roeske, N. C. A.: Quality of life and factors affecting the response to hysterectomy. *J. Fam. Pract.,* 7:483–438, 1978.

Rosner, F., and Tendler, M. D.: Practical medical halacha. *Association of Orthodox Jewish Scientists,* 10–12, 1974.

Sadigh, H.; Naples, J. D. Jr.; and Batt, R. E.: Conservative surgery for endometriosis in the infertile couple. *Obstet. Gynecol.,* 49:562, 1977.

Sampson, J. A.: The development of the implantation theory for the origin of peritoneal endometriosis. *Am. J. Obstet. Gynecol.,* 40:549, 1940.

Sarrel, P.; Steege, J.; Maltzer, M.; and Bolinsky, D.: Pain during sex response due to occlusion of the Bartholin's gland duct. *Obstet. Gynecol.,* 62:261–264, 1983.

Schifrin, B. S.; Erez, S.; and Moore, J. G.: Teenage endometriosis. *Am. J. Obstet. Gynecol.,* 116:973, 1973.

Sheinfeld, M.: Helping the infertile orthodox Jewish couple. *Contemp. OB/GYN,* 137–139, 1983.

Spangler, D. B.; Jones, G. S.; and Jones, H. W.: Infertility due to endometriosis. *Am. J. Obstet. Gynecol.,* 109:850, 1971.

Turpin, T. J., and Heath, D. S.: The link between hysterectomy and depression. *Can. J. Psychiatry,* 24:247–254, 1979.

Weddington, W. W., Jr.: Psychiatric aspects of chronic abdominal pain. *Drug Ther.,* 12:97–111, 1982.

Westrom, L: Effect of acute pelvic inflammatory disease on fertility. *Am. J. Obstet. Gynecol.,* 121:707, 1975.

# CHAPTER 15 MALIGNANT NEOPLASIA

*Barrie Anderson, M.D.*

## INTRODUCTION

Women facing the specter of gynecologic malignancy are in double jeopardy. Not only are their very lives in danger, but even in the event of cure or control of malignancy, daily functioning can be profoundly affected. The stress of diagnosis and treatment is severe, pervasive, and long-lasting.

The long-term survival of one-half to two-thirds of all gynecologic cancer patients (International Federation of Gynecology and Obstetrics, 1982) means that a large number of women must be assisted in returning to normal psychosexual functioning. The physical handicaps to be faced in survival may be minimal or great, but there is an unfortunately large and consistent emotional burden shared by the majority of cancer patients. Understanding of the stresses to be faced by the patient can enable the physician to ease emotional and physical pain. At the very least, the patient can be sustained through an arduous course of treatment and a prolonged and uncertain follow-up. At best, she can grow to a new and deeper level of understanding and awareness that can enhance her life immeasurably and can be inspirational to those around her, including family and medical personnel.

## STRESS AND THE CANCER PATIENT

The stages of dealing with serious illness have been described as denial, anger, bargaining, depression, and acceptance (Kubler-Ross, 1969). Specific emotional responses to stress include anxiety, depression, guilt, and anger (Peck, 1972). During the course of the illness, an individual moves back and forth through these stages, exhibiting various emotional responses, with temporary regression to an earlier stage, even after the resolution of a particular crisis.

Helplessness and loss of self-esteem are the most pervasive feelings reported by investigators of the psychological differences between cancer patients and controls. The diagnosis of cancer apparently adds a special kind of stress beyond that of surgery alone (Gottesman and Lewis, 1982). Cancer patients experience significantly greater feelings of helplessness than do patients undergoing surgery but not for cancer or controls in a noncrisis state. This sense of helplessness is more persistent and is still present six months after surgery, at a time when other crisis stress reactions have achieved resolution (Lewis *et al.*, 1979). Early stage cancer patients whose return to work after completion of radiation therapy is delayed show a significantly lower sense of well-being and a greater morale loss, as indicated prospectively by subtests of the Minnesota Multiphasic Personality Inventory (MMPI; Schonfield, 1972).

In an ongoing study using the Profile of Mood States (McNair *et al.*, 1971), patients with early stage gynecologic malignancies are being compared at the time of their first visit for work-up with patients one day prior to non-cancer gynecologic surgery and a third group making a routine gynecologic office visit (Andersen *et al.*, 1985 unpublished manuscript). Preliminary data shows the gynecologic cancer patients to be significantly more depressed, confused, and fatigued. The cancer patients and the non-cancer surgical patients had comparable levels of anxiety, with both significantly more anxious than the outpatients. For the cancer patients this state is prolonged—at four months follow-up there is a decline in anxiety and confusion, but not in depression and fatigue. In addition, about one-third experience significant sexual difficulties at four month follow-up.

Failure of resolution of these feelings of helplessness and depression can lead to difficulties in psychological and sexual rehabilitation. Efforts directed at restoring a sense of control and self-determination can begin to dispel depression and promote integrative and adaptive behavior.

## SPECIFIC STRESS AREAS

Stress for the cancer patient is ongoing and repetitive, with new components being added all the time (*e.g.*, cancer diagnosis yesterday, barium enema today, surgery next week, radiation therapy next month, maybe chemotherapy next year). The process of dealing with and adjusting to stress is a dynamic one proceeding simultaneously on many fronts. One can identify six general stress areas for the gynecologic cancer patient: prediagnostic, diagnostic, treatment, follow-up and rehabilitation, recurrence, and terminal phases.

### PREDIAGNOSTIC PHASE

The prediagnostic phase can be described as that time during which symptoms and signs of the disease are present but the diagnosis of cancer has not yet been made. This period will include a time prior to medical consultation and a time of early diagnostic testing. Individual personality patterns often exert themselves now, and an evaluation of how the patient has dealt with this particular area can be helpful in predicting future responses to stress and individual ways of coping. With the American Cancer Society's publicity regarding the seven early warning signs of cancer, many women are alert to the need for medical consultation immediately upon the first episode of abnormal vaginal bleeding. In addition, the well-publicized need for Papanicolaou smear screening for early cervical cancer commonly leads women to the physician early in the development of cervical malignancy. Excessive denial may lead to procrastination of medical consultation often seen in vulvar carcinoma. With the diffuse, nonspecific and often nongynecologic presenting symptoms of ovarian cancer, the patient may seek medical help but symptoms may be misinterpreted or minimized by the physician (Lennane and Lennane, 1973). A subsequent diagnosis of cancer as the cause of these symptoms, which may have gone on for many months, may lead to anger directed at the original physician. Finally, the conscious acknowledgment of symptomatology may produce anxiety by raising the fear of the diagnosis of cancer.

During the initial phase of testing, the patient is poked and prodded, and her bodily cavities are invaded for Papanicolaou smears, rectovaginal exams, endoscopic examinations, and X-rays. These tests are uncomfortable and are a gross invasion of the privacy and bodily integrity of the patient. In addition, the stress of waiting for the test results adds to the anxiety already produced by the symptoms and the possibility of a serious diagnosis.

### DIAGNOSTIC PHASE

In the diagnostic phase, stress reactions become more apparent, with denial, depression, and anger beginning to overlap. The diagnosis of cancer is inevitably associated with pain and death; to many it is virtually a death sentence. In those with personal experience with friends and relatives who have undergone cancer treatment, this diagnosis calls to mind endless suffering that is purposeless, since life is lost despite all efforts.

Cancer is a disease that most people would prefer not to talk about. The patient who is cured prefers to "put all that behind" her and get on with living. Thus, cancer patients, who are willing to admit their diagnosis to friends and family, frequently discover that many of these confidantes have had cancer, but the patient never knew. Finding the evidence of such curative possibilities can be heartening. But the first reaction occurs in a milieu of ignorance.

The fear of death is followed quickly by the fear of pain and mutilation and the fear of losing normal role functioning. Specific reactions will relate to the patient's usual way of dealing with stress and her own personal way of approaching life. Guilt may play a role here, especially if the patient delayed consultation. However, if others were responsible for the delay, then anger may supervene. A patient's responses will also be colored by the personal meaning of the organ involved (uterus, ovary, clitoris).

During the diagnostic phase the rather extensive work-up for metastatic disease proceeds unabated, and again involves invasion of body orifices and a strong sense of personal violation. A sense of loss of control begins to become apparent; the patient no longer is in charge of her schedule. She feels that even her own body has turned against her.

### Treatment Phase

During the treatment phase the sense of loss of control becomes even more overwhelming. The patient's body and daily schedule are controlled by people who until a short time before were strangers. Her professional role or family role is disrupted and may be permanently threatened. In addition to the general stresses of treatment, each of the various modalities of cancer therapy—surgery, radiation, and drugs—has its own unique stresses.

**Surgery.** Surgery entails the greatest and most focused physical and emotional stress. Fear of death may be heightened by the need for anesthesia and "being put to sleep." Anesthesia, surgery, and the possible complications of surgery are major physical stresses. The emotional reaction to the surgery is compounded by the physical letdown commonly observed postoperatively—the so-called third day blues—which can occur up to two weeks postoperatively. Lack of understanding of anatomy and physiology due to ignorance about internal organs and their function, and denial of even external organs, leads to confusion and anxiety regarding surgical procedures to be performed. A change in body image is caused by the presence of surgical scars, drains, and removal of organs, each of which has its own personal significance to the individual. Drugs used to control pain, promote sleep, combat infection, and decrease gastric secretions have side effects, many of which may be psychotropic in nature. Use of combinations of these drugs can lead to synergistic side effects that can be frightening and confusing to the patient.

The length of hospital stay and dosage of postoperative analgesics are influenced by perception of the relationship between one's actions and one's experience (Johnson and Leventhal, 1971). Individuals who believe that their actions, skills, and efforts determine their fate exert more control over the environment. In nonsurgical settings this trait has an enhancing effect on learning and performance. A negative effect is seen in those who believe they cannot influence what is happening to them and that outcome is determined by luck, outside forces, or other persons. Postoperative patients with a strong sense of internal control manipulate their environments to obtain higher doses of analgesics and longer hospital stays than do patients with a belief in external control. However, Johnson and Leventhal point out that these increases are not to extreme levels and could well be viewed as adaptive, with the strong possibility that externally controlled patients are undermedicated. Identification of this aspect of personality can help care givers deal more effectively with the patient's needs at this time.

Following an acute loss, a mourning period

lasting about six to eight weeks has been described (Brown and Stoudemire, 1983). This grieving period is generally completed within about six months. Loss and grief reactions are also seen after surgical removal of body parts. Problems delaying the normal response can be anticipated when the patient's reactions to prior stresses in her life indicate that she may have difficulty expressing her sadness at this time.

Hysterectomy alone can have a positive or negative effect on sexual functioning. Many women report a feeling of liberation from the concerns of possible pregnancy and a subsequent increased enjoyment of sex. When the surgery is performed to relieve a problem with noxious symptomatology, such as heavy or irregular bleeding, pelvic pain, or persistent discharge, relief of symptoms that themselves have decreased sexual functioning allows a return to a prior level of enjoyment. However, some women, and particularly those in certain subcultures, may have a strong belief that sexual identity and desirability is provided by the uterus, or that orgasm is a uterine function. This may be a self-fulfilling prophecy with subsequent loss of sexual desire. These women may also report rejection by their sexual partners. Still other women who have had suboptimal sexual experiences prior to surgery may use hysterectomy as an excuse for escape from an unpleasant duty.

Although hysterectomy for cancer is more likely to involve an older population with a decreased frequency of coitus, sexual functioning may remain an important and meaningful part of relationships that is valued highly (Newman and Nichols, 1960; Pfeiffer and Davis, 1972). Age *per se* should not lessen the care giver's concern for posttreatment sexual adjustment.

Patients who have undergone a vulvectomy experience more severe changes in body image as well as function. It is especially critical to clarify anatomy for these patients, both pre- and postoperatively. The learned aspect of orgasm makes it possible to have satisfactory sex after such deforming surgery, even if the clitoris has been removed (Andersen and Hacker, 1983b). However, numbness may interfere with sexual response. Other coital problems postoperatively may be due to contraction or cicatrization of the introital portion of the scar. Relaxing incisions can surgically alleviate such stricture.

As part of ultraradical pelvic surgery, such as exenteration, it is technically useful in supporting the pelvic floor to perform a vaginal reconstruction (Becker *et al.*, 1979; Delgado, 1978; Hatch, 1984; Perticucci, 1977; Trelford *et al.*, 1973; Webb and Symmonds, 1977). This technique can also have a positive psychological effect, since it can reassure the patient that sexual functioning will be possible for her in the future. Also it makes the statement that a future is expected.

Caution should be used in describing sexual functioning with the neovagina, since it has been reported that coitus does not "feel just like it did before" and many women with expectations of resuming prior functioning are disappointed (Andersen and Hacker, 1983a). However many different surgical techniques have been successful in allowing satisfactory sexual function (Berek *et al.*, 1983; Pratt, 1972; Williams, 1964).

The presence of urinary or fecal diversion, whether as a result of primary treatment as in a pelvic exenteration or for management of complications of prior treatment, presents special problems. Stomas contribute particularly to a loss of body image and, because of conditioning from early childhood, may be interpreted as despicable and dirty. It is important to emphasize the life-saving aspects of these diversions as allowing the body a natural way of functioning. Full skirts rather than formfitting slacks can help mask the presence of a stoma. Bags made of crinkly or crunchy material can be replaced with those made from soft plastic. Inadvertent flatulence during sex can be masked with background music as a counterirritant. The stomas themselves can be hidden with a cummerbund, clothes, or nightgowns. And the sexual focus can be shifted to other areas such as the breasts or clitoris.

Pelvic exenteration with or without vaginal reconstruction is associated with long-term depression and disruption of sexuality (Andersen and Hacker, 1983a; Brown et al., 1972; Dempsey et al., 1975). Adjustment of sexual techniques can provide satisfactory functioning, but counseling will always be a requirement for these patients and their partners. Again, the major emphasis is one of integration rather than denial of the experience.

**Radiation Therapy.** The initial reaction to radiation therapy is commonly fear (Peck and Boland, 1977): the fear of advanced or incurable disease; concerns about body damage or future cancer-causing effects; and lack of understanding of the rather mysterious nature of radiation, which raises the question of whether or not it really works. The physical stress associated with radiation therapy is somewhat less concentrated, but on the whole equally great, as with surgery. The trauma of side effects, such as diarrhea, dysuria, and nausea, and of regular diagnostic blood "letting" is great. Drugs used to control the side effects of radiation therapy, such as antispasmodics and opiates, may produce troublesome side effects.

However, radiation therapy may also have a positive benefit, in that it provides an "opportunity" to see other cancer patients, many of whom may be much sicker or have more apparent side effects, such as hair loss. A more prolonged contact with other patients, physicians, and treatment personnel may allow a more open discussion of diagnosis and provide an outlet for many feelings that may otherwise be unexpressed.

Inflammation in the acute reaction to radiation can lead to vaginal agglutination. This tendency is aggravated by atrophy secondary to loss of estrogen, whether pre-existent as in the postmenopausal woman or when secondary to radiation-induced ovarian failure. Physical consequences of the loss of estrogen, whether secondary to surgical extirpation, radiation, or chemotherapy, include loss of vaginal lubrication and eventually decreased pliability of the vaginal wall with decreased caliber in particular. Hot flashes are a systemic manifestation of estrogen deprivation that can be distressing. Estrogen replacement, whether oral or via vaginal insertion, can control these symptoms but may be contraindicated in patients in whom an estrogen-sensitive cancer exists. In patients with an intact uterus, with or without radiation therapy, progestational agents should be included in the second half of the replacement cycle.

Although patients undergoing radiation therapy have traditionally been counseled to avoid coitus during and immediately after the course of treatment and, in fact, local irritative symptoms may preclude comfortable sex, the early use of vaginal dilators can aid in prevention of coaptation of the vagina and lessen unfounded fears of pain or damage from subsequent coital activity (Pitkin et al., 1975). The use of vaginal estrogen containing creams, when not contraindicated, can aid in epithelialization and decreasing inflammation secondary to atrophy.

The long-term side effects of radiation therapy are related to atrophy, fibrosis, and cicatrization. Narrowing and decreased distensibility can lead to sexual dysfunction (Abitol and Davenport, 1974a, 1974b; Seibel et al., 1980; Weinberg, 1974). Patients with atrophy and fibrosis may be at greater risk for coital vaginal vault lacerations (Daw, 1972). The regular use of vaginal dilators or coitus can prevent or minimize major functional limitations. Even after complete vaginal agglutination it may be possible to perform vaginal reconstruction (Berek et al., 1983; Day and Stanhope, 1977; Jafari et al., 1980).

While changes in the lower genital tract that can adversely affect coital function are greatest after radiation therapy, it should be noted that surgically treated patients and those undergoing chemotherapy often have nearly as great limitations of function. This phenomenon may be related to the pervasive feelings of helplessness and loss of self-esteem with resultant depression that have been described in cancer patients treated with all three modalities. However, counseling and support can alleviate psychological symptoms in surgically treated patients but cannot alter the fibrosis that causes decreased vaginal caliber, length, and distensibility in the irradiated patient. This regaining of function may be a reason for choosing surgery over radiation therapy for the younger, sexually active patient, since vaginal and ovarian function can be more satisfactorily maintained (Abitol and Davenport, 1974a, 1974b; Seibel et al., 1980; Weinberg, 1974).

With the use of preradiation laparotomies and lymphadenectomies for determination of extent of disease in planning of treatment fields in cervical cancer, it is possible to perform ovarian transposition, moving the ovary out of the irradiated field, and thus allowing preservation of ovarian function in the young patient who must receive radiation for advanced disease. Metallic clips can be used as markers to allow shielding of the ovary during radiation treatment.

**Chemotherapy.** The use of chemotherapy, whether as primary treatment or as secondary therapy, is often associated with the fear of death, as it is seen as the "last chance" treatment or only used when other curative treatments have failed. In addition, it is well known among the lay population that the drugs used in chemotherapy are highly toxic and produce noxious side effects. Nausea and vomiting further the sense of loss of control over body functions. Hair loss and skin changes threaten body image. Fatigue and lassitude threaten normal lifestyle (Meyerowitz et al., 1979). Because patients who are receiving chemotherapy often do have more advanced disease, the disease itself may contribute to fatigue and may produce other symptoms that interfere with normal functioning.

The stress of chemotherapy occurs in repetitive episodes, producing a more chronic stress situation. As therapy continues, negative conditioning can lead to anticipatory vomiting. Again, the sense of loss of control over lifestyle and time schedule, is troublesome. Drugs used to control symptoms and side effects, such as antiemetics and tranquilizers, can be disorienting and produce symptoms even more bothersome to the patient than those they are intended to control.

Chemotherapy is often employed in older women who no longer have functioning ovaries or an interest in reproduction. In these patients the major effects on sexual functioning are those of the stresses of cancer diagnosis and treatment and the fatigue and side effects produced by the drugs themselves. Often these symptoms are limited to the immediate peritreatment time, and normal functioning can go on in between treatments.

However, in the younger, ovulating patient, ovarian failure is quite common. Women undergoing chemotherapy for nongynecologic cancer, such as Hodgkin's disease, experience markedly decreased libido, amenorrhea, hot flashes, vaginal dryness, and poor self-image (Chapman et al., 1979a, 1979b). These symptoms are dramatically relieved by hormone replacement. Ovarian failure is more commonly associated with age greater than 36, but is great in all age groups (Whitehead et al., 1983). Only 12 percent of patients with normal ovarian function prior to treatment retained ovarian function at three years after cessation of treatment. Sexual dysfunction, evidenced by loss of libido, painful coitus, and disruption of relationship, mirrored ovarian function and often responded to hormonal replacement.

It has been theorized that suppression of the hypothalamic-pituitary-ovarian axis with combined estrogen–progesterone medications in the form of birth control pills might prevent ovarian failure by keeping the ovary in an essentially dormant state during chemotherapy treatments (Sutcliffe, 1979). Results have been mixed, but successful pregnancy, while rare, has also been reported in patients without the use of oral contraceptives (Forney, 1978).

As with radiotherapy, the repetitive and prolonged character of chemotherapy treatments can lead to a closer relationship between the patient and care givers. Frequent contacts allow opportunities to provide support and to complete the emotional dealing with the illness and its stresses.

## FOLLOW-UP PHASE

The follow-up phase is largely dominated by uncertainty regarding the future and by gradual re-establishment of the patient's role in her family and/or profession. Delayed reactions from the patient who has "toughed it out" up to this point will begin to appear and may be associated with dates that are significant to the patient. Self-established goals such as the return of the pathology report ("the diagnosis is not real until the organ is out and the diagnosis is confirmed") or the six-week postoperative office visit (at that time she expects to be back to normal, but the cancer diagnosis is still there), or on the anniversary of the diagnosis and/or treatment are very meaningful. Visits to the doctor or hospital serve as continuing reminders of the diagnosis and are usually associated with anticipatory anxiety, which can be severe. Anniversaries of deaths of significant others, such as parent, child, or spouse, may also serve as a focus of recurrent anxiety or depression.

As the patient re-establishes her role in her family, profession, and community, she may begin to have problems with financial matters, particularly with life and/or disability insurance, based on the prejudices of a society that also considers cancer a death sentence. Such reminders may cast a pall on an otherwise justifiable optimism for the future.

### Recurrence Phase

In the event of recurrence, the fears and stresses of the prediagnostic and diagnostic phases are reignited. The patient who has never resolved her feelings about her diagnosis may have a particularly difficult time. However, when resolution has occurred during the original diagnosis and treatment phases, the patient will usually move through the phases rapidly and effectively. In fact, it is not uncommon to see a reaction of almost relief—the long-feared devil can finally be seen and fought in the open.

Treatment for recurrence generally has more profound effects on functioning than does primary therapy. Extended surgery and urinary and fecal diversions challenge reserves of physical and emotional strength. Chemotherapy gradually saps remaining energies. Physical stress is at its greatest since these demands may be made of a body and psyche already weakened by illness and treatment. The expectation is that death is imminent; many patients (and even some doctors) do not realize that treatment for recurrence can often be successful.

### Terminal Phase

For the patient who will not survive her cancer, the terminal phase again rekindles the fear of death, pain, and body image changes. Change in bodily functions, dietary habits, and activity, combined with weight loss and the need for supportive measures, such as IVs, catheters, and nasogastric tubes, serve to emphasize the sense of loss of control and lead to anger and depression. Concerns for the financial and emotional future of loved ones contribute to anxiety. Pain medications may lead to a loss of mental clarity and to confusion and even hallucinations that can, in themselves, be a threat to the well-being of the patient.

## INTERVENTIONS

Easing the progress of the gynecologic cancer patient through this maze of terrors and challenges requires much of the person who is willing to undertake the task, but also offers great personal rewards. In a society that spends much time denying the discussion of death (Becker, 1973), the diagnosis of a disease that symbolizes death or is inextricably involved with death produces great stress. Not only the patient but also the physician is reminded of the existence of mortality, specifically one's own. The first requirement, therefore, is exploration of one's own feelings, self-expectations, and knowledge of limitations. This phase is critical in order to avoid projecting personal fears and prejudices on to the patient. While we may be wondering how to tell the patient the long-term side effects of radiation therapy, she may only need to hear that radiation therapy can actually work; while we are trying to figure out how to tell her she may not be cured, she may be afraid she will die within the next few days or that death will be unbearably painful or that we will abandon her and not continue to keep her pain-free. We must free ourselves from our own personal agendas and, in so doing, attune ourselves to the needs of the patient.

It is well-documented that anxiety is greatly alleviated by increasing knowledge of what is to come (Mitchell and Glicksman, 1977; Rotman et al., 1977). In the diagnostic phase it is important to be honest without sacrificing hope. The patient can, in honesty, be told that "there is treatment available," that "not all patients are cured, but that the chances are good to excellent," or that "many are cured." A sense of control can be imparted by alerting the patient to the need for testing and by describing those tests in advance of their performance. Acknowledgment of the loss of dignity involved in a pelvic exam and proctosigmoidoscopy can be the first step in restoring that sense of personal dignity. Insofar as it is possible, discomfort should be anticipated and a reasonable estimate of the amount and duration should be given. Honesty at this stage begins to build a foundation of confidence in the care giver. A patient who feels this active and ongoing concern and support will have an easier passage through the trials to come. Time given early in the relationship to establishing good communication is time well spent.

Pre-existing personality characteristics strongly influence response to stress and both adaptive and maladaptive reactions in the perioperative period. It is helpful to identify the patient's unique way of dealing with stress and the personal significance of particular body organs and areas. This personal history can be elicited through the identification of past stress situations, such as surgery or death of a parent or spouse, and the patient's reactions to these stresses.

Information regarding cancer comes from many sources—personal experience, media communication, cultural taboos, and the like. This information will determine the patient's expectations of what is and will be happening to her. Particular fears, often without foundation, can lead to great anxiety and subsequent compliance problems. Acknowledging the presence of these fears allows the patient a sense that she will be taken seriously and begins to reinstitute some of her lost sense of control and self-determination. Exploring fears and beliefs in a nonjudgmental way can uncover myths (operating on cancer and exposing it to air leads to its spread) and misperceptions (loss of the uterus is loss of femaleness) that can then be dealt with realistically. Drawings and three dimensional models of pelvic organs can be used to teach anatomy and to explain tests and surgery. It is important to be specific in what is and what is not removed.

After surgery removing significant organs such as the uterus, ovaries, or vulva, allowing expression of the sense of loss can be liberating and can facilitate resolution of grief. In both the acute and long-term phases, it is helpful to emphasize gains from treatment, as well as the toleration of loss. Care givers should avoid denying the significance of the patient's feelings, rather the emphasis is on promoting the integration of her feelings into her current and future life.

Consistency in presentation of information is critical. Verbal and written descriptions should use the same language. Those care givers who impart information should actively consult each other so that they use the same words as each other, and, in turn, all use the same words as the patient. Confusion may result if the word is changed from "cancer" to "tumor" or "malignant tumor," from "vagina" to "birth canal," or from "uterus" to "womb."

Most cancer treatment centers now acknowledge the importance of a multidisciplinary approach to cancer. This concept has grown to include not only physicians who employ surgery, radiation, or drugs, but also individuals with expertise in many other areas, such as nursing, counseling, and social services (Mays, 1981; Mitchell and Glicksman, 1977; Smith and McNamara, 1977; Young-Brockopp, 1982). A still larger concept of the team approach is one that includes as many individuals who come into contact with the patient as possible: inpatient and outpatient nursing staff, secretaries and scheduling personnel, radiation technicians, dieticians, stoma therapists, chaplains (Dayringer, 1982), and many others. Whether or not these individuals are actually identified as team members, their active participation in the care-giving process is an influence that can be a very positive one if utilized effectively.

Regular conferences between the members of the team are necessary to identify the needs and specific problems of each patient. Information may come from contact with any member of the team and specific roles often overlap.

At all stages the patient should be allowed to participate in her care as much as she desires and as much as is possible. Alternative treatments and rationale for the recommended treatment should be presented, and the patient should be given time to assimilate information whenever possible, which should be most of the time. A sense of control can be greatly enhanced by allowing the patient the option of no further treatment if at any time she so desires.

If radiation therapy is used, there is an equal need to understand anatomy. Following treatment, the use of vaginal obturators to prevent vaginal adhesions can also be instructive to the patient and to her partner regarding future coital possibilities. Estrogen cream can be used to increase epithelialization in the irradiated vagina, but systemic absorption must be remembered and oral progesterone added to the regimen when the uterus remains in place.

In patients who have had more extensive vaginal irradiation, such as those with more advanced carcinoma of the cervix or vaginal carcinoma, decreased caliber and/or length may make old methods of sexual functioning impossible. In such situations, manual control by the patient of the direction and degree of penetration of the penis can be taught and alternate methods of sexual gratification, such as mutual masturbation, oral sex, and anal sex, can increase the sense of control and self-esteem.

Throughout this entire process, it is critical to involve the patient's life partner; he is all too easy to exclude, since he may also contribute to this exclusion by denial and avoidance. Both the patient and the partner should be allowed to have time alone with the physician to express their fears and needs. The partner should be included in the educational process with the patient. Sexual rehabilitation is greatly facilitated by including the partner, thus giving him a sense of control by letting him help.

In the ongoing management of the cancer patient, physicians must recognize their time and expertise limitations. One person cannot possibly meet all the needs of every patient. Paramedical personnel can be used extensively at all levels and during all phases. It is especially important that these personnel have wide experience in the management of gynecologic malignancy and the specific problems that such patients encounter. The person's background (e.g., nurse, physician's assistant, psychologist, pastoral counselor, or secretary) is not as critical as is the experience of the individual and the integration of that individual into the overall management process. Such personnel are often in a better position than the physician to identify problem areas in coping. The patient may not express her needs or fears to the physician because of fear of the medical establishment. Instead she may feel that only if she is a good patient will the doctors continue to treat her or relieve her pain. Other difficulties with compliance may be related to a sense of hopelessness that may or may not be justified, or to an inability to read and, therefore, understand certain instructions and patient information materials or prescriptions (Applebaum and Roth, 1983).

## CONCLUSION

The gynecologic cancer patient is confronted not only with a very real threat to her life, but also with the loss of bodily functions and organs that have great meaning, both psychologically and in terms of role functioning. Her reactions are first and foremost those related to stress, but the diagnosis of cancer itself adds a dimension of helplessness that is persistent for many months after completion of treatment. Sexual functioning is particularly vulnerable in patients with gynecologic cancer. Stress can be reduced by consistent, honest, and accurate communication of information regarding diagnosis, testing, treatment, and prognosis. Support must be extensive and long-term. Integration of the experience can be promoted by careful attention to the concerns of the patient herself. In order to accomplish these goals, it is critical that a personal understanding of one's own feelings regarding serious illness and death be understood and set aside so that they are not projected on to the patient where they will interfere with meaningful communication.

Finally, a multidisciplinary approach to the management of cancer patients includes physicians, nurses, social workers, psychologists, psychiatrists, physician assistants, patient advocates, secretaries, and any other individual trained and experienced in the approach used by the team. Through active participation of all such individuals, the patient with gynecologic cancer can receive optimal medical treatment and the impact on her life and that of her family and community can be one of integration rather than disruption.

## REFERENCES

Abitol, M. M., and Davenport, J. H.: Sexual dysfunction after therapy for cervical carcinoma. *Am. J. Obstet. Gynecol.*, 119:181–189, 1974a.

Abitol, M. M., and Davenport, J. H.: The irradiated vagina. *Obstet. Gynecol.*, 44:249–256, 1974b.

Andersen, B.; Anderson, B., and deProsse, C. A.: Unpublished manuscript, 1985.

Andersen, B., and Hacker, N. F.: Psychosexual adjustment following pelvic exenteration. *Obstet. Gynecol.*, 61:331–338, 1983a.

Andersen, B., and Hacker, N. F.: Psychosexual adjustment after vulvar surgery. *Obstet. Gynecol.*, 62:457–462, 1983b.

Appelbaum, P. S., and Roth, L. H.: Patients who refuse treatment in medical hospitals. *JAMA*, 250:1296–1301 1983.

Becker, D. W.; Massey, F. M.; and McCraw, J. B.: Musculocutaneous flaps in reconstructive pelvic surgery. *Obstet. Gynecol.*, 54:178–183, 1979.

Becker, E.: *The Denial of Death*. Macmillan Publishing, New York, 1973.

Berek, J. S.; Hacker, N. F.; Lagasse, L. D.; and Smith, M. L: Delayed vaginal reconstruction in the fibrotic pelvis following radiation or previous reconstruction. *Obstet. Gynecol.*, 61:743–748, 1983.

Brown, J. T., and Stoudemire, G. A.: Normal and pathologic grief. *JAMA*, 250:378–382, 1983.

Brown, R. S.; Haddox, V.; Posada, A.; and Rubio, A.: Social and psychologic adjustment following pelvic exenteration. *Am. J. Obstet. Gynecol.* 114:162–171, 1972.

Chapman, R. M.; Sutcliffe, S. B.; and Malpas, J. S.: Cytotoxic-induced ovarian failure in women with Hodgkin's disease. I. Hormone function. *JAMA*, 242:1877–1881, 1979a.

Chapman, R. M.; Sutcliffe, S. B.; and Malpas, J. S.: Cytotoxic-induced ovarian failure in Hodgkin's disease. II. Effects on sexual function. *JAMA*, 242:1882–1884, 1979b.

Daw, E.: Coital vaginal vault laceration. *Obstet. Gynecol.*, 40:451–452, 1972.

Day, T. G., and Stanhope, R.: Vulvovaginoplasty in gynecologic oncology. *Obstet. Gynecol.*, 50:361–364, 1977.

Dayringer, R.: *Pastor and Patient*. Jason Aronson, New York, 1982.

Delgado, G.: Plastic procedures in cancer of the lower genital tract. *Am. J. Obstet. Gynecol.*, 131:775–777, 1978.

Dempsey, G. M.; Buchsbaum, H. J.; and Morrison, J.: Psychosocial adjustment to pelvic exenteration. *Gynecol. Oncol.*, 3:325–334, 1975.

Forney, J. P.: Pregnancy following removal and chemotherapy of ovarian endodermal sinus tumor. *Obstet. Gynecol.*, 52:360–362, 1978.

Gottesman, D., and Lewis, M. S.: Differences in crisis reactions among cancer and surgery patients. *J. Consul. Clin. Psychol.*, 50:381–388, 1982.

Hatch, K.: Construction of a neovagina after exenteration using the bulbocavernosus myocutaneous graft. *Obstet. Gynecol.*, 63:108–114, 1984.

International Federation of Gynecology and Obstetrics. Annual report on the results of treatment in gynecologic cancer. Vol. 18, 1982.

Jafari, K.; Thaker, P.; and Jayaraun, B.: Vaginal reconstruction following irradiation complication for cervical cancer. *Gynecol. Oncol.*, 9:247–250, 1980.

Johnson, J. E., and Leventhal, H.: Contribution of emotional and instrumental response processes in adaptation to surgery. *J. Pers. Soc. Psychol.*, 20:55–64, 1971.

Kubler-Ross, E.: *On Death and Dying*. Macmillan Publishing, New York, 1969.

Lennane, K. J., and Lennane, R. J.: Alleged psychogenic disorders in women—A possible manifestation of sexual prejudice. *N. Engl. J. Med.*, 288:288–292, 1973.

Lewis, J.; Gottesman, D.; and Gutstein, S.: The course and duration of crisis. *J. Consul. Clin. Psychol.,* 47:128–134, 1979.

Mays, L. H.: Cancer management, the clergy and the human spirit. *CA—A Cancer Journal for Clinicians,* 31:51–54, 1981.

McNair, D.; Lorr, M.; and Droppleman, L.: *Manual for the Profile of Mood States.* Educational and Industrial Testing Service, San Diego, Calif., 1971.

Meyerowitz, B. E.; Sparks, F. C.; and Spears, I. K.: Adjuvant chemotherapy for breast carcinoma. Psychosocial Implications. *Cancer,* 43:1613–1618, 1979.

Mitchell, G. W., and Glicksman, A. S.: Cancer patients: Knowledge and attitudes. *Cancer,* 40:61–66, 1977.

Newman, G., and Nichols, C. R.: Sexual activities and attitudes in older persons. *JAMA,* 173:33, 1960.

Peck, A.: Emotional reactions to having cancer. *Am. J. Roentgenol. Radium Ther. Nucl. Med.,* 144:591–599, 1972.

Peck, A., and Boland, J.: Emotional reactions to radiation treatment. *Cancer,* 40:180–184, 1977.

Perticucci, S.: Pelvic floor reconstruction following gynecologic exenterative surgery. *Obstet. Gynecol.,* 50:31–34, 1977.

Pfeiffer, E., and Davis, G.: Determinants of sexual behavior in middle and old age. *J. Am. Geriatr. Soc.,* 20:151, 1972.

Pitkin, R. M.; Buchsbaum, H. J.; and Lenz, H.: Estrogen and the irradiated vagina. *Obstet. Gynecol.,* 46:243–244, 1975.

Pratt, J. H.: Vaginal atresia corrected by use of small and large bowel. *Clin. Obstet. Gynecol.,* 15:639–649, 1972.

Rotman, M.; Rogow, L.; DeLeon, G.; and Haskel, N.: Supportive therapy in radiation oncology. *Cancer,* 39:744–750, 1977.

Schonfield, J.: Psychological factors related to delayed return to an earlier life-style in successfully treated cancer patients. *J. Psychosom. Res.,* 16:41–46, 1972.

Seibel, M. M.; Freeman, M. G.; and Graves, W. L.: Carcinoma of the cervix and sexual function. *Obstet. Gynecol.,* 55:484–487, 1980.

Smith, L. L., and McNamara, J. J.: Social work services for radiation therapy patients and their families. *Hosp. Community Psychiatry,* 28:752–754, 1977.

Sutcliffe, S. B.: Cytotoxic chemotherapy and gonadal function in patients with Hodgkin's disease. Facts and thoughts. *JAMA,* 242:1898–1899, 1979.

Trelford, J. D.; Hanson, F. W.; and Anderson, D. G.: The feasibility of making an artificial vagina at the time of anterior exenteration. *Oncology,* 28:398–401, 1973.

Webb, M. J., and Symmonds, R. E.: Management of the pelvic floor after pelvic exenteration. *Obstet. Gynecol.,* 50:166–171, 1977.

Weinberg, P. C.: Psychosexual impact of treatment in female genital cancer. *J. Sex Marital Ther.,* 1:155–157, 1974.

Whitehead, E.; Shalet, S. M.; Blackledge, G.; Todd, I.; Crowther, D.; and Beardwell, C. G.: The effect of combination chemotherapy on ovarian function in women treated for Hodgkin's disease. *Cancer,* 52:988–995, 1983.

Williams, E. A.: Congenital absence of the vagina: A single operation for its relief. *Br. J. Obstet. Gynaecol.,* 71:511, 1964.

Young-Brockopp, D.: Cancer patients' perceptions of five psychosocial needs. *Oncol. Nurs. For.,* 9:31–35, 1982.

# CHAPTER 16 BREAST DISEASE

*Elisabeth C. Small, M.D.*

## INTRODUCTION: GENERAL CULTURAL ATTITUDES

The breasts are not primarily sexual organs, but apparently have secondary effects on sexual function. The medical definitions of the breasts usually describe the organs as: (1) bilateral hemispheric projections in the superficial fascia over the pectoralis major on either side of the anterior thorax; or (2) the mamma; mammary gland; the organ of milk secretion. Basically the breasts are designed for feeding the young.

The anatomic and physiological definitions are frequently obscured by the cultural and emotional value placed on the breasts. The psychosocial definitions include the following: (1) Breasts represent nurturance as milk bearing organs. The lactating breast, available to the infant, offers physical and emotional gratification to both child and mother. (2) As a function of cultural expectations the breast represents sexuality and femininity. The cultural factors are often subjected to the whims and values of a given era, and are thus, especially relevant in assessing and managing a patient with breast problems in gynecological practice.

In American society, the psychosocial attitudes related to breast disease are a reflection of the role that has been assigned to the breast. Though interest in the female breast is universal, anthropologists have remarked that there is no society more obsessed with the breast than that of the United States. Margaret Mead stated that the female breast has become so idealized that it is the primary focus of a woman's identification with the feminine role (Mead, 1975). *Time* Magazine, in an editorial on feminine beauty, makes this comment: "Breasts have been strapped down, cantilevered up, pushed together and apart, oiled and siliconed—and in 16th century Venice, fitted with wool or hair padding for a sexy 'duck breast' look, curving from bodice to groin" (Leo, 1978). The attitudes have fluctuated with the whims and values of the times, and, "every delicate detail of the female body may of course be reinterpreted by the culture" (Mead, 1975).

Historically, due to the lack of information, there has been a general confusion between the sexual and reproductive–nurturing functions of the breast. Psychoanalytic literature has contributed to an overvaluation of the sexual function of the female breasts by equating them in importance with the male penis. This analogy seems to be an inaccurate assignment since research data in human sexuality have established that it is the clitoris which is the analogue of the penis (Lowry and Lowry, 1976). If only from the point of view of appearance as bilateral pendants, the breasts would be better compared with the testes, and thus fit into more of a reproductive, nurturing role rather than a purely sexual one.

The data regarding the role of the female breast in the sexual response has been inconclusive. Although the organ is capable of vascular engorgement during the sexual response cycle, studies generally agree that although breast eroticism is potentially present, not all women find the breasts of sexual importance (Kinsey *et al.*, 1953; Pion and Reich, 1975). The wide range of women's responses to breast stimulation suggests that the sexual behavior may be acquired by sociopsychologic learning rather than by physiology alone.

Learning sexual values from the culture occurs through the influence of art, advertisements, theatre, film, television, and popular literature. The individual is subjected to overt and covert stimuli which idealize the female breast as erotic and feminine, frequently to the exclusion of its nurturing value. Naked breasts are seen not only in erotic publications hidden behind the counter, but are seen on the covers of women's magazines, sports magazines, and general periodicals displayed in the supermarket.

The strong emphasis on idealized breasts affects both the developing girl and boy. For the girl, there is an early awareness that the appearance of the breasts is an important criterion of her desirability and acceptability as a woman. She feels her value is measured by the size and shape of her breasts. Whatever the actual physical state of her breasts, the girl will subliminally interpret her own development in terms of the social expectations. The usual message implies that larger breasts are equated with greater femininity. Recently, with the movement toward physical fitness and exercise, smaller breasts are now also valued. A humorous article in a popular magazine in praise of smaller breasts speaks of a "critical erotic mass" (Leonard, 1983) and assigns positive values to small breasts and negative values to large ones. Dissatisfaction with size and shape supports a large industry which produces devices or techniques to increase or decrease breast size or to alter the shape. Plastic surgery, offering augmentation or reduction mammoplasty, can affect the ultimate in body image change.

The American male, having been subjected to the same stimuli, is also affected. How much male interest in the female breast is culturally determined and how much is biologically remains unclear. The sight of a woman's breast is often reported as a greater sexual stimulus than that of the female genitalia. Sexual behaviors, acquired through general sociopsychologic learning, can explain a range of behaviors. Thus, it can be understood that if a man places a high sexual valuation on his female partner's breasts, the loss of the breast of his partner may be perceived as a serious loss for the man as well.

Surprisingly, the female breasts were also assigned a sociopolitical role during the 60s, associated with the women's liberation movement. The occasion of burning brassieres was construed as a symbolic gesture of freedom from the constraints of male domination. For a short period, wearing a bra connoted submission to male dominance. With improvement in social and economic opportunities, the brassiere was construed to be more of a natural support than as a binder, and the stigma of the brassiere has now been removed.

## ISSUES IN BREAST-FEEDING

Fascination with the breast in sexual and feminine aspects is contrasted with the general lack of interest and support for the nursing mother. An article in a woman's magazine offering advice to a hostess who had been uncomfortable with a dinner guest who had publicly nursed her baby, suggested that she avoid entertaining that couple again until the baby was past the nursing stage (Post, 1978). The custom of breast-feeding had actually been prevalent in early American history, where wealthier families had even employed "wet nurses" to suckle the young. With industrialization, women increasingly sought work outside the home and the practice became less common. While the pattern of breast-feeding declined in popularity, the use and sale of proprietary infant formulas grew in developed countries and, for decades, the sight of a nursing mother in America was rare.

In spite of the minimal risks of transmission

of pathogens and pollutants through breast milk and some nutritional deficiency states resulting from poor maternal instruction and support, human milk provides distinct advantages over bottle feeding in immunological, metabolic, and nutritional properties (Glass, 1983; Hambraeus, 1977; Rogan, 1980; Rowland et al., 1982; Stagno et al., 1980). Yet, medical approval of breast-feeding has tended to be lukewarm and ill-informed as to the psychoneurophysiology of lactation and the properties of human milk. The infant formula industry, on the other hand, has filled the gap with media saturation affecting both the medical and public sectors. Decline in breast-feeding, in both Europe and the United States, has been noted between the 1930s and the mid-1970s, with a moderate resurgence since then. Following suit, low income countries have shown some decline in the more recent years from the 1950s to the mid-1970s. The evidence from studies of breast-feeding patterns from the World Fertility Surveys and secondary sources suggest that in these countries, the practice is still nearly universal, particularly in Asia and Africa, but that earlier weaning is more common in Latin America. These patterns are of social and economic consequence since breast feeding not only provides superior nutrition and immunologic protection, but also affects fertility control through prolongation of postpartum amenorrhea and increases the interval between births (Jellife and Jellife, 1977; Martinez and Dodd, 1983; Popkin et al., 1982).

One can strongly dispute the inference that bottle feeding and breast-feeding are interchangeable phenomena, emotionally or psychophysiologically: The interaction between mother and infant is very different in each situation. Maternal bonding in the neonatal period has been demonstrated to relate to that sensitive time during the first day of life and proceeds into a mutually reinforcing reflex behavior, particularly during biological breast-feeding. The likelihood of "disorders of mothering," including child abuse and psychosocial maladjustments in childhood are considered to be more prevalent in situations of bonding failure. The maternal hormonal status and the neonatal somatosensory stimulations in breast feeding results in a quality of contact that is more direct and biologically intimate. The consequences of Western-style neonatal practices of separating the mother and newborn, and the use of bottle feeding may be factors in the development of psychosocial abnormalities (Cole, 1977; Lynch, 1975).

RESISTANCE TO BREAST-FEEDING

Resistance to breast-feeding often appears to be directly related to sexualization of the female breasts, resulting in feelings of guilt, shame, repugnance, or male resentment. If the breasts are given a sexual role, exposure of the breasts may be an infringement on modesty. This paradox is evident in a society that permits sexual explicitness, but is hostile to the public display of nursing. The woman and her partner may be embarrassed at the exposure of breasts which are not the idealized shape, or fear that breast-feeding may cause disfigurement.

Some physiological factors may also affect resistance to breast-feeding. During sexual arousal, even if the breasts are not stimulated directly, vascular engorgement occurs as a reflex response to the changes with pelvic congestion involving the clitoris and vagina. As the sexual response cycle continues, the size of the breasts enlarges, the nipples become erect, followed by areolar engorgement, and a generalized hyperemia in the skin (the "sex flush") appears on the breasts as elsewhere. During resolution of the sexual response, with vascular decongestion, there is a gradual return of the breasts to normal size and detumescence of the areolae and nipples with disappearance of the "sex flush" (Masters and Johnson, 1966).

In lactating and nonlactating women, direct breast stimulation either by mechanical contact or suckling will also result in increased serum prolactin.

Suckling in the nursing woman evokes both prolactin and oxytocin release. Oxytocin is believed to be released as part of the milk ejection reflex, essential for milk transfer to the infant, which can be conditioned by not only suckling, but by psychic stimulus such as the cry of the infant occurring prior to the suckling. This reflex may be inhibited by both physical and psychological stress and underscores the necessity of mothers to avoid stress immediately before and during suckling (Lucas et al., 1980; McNeilly et al., 1983). Oxytocin not only initiates the milk ejection reflex, but also has a direct effect on uterine contractions. Some women interpret these contractions as orgasmic. An association of an experience construed as erotic with the feeding of one's child may evoke fears of incest and be repugnant and unacceptable and, therefore, may be avoided.

If women are poorly educated regarding the value of breast-feeding, many men are also uninformed and refuse to allow their wives to breast-feed. Some psychologists also believe that men may feel competition with the child for the exclusive possession of the woman's breasts, or fear that the breasts would lose their erotically arousing shape and thus reduce the man's sexual pleasure. These feelings are not usually directly expressed, for the male may be embarrassed to let the real reasons be known. In such a situation, it would be difficult, if not impossible, for a woman who desires to breast-feed to communicate her wishes to her partner.

Many women simply do not know how to breast-feed. Inadequate preparation, lack of role models and permission, and insufficient support in the efforts at breast feeding leave them without the emotional and social support required for successful lactation, resulting in the "anxiety-nursing failure syndrome" (Jellife and Jellife, 1977).

### PATTERNS IN BREAST-FEEDING

Studies of prevalence of breast feeding in Western countries have described some general features. The decision to breast or bottle feed is usually made before pregnancy and delivery. Women who choose to breast-feed are likely to be better educated and relatively more affluent. Usually they have witnessed a mother who breast-fed and have been breast-fed themselves. They usually have given a good deal of thought to breast-feeding and have attended prenatal courses (Llewellyn-Jones, 1982; Martinez and Dodd, 1983). Attitudes toward nursing involve complex variables including early life experiences, feelings about nudity, sexuality, pregnancy, relationship with the father of the child, the quality and quantity of contact with one's own mother, the resolution of one's own developmental crises, and the availability of support systems. Geography, education, social class, and historical period also play a significant role.

## ISSUES IN BREAST PATHOLOGY

### SEXUAL CONCERNS AND THE IMPORTANCE OF THE SEXUAL HISTORY

The sexual meaning of the breast extends into medical management. Although the teaching of human sexuality has still not been universally accepted into medical curriculum, the importance of a relevant sexual history as part of the total medical history does need emphasis. The omission of relevant sexual data leaves the physician with only a partial data base upon which to make a diagnosis and to plan treatment. Given an attitude of serious professional concern, the physician can, tactfully and with candor, question the patient at the appropriate juncture during the routine history and review of systems to ascertain what her sexual concerns are and what her sexual practices are in relation to her presenting problem. The success of adequate data gathering depends a great deal on the physician's openness and nonjudgmental attitude toward sexual issues, fund of information in the sexual aspects of pathological states, and skill in integrating the sexual information from the patient into the treatment plan and management.

With breast problems, the entry of the sexual history is readily facilitated. The physician can query the patient in questions such as:

"What does this problem mean to you?" "How has this affected your sexual functioning?" "How has it affected your relationship with your sexual partner?" "What is the attitude of your partner to the problem (or the planned treatment)?"

Often it is not necessary to go into explicit detail of a patient's sexual life, but some basic data are essential. It is relevant to know:

1. If the patient is sexually active?
2. If so, is her sexual functioning presenting any difficulty?

"Sexual activity" does not describe any specifics as to whether her activity is heterosexual, homosexual or self-stimulatory. This aspect may not be relevant, depending on the problem, and can be omitted, *but should be explored if her pathology and treatment are related to any specific practices important in her sexual experience.*

3. Will her pathology and/or treatment affect specific practices?

If so, then not only a more detailed history is needed, but the physician is responsible for preparing the patient for the need for any changes in her sexual activities and this may even require the physician to give sexual counsel or to refer the patient to a well-trained sexual counselor at some later date.

In the case of breast disease, the meaning of the breast to the woman and to her partner is important, both in terms of her self-esteem and her sexuality. If there is high sexual valuation of the breast to either, then any changes in breast appearance, as in surgical alteration—by biopsy, mastectomy or plastic change—will require information from the couple on how the breasts are perceived by them and what role do they have in their sexual experiences. The usual expectation of the man to stimulate the woman by fondling, caressing, and suckling the female breasts may not always hold true as sexually arousing to the woman. Studies have shown that a very low percentage of women were actually aroused by breast stimulation (Kinsey, 1953; Pion, 1975). On the other hand, the male's needs are important to consider. If he has learned that breast stimulation of the female enhances his male proclivities and if he himself is aroused and gratified by breast petting, then his concerns must necessarily be addressed and dealt with as part of the management.

## Pain and Discomfort: Mastodynia, Mastalgia

Pain in the breast is commonly encountered in situations of benign breast disease. The terms "fibrocystic disease of the breast," "chronic cystic mastitis," "fibrous mastopathy," and "mammary dysplasia" are some of the catch-all names for several types of histologic patterns including cyst formation, apocrine metaplasia, adenosing and sclerosing adenosis, papillomatosis and various degrees of hyperplasia of the ducts and lobules. This discussion will be limited to that clinical syndrome of mammary dysplasia which is benign, *cyclic,* with histologic changes on the terminal ducts and lobules of the breast in both epithelial and connective tissue, usually accompanied by pain in the breast. The symptoms occur in 50 percent of women during their reproductive lifetime, and are exacerbated prior to or during menses and progressively worsen until menopause. Its occurrence is more frequent in ovulatory women, and, though its precise etiology is uncertain, it is believed to be caused by an exaggerated or inappropriate tissue response to other cyclic changes of the ovarian hormones. Whether the clinical state is to be considered "disease" or a normal variant because of its frequency is still disputed; and whether its general presence or whether the presence of particular histologic types predisposes the patient to high risk of cancer is still unclear (Greenblatt et al., 1982; Livolsi et al., 1978; London et al., 1982; Love et al., 1982).

Nonetheless, painful, tender, nodular, lumpy breasts which recur monthly do have an effect on a woman's sexual function, if only for the fact that any touch or contact produces a noxious stimulus that affects the pleasurable response to sexual arousal. As a result, the pain can set up a negative response to sexual overtures and a dysfunctional state results.

Unexplained mastalgia has traditionally been considered a psychosomatic complaint and should be considered in some circumstances. Eliciting a previous history of sexual abuse or assault as a child or adult sometimes can explain the focus of pain on the breasts or other areas of the body with symbolic meaning. However, results of a recent study of women with breast pain does not indicate that there is any greater incidence of neurotic or personality disorder in women with breast pain (Preece, 1978). The best treatment for mild to moderate pain is a careful evaluation and confident reassurance by an experienced physician.

## Cancer Anxiety

Despite the fact that American women are more knowledgeable about breast cancer than others, their concern regarding cancer of the breast as a threat to life and to femininity and sexuality is no less. The National Cancer Institute, in a national survey conducted in 1979, including black and Hispanic women and their sexual partners, revealed that the greatest health concern of the women was breast cancer (National Institute of Health, 1981). The data show that many women wanted to play an active role in their health care and did not want to rely solely on their physicians for decision making and health information. If ever given a diagnosis of breast cancer, most would seek a second medical opinion. There was preference for a two-step surgical procedure since there was a belief expressed that unnecessary mastectomies were sometimes performed. A majority of the women felt that they were more likely to discover a breast lump before their physicians.

Nearly the whole sample (96 percent) had heard of the breast self-examination (BSE), but fewer (83 percent) reported that they examined their breasts in the past year. While BSE may be an effective method for early detection, a small number (29 percent) said that they actually did monthly examinations. Many women who said they regularly practiced BSE could not give adequate descriptions of steps in doing a proper BSE. Women who received individual training from a nurse or physician reported more confidence in their BSE skills and a greater frequency of examination than those who had not received individual help.

A majority of the women were aware of the increased risk of breast cancer in women who have a positive family history; a third of the women knew of the increased risk of advanced age and later parity.

Misconceptions about the etiology of breast cancer were shown to persist. Half of the women felt that bumping or bruising the breasts causes cancer. Black and Hispanic women were more likely to believe that caressing and fondling the breasts causes cancer. Although nearly all the women realized that lumps in the breasts may signal cancer, fewer realized that nipple changes or breast appearance were significant. There was much less awareness of the variations of diagnostic procedures to be followed when a lump is discovered, and few women realized that there are treatment options for breast cancer outside of surgery. While 75 percent of the women discussed surgery, only 15 percent mentioned mastectomy specifically.

Generally, the women viewed breast cancer as a medical rather than a social or emotional issue, although the Hispanic women focused more on the emotional aspects. If mastectomy resulted, the major concern would be whether the cancer was entirely removed and whether it may recur. The women were more worried about high medical costs than the physical changes in appearance. Only two in ten women knew of breast reconstruction; once informed, one in ten said that they wished breast reconstruction in the event of a mastectomy mainly to improve self-esteem and appearance. Hispanic women were more desirous of breast reconstruction.

## Breast Self-Examination: Factors in Resistance

The value of the monthly breast self-examination as an integral aspect of early screening of cancer of the breast has been accepted for many years (Foster et al., 1978; Greenwald et al., 1978; Marchant, 1979). Yet, studies consistently report a low percentage of American women actually practicing monthly examinations. The Breast Cancer Detection Demonstration Project reported in 1982 (Baker, 1982) that of their sample population of over 280,000 women, 18.3 percent did not perform the BSE, and while 80.5 percent had practiced BSE prior to entry into the study, only 35.9 percent did so on a regular basis. This figure is consistent with a 1977 Gallup poll study that reported 35 percent monthly BSE participants (Baker, 1982). In spite of national efforts at educating women in self-examination, women appear unwilling to engage in self-examination. In a Boston study, the profile of the woman who was likely to practice monthly examinations was a woman who was living with a sexual partner (who often may be the breast examiner), who had been shown how to do the BSE, and who was confident in her examination technique. The study showed that women who had a history of maternal breast cancer were more likely to practice BSE, though there were no associations with educational level or other health practices.

The BSE is an examination of an intimate nature, not only anxiety-provoking because of apprehensions of cancer, pain and dying, but also because of its possible sexual nature. It can be compared to a testicular self-examination in the male, which can also be uncomfortable if performed rigorously and carefully. It may be the sexualization of the process that sets up the inhibition to self-examine, since many persons in this culture may still have attitudes prohibiting self-stimulation so that the act of touching oneself in assigned erogenous areas is, again, not acceptable—even in the service of health.

Realizing this attitude, the physician who wishes to educate the patient in the BSE can give permission to touch by a supportive and positive attitude in teaching a woman how to properly conduct a BSE and to encourage her to do so throughout the course of her clinical visits.

## MANAGEMENT STRATEGIES

### Reassurance and Education

Although American men and women are more knowledgeable and open about sexual matters in current times, an accurate fund of information regarding the separation of sexual and reproductive functions is still generally lacking. A clear understanding of the separation of sex and reproduction in anatomic and physiological terms sometimes even eludes the medical practitioner. However, the clarification of where the sexual component is essential in the treatment and management of breast pathology is of primary importance to the physician. With a good sexual history, and with its correlation to the presenting problem, a physician can then move on to inform, instruct, and allay unnecessary fear and anxiety. As was stated initially, if the breast is accepted as secondary to sexual function, and a woman (and her partner) realizes that the core of the sexual response is genital, then any threat to breast integrity can be diminished by the awareness that basic feminine sexuality is not at stake. This observer's experience has been that, in general, patients are not well-informed about anatomy or physiology, and few women, when directly questioned about it, say they have viewed their own perineum, even out of curiosity. This observation cuts across class, education, and age lines.

Fear of the unknown is worse than the known. Knowledge is power and can be used as a therapeutic tool to help the patient gain a sense of control, as well as engender a collaboration with the physician. If possible, include the sexual partner. Simple explanation of the anatomy and physiology of the breast, using audiovisuals, such as pictures and diagrams pointing out normal anatomy and physiology can be performed first, then the pathology and treatments can be considered. This technique is helpful to both the patient and her partner. This need not be overly extensive and time consuming, but can be incorporated into the office visit, just as the sexual history need not be time consuming, but simply added to the routine history interview. In the course of follow-up, the information can be augmented as the workup and treatment continues. In this way the patient (and partner) has a baseline of information upon which she can build; the physician, having instructed her initially, is also reassured that the patient understands what the issues are. If such a technique overwhelms the physician because of time constraints, then a member of the staff can teach the initial level of basic anatomy and physiology with the physician adding information in matters of pathology and treatment.

It cannot be emphasized enough how much therapeutic value the attending physician's investment of time has in handling this aspect of teaching and reassurance. It not only cements the physician–patient relationship, but can reduce complications, psychological and otherwise, and enhance patient cooperation in later management. The patient feels that the physician is concerned and sensitive to her needs and thus, a well-informed patient can also be considered as a colleague in the treatment phase. As an added advantage, the likelihood of malpractice suits diminishes the more the patient sees and relates to the physician as a caretaker (Hirsch and White, 1978).

## Treatment Issues in Benign Disease

The alleviation of pain and discomfort is the obvious goal in treatment for mastalgia. In the past, treatment for mammary dysplasia had primarily focused on surgery and the use of analgesics. More recently, medical management using diuretics, oral estrogens and/or progestogens as well as androgens has been found to be effective. Danazol, a new synthetic derivative of 17-alphaethinyltestosterone, an impeded androgen, has been effective in relief of symptoms. Danazol suppresses ovarian function by abolishing the surge of luteinizing hormones and blocks ovarian steroidogenesis. The result is a decrease in ovarian hormone secretion, which some believe is cause for the dysplasia. Because of a correlation between hypothyroidism and mammary dysplasia, thyroid hormone has provided improvement in some patients, but caution is suggested in its use in euthyroid patients (Estes, 1981; Greenblatt et al., 1982; LiVolsi et al., 1978; London et al., 1982; Love et al., 1982).

Since benign breast lesions contain estrogen receptors, blocking receptor sites has been tried with drugs such as tamoxifen, a synthetic antiestrogen which competes with estradiol for estrogen receptors in target tissues and lowers serum prolactin. The specific role of prolactin in benign breast disease is not yet clear, but dopamine agonists such as bromocriptine inhibit prolactin and appear to bring relief (Durning and Sellwood, 1982).

Vitamin E supplementation has relieved some women and causes regression of the dysplasia in others (Abrams, 1965; London et al., 1982). It is believed that Vitamin E has some effect on steroidogenesis and causes an alteration in lipoproteins, but the exact mechanism is still unclear.

The withdrawal of methylxanthines (caffeine, theophylline, and theobromine) from the diet has been suggested. It is believed that the methylxanthines block the action of the catabolic enzyme phosphodiesterase, which degrades cyclic adenosine monophosphate (cAMP) to adenosine monophosphate (AMP), and cyclic guanosine monophosphate (cGMP) to guanosine monophosphate (GMP). This action results in an intracellular increase of cAMP and cGMP which then promotes cellular growth and metabolism ending in fibrous formation and cystic fluid accumulation. Thus, avoidance of coffee, tea, colas, cocoa, chocolate, and drugs containing methylxanthines has been found effective in treatment of some. Since nicotine also increases intracellular cyclic nucleotides by stimulating epinephrine, women are also advised not to smoke (Minton et al., 1979).

The effects on sexual functioning of the various treatments are determined by the side effects of each modality. For instance, a concern in the use of the androgenic treatments may include symptoms of weight gain, hirsutism, nervousness, depression, nausea, hot flashes, amenorrhea, or menstrual irregularities. These symptoms have obvious bearing on a woman's interest in sex. It suffices to say that it is the clinician's awareness of which side effects of a given modality of treatment can affect a patient's sexuality that determines whether reassurance or alteration in treatment will best serve the patient's need for effective sexual function.

TREATMENT ISSUES IN MALIGNANT DISEASE

At all levels of management, it is useful to have the patient's partner present during discussion and counseling as the partner can play an important role in the rehabilitation by lending much needed emotional and physical support to the patient. Furthermore, the anxieties of both the patient and partner can be dealt with simultaneously. In the situation of cancer, this is especially relevant since the disease and its treatment have serious ramifications, not only for the patient, but also to her family and those close to her. The meaning of the diagnosis and preparation for the planned work-up and treatment are issues that need to be clarified and explained.

At diagnosis, the fear of imminent death associated with the word "cancer" should be dispelled. Verbal reassurance that she will not die "tomorrow" and that treatment will be available is helpful in reducing anxiety and tension. If the physician is not fearful of saying the words "cancer" and "death," then the disease may not be so fearful to the patient when she realizes that help and hope are available. Moreover, in verbalizing what is the usual fear in a diagnosis of cancer for the patient and family, the physician is perceived by the patient as someone who not only understands the medical problems, but also her feelings.

Lack of knowledge about the anatomy and physiology of the thorax, and lack of understanding of hospital procedures, often can give rise to myths and fears. A simple but graphic description of chest anatomy and the axilla, incorporating a discussion of work-up procedure and modalities of treatment, is very reassuring. In the discussion visual aids are helpful, as is giving the patient and partner an idea of what anatomic or functional changes to expect. A common misconception is that the breast is like an orange pressed into the chest wall, and if removed would leave a concave deformity. If mastectomy is planned, a simple line drawing of the expected surgical scar will give the couple a preparation for the postoperative body image change. In some states, a full discussion by the physician of the risks and benefits of treatment options is required to fulfill the legal obligation of preparing the patient for an informed consent.

A de-emphasis of the breast as an overvalued sex or maternal symbol is necessary in the early diagnostic phase as a preparation for the patient to accept the changes or the loss of breast integrity in treatment. It is essential to clarify the reality that the breast is now a *diseased* portion of the body that serves no purpose in sustaining health and is a threat to life. In this matter, preparation for breast loss, such as devaluation of the diseased organ, and separation of the diseased part from its sexual value may be the first therapeutic move in helping the couple to give up the affected breast, if it is necessary. Emphasis on the lifesaving aspect sometimes is not heard initially because the fear of defeminization and disfigurement is more threatening. Revaluation of the surgical site as "healthy" tissue, with a well-healed scar as a positive replacement, also aids in the acceptance of the altered body image.

Among the distressing myths which will require clarification are that: (1) cancer always recurs or kills; (2) cancer is communicable and the patient may spread the disease; (3) she has caused the cancer by some past misdeed, or had done so by not taking proper health precautions; and (4) she will no longer have sexual interest, or may be changed so that she is not sexually acceptable.

Many women claim that the most stressful time in the whole treatment process is the time between biopsy of the lesion and the definitive diagnosis. The waiting period sometimes initiates the process of adjusting to the reality of death, and the process of reorganizing and reviewing the priorities of living.

**Surgery.** In the case of mastectomy, the patient is met with the task of adaptation to hospitalization, loss of a body part, and the building of physical resources to return to normal functioning with self-esteem. Initial response to body change is an expected depressive or postoperative "fatigue" state (Rose and King, 1978). This response usually is seen within the first week after surgery. Symptoms of lassitude, anxiety, irritability, spontaneous crying spells, anorexia, insomnia, and feelings of worthlessness and shame may occur about the fourth day. These symptoms last about a week and, ordinarily, should not extend beyond a month. If symptoms persist longer, factors other than breast loss may be present, and a psychiatric consultation is indicated.

Restoration of body image and functioning as soon after surgery as possible is suggested. First, the patient needs to feel that although she has changed, she is not lessened or devalued. At the time of the first dressing change, she can be invited to see the site. If she is not emotionally able to look directly at the wound, allow her some time to adapt and encourage her to look again at a later time. Commonly, the first view of the site results in a sense of the reality of the loss and a response of tears and anxiety is a normal part of the grief reaction. A woman who has refused to look by the time of discharge may be at high risk for problems in adjusting to the change.

Tactile changes perceived by the patient and partner are part of the adaptation. When the wound is adequately healed, the patient and partner are encouraged to touch the unaffected site, and then gently to move the fingers over the affected area to learn the subjective and objective sensations. Changes in skin sensation, particularly paresthesias, are then noted and, in advance of discharge, the patient can be reassured as to whether these feelings are to be expected or not. Again, recalling that women sometimes are inhibited about touching themselves, the physician may need to give permission and encouragement to the patient not only to relearn how her body feels, but also to allow her partner to touch and relearn.

The couple should also be encouraged to resume sexual activity as soon as the woman is emotionally ready, and to use the breast area if it had been of importance in their previous sexual practice. This maneuver restores not only a sense of body integrity, but integrates the feminine sexuality component as well.

Balance and symmetry may be of concern. Patients should have the option of the use of a temporary prosthetic cotton puff to give a symmetric appearance at time of discharge. The Reach to Recovery volunteer group of postmastectomees, sponsored by the American Cancer Society, can be helpful to patients near discharge by providing counsel on practical issues in dress, appearance, and return to family and the community. Identification with a woman who has successfully adapted is also supportive.

**Phantom Breast Syndrome.** Some women after mastectomy report feelings of having a replacement of a breast or part of a breast at the space where the removed breast had been. This phantom breast syndrome (PBS) phenomena has been known for some time and has been reported to occur among all types of mastectomy patients, radical, modified radical, and simple, and range from one-fourth to over one-half of women so operated, depending on the study. The symptoms range from an awareness of a breast to discomfort from itching, ache, tightness, numbness, burning, tingling, and heaviness. There is no defined pattern of onset, frequency, or relationship to exhaustion, mood, sexual state or mere looking at the operative site. Although some studies suggest that psychological factors such as sexual attitudes towards the breast or maternal identification are relevant (Jamison et al., 1979), others show no significant difference (Ackerly et al., 1955; Jarvis, 1967). The symptoms have varying effects on rehabilitation. The high-risk group appears to be younger, premenopausal women who were subject to postoperative depression, who evaluated themselves as having a poor relationship with their partners, or who experienced a poor relationship with their surgeons, again emphasizing the importance of the physician's role in the education and support of the patient in the preoperative and rehabilitative stages.

**External Prosthesis and Breast Reconstruction.** For some women, an external prosthesis may be adequate to achieve the feelings of restoration and integrity, while for others the sense of deformity is psychologically crippling. Since body image and self-esteem are directly related to personal identity, any sudden change of appearance can disrupt self-integrity and result in feelings of panic, depersonalization, and confusion. For women who cannot feel intact without a replacement of a "mound," breast reconstruction is therapeutically necessary. For these women, it is necessary to set realistic goals, that is, a normal appearance can be achieved when clothed, but that obliteration of scars or a perfect replacement may not be possible. Women who cannot specify their wishes may need psychological evaluation to rule out any serious underlying emotional conflicts.

**Radiotherapy and Chemotherapy.** If the primary treatment is radiotherapy, breast loss is not an issue. However, skin changes due to radiation and fear of recurrence are the major concerns. Women not having a mastectomy may have less social supports available because there are fewer lay support groups, and they may be the object of envy from mastectomized women. Their sense of loss is considerably less and sexual function should not be as markedly directly affected. However, the response to radiotherapy and/or depression may affect libido. In the case of chemotherapy, the physiological response to the chemotherapeutic agent and its side effects frequently not only result in fatigue, debilitation, and depression, but also the chemotherapeutic agent often directly affects libido as well. Symptomatic treatment and support to increase a patient's physical strength is important to maintain her sense of integrity and self-esteem first, and the sexual aspect may, in turn, also be enhanced.

The effects of having cancer, with the concomitant debilitating states during surgery, irradiation, or adjuvant therapy necessarily affect the sexual interests of the patient. Decreased libidinal interest also results as a side effect of the drugs, other than cytotoxics, used in treatment. However, as soon as the patient is physically and emotionally ready, return to sexual activity is encouraged, since, from an anatomic point of view, there has been no major change in her genital capacity. Except for emotional factors, she should enjoy sexual activity again, however, the emotional factors affecting her sense of womanliness, attractiveness, and desirability do play a large role in her ability to relate to her partner and to allow the partner to be intimate. Many studies suggest that the response to mastectomy is less of a problem for the male than is expected and that love and communication are more important in the sexual rehabilitation. Sexual partners are encouraged to be especially attentive and openly expressive of their love and desire and to reassure the patient of their continuing love and support. An inability of a woman to return to sexual activity, when she has a concerned, caring, and willing partner, suggests serious psychological conflict and may require therapeutic intervention.

Awareness of the specific cultural and emotional factors and attitudes toward the female breast, and the inclusion of these factors in the care of the patient with breast problems, facilitates the overall management of the patient afflicted with breast disease.

## REFERENCES

Abrams, A. A.: Use of Vitamin E in chronic cystic mastitis. *N. Engl. J. Med.*, 272:1080–1081, 1965.

Ackerly, W.; Lhamon, W.; and Fitts, W. T.: Phantom breast. *J. Nerv. Ment. Dis.*, 121:177–178, 1955.

Baker, L. H.: Breast Cancer Detection Demonstration Project: Five-year summary report. *Cancer*, 32:194–225, 1982.

Bard, M. and Sutherland, A. M.: Psychological impact of cancer and its treatment: IV. Adaptation to mastectomy. *Cancer*, 8:656–672, 1955.

Bennett, S. E.; Lawrence, R. S.; Fleischmann, K. H.; Gifford, C. S.; and Slack, W. V.: Profile of women practicing breast self-examination. *JAMA*, 249:488–491, 1983.

Cole, J. P.: Breast feeding in the Boston suburbs in relation to personal-social factors. *Clin. Pediatr.*, 16:352–356, 1977.

Durning, P., and Sellwood, R. A.: Bromocryptine in severe cyclical breast pain. *Br. J. Surg.*, 69:248–249, 1982.

Estes, N. C.: Mastodynia due to fibrocystic disease of the breast controlled with thyroid hormone. *Am. J. Surg.*, 142:764–766, 1981.

Foster, R. S.; Lang, S. P.; Costanza, M. C.; Worden, J. K.; Haines, C. R.; and Yates, J. W.: Breast self-examination practices and breast cancer stage. *N. Engl. J. Med.*, 299:265–270, 1978.

Glass, R. I.; Svennerholm, A. M.; Stoll, B. J.; Khan, M. R.; Belayet Hossain, K. M.; Imdadul Huq, M.; and Holmgren, J.: Protection against cholera in breast-fed children by antibodies in breast milk. *N. Engl. J. Med.*, 308:1389–1392, 1983.

Greenblatt, R. B.; Vasquez, J.; and Samaras, C.: Fibrocystic breast disease: current status of diagnosis and treatment. *Postgrad. Med.*, 71:159–168, 1982.

Greenwald, P.; Nasca, P. C.; Lawrence, C. E.; Horton, J.; McGarrah, R. P.; Gabriele; and Carlton, K.: Estimated effect of breast self-examination and routine physician examinations on breast-cancer mortality. *N. Engl. J. Med.* 299:271–273, 1978.

Hambraeus, L.: Proprietary milk versus human breast milk in infant feeding. *Pediatr. Clin. North Am.*, 24:17–36, 1977.

Hirsch, H. L., and White, E. R.: The pathologic anatomy of medical malpractice claims. *Legal Aspects of Medical Practice*, 6:25–32, 1978.

Jamison, K.; Wellisch, D. K.; Katz, R. L.; and Pasnau, R. O.: Phantom breast syndrome. *Arch. Surg.*, 114:93–95, 1979.

Jarvis, J. H.: Post-mastectomy breast phantoms. *J. Nerv. Ment. Dis.*, 144:266–272, 1967.

Jelliffe, D. B., and Jelliffe, E. F. P.: Breast is best, modern meanings. *N. Engl. J. Med.*, 297:912–915, 1977.

Kinsey, A. C.; Pomeroy, W. B.; and Martin, C. E.: *Sexual Behavior in the Human Female*. W. B. Saunders, Philadelphia, 1953.

Leo, J.: "Mirror, mirror on the wall . . ." *Time*, March 6, 1978:54.

Leonard, A.: In praise of small breasts. *Forum*, 12:27–37, 1983.

Lewellyn-Jones, D.: The psychosocial aspects of breast feeding. In: Dennerstein, L.; Burrows, G. D.: (eds.): *Proceedings of the Ninth Annual Congress of the Australian Society for Psychosomatic Obstetrics/Gynecology*. York Press Property, Ltd., Victoria, Australia, 1982.

LiVolsi, V. A.; Stadel, B. V.; Kelsey, J. L.; Holford, T. R.; and White, C.: Fibrocystic breast disease in oral contraceptive users. *N. Engl. J. Med.*, 299:381–385, 1978.

London, R. S.; Sundaram, G. S.; and Goldstein, P. J.: Medical management of mammary dysplasia. *Obstet. Gynecol.*, 59:519–523, 1982.

Love, S. M.; Gelman, R. S.; and Silen, W.: Fibrocystic "disease" of the breast—a nondisease? *N. Engl. J. Med.*, 307:1010–1014, 1982.

Lowry, T. P.; Lowry, T. S.: *The Clitoris*. Warren H. Green, St. Louis, 1976.

Lucas, A.; Drewett, R. B.; and Mitchell, M. D.: Breast feeding and plasma oxytocin concentrations. *Br. Med. J.*, 281:834–835, 1980.

Lynch, M. A.: Ill health and child abuse. *Lancet*, 2:317–319, 1975.

Marchant, D. J.: Screening for breast cancer. *Clin. Obstet. Gynecol.*, 22:759–776, 1979.

Martinez, G. A., and Dodd, D. A.: 1981 milk feeding patterns in the U.S. during the first 12 months of life. *Pediatrics*, 71:166–170, 1983.

Masters, W. H.; Johnson, V. E.: *Human Sexual Response*. Little, Brown, Boston, 1966.

McNeilly, A. S.; Robinson, I. C. A. F.; Houston, M. J.; and Howie, P. W.: Release of oxytocin and prolactin in response to suckling. *Br. Med. J.*, 286:257–259, 1983.

Mead, M.: *Male and Female*. William Morrow, New York, 1975.

Minton, J. P.; Foecking, M. K.; Webster, D. J. T.; and Matthews, R. H.: Caffeine, cyclic nucleotides and breast disease. *Surgery*, 86:105–109, 1979.

National Institutes of Health: Survey finds U.S. women knowledgeable about breast cancer. *JAMA*, 245:918, 1981.

Pion, R. J., and Reich, L. A.: Role of the breast in female sexual response. *Med. Aspects Hum. Sex.*, 9:103–109, 1975.

Popkin, B. M.; Bilsborrow, R. E.; and Akin, J. S.: Breast feeding patterns in low-income countries. *Science*, 218:1088–1093, 1982.

Post, E. L.: Etiquette for everyday: The new Emily Post. *Good Housekeeping*, June 1978:70.

Preece, P. E.; Mansel, R. E.; and Hughes, L. E.: Mastalgia: Psychoneurosis or organic disease? *Br. Med. J.*, 1:29–30, 1978.

Rogan, W. J.; Bagniewska, A.; and Damstra, T.: Pollutants in breast milk. *N. Engl. J. Med.*, 302:1450–1453, 1980.

Rose, E. A., and King, T. C.: Understanding postoperative fatigue. *Surg. Gynecol. Obstet.*, 147:97–102, 1978.

Rowland, T. W.; Zori, R. T.; Lafleur, W. R.; and Reiter, E. O.: Malnutrition and hypernatremic dehydration in breast fed infants. *JAMA*, 247:1016–1017, 1982.

Stagno, S.; Reynolds, D. W.; Pass, R. F.; and Alford, C. A.: Breast milk and the risk of cytomegalovirus infection. *N. Engl. J. Med.*, 302:1073–1076, 1980.

# CHAPTER 17 PSYCHOSOMATIC ASPECTS OF HIGH-RISK PREGNANCY

*Robert C. Goodlin, M.D.*

## INTRODUCTION

The focus of this chapter will be sexual activity and anxiety during pregnancy. Admittedly, this restriction eliminates important psychosomatic factors affecting pregnancy. However, after reviewing the records of 650 families who elected to give birth in an alternate birth center and attempting to determine why their obstetrical performance was so superior to those deliveries in the standard delivery suite (Goodlin, 1980), I have concluded that psychosomatic aspects other than sexual activity and anxiety are too diffuse to be discussed in a single chapter. By contrast, sexual activity and anxiety levels during pregnancy are easily studied and have been the topic of numerous recent papers. In keeping with recent trends, emphasis will be placed on fetal development and *in utero* effects.

## SEXUAL ACTIVITY DURING PREGNANCY

Numerous studies have indicated that there is a decline in overall sexual activity during normal pregnancy (see Chapter 5; Goodlin *et al.,* 1971; Limner, 1970; Masters and Johnson, 1966; Mills *et al.,* 1981; Naeye, 1980; Naeye and Ross, 1982, Nuckolls *et al.,* 1972). This reduction is related to declining interest and to maternal positional difficulties. Much of this reduced maternal interest can be ascribed to social attitudes as women generally report no lack of decline of positive feelings regarding sex with their partners as a result of pregnancy. Sometimes pregnant women will engage in sexual activity in consideration of the sexual needs of their partners. Rarely is the male responsible for the decline in sexual activity except those who, for religious or medical attitudes, believe that sexual activity should be eliminated or reduced during pregnancy.

In a 1973 study, Solberg, Butler, and Wagner differed from the general consensus regarding sex in pregnancy. They found through a retrospective study of 260 postpartum women that the decrease in sexual performance during pregnancy was due predominantly to increase in physical discomfort, anxiety over fetal well-being, and reduced libido—as well as medical advice. Their interviews suggested that noncoital activity, such as masturbation and mutual oral–genital contact were also used less frequently. Coital position changed gradually from the popular male-superior position before pregnancy to side-by-side and, to a lesser extent, the female-superior and rear-entry positions during pregnancy.

## Fetal Effects of Maternal Sexual Activity

From a physiological standpoint, maternal sexual relations or orgasm may be detrimental to the fetus for the following reasons. Maternal sexual activity is associated with increased blood levels of oxytocin, prolactin, catecholamines, and prostaglandins—all of which may produce increased uterine tone and/or contractions. It has been suggested that sexual activity may be associated with decrease in uterine blood flow (Freud, 1926; Goodlin, 1979, 1980; Goodlin et al., 1972). The fetus may respond to uterine contractions induced by maternal orgasm with fetal heart rate recording as shown in Figure 17–1. We originally interpreted this recording to show an abnormal fetal heart rate response (Goodlin et al., 1971), but today we regard the records as showing only excessive fetal vagal activity. Numerous cases of abruptio placenta, which apparently began with maternal sex relations or orgasm, have been reported (Freud, 1926).

## Fetal Affects of Maternal Anxiety

Talbert, Benson, and Dewhurst (1982) studied women in late pregnancy who were subjected to mild psychological stress by listening to prerecorded sounds of babies crying. A positive maternal reaction was indicated by changes in heart rate and skin resistance. They found that when the mothers responded with signs of stress the fetus often had coincidental changes in its fetal heart rate patterns. The authors also showed that it is possible to modify apparently normal antenatal fetal heart rate patterns (nonstress tests) with sounds of babies crying, presumably involving maternal sympathetic nervous control affecting uterine blood flow. Fetal responses during *in utero* life and birth have been considered, both by Freud and his student, Otto Rank, as basic models for later attacks of fear. Freud (1926) stated: "All anxiety goes back originally to the anxiety of birth," and Rank (1952) expressed the traumatic effect of separation of mother and her newborn child with the phrase "the primal castration." Rene Dubos (1965) expressed the view that subtle variations in the *in utero* environment relative to the environmental changes of the mother can have profound effects on fetal growth and development and even the personality of the child.

In the primal union described by Grof (1976), the fetus floats in its amniotic sac, its needs provided through the umbilical cord, moving in symbiotic harmony with its mother. He suggested that a fetal feeling of oceanic ecstasy prevails. The mother's activities can affect this tranquil environment with disturbances upsetting this fetal universe. According to Grof, if *in utero* assaults such as maternal anxiety, drinking, and sexual relations are con-

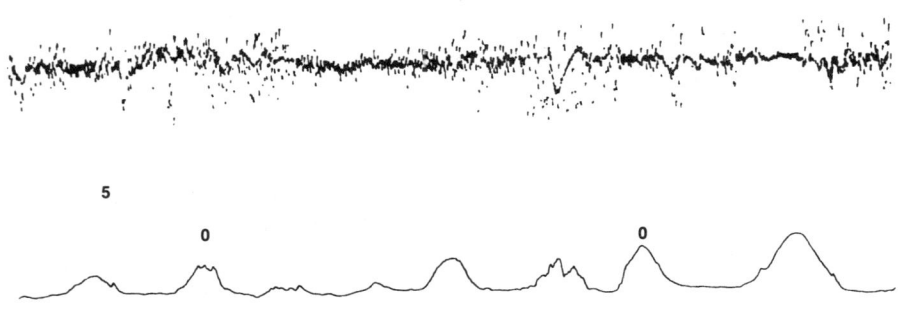

**FIGURE 17–1.** External fetal heart rate recording. O = Painful orgasmic episode. (Reprinted with permission from Goodlin, R. C.; Schmidt, W.; and Creevy D. C.: Uterine tension and fetal heart rate during maternal orgasm. *Obstet. Gynecol.* 39:125, 1972.)

tinual, they create the fetal impression of a "bad womb" with lasting effects.

## MATERNAL PROBLEMS WITH SEXUAL ACTIVITY

During normal pregnancy there are at least five possible maternal problems related to sexual activity during the third trimester of pregnancy. These include: (1) the possible uterine contractile effects of semen prostaglandin introduced into the vagina; (2) the related maternal systemic effects associated with orgasm (elevated prostaglandins, oxytocin, prolactin, etc.); (3) the possibilities of vaginal and cervical infections being exacerbated following general or local sexual stimulation introducing amniotic fluid infection or bacterial production of prostaglandin; (4) the possibility of transmitting venereal disease such as herpes simplex, gonorrhea, or the like; and (5) the associated maternal problems associated with trauma such as vaginal lacerations or air embolism.

**Vaginal Introduction to Prostaglandins.** There has been speculation that semen prostaglandins may induce sufficient uterine activity so as to initiate labor. Several reviews have independently concluded that, given the amounts of prostaglandin found in semen, semen prostaglandins by themselves are insufficient to initiate uterine activity sufficient for labor in normal pregnancy (Fox et al., 1970; Goodlin, 1980; Naeye, 1979; Nuckolls et al., 1972).

**Maternal Orgasm.** Orgasm was shown by our studies to evoke powerful uterine contractions in some pregnant women who were near term. Many pregnant women agree that orgasm does elicit strong uterine contractions, and old wives tales suggest that orgasm or breast stimulation can be a technique for inducing labor. Maternal blood levels of oxytocin, prostaglandin, prolactin, and catecholamines are elevated during or after orgasm.

Using a photoelectric plethysmographic probe placed in the lateral fornix of the vagina of pregnant women, we found that during uterine contractions a significant decrease in vaginal apex blood flow was initiated by maternal orgasm (Goodlin, 1979). Since the apex of the vagina has the same blood supply as the uterus, we reasoned that during maternal orgasm, uterine blood flow may be diminished. This observation offered an explanation for the apparent association between fetal bradycardia and/or abruptio placenta associated with uterine activity that was evoked by maternal orgasm.

The above considerations should be considered mostly theoretical, yet there are a few objective observations concerning the detrimental effects of sexual activity.

In our study, we found that there was a higher incidence of premature labor and premature rupture of membranes associated with vaginal coitus and orgasm (Goodlin, 1979). Others have failed to substantiate this finding (Table 17-1). In particular, Rayburn and Wilson (1980) studied the coital activity of pregnant women who delivered prematurely. They were compared with a subsequent number who did not. However, these investigators conclude that coital activity in the group delivering prematurely was significantly greater only when there was no obvious reason for premature labor. Rayburn and Wilson (1980) suggest that in most cases normal coital activity does not result in premature delivery and should not be discouraged during pregnancy in the absence of complications. A similar conclusion concerning sexual activity during pregnancy had been reached previously by Perkins (1979). He found that orgasmic pregnant women actually had a lower percentage of premature deliveries than those without orgasm. Perkins observed that in the absence of adequate sexual satisfaction and the presence of a need, patients were more predisposed to premature labor than those who engaged in regular satisfying sexual relationships (Naeye, 1979). Naeye, in several publications, demonstrated that among high-risk pregnant women, maternal coitus is associated with antenatal hemorrhage independent of other factors that predispose to third trimester bleeding (Naeye, 1979, 1980, 1981; Naeye and Peters, 1978; Naeye and Ross, 1982).

TABLE 17-1 **The Change in Attitude Regarding Possible Deleterious Effects of Maternal Coitus/Orgasm during Pregnancy**

| Investigator | Year | Finding |
| --- | --- | --- |
| Taussig | 1936 | Causes uterine contractions |
| Pugh and Fernandez | 1936 | No deleterious effects |
| Javert | 1957 | Increased spontaneous abortion rate |
| Fox, Wolff, and Baker | 1971 | Causes uterine contractions |
| Goodlin, Keller, and Raffin | 1971 | Increased premature labor |
| Solberg, Butler, and Wagner | 1973 | Decreased occurrence during pregnancy, no detrimental effects |
| Wagner, Butler, and Sanders | 1976 | Increased orgasm associated with premature labor |
| Perkins | 1979 | No deleterious effects of sexual activity |
| Grudzinskas, Watson, and Chard | 1979 | No deleterious fetal effects |
| Naeye | 1979 | Coitus associated with decidual chorioamnionitis |
| Naeye | 1980 | Perinatal mortality rate associated with frequency of coitus |
| Rayburn and Wilson | 1980 | Coital activity should not be discouraged |
| Naeye | 1981 | Recent coitus increased antepartum hemorrhage |
| Naeye and Ross | 1981 | Premature labor increased 4 times with recent coitus. Spontaneous rupture of membranes increased after coitus |
| Mills, Harlap, and Harley | 1981 | Coitus in late pregnancy not harmful |
| Reamy, White, Daniell, and LeVine | 1982 | Guidance should be provided for satisfactory coitus |
| Zlatnik and Burmeister | 1982 | Coitus not deleterious |

**Chorioamnionitis and/or Cervicitis.** Naeye (Naeye, 1979; Naeye and Ross, 1982) also showed a strong association between coitus and decidual chorioamnionitis. Bejar and colleagues (1981) in addition have demonstrated that cervical and vaginal bacteria produced considerable prostaglandins. They suggested that coitus may initiate a cervicitis which results in production of increased prostaglandins. Others have noted that patients with heavily infected cervices are more likely to go into premature labor, especially if maternal coitus and/or orgasm are common (Naeye and Ross, 1982; VandenBerg and Yerushalmy, 1966).

**Venereal Disease.** The relationship of coitus to venereal disease is obvious. At the present time, there is considerable concern regarding herpes and, indeed, vaginal herpes is one of the more common indications on our service for primary cesarean section. Abstinence does not appear to prevent secondary vaginal herpes.

**Maternal Trauma.** Deleterious maternal effects associated with coitus include vaginal laceration and air embolism. Numerous reports suggest that maternal air embolism, usually the result of sexual foreplay associated with the increased incidence of oral–genital relations (Goodlin, 1979), is a factor in recent causes of maternal mortality.

The argument continues with those challenging Naeye's and Goodlin's observations. After reviewing the records of 10,981 low-risk pregnancies who had been interviewed concerning their sexual activity, Mills and colleagues (1981) concluded that coitus in late pregnancy had no deleterious effects. Perkins in a 1983 "Letter to the Editor" over Naeye's latest report of deleterious effects of orgasm and/or coitus, suggested that "a non-problem had been extensively attributed to a non-disease."

## THE FETAL RESPONSES IN UTERO

When dealing with pregnant women, there are always at least two patients or subjects, the mother and her *in utero* fetus(es). *In utero* fetal responses would be expected to be, in part, dependent upon the fetus's sensory and neurological development. *In utero* human sensory response has been extensively studied, suggesting that birth is only a minor interlude in terms of development of acquired responses. Maternal sexual responses probably modify these milestones of development.

### TASTE

Bradley and Stern (1967) in their studies of human embryos found taste buds at approximately 8 weeks, with hair cells in place from 14 weeks on. They concluded that taste buds are functional at approximately the 14th week of gestation. Fetal swallowing begins as early as 12 weeks, perhaps explaining the older observations that *in utero* fetuses respond to injections of sugar into the amniotic fluid with increased swallowing, or to injections of quinine or citric acid with decreased swallowing or sucking (Chamberlain, 1983). Fetal swallowing is considered a significant source of nutrients for the large fetus, as they swallow more than the small fetus. Whether they are larger because of this *in utero* bulimia or whether larger fetuses swallow more because they are big is unknown. Sir Albert Liley (1972) suggested that *in utero* nutrition could be influenced by induced tranquility or hyperactivity and associated fetal bulimia.

### VISION

Those performing fetoscopy report that from 12 weeks on the human fetus will turn its head away from a bright *in utero* light. Smyth (1965) used a bright extrauterine light to test fetal heart rate responses to external stimuli. Most fetuses have circadian rhythm patterns of fetal activity. Absence of such activity suggests absence of a functioning fetal cerebral cortex or visual system. Lack of circadian activity is also characteristic of the hyperactive fetus who might benefit from maternal tranquility and reduced stress.

### HEARING

Clements (1982, quoted in Chamberlain, 1983) described 4–5 month-old *in utero* human fetuses as being quieted by the playing of certain music and disturbed by others. Goodlin (1979) suggested that hyperactive *in utero* human fetuses could be habituated to high frequency music. Bernard and Sontag (1947) demonstrated that third trimester human fetuses responded to tone stimulation with varying degrees of acceleration of fetal heart rate and body movements.

### NEUROLOGICAL DEVELOPMENT

*In Vitro* **Studies.** The neurological milestones of the human fetus were described extensively by Davenport Hooker (1959) who worked with more than 140 human embryos and fetuses of various gestational ages obtained by hysterotomy performed for therapeutic abortions. Within two minutes of delivery, the specimen was placed in a warm saline bath and stroked gently with a fine hair to test for reactions.

By the 19th week of gestation the first reflex appears, the contralateral (moving away) head flexion. By the 20th week more complex reflexes can be elicited. Swallowing and tongue movements are noted as early as 12 weeks and sucking at 22 weeks. Audible crying occurs between 21–24 weeks of fetal development. The vestibular, gustatory, and auditory reflex circuits first manifest themselves at about 10 weeks (Hooker, 1959).

Sontag and Wallace (1934) demonstrated that 8–10 minutes after the mother finished a cigarette, the fetal heart beat increased as did the beat-to-beat variability. Leiberman and associates with the modification of the Sontag study, showed in 1980 that even before the mother lit her cigarette, the baby's heart beat increased in anticipation of the event. Lieberman (1980) suggested that it was the sympathetic innervation, as well as the mother's catacholamine upsurge, which were responsible for the fetal heart rate's response of anticipation of maternal smoking.

**Real Time *In Utero* Ultrasound Studies.** In general, present-day real time ultrasonic studies confirm Hooker's *in vitro* observation on fetal milestones of motor development. The ultrasonic examination of the human fetus by Ianniruberto and Tajani (1980) showed that at 6–7 weeks of gestation there are smooth vermicular motions of the embryonic body. By 9 weeks there are sudden small spasms of trunk extension. At 12–13 weeks there is rotation of the fetal head and extension of the head and lower limbs while the upper limbs are often extended and brought downward in a flexed motion. At this time the fetal hands are frequently brought to the head and the mouth. After 13–14 weeks the fetus will show a startle response and a creeping or climbing motion representing symmetrical limb movements. At 15 weeks the fetus has coordinated movements with its hands as if exploring the uterine cavity. At 22 weeks it is engaging in regular breathing activity and its legs often move in a scissoring fashion. Thus, there are definite milestones in fetal neurological and muscular development that enable the observer to place the fetus at a retarded, normal, or advanced level of neurological development.

The ultrasound also shows that the fetus, in addition to these evoked reflexes, usually floats peacefully in the amniotic fluid from 12–24 weeks of gestation and occasionally kicks, hiccups, sighs, urinates, swallows, and breathes amniotic fluid as well as sucks its thumbs, fingers, and toes, and grabs its umbilicus. It appears to become calm when the mother talks quietly, but moves rapidly when strangers or loud noises are present (Chamberlain, 1983).

Milani-Comparetti (1981) has demonstrated from real time ultrasonic studies that the fetus has definite *in utero* patterns such as fetal locomotion, fetal propulsion, and what he terms "competence for survival," which includes the Moro reaction. He believes that the fetus develops other abilities called "emerging competence" that prepare it for extrauterine life. He considers that each fetus through its activities gives *in utero* suggestions as to its future development. These indications may have prognostic value, but only if one is able to recognize the features of the normal fetal developmental process. For example, when the mother is emotionally disturbed, both Ianniruberto and Tajani (1981) and Milani-Comparetti (1981) describe her fetus as often having a phase of hyperkinesia, then a phase of akinesia, followed by recovery to normal motor activity. During times of stress, which include maternal emotional upsets as well as maternal hypoxia, these researchers further described regression in fetal motor behavior to stages behind that considered normal for gestational age. These authors describe various "regression" syndromes of earlier fetal motor patterns which, in their experience, was correlated with cerebral dysfunction after birth. These Italian investigators also believe that observation of fetal movements may suggest harmful *in utero* conditions such as those associated with maternal drug consumption, emotional stress, sexual relations, or illness.

**Rapid Eye Movements as Seen with Ultrasound.** According to Birnholz (1981), the fetal eyes begin to move sporadically at 16 weeks gestation. They become more brisk between 20 and 24 weeks, and after the 24th week there is the pattern of three or more darting movements. Between weeks 25–35, episodes of rapid eye movements increase and nystagmoid rapid eye movements become more frequent. Along with fetal breathing activity, which is usually seen on ultrasound, the fetus's rapid eye movements provide an indication of fetal state. It has been observed that as a mother has rapid eye movements, so does the fetus, suggesting that a substance involved is transported across the placenta. At any rate, the mother's emotions and activities do influence the fetus's state in many ways. Whether these *in utero* "states" have lasting effects is the argument (Goodlin, 1979).

## FETAL PERSONALITY

In 1972, Sir Albert Liley, who introduced *in utero* fetal transfusions, asked in an editorial whether the fetus had a personality: He answered with a qualified "yes." Freud (1926) believed that the fetus was born with an ego and id which reflected development of an *in utero* fetal personality. In 1981, Mancia reviewed the psychoanalytic literature on the beginning of mental life for the human fetus. He paid particular attention to the motor function present in the fetus and fetal stages in development as well as the development of sensory functions. He further analyzed the integrative central nervous system (CNS) functions of the human fetus as illustrated by the stages of active sleep with rapid eye movements. Mancia concluded that active fetal sleep constitutes a biological framework within which the sensory experiences coming through the mother are transformed into "internal representations." Mancia further suggested that this fetal activity constitutes the beginning of fetal protomental activity that builds itself around a nucleus of material transmitted genetically from the parents. The role of active fetal sleep in the maturation of psychological function is in the development of the "skin," which in turn may be able to contain the Self of the fetus. The fetal skin may protect the Self from disintegration under the pressures of impulses that arise from maternal stress and at the moment of birth (Mancia, 1981). For those who believe in the *in utero* personality, the fetal period is important in development of the individual (Feher, 1980). An adverse *in utero* experience due to maternal stress can have major implications.

Ellis (1940) has described how more than ten centuries ago, the Chinese had "prenatal clinic," not for the purposes of dispensing vitamins, but to attempt to ensure maternal tranquility for its presumed benefits for the fetus. Stott (1977) has recommended that society should assure women an undisturbed pregnancy. He found from a study in Glasgow, Scotland, that the majority of women who had suffered from interpersonal tension during their pregnancies had "unhealthy" children.

## FETAL LEARNING *IN UTERO* AND SEXUAL ACTIVITY

Since the advent of electronic fetal monitoring, it has been noted that fetal heart rate accelerations are associated with fetal movement. Lauersen and Hochberg (1982) claim that the fetal heart rate acceleration begins before the fetal movements which, to them, suggests that the fetus is contemplating its movement before the action. They also suggest that this movement constitutes some sort of fetal thought and planning. Leader and colleagues (1982) have ascribed fetal habituation to external stimuli. These researchers claim that habituation is a basic form of learning and probably requires an intact central nervous system. They found that high-risk fetuses had significant differences in their habituation pattern when compared with fetuses of normal pregnancies. While they suggested studies of fetal habituation to vibration or sound as a means of monitoring fetal health, their findings also suggest that maternal high-risk conditions affect the fetal thought processes. Similarly, maternal sexual activity may produce habituation *in utero,* while the psychoanalytic literature suggests imprinting of untoward fetal events associated with maternal orgasm and uterine activity (Mancia, 1981). Limner (1970) suggests that maternal sexual activity has a lasting deleterious effect on the developing fetus, both from a physiological standpoint and a psychological one.

## MATERNAL BONDING WITH THE FETUS

A woman's appreciation of fetal movements frequently results in significant bonding with her unborn fetus. Since the advent of the ultrasound, both the Doppler apparatus, which allows the parents the ability to hear the fetus' heart beat, and the real time ultrasonic scanner, which provides observation of fetal movements, have increased maternal and paternal bonding to the *in utero* fetus. A recent study by Fletcher and Evans (1983) suggested that when the mother views the ultrasound image in early pregnancy, she immediately begins to bond with her fetus. This, of course, can have untoward maternal effects if the fetus is abnormal, but in general is a very positive event in the development of parental bonding. Braslow (1983) showed that there was increased compliance with obstetric care when the mother views the ultrasonic image in early pregnancy.

In the discussion of the relationship of parents with their unborn, Cranley (1981) noted that many high-risk pregnant women derive a keener sense of bonding to the fetus from the various kinds of antenatal fetal assessment studies. When performing these studies, both the nurses and the mother often "talk" to the fetus and request that it "be still" or "move" which may well enhance perception of a real person within the uterus. This sort of maternal attachment, of course, is further enhanced by viewing the fetus on real time ultrasound.

After bonding with their fetus, the prospective parents are more prone to express added concern about the fetus's welfare, particularly if the mother is ill, takes drugs, or is under added stress. In our experience with development of significant fetal bonding, the couples often report decreased interest in sexual activity (Goodlin, 1979, 1984). When asked *why* these couples commonly used terms similar to those used by Stanislav Grof (womb life is either harmonious or threatening; 1976) that maternal sexual activity might well disrupt their fetus's blissful *in utero* life. Much of these same paternal concerns are expressed during amniocentesis, drug usage, and during labor. Indeed, it is common to have prospective parents wonder if cesarean section without labor is preferred in order to avoid birth pain and untoward feelings as described by Janov's primal therapy concepts (1970). In high-risk pregnancies, these parental concerns about the fetal personality are often increased. On the other hand, one occasionally is forced to deal with the high-risk patient who very much resents that she is forced to be "an incubator" for her unwanted fetus. In our experiences, such pregnancies are filled with hostility and often increased sexual activity.

## FETAL PSYCHOLOGICAL PROBLEMS ASSOCIATED WITH BIRTH

If the beliefs of advocates of maximum obstetrical interferences as well as the psychologist's concern about the pain of birth are valid, it should be possible to demonstrate the subsequent benefits of elective cesarean section (without labor) on a child's development. Surprisingly, studies completed when cesarean section rates were less than 2 percent (instead of today's greater than 20 percent) show that the first born is more likely to be the greatest achiever and with no increase in maldevelopment (Goodlin, 1979). This is an important consideration, as the first born's labor is almost always longer and presumably more stressful than his or her sibling's. Given todays high birth rate by elective cesarean section, it should soon be possible to compare the sufferers (vaginal birth) with those with atraumatic birth (delivered without labor).

## PROBLEMS WITH RECOMMENDING SEXUAL ABSTINENCE

Maternal orgasm itself may be deleterious to the fetus's welfare and, therefore, the pregnant woman should perhaps be warned against any sexual activities if they lead to orgasm. To a large degree, however, the problems of such recommended abstinence during pregnancy is culturally determined. Many Asian and Central American cultures believe that coitus is deleterious during pregnancy. On the other hand, North Americans, who have their sexual activities restricted because they follow natural birth control methods, view pregnancy as an opportunity for frequent sexual relations. Whenever abstinence is recommended, the health practitioner should discuss the situation thoroughly both with the pregnant woman and her partner. Recommended abstinence has caused many a faithful lover or husband to establish sexual contacts elsewhere, sometimes for the first time. Perkins (1979) has suggested, and others have referred to the concept, that heightened sexual needs may, in themselves, be deleterious to the pregnant woman if she is not allowed "relief" during her pregnancy. Pregnant women attempting abstinence may still "dream orgasm" with apparently the same physiologic responses as during the actual event (Nuckolls et al., 1972). Given the importance of sexual activity to some couples, it may be reasonable that abstinence is more deleterious to the pregnancy outcome than is sexual activity.

An important attribute of normal pregnancy is tranquility and relaxation. Normal pregnancy outcome is associated with normal plasma volume expansion and, indeed, most women with pregnancy complications have, for one reason or another, failed to expand their plasma volumes. Therapy for plasma volume expansion is very limited, except for the recommendation of the recumbent lateral position for prolonged periods of time, relaxation, and the achievement of tranquility. It has been demonstrated that individuals who can relax can lower their hematocrit 10 to 15 percent over an 8-hour period. Pregnant women likewise lower their hematocrits when they are relaxed and tranquil because of the associated vascular relaxation and the mobilization of extravascular fluids. Under these circumstances, anything that increases stress, such as unfulfilled sexual gratification, could reduce plasma volume (Goodlin, 1984).

## HIGH-RISK PREGNANCY

Clinical investigators of sexual activity and/or orgasm during pregnancy uniformly caution that high-risk pregnant women should abstain from sexual activity, especially during the last trimester (Goodlin, 1979, 1984; Limner, 1970; Masters and Johnson, 1966; Naeye, 1979, 1980; Nuckolls et al., 1972; Reamy et al., 1982; Solberg et al., 1973; Wagner et al., 1976; Zlatnik and Burmeister, 1982). Apparently no debate exists on this issue. In all our high-risk pregnant women, cervical examinations are done at each visit starting at approximately the middle of the second trimester. If there appears to be any cervical dilatation greater than 2 cm, particularly if the woman has had a past history of premature labor, she is asked to abstain from sex relations and/or orgasm (Goodlin, 1979, 1980). Since there is an apparent association between severe cervicitis and amniotic fluid infection syndrome, we also attempt to eradicate any cervicitis in these high-risk pregnant women.

We do not question extensively concerning sexual activity "after the fact" of pregnancy complications as this often leads to guilt in both the patient and her partner. However, it occurs with sufficient frequency that we continue to recommend abstinence in all but low-risk gravidas. In women who deliver prematurely or who have abruptio placenta, we continue to find a high incidence of apparent association with sexual relations and/or orgasm.

CASE HISTORY

A 33-year-old gravida had one premature infant who survived, then three early, spontaneous miscarriages, and then a fourth midtrimester spontaneous abortion who did not survive. A hysterogram in the interval between pregnancies had been normal and the patient's last two pregnancies had been unsuccessfully treated with cervical cerclage. Upon questioning, the patient related that she had experienced frequent postcoital orgasm with her past pregnancies, but that her obstetrician had suggested that "sex" was not harmful. During the current pregnancy, she was given the standard care for prevention of premature labor which included increased bed rest, forced fluids, and abstinence. The patient said that she avoided orgasm from the 18–28th week, but then she claimed to have "dreamed" an orgasm which was followed by coitus which was followed by further orgasm. Within a 30-minute interval, the patient began having painful uterine contractions that we were unable to inhibit with tocolysis, and two days later she delivered an 820 g male infant who survived.

**Recommendations to High-Risk Pregnant Women Concerning Sexual Relations.** Try to explain to patients what the relative risks of coitus are, including the possibility that many pregnant women have postorgasmic pelvic discomfort. Such a discomfort is sometimes diagnosed as "round ligament pain" or as weakened joints or pelvic congestion syndrome. Whether this sort of discomfort reflects orgasm or the lack of orgasm with sexual activity is unknown. At any rate, true abstinence can have its value to the pregnant woman. In the event that the pregnant woman has a poor obstetric history and a strong orgasmic response and continues to have vaginal coitus, recommend the use of vaginal antibacterial suppositories precoitus. One of the problems related to cervical infection and the deciduitis or chorioamniotis, is amniotic fluid infection syndrome arising from orgasmically induced uterine contractions. Try to explain to the couples that orgasm is a natural function and that its occurrence is sometimes not under the couple's absolute control. The last thing a physician wishes to do is to increase the anxiety level of the pregnant patient, especially the high-risk one.

### Suggestions Concerning Maternal Support of In Utero Development

Considerable scientific literature exists outside the usual medical journals that indicates that maternal attitudes do affect fetal development and that fetuses can be habituated to various *in utero* stimuli, such as sounds or light, and that stressful maternal environments have an adverse effect on fetal development (Leader *et al.*, 1982; Mancia, 1981). The latter can be demonstrated especially in rodents (Chamberlain, 1983). At the same time, however, studies of pregnancies and children from women who had opted for therapeutic abortions, but for one reason or another did not obtain one and instead carried the pregnancy to viability, have failed to indicate any adverse effects of such a hostile maternal attitude. In other words, while there is literature that supports the positive effects of parental support for *in utero* development through the assurance of maternal tranquility, no evidence suggests that when there is particular maternal stress, the pregnancy will necessarily be adversely affected in a particular manner. Given this type of information, the usual advice to pregnant women is to be as tranquil as possible.

Several studies (Grof, 1976; Janov, 1970) have suggested that anxiety or stress may increase the incidence of toxemia, forceps delivery, and fetal distress. Those clinics with techniques for measuring anxiety levels in pregnancy may wish to identify those gravidas at risk and attempt to determine what are the contributing emotional factors. It is possible that these anxious pregnant women and their fetuses may benefit from special supportive care or management during the antenatal period. It is probable that much of the benefits of antenatal care come from generalized supportive care from the clinic personnel, even without special tests or diagnostic procedures, rather than the performance of complicated fetal heart rate analysis and ultrasonic examination.

## PSYCHOSOMATIC ASPECTS OF THE PERIPARTUM PERIOD

Rosenberg and Darby (in press) found that in the month prior to the onset of labor, positive maternal emotions are at a low level and negative emotions are at a peak. Shortly after her child's birth, however, a woman's positive emotions reach their highest level and negative emotions are at their lowest. For two to three months postpartum, these extremes in emotions are moderated considerably, with many women having long periods of low emotional feelings. The ratio of positive to negative emotions is influenced to a large extent by availability of family support and whether the women were primigravidas, as the presence of a new baby is considerably more stressful than if mothers and families already had children (Nuckoll, et al., 1972).

Nisbett and Ross (1980) suggested that a new mother's positive emotional state at the time when she first encounters her newborn, predisposes her to interpret her infant in a positive light, and such feelings are important for the foundation of future positive exchanges between mother and newborn. Robson and Kumar (1980) also report that mothers who had had difficult deliveries or who were heavily medicated were more likely to respond to their infants with initial indifference. While further studies are required, it would appear that "optimal" deliveries are associated with very positive maternal feelings in the postpartum period and positive maternal infant bonding (Goodlin, 1980). What constitutes "an optimal" delivery is uncertain, but family support, maternal age and parity, circumstances of delivery, and prenatal preparation for labor and the newborn all are factors in determining the degree of the new mother's positive feelings in the immediate postpartum period. We found that the presence of the labor room nurses in the prenatal clinics contributed to a positive family experience with birthing. Indeed, our study suggested that knowing their labor room or birthing nurse was more reassuring to most pregnant women than knowing their obstetrician prior to onset of labor.

Kimball and coworkers (1981) have shown that, in part, these "positive feelings" are related to the new mothers' endorphin levels and such positive feelings may be at least blunted by the use of Narcan (naloxone). Since endorphins are natural opiates, it is interesting that they increase the positive maternal feelings, whereas exogenous opiates, such as morphine or meperidine hydrochloride, apparently decrease maternal positive feelings. An interesting study would be the use of opiates in mothers in the postpartum period who are exhibiting negative feelings. It is a common experience that women who are enduring considerable postpartum pain are more likely to have negative feelings about their newborn than those who are without significant pain or discomfort. Considerably more research on how to bring about the maximum positive feelings on the part of the new mother is required.

## CONCLUSION

A recent tendency has been to direct our obstetrical efforts toward the development of high-tech procedures for detection and treatment of high-risk pregnancies. The available studies suggest that the psychosomatic factors influence all pregnant women and their fetuses (Nuckolls et al., 1972), not just high-risk ones. While a consistent pattern has not yet emerged, several studies indicate that development of improved skills and research techniques in psychosomatic aspects would benefit all pregnancies, providing a much higher benefits to cost ratio than could be achieved through improved technology (Goodlin, 1979).

## REFERENCES

Bejar, R.; Curgello, V.; Davis, C.; and Gluck, L.: Premature labor. II: Bacterial sources of phosphotipase. Obstet. Gynecol., 57:479, 1981.

Bernard, J., and Sontag, L. W.: Fetal reactivity to tonal stimulation. J. Gen. Psych., 70:205, 1947.

Birnholtz, J. The development of human fetal eye movement patterns. Science, 213:679, 1981.

Bradley, R. M., and Stern, L. B.: The development of the human taste bud during the foetal period. J. Anat., 101:743, 1967.

Braslow, L.: To the Editor. N. Engl. J. Med., 303:114, 1983

Chamberlain. D. B.: Consciousness at birth: A review of the empirical evidence. Chamberlain Publication, San Diego, Calif., 1983.

Clements, M.: Observations on certain aspects of neonatal behavior response to auditory stimuli. I: quoted by Chamberlain D. B., Consciousness at birth. Chamberlain Publications, San Diego, Calif., 1982.

Cranley, M. S.: Roots of attachment: The relationship of parents with their unborn. *Birth Defects Original Article Series,* 18:59, 1981.

Dubos, R.: *Man Adapting.* Yale University Press, New Haven, 1965.

Ellis, H.: *Studies in the Psychology of Sex.* Random House, New York, 1940.

Feher, L.: *Psychology of Birth.* Souvenir Press, London, 1980.

Fletcher, J. C., and Evans, M. I.: Maternal bonding in early fetal ultrasound examinations. *N. Engl. J. Med.,* 308:392, 1983.

Fox, C. A.; Wolff, H. S.; and Baker, J. A.: Measurement of intra-vaginal and intra-uterine pressures during human coitus by radio-telemetry. *J. Reprod. Fertil.,* 22:243, 1970.

Goodlin, R. C.: *Care of the Fetus.* Masson Publishing USA, Inc., New York, 1979.

Goodlin, R. C.: Low risk obstetric care for low risk mothers. *Lancet,* 1:1017, 1980.

Goodlin, R. C.: *Orgasm and Coitus in Pregnancy: Possible Deleterious Effects.* Edizione Libreria, Verona, Italy, 1984.

Goodlin, R. C.; Keller, D. W.; and Raffin, M.: Orgasmic response during pregnancy: Its possible deleterious effects. *Obstet. Gynecol.,* 38:916, 1971.

Goodlin, R. C.; Schmidt, W.; and Creevy, D. C.: Uterine tension and fetal heart rate during maternal orgasm. *Obstet. Gynecol.,* 39:125, 1972.

Grof, S. *Realms of Human Unconscious.* Dutton, New York, 1976.

Grudzinskas, J. G.; Watson, C.; and Chard, T.: Does sexual intercourse cause fetal distress? *Lancet,* 2:692, 1979.

Hooker, D.: *The Prenatal Origin of Behavior.* University of Kansas Press, Lawrence, 1959.

Ianniruberto, A., and Tajani, E.: Ultrasonographic study of fetal movements. *Semin. Perinatol.,* 5:175, 1981.

Javert, C. T.: *Spontaneous and habitual abortion* McGraw-Hill, New York, 1957.

Janov, A. *The Primal Scream: Primal Therapy the Cure for Neurosis.* Putnam, New York 1970.

Kimball, C. D.; Chang, C. M.; Haung, S. M.; and Houch, C.: Endorphin peptides in umbilical vein and maternal blood. *Am. J. Obstet. Gynecol.,* 140:157, 1981.

Lauersen, N. H., and Hochberg, H. M.: Letter to the Editor. *JAMA,* 247:3185, 1982.

Leader, L. R.; Baillie, P.; Martin, B.; and Vermeuler, E.: Fetal habituation in high-risk pregnancies. *Br. J. Obstet. Gynaecol.,* 89:441, 1982.

Lieberman, A.: Smoking for two: cigarettes and pregnancy. In Fried, P. A., and Oxora, H.: (eds.): *Fetal Well Being.* Free Press, New York, 1980.

Liley, A. W.: The foetus as a personality. *Aust. NZ. J. Psychiatry,* 6:99, 1972.

Limner, R.: *Sex and the Unborn Child.* Julian Press, New York, 1970.

Mancia, M.: On the beginning of mental life in the foetus. *Int. J. Psychoanal.,* 62:351, 1981.

Masters, W. H., and Johnson, V. E.: *Human Sexual Response.* Little, Brown, Boston, 1966.

Milani-Comparetti, A.: The neurophysiologic and clinical implications of studies on fetal motor behavior. *Semin. Perinatol.,* 5:183, 1981.

Mills, J. L.; Harlap, S., and Harley, E. E.: Should coitus late in pregnancy be discouraged. *Lancet,* 2:136, 1981.

Naeye, R. L.: Coitus and associated amniotic fluid infection. *N. Engl. J. Med.,* 301:1198, 1979.

Naeye, R. L.: Seasonal variation in coitus and other risk factors, and the outcome of pregnancy. *Early Hum. Dev.,* 4:61, 1980.

Naeye, R. L.: Coitus and antepartum haemorrhage. *Br. J. Obstet. Gynaecol.,* 88:765, 1981.

Naeye, R. L., and Peters, E. C.: Amniotic fluid infections with intact membranes leading to perinatal death. *Pediatrics,* 61:171, 1978.

Naeye, R. L., and Ross, S.: Coitus and chorioamnionitis. *Early Hum. Dev.,* 6:91, 1982.

Nisbett, R., and Ross, L.: *Human Inference Strategies and Shortcomings of Social Judgment.* Prentice-Hall, Englewood Cliffs, N.J., 1980.

Nuckolls, K. B.; Cassel, J.; and Kaplan, B. H.: Psychosocial assets, life crisis and the prognosis of pregnancy. *Am. J. Epidemiol.,* 95:431, 1972.

Perkins, R. P.: Sexual behavior and response in relation to complication of pregnancy. *Am. J. Obstet. Gynecol.* 134:498, 1979.

Perkins, R. P.: Letter to the editor. *Am. J. Obstet. Gynecol.,* 62:399, 1983.

Pugh, W. E., and Fernandez, F. L.: Coitus in late pregnancy. *Obstet. Gynecol.,* 2:636, 1953.

Rank, O.: *The Trauma of Birth.* New York, Richard Brummen, 1952.

Rayburn, W. F., and Wilson, E. A.: Coital activity and premature delivery. *Am. J. Obstet. Gynecol.,* 137:972, 1980.

Reamy, K.; White, S.; Daniell, W.; and LeVine, E.: Sexuality and Pregnancy. *J. Reprod. Med.,* 27:321, 1982.

Robson, K., and Kumar, R.: Delayed onset of maternal affection after childbirth. *Br. J. Psychiatry,* 136:347, 1980.

Rosenberg, J., and Darby, K.: Responses to pregnancy and delivery (in press).

Smyth, E. N.: Exploratory methods for testing the integrity of the foetus and the neonate. *Br. J. Obstet. Gynaecol.,* 72:920, 1965.

Solberg, D. A.; Butler, J., and Wagner, N. N.: Sexual behavior in pregnancy. *N. Engl. J. Med.,* 288:1098, 1973.

Sontag, L., and Wallace, R. F.: Preliminary report of the Fels Fund. *Am. J. Dis. Child.,* 48:1050, 1934.

Stott, D. H.: Maternal anxiety. *New Society,* 19:329, 1977.

Talbert, D. G.; Benson, P.; and Dewhurst, J.: Fetal response to maternal anxiety: a factor in antepartum heart rate monitoring. *J. Obstet. Gynecol.,* 3:34, 1982.

Taussig, F. J.: *Abortions—spontaneous and induced. Medical and Social Aspects.* H. Kimpton, London, 1936.

Vandenberg, B. J., and Yerushalmy, J.: The relationship of the rate of intrauterine growth of infants of low birth weight to mortality, morbidity and congenital anomalies. *J. Pediatr.,* 69:531, 1966.

Wagner, N. N.; Butler, J. C.; Saunders, J. P.: Prematurity and orgasmic coitus during pregnancy: data on a small sample. *Fertil. Steril.,* 27:911, 1976.

Zlatnik, F. J., and Burmeister, L. F.: Reported sexual behavior in late pregnancy. *J. Reprod. Med.,* 27:627, 1982.

# CHAPTER 18 THE PUERPERIUM

*Ruth York, Ph.D., R.N., Jane Berry, M.S.N., R.N., and Steven G. Gabbe, M.D.*

## INTRODUCTION

Pregnancy and childbirth are usually anticipated by the mother-to-be as positive physiological and psychological events. However, the new baby's presence may represent a reality much different from maternal expectations. This difference may result in mood changes, depression, and, rarely, in postpartum psychosis. Should the pregnancy fail, the resulting grief response must be understood and skillfully managed if serious psychologic consequences are to be prevented.

## MOOD DISTURBANCE IN THE PUERPERIUM

Puerperal mood disturbances were first described by Hippocrates. He speculated that suppressed lochial discharge was carried to the head, resulting in agitation, delirium, and attacks of mania (Steiner, 1979). Contemporary medical literature discusses hormonal and psychosocial causes of postpartum mood disturbances. However, no evidence relating social factors (Cox et al., 1982) or hormonal factors (Nott et al., 1976) to puerperal mood disturbances has been conclusive.

Although only 10 percent of women have postpartum depression severe enough to require treatment (Pitt, 1968), it has been estimated that as many as 50 to 80 percent of new mothers experience transitory but identifiable levels of depression or lability of mood (Kendell et al., 1981; Pitt, 1968; Tod, 1964; Yalom et al., 1968) which generally improve by the tenth postpartum day (Cox et al., 1982; Vandenberg, 1980). While this depression is relatively brief, its common occurrence and disruptive consequences constitute a problem for the mother of a new infant and her family. Although these women are depressed because they feel unable to cope with their new responsibilities, they rarely report such depression to their physician (Clarke, 1979; Cox et al., 1982; Vandenberg, 1980). At times, their depressive moods are denied, since by societal standards, childbirth is considered a joyous occasion. As a result of their denial, patients fail to learn new coping skills (Lesh, 1978). Depression in the early puerperal period, though transient, can also identify those women who are at-risk for prolonged depression (Cox et al., 1982).

Psychological reactions to childbirth have been classified by several investigators into three types: transitory depression ("blues"), puerperal depression, and puerperal psychosis.

*Transitory depression* has an early onset; it occurs in the first few days after delivery and lasts for approximately ten days (Cox et al., 1982; Nott et al., 1976; Vandenberg, 1980). Its symptoms include mild depression, anxiety, minimal intellectual clouding, despondency, poor concentration, and forgetfulness (Howells, 1972; Pitt, 1975). Transitory depression, although considered short-lived, is not easily differentiated from other depressed moods (Handley et al., 1980).

*Puerperal depression,* on the other hand, has a delayed onset or may follow a transitory depression. The symptoms of postpartum depression are more severe than those of transitory depression and may persist for several weeks or months (Howells, 1972; Pitt, 1975). Symptoms include moderate depression, anxiety, irritability, insomnia, loss of libido, concern for the child's health, feelings of inadequacy and inability to cope with the infant (Kendell et al., 1981). Puerperal depression may be an extension of transitory depression (Cox et al., 1982; Playfair and Gowers, 1981) or it may occur as a separate entity characterized by its later onset and longer duration.

*Puerperal psychosis,* which occurs in approximately three women per 1000, delivered is marked by episodes of extreme depression or elation. It may last a year or more and may require hospitalization. Puerperal psychosis has its onset in the third to the sixth postpartum day, reaching a peak in the first puerperal month. The following symptoms may occur: hallucinations involving all sensory modalities; delusions; distorted thought processes involving preoccupation with death, mutilation, and other imaginary dangers; altered perceptions of reality; distorted interrelationships exhibiting extreme dependency and a demanding attitude upon those close to the woman (Kaij and Nilsson, 1972). Approximately half of the women who experience postpartum psychosis will subsequently manifest another serious mental disorder.

Although women who experience puerperal mood disturbances are not prone to depression at other times in their lives (Dalton, 1971; Jansson, 1964; Pitt, 1975; Reich and Winokur, 1970), women with a history of depression are predisposed to a 10 to 40 percent incidence of postpartum depression (Bratfos and Haug, 1966; Playfair and Gowers, 1981; Reich and Winokurm, 1970; Tentoni and High, 1980). Moreover, a woman who experienced puerperal depression is very likely to experience depression with subsequent births (Braverman and Roux, 1978). While the causes of puerperal mood changes in women have been widely explored, the etiology of puerperal mood disturbances in men have received little attention. Since there is some evidence that men as well as women experience mood disturbances after childbirth, both spouses will be discussed in this chapter. In addition to reviewing physiological factors that may influence maternal mood disturbances, the possible relationship of psychosocial events to puerperal mood disturbances for both men and women will be examined. Interventions that may help a couple cope and understand their emotions will also be described.

PHYSIOLOGICAL FACTORS

Many emotionally labile periods occur during a woman's life that suggest a relationship between hormonal levels and mood changes. There is a concurrence of mood changes and alterations in hormonal levels premenstrually, during the menopause, and in association with the use of oral contraceptives. Hormones such as estrogen and progesterone return to prepregnancy levels six to eight days after delivery. The greatest drop occurs during the first three puerperal days, a time when a combination of psychosocial factors also surface. The continuous demands of the new baby will cause anxiety and fatigue. Early puerperal mood changes produce additional anxiety, stressing the new mother and draining her of energy needed to deal with her child.

Hormonal changes may contribute to transitory depression (Table 18–1). The stresses of parturition produce significant increases in maternal cortisol levels, which fall rapidly after delivery and return to normal within three days. High levels of cortisol have been correlated with depressive illness (Hullen et al., 1967). An association between elevated cortisol levels at 38 weeks gestation and puerperal transitory depression peaking on the fourth puerperal day (Handley et al., 1980) has also been reported. However, high cortisol levels were thought to be an etiologic factor in re-

TABLE 18-1 **Possible Mediators of Mood Disturbances in the Puerperium**

Cortisol
Estrogen
Progesterone
Catecholamines
Prolactin
Tryptophan
Tyramine

cently delivered women who exhibited mood elevation (Handley et al., 1977).

The relationships of progesterone and estrogen to puerperal mood changes are not clear. However, three hypotheses have been proposed.

1. The level of progesterone before delivery is exceedingly high in women who develop puerperal mood disturbances.
2. The decrease in progesterone may be too rapid in women who develop puerperal mood disturbance.
3. The changes in progesterone and estrogen may produce an abnormal estrogen to progesterone ratio, possibly causing mood changes.

Because progesterone has a tranquilizing effect, it is tempting to implicate its precipitous drop during parturition, the largest change in progesterone in a woman's lifetime, to the early mood changes that occur in the puerperium (Dalton, 1971; Yalom, 1968). To assess the relationship of progesterone and estrogen to puerperal mood changes, Nott and coworkers (1976) measured progesterone and estrogen blood concentrations both before and after delivery. These researchers then compared the levels of the two hormones to an inventory of 30 symptoms of depression in 27 women. Only four symptoms could be significantly correlated with hormonal changes. Specifically, the study showed.

1. Predelivery estrogen blood levels were higher in those women who reported more irritability.
2. Postdelivery estrogen blood levels were lower in women who reported more sleep disturbances.
3. The progesterone drop was greater in women who experienced depression in the first ten puerperal days.
4. The progesterone drop was also greater in new mothers who reported minimal sleep disturbances.

Kuevi noted that lower levels of estrogen and progesterone were always present in women with mood disturbances during the second through the fifth day of the puerperium (Kuevi et al., 1983). It has been suggested that the rapid drop in estrogen after delivery of the placenta may cause puerperal depression. However, the effect of estrogen on transitory depression may well be related to predelivery plasma concentrations. Women who experienced puerperal transitory depression had lower predelivery estrogen blood levels (Nott et al., 1976).

Changes in catecholamine secretion have been related to postpartum mood disturbances. As early as 1969, decreased urinary catecholamine excretion was found to be significantly correlated with the severity of puerperal depression (Treadway et al., 1969). More recently, Kuevi observed decreased plasma levels of norepinephrine and epinephrine on the day transient depression was recorded (Kuevi et al., 1983).

Throughout pregnancy, plasma levels of prolactin increase progressively. Estrogen is thought to block the action of prolactin during pregnancy and prevents the initiation of lactation. Plasma prolactin levels decrease rapidly in women who bottle feed their infants, reaching the prepregnancy range by the third puerperal week. In breast-feeding mothers, however, prolactin levels remain significantly elevated. Furthermore, three days after delivery, at the onset of lactation, prolactin levels are significantly higher in mothers who are breast-feeding when compared to mothers who are bottle feeding. These findings have led to the hypothesis that puerperal depression could be due to increased plasma prolactin. Women who breast-fed only and did not introduce any other food or formula and who most likely had a higher level of prolactin reported more depressive symptoms (Adler and Cox, 1983). George, Copeland, and Wilson (1980) reported evidence of elevated prolactin levels and symptoms of transitory depression such as anxiety, tension, and depression.

Premenstrual syndrome has been associated with many symptoms which have also been observed in transitory depression including anxiety, irritability, crying, and extreme fatigue. Women who experience difficulties in adjusting to the changing hormonal levels demonstrated during the menstrual cycle have a predisposition to depression in the puerperium (Dalton, 1971). Although, the hormonal changes in the early puerperium are more complex and occur more rapidly than those in the luteal phase, the same hormonal mediators may be involved. Depressive illness has been related to a deficiency in plasma free tryptophan (Coppen et al., 1973). Low concentrations of free tryptophan have been found in women with transitory puerperal depression (Handley et al., 1977; Stein et al., 1976). More recently Hanley and colleagues (1980) observed that free tryptophan levels fluctuated seasonally and were reduced in women who experienced transitory depression only at a certain time of year (June–December) when tryptophan levels were normally high.

A decrease in conjugated tyramine may play a role in producing affective disorders. This deficiency persists even after the patient has recovered (Sandler et al., 1980) and may be associated with a vulnerability to subsequent depression. A tyramine loading test could not distinguish between women with depressive moods and a control group during the puerperium. Of note, all women with a history of postpartum depression fell into the low tyramine group (Carter et al., 1980).

After delivery, the fall in circulating estrogen and progesterone can be associated with a fall in platelet $\alpha_2$-adrenoreceptors. However, women who reported an episode of transitory depression had significantly higher platelet $\alpha_2$-adrenoreceptor capacity than women who were not depressed. Such changes in platelet $\alpha_2$-adrenoreceptors may reflect $\alpha_2$-adrenoreceptor capacity in the brain. Although the symptoms of transitory depression occurred four to six days after childbirth, the difference in platelet $\alpha_2$-adrenoreceptor capacity was documented on the seventh to tenth postpartum day. Platelet $\alpha_2$-adrenoreceptor binding capacity of women who did not experience puerperal mood changes returned to normal by day ten. This study suggests that women with higher $\alpha_2$-adrenoreceptor capacity may be predisposed to transitory depression (Metz et al., 1983).

Although the causes of early puerperal mood disturbances have not been conclusively defined, the marked hormonal changes that take place during parturition and the first few puerperal days may play an important role in transitory depression. In addition, the effects of the hormonal changes in the early puerperium may serve as catalysts for other biochemical sequelae, that is, alterations in $\alpha_2$-adrenoreceptor capacity, which then produce depressive reactions. However, it is unlikely that mood disturbances in the puerperium are solely the result of hormonal changes. It is more likely that the biochemical milieu heightens a woman's responses to her new parental role.

## Psychosocial Factors

From the moment a woman discovers she is pregnant and throughout the transition period following delivery she experiences various emotional, as well as physiological, changes. Gradually the realization of the need for an integration of identities occurs. The woman is no longer viewed solely as a wife, daughter, professional, or friend—roles in which she has felt secure, independent, and assertive. While these roles are still maintained, her life will take on new dimensions as the role of mother is initially perceived and later actualized.

A woman anticipates the birth of her child will fulfill her role as an active parent. Most parents form mental images of the child they are expecting—its sex, physical characteristics, temperament, personality development, and life-long accomplishments. If the reality of the child's appearance and temperament falls short of these expectations, disappointment may result. The new mother may envision herself as the loving parent, able to soothe her child's discomforts. In reality, she may be unable to understand why her infant is crying. Spontaneous outflowing of love for the baby may be absent, causing the parent to feel guilt, anxiety, and stress. Mothering is not an instinct, but a major role that must be learned. Thus, maternal feelings may develop considerably later than biological motherhood. New mothers, ill-prepared for the reality of motherhood, have the added trauma of the sudden withdrawal of all assistance from the health care team at discharge from the hospital. However, on returning home with the baby, the woman is expected to resume her life as usual and, in addition, take on the responsibility of the newborn. If a gap exists between her aspirations and her actual capabilities, she may see herself as a failure. As a result, she may experience lowered self-esteem and depression (Lesh, 1978).

The first few months after delivery encompass a period of major hormonal and psychosocial adjustments. This puerperal period is considered by some as a maturational period, a time for adaptation to the mothering role. The smoothness of the transition from pregnancy and biological motherhood to the puerperium and its reality of parenthood depends on maternal role adjustment. This adaptation is dependent on the available support systems, on past life experiences, and on present expectations.

A woman's identification with her new maternal role encompasses a transformation from her predelivery to her postdelivery role attachment and self-identity. Coming home from the hospital, the new mother is primarily concerned with the feeding and comfort of her baby. She soon learns that the care of the baby takes up more of her time than she had anticipated, leaving little time for her spouse and almost none for herself. Figures 18–1 and 18–2 illustrate how one woman viewed the changes in her role and self-identity before and after delivery (Eheart and Martel, 1983). Each of the four circles is divided into sections that represent a major role or a major identity.

How well a woman adapts to the maternal role depends in part on the temperament of the newborn. The baby may be tranquil and easy to comfort or active, responding with crying to intrusions of sounds and movements, or even passive, rarely expressing an emotion (Eheart and Martel, 1983). Most new mothers who experience mood changes in the puerperium will also report that they have crying babies and wakeful nights with their children (Dalton, 1971). The resulting fatigue had its inception during pregnancy with its physical

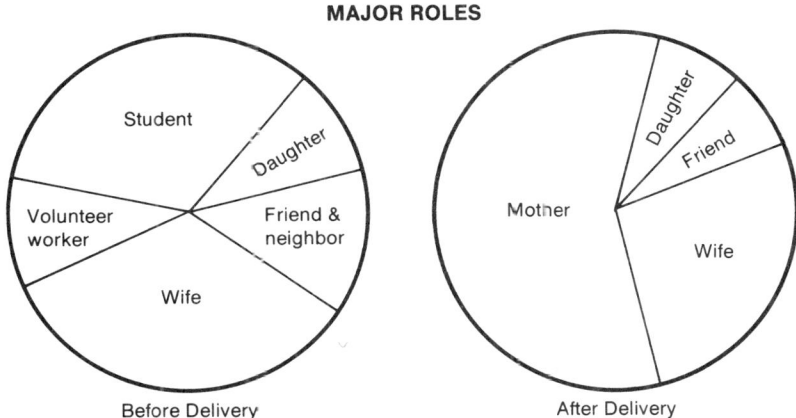

**FIGURE 18–1.** The sections in these circles represent the way one woman may view her various major roles before and after delivery. (Reprinted with permission from Eheart, B. K., and Matrel, S. K.: *The Fourth Trimester: On Becoming a Mother*. Appleton-Century-Crofts, Norwalk, Conn., 1983.)

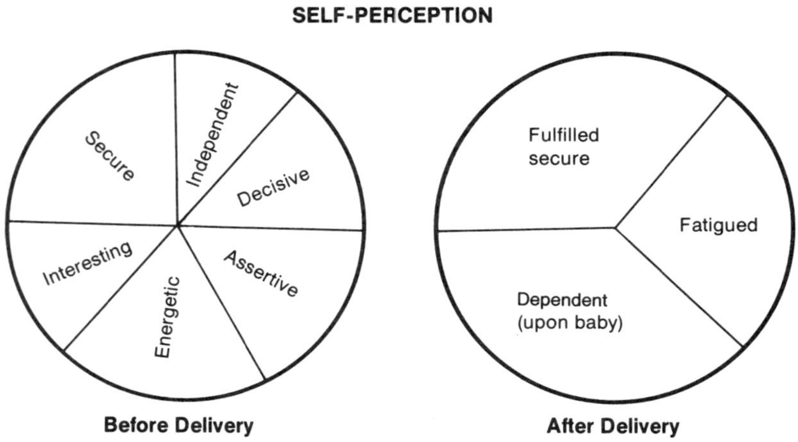

**SELF-PERCEPTION**

**FIGURE 18–2.** The sections in these circles represent one woman's self-perception before and after delivery. (Reprinted with permission from Eheart, B. K., and Matrel, S. K.: *The Fourth Trimester: On Becoming a Mother.* Appleton-Century-Crofts, Norwalk, Conn., 1983.)

discomforts and sleeplessness. Fatigue is a stress factor that drains the woman of the psychological and physical reserves needed to deal with her immediate environment. Her energy depleted, the woman may be unable to concentrate effectively. Everything she undertakes may require a great effort. As a result, the new mother may experience tension, irritability, anxiety, frequent crying, loss of libido, and depression.

During her adjustment period, the new mother may feel anger, ambivalence, and loneliness (Eheart and Martel, 1983). Some women have difficulty in acknowledging these emotions, and the new mother may not understand why these feelings are present. She may question her capabilities as a loving parent, and, as a result, she may experience depressive symptoms. Her anger could be directed at the child who has interrupted her life or at her husband who goes to work each day leaving her alone and who may be jealous of the attention required by the dependent newborn. Fatigue, loneliness, and boredom contribute to the new mother's ambivalent feelings about her child. If she has disrupted her career, the woman's ambivalent feelings may be generated by the boredom of her daily routines. These ambivalent feelings toward her child may be frightening, especially if the woman has expected motherhood to be characterized only by joy, warmth, and love.

Although a woman may not be aware of all those factors which influence her moods after childbirth, her past experiences and present situation play an important part in her emotional reactions. As noted, the extent of maternal sleep disturbance and resulting maternal fatigue will influence the woman's coping skills and the degree of puerperal depression experienced. In addition, the new mother's past relationship with her own mother is of great importance in the early puerperium. Women whose mothers have died are more likely to experience transitory depression (Cox et al., 1982). Women who lack identification with their mothers and their mothering role model, will more often experience puerperal mood disturbances.

Childbirth may be a significant stress factor in an already unstable marriage. A woman who perceives mothering as a full-time role, but who must return to work for economic reasons may feel unfulfilled and guilty. A change in life situations, such as a domestic move away from family and friends or the death of a loved one, can at the best of times require significant adjustments. After childbirth, when the mother must develop new coping skills, such additional stress can trigger undue withdrawal, mood swings, and other depressive symptoms. A mother who feels unloved or unsupported may exhibit depressive symptoms three to five months after childbirth (Cox et al., 1982).

With the advent of family centered maternity care, fathers have been able to share in the birth experience more completely. Childbirth has important psychologic manifestations for men as well as women (Wainwright, 1966). During pregnancy, men will fantasize about their role as a father. The new father views himself as a companion, counselor, and disciplinarian. Yet, these are not roles that a new father can easily assume with his newborn child. Seeing a helpless, dependent infant, the new father has difficulty in understanding how to approach the infant and may relinquish total care of the child to his partner.

The puerperium is an important maturational period for the father. Therefore, the first few months after delivery are a time of significant psychosocial adjustment to the reality of parenthood and its associated stresses. The new father may feel the pressures of his added financial responsibilities and may suffer the loss of his mate's companionship. He may react with resentment toward his child while not understanding the cause of these feelings. Symptoms exhibited at this time can include anxiety, depression, tension, insomnia, irritability, and nervousness (Trethowan, 1972). Unresolved past conflicts may be instrumental in causing paternal depression. Some new fathers may have an unconscious envy of their partner's reproductive capacity. In addition, the birth of a male child may reactivate a latent or overt homosexual conflict, heightened by lack of heterosexual experiences prior to childbirth (Wainwright, 1966). Many of these factors, while present to some degree in most new fathers, are rarely sufficient to cause significant psychiatric pathology.

## INTERVENTIONS

Most women exhibit depressive and stressful periods in the early puerperium. This predictive knowledge influences the anticipatory guidance that will allow new parents to understand their emotions and have more control over their new situation. Braverman and Roux (1978) documented seven items that could be identified during antepartum care which were predictive of puerperal depression:

1. depression with a previous birth
2. single parenthood
3. marital problems
4. pregnancy was unplanned
5. child is not desired
6. woman regrets pregnancy
7. woman feels unloved by father of child.

Identifying these seven factors during the pregnancy may alert the health team to women at high risk for puerperal depression.

Puerperal care involves monitoring physical parameters such as involution, breast tenderness, and lochial flow. However, there is usually little attention paid to psychological symptoms. During their stay in the hospital, women should be assessed for high-risk factors that may lead to puerperal mood disturbances. Some of these factors are:

- low parity
- depression with previous birth
- poor relationship with her mother
- lack of support system
- lack of financial support
- level of fatigue
- restlessness
- sleep disturbance
- low hemoglobin
- poor nutritional status
- lack of self-confidence in the care of the child.

Fatigue is a major stress factor that accounts for maternal vulnerability to depression and an inability for the development of psychological coping skills in the puerperium. Deep sleep patterns are markedly reduced approximately two weeks prior to delivery and do not return to normal until the second week of the puerperium (Karacan and Williams, 1970). Women must be alerted to the impending changes in sleep patterns and the resulting fatigue. Adequate rest must be ensured during the antepartum period. In the puerperium, the mother's rest periods should coincide, when possible, with her infant's sleeping patterns. Arrangements for meals and housekeeping should be planned prior to delivery; these chores should be shared by the couple and other members of their support system. The new mother's confidence and self-esteem can be strengthened by appropriate remarks and assistance with her mothering skills, which emphasize that infant care is a learned skill.

During the puerperium, parents often lack an understanding of their own feelings. For example, the new parents may not have a spontaneous outflow of love for their newborn. Through anticipatory guidance, they will understand that this can be a normal reaction and that their affection for their infant will increase over time. Dealing with emotions is dependent on past role modeling and coping skills. For the new parents, this means having the knowledge of the normality of the emotions that they are feeling. New mothers can have angry feelings and must understand that this does not threaten the love they have for their husbands or their infants. To resolve this anger, it is imperative that the new mother discuss the reasons for her feelings with her partner.

The new mother must remember that ambivalence exists in most life situations. Therefore, her ambivalent feelings about her child are not abnormal, nor should they be unexpected. For the first few puerperal months, the new mother is separated from previous enjoyable activities, and diminished adult contact can cause her to feel lonely. To prevent this response, new hobbies may be undertaken. A support group of new and expectant mothers in her neighborhood can be formed. Planning short excursions with other new mothers to a park or sharing experiences over a cup of tea may alleviate loneliness.

How new mothers deal with their emotions is in part dependent on their support systems. Many women have difficulty in verbalizing feelings and need someone to help them deal with their seemingly overwhelming responsibilities. The new mother needs time to rest, to get to know her child, to understand its cries. It is especially important for the new mother to have time for herself—a grandparent or friend should be enlisted to stay with the baby for a few hours. In addition, sharing the responsibilities of parenthood will help the new father to identify his fathering role. The new mother's ability to express herself will greatly influence her ability to deal with her puerperal adjustment. Expressions of feelings leads to their acceptance and their resolution. A woman who has been brought up to control her emotions may lack the ability to express her thoughts and her fears. This failure to communicate may, more than any single factor, lead to depression.

The health care team should play a significant role in alleviating maternal anxiety during the puerperium. Childbirth classes, which include sessions in parenting, help to develop coping skills and confidence in creating a new parenting role. During the short hospital stay, the new mother's physical and psychological reserves must be protected and her confidence in mothering skills enhanced. In addition, telephone calls should be made by health care professionals in the puerperium to reinforce anticipatory guidance. The frequency of these calls will depend on maternal needs for reassurance. The first phone call after hospital discharge should be made on the fourth or fifth puerperal day. Research has revealed the fifth puerperal day as a vulnerable time for depressive symptoms. Furthermore, women who are bottle feeding report most of their breast discomfort on the fifth day after delivery (Brooten *et al.,* 1983). Mothers who are breast-feeding may need additional guidance and support to ensure that this experience will be successful. Weekly calls may be continued after the initial contact. In addition, the new mother should have a telephone number available to her if a concern arises. By six weeks after childbirth, mothers have fewer questions, more confidence and are coping well with the realities of parenting.

PERINATAL LOSS

*Give sorrow words; the grief that does not speak Whispers the o'er-fraught heart and bids it break.*
*Macbeth*—Shakespeare (Act IV, Scene 3)

It is most natural for a woman to fantasize about her child and what motherhood will be like. Such fantasies include the sex of the infant, who it will resemble, plans for its future, mode of delivery, and method of feeding. This process encourages the formation of bonds and attachments between mother and child that continue to develop as the pregnancy progresses.

When a significant loss occurs, fantasies and expectations are not realized. Although the severity of a loss may range from minor to extreme, one must never assume a so-called minor loss to be inconsequential. For example, the fantasy of dressing up a little girl in frilly clothes is quickly dispelled when the baby turns out to be a boy. A mother may be equally disappointed when her plans to breast-feed are thwarted by an inadequate flow of milk. Some complications of pregnancy including premature labor, placenta previa, and hypertension will necessitate an alteration in lifestyle. Activities may be restricted, hospitalization required, or an early delivery planned.

When the pregnancy is at high risk, the labor and delivery experience may be particularly stressful. Some complications coupled with fetal distress necessitate delivery by cesarean section. A woman who has prepared for months to have natural childbirth may be denied this wish and she may feel frustrated and angry over her inability to meet the expectations she has set for herself. In effect, she views herself as a failure. This mother has indeed experienced a form of loss, and it is essential that those caring for her recognize and acknowledge her needs. Since much of nursing and medical care is directed toward the delivery of a healthy baby, the mother may lose her own sense of self-worth. Feeling that she is not as important as her baby may result in subsequent neglect of her own health care after the pregnancy (Johnson, 1979).

Premature birth, serious neonatal illness, and fetal malformation represent more severe forms of loss. The mother of an infant who must spend extended time in the intensive care nursery often faces a temporary loss of the opportunity to parent effectively. The infant may be confined to an isolette or require ventilatory assistance and/or connection to monitors. In some instances, the infant may even be transferred to a different facility for acute management, further intensifying the separation. As a means of defense in the event of a more permanent loss, a mother may withdraw and become fearful of attachment to her infant. Such detachment represents anticipatory grieving. During this critical period, both mother and father will need answers to questions about the baby's condition and emotional support and assistance in forming attachments. Photographs of the baby, a direct telephone line to the intensive care nursery, and regular meetings with members of the neonatal team are all means of satisfying these needs.

Discovery that one's baby has special and unexpected problems results in shock, confusion, and the realization that the perfect child has been lost. The mother's guilt is intensified as she wonders what she has done to contribute to the condition. When the defect is a permanent one, as in the case of fetal anomalies, the feelings of loss and guilt are more complex. The realization that the situation will not improve increases the hopelessness. For parents to cope effectively with the reality of their situation, they must be encouraged to ask questions and seek information. The health care team must be open and honest in their answers concerning the child's prognosis.

PERINATAL DEATH

Perinatal death, the ultimate loss for the new mother and father, may be experienced as a miscarriage, stillbirth, or neonatal death. According to Borg and Lasker (1981) a common reaction to miscarriage is the fear of being responsible for its occurrence, especially when the pregnancy is unplanned or if there were feelings of ambivalence regarding the parenting role. Miscarriage following sexual intercourse often results in feelings of guilt, despite reassurance that the loss was neither induced nor preventable. Stillbirth, the sudden death of the fetus *in utero,* strikes the heart like a thunder bolt. This unexpected blow shatters all fantasies: The wished for child is lost forever; the dream will be unfulfilled. While for some the loss is experienced as a stillbirth, others realize the joy of childbirth but must watch in agony as their baby struggles for survival and finally succumbs to complications of prematurity or other neonatal disease. A recent study confirmed that the presence of a living twin does not lessen the grief of parents who have lost one premature twin (Wilson *et al.,* 1982).

The pain of loss at any of these stages is intense. Thus, the death of a longed-for child cannot be brushed aside by pat phrases such as "you are young, you can have other children" or "it was God's will." As Peppers and Knapp (1980) point out, while the tragedy surrounding the death of an older child or adult is experienced and shared by everyone with whom they were associated, the loss of an infant is limited to the immediate family, parents and, perhaps, grandparents. One might ask how the loss of a fetus or newborn can be as great as that associated with the death of an adult? Why is the grief so intense? A wise pastor once counseled a bereaved parishioner: "Treasure your grief, for many people never love enough to ever know deep grief." The impact of love on life cannot be underestimated. According to Phillips (1981) "Anything that holds such possibilities for joy, fulfillment and natural strength must have roots that go so deep that its loss will inevitably produce overwhelming pain and grief" (p. 1). Consequently, the loss of a child, no matter how young, will result in a classic grief response characterized by somatic distress, preoccupation with the image of the deceased, guilt, hostile reactions, and loss of normal patterns of conduct. Lewis (1976) has emphasized that even with a live birth the mother feels a sense of loss of her "inner" baby but is consoled by her surviving "outside" baby. After a stillbirth, there is an outer, as well as an inner, void.

The grief response tends to follow a specific pattern as the individual progresses through the phases of shock, suffering, and recovery. The phases often overlap and periods of regression are not uncommon.

**Conceived But Not Cradled: Shock.** This phase commences with the initial knowledge that the infant is abnormal or that it has died. It is a time of disbelief that such a tragedy has occurred. Disorientation is overwhelming, and the emotions range from denial, anger, and guilt to depression and hopelessness. Accompanying these feelings, the physical response to loss includes restlessness or exhaustion, loss of appetite, as well as vague somatic complaints such as exhaustion, chest pain, and headaches. This phase usually lasts for six to eight weeks (Willis, 1982).

**Why is This Happening? Suffering.** The second phase in the grief pattern is that of suffering. This slow period of adjustment is often referred to as a time of searching and yearning. Outwardly life appears to go on as usual as the individual returns to work or goes about his or her daily routine. However, the loss continues to have an impact on the bereaved parents and is expressed in diverse ways. It is essential that lines of communication between the couple remain open at this time to eliminate misconceptions regarding unusual behavior or reactions to the loss. Fathers may find it especially difficult to express their true feelings since society places such emphasis on the strong and controlled male image. Consequently, the father may need additional support and counseling to facilitate his grieving process.

**Feel the Pain and Let It Go: Recovery.** This constitutes the third phase of the grief process. This period of reorganization occurs between 12 to 24 months after the loss. The future appears brighter as the individual feels a sense of release and renewal of energy. Eating and sleeping habits will stabilize, social relationships are reactivated and judgment becomes clearer and more efficient. The infant that was lost is not forgotten, but the pain is now bearable and life goes on.

## ROLE OF THE HEALTH PROFESSIONAL IN FACILITATING THE GRIEF PROCESS

Assessment of the individual's needs following perinatal loss involves a distinct process. It is important for the care giver to realize that the newly bereaved parents have not thought through their grief behavior. Their responses are automatic. The degree of denial, as well as their need to protect each other, will significantly influence the behavior of the parents. As a result the mother and/or father may need gentle questioning before feeling free to express grief. It is essential that the well-meaning "conspiracy of silence" and denial imposed by most health care personnel be broken (Lewis, 1976).

The sensitive care giver will solicit interpretations and perceptions of the loss experience. Although some individuals may be reluctant to reveal their feelings, most will take the opportunity to ventilate. Since family and friends often distract the grieving parent, drawing attention away from the loss or avoiding the situation altogether, the health professional may indeed be the sole facilitator in the grief process.

It is important to remember that each person grieves in his or her own unique way. Therefore, one may not necessarily observe the five stages (denial, anger, bargaining, depression, and acceptance) observed by Kubler-Ross (1969). Many individuals may experience only three or four of these stages. For others, the sequence may be altered. Regression to an earlier stage is not infrequent. Therefore, it is essential for the health professional to identify the direction of the grief process and respond to the individual's needs. The support rendered to the mother frequently may be dramatically different from that needed for the father. As noted above, men, as a result of societal expectations, often fail to let down their defenses. In addition, the mother may be so obviously overwrought that her partner feels compelled to hold back his true feelings to protect her. The father may displace his grief by maintaining a daily work routine and he can be either ignored or looked upon as cold and unconcerned. Recognition of such "incongruent grieving" and prompt intervention will help the couple understand their individual needs and maintain their communication (Peppers and Knapp, 1980).

Because grief following a loss is an appropriate and therapeutic process, administration of sedatives is generally contraindicated. Memory facilitates mourning (Lewis, 1976), and sedation will impair the patient's ability to deal with her loss. In addition, consolation in the form of cliches and platitudes such as "I know just how you feel" only serve to deny the uniqueness of the loss and further exacerbate the pain.

The health care team has three major tasks: (1) to help the parents digest the loss and make it real; (2) to ensure that normal grief reactions will begin and that both parents will go through the entire process; and (3) to meet the individual needs of specific parents (Klaus and Kennell, 1976). In addition to providing direct emotional support, the health care team should follow some practical guidelines when dealing with perinatal loss (Lake et al., 1983).

A. *The acutely ill or dying infant*
   1. Allow the parents to see and touch the infant as soon as possible. Special arrangements may be needed for those mothers who have medical or surgical complications, for example, transport to the nursery via litter or transport of the infant to the mother's bedside.
   2. Explain treatment measures and procedures (*i.e.*, medications, intravenous lines, catheters, ventilators, monitors).
   3. Be honest regarding the prognosis.
B. *Fetal death, stillbirth*
   1. Provide parents the opportunity to spend time alone with the infant. En-

courage them to view, touch and hold the infant. Focus on positive features, that is, hair, fingers and toes, family resemblance.
2. Encourage the parents to name the infant. This is an optional decision. However, this acknowledgement of the baby as a unique individual will further facilitate achievement of resolution.
3. Provide momentos: photographs, footprints, name bracelet, locks of hair.
4. Arrange for baptism if desired.
5. Discuss burial options. Parents are often unaware of their rights in this matter as well as ill-prepared with regard to funeral arrangements. Information concerning hospital disposal or private burial is especially helpful. A funeral formalizes the loss and may facilitate mourning. The baby's grave provides a special place the parents can visit when they wish to be with their baby. (Speck and Kennell, 1980)

Hesitation on the part of the parents regarding viewing and naming the infant is not uncommon. Thus, it is important to stress the long-term value in relation to the grieving process. Nevertheless, there will be, on occasion, those parents who steadfastly refuse all offers of support. It is their right to do so and their wishes must be honored.

The health care team should meet with the family throughout the grieving process (Speck and Kennell, 1980). Parents should be seen immediately following the death, and the mourning process explained at this time. A meeting several days later will provide the opportunity to review again what the couple can expect in the coming weeks and to stress the support of the health care team. At the postpartum visit in four to six weeks, results of the autopsy findings and placental pathology may be reviewed and plans for future pregnancies explored. During the following weeks and months, telephone contact may be maintained to determine if the couple has resumed normal social interactions or if a pathological mourning response has resulted. Some groups encourage a meeting at the first year anniversary of the baby's death, a time of resurgence of grief.

## "I Had a Baby Sister But She Only Lasted One Day"* —Sibling Response to Perinatal Loss

It is important for the health care team to be sensitive to less obvious problems affecting the bereaved family. One such dilemma involves relaying the news of the loss to other children.

The younger child who is not yet able to fully understand the meaning of death may benefit from the use of illustrations, for example, fading flowers, a dead pet, or a reminder of a previous experience with death. The parents should be advised against equating death with sleeping as sleep disturbances in the child can result. Furthermore, illness should not be overly emphasized as this may lead to fearfulness when a minor illness occurs. Experts agree that it is preferable for children to be told of the death as soon as possible. They may also be included in the funeral arrangements made for the baby. Regardless of the age of the surviving child, it is essential for parents to maintain open and honest communication. All too often, the child, having had mixed feelings concerning the anticipated new arrival, will assume responsibility for the death. Failure to recognize this misconception may result in more serious psychological difficulties in the future.

In general, when there is a death in the family, the child needs to be:

- assured that basic needs will be met
- allowed to express sadness and to observe others doing so
- allowed to ask questions and to receive honest answers
- accepted despite regression

*See Scrimshaw (1984).

- reassured that death is not the result of someone's wishes
- reassured that he or she will not also die.

In essence, the child, as an integral part of the family unit, must be permitted to share in times of sorrow as well as joy (Scrimshaw, 1984). A coloring book *The Frog Family's Baby Dies* developed by Jerri Oehler, a nurse educator, may help communicate with the child during this difficult time (Oehler, 1981).

### PROBLEMS CONCERNING SEXUALITY

Perinatal loss often brings about abrupt changes in the sexual relationship of the husband and wife. While for some couples this intimate aspect of their sexuality may be enriched, for others significant deterioration occurs. The change in sexuality often appears shortly after the loss and lasts for a brief time. However, it is not uncommon for several months to pass before sexual problems surface, leading to more complex marital discord.

According to Peppers and Knapp (1980), both men and women can experience diminished sex drive secondary to the grief reaction. Loss of self-esteem on the part of the mother results in decreased sexuality. In addition, guilt may dispose either partner to deny themselves the pleasure of sexual intimacy.

Peppers and Knapp (1980, p. 81) summarize the most common alterations to sexual activity in the grieving parents as follows:

| *Type of Change* | *Reasons for Change* |
|---|---|
| POSITIVE (Increase in sexual response and activity) | Expression of affection and intimacy |
| | Compensation for the loss |
| | Desire to conceive another child |
| NEGATIVE (Decrease in sexual response and activity) | Fear of pregnancy |
| | Obsession with getting pregnant |
| | Loss of self-confidence |
| | Disallowance of personal pleasure |
| | Loss of sex drive |

The health professional will be better able to assist the couple in the area of sexual function if consideration is given to the following points.

1. Provide information about contraception.
2. Help the couple to understand the basis for their fears of a subsequent pregnancy.
3. Refer the couple for genetic counseling if indicated.
4. Encourage the couple to allow time for resolution.
5. Emphasize that temporary changes in sex drive are normal during depression.
6. Recommend professional psychiatric help if needed.
7. Stress the importance of maintaining open channels of communication.

### SUPPORT GROUPS

Parents who have experienced a perinatal loss find they must cope not only with their own emotions, but also with the distress of relatives and friends. Yet, unless those individuals have experienced a similar loss they will not truly comprehend the anguish of the bereaved parents. Consequently, it is with good reason that many parents seek out the support of others with whom they can openly share their feelings and in doing so find comfort.

In recent years, hospitals and communities across the country have established groups to assist parents in coping with infant death. Although the objectives are similar, support groups may utilize different approaches. There are three basic types of groups:

1. *Educational.* These groups are designed to assist parents in finding answers to their many questions. In essence, knowledge facilitates self-help. Groups are led by trained professionals or parents. HOPE is an example of such an educational group.

2. *Lay Counseling.* This approach is offered by organizations such as AMEN. Trained counselors who have experienced a similar loss provide moral support and encouragement through telephone or personal contact.

3. *Professionally Facilitated Small Groups.* This popular approach encourages regular

monthly meetings of small groups of parents for the purpose of discussing the grief experience. The facilitator is either a trained professional or parents who have attained resolution and are therefore knowledgeable regarding the subject matter. SHARE and UNITE are two such groups.

The decision to participate in a support group must be the choice of the individual or couple. An approach that works well for one person may be unsuitable for another. Consequently, some parents will prefer private sessions with a clergyman or counselor rather than group interaction. Nevertheless, the care giver should be familiar with the support services in the community so that appropriate referrals can be made. Parents will then be free to choose the most comfortable means of support.

THOUGHTS ABOUT ANOTHER PREGNANCY

As each individual will experience the resolution of grief in his or her time, so too a renewal of hope signified by plans for subsequent pregnancies must evolve in a gradual manner. The period immediately following the loss of a child is not the appropriate time for making future plans. Emotions are fragile and thought processes are too unstable to cope with the stresses of decision making. The bereaved couple will undoubtedly receive unsolicited advice from family and friends regarding future pregnancies. If there are medical concerns including the need for a repeat cesarean section or initiation of a work-up to determine the etiology of the perinatal death, the counsel of the physician is vital. Beyond this point, the decision if and when to undertake another pregnancy should be left entirely up to the couple. Discussion of this subject will be most valuable if emphasis is focused on the question *why* and not if or when. All too often a subsequent pregnancy is begun as a means of negating the loss. The infant born of this pregnancy is then perceived as a replacement rather than as a uniquely different, but equally special, child. Consequently, it is essential for any couple considering a future pregnancy to recognize and understand their motivations clearly and to continue to work through the grief process until resolution is attained (Szybist, 1973).

## CONCLUSION

Care of the pregnant woman must not end after labor and delivery. The puerperium represents a period of marked psychosexual adjustment. The health care team must prepare the patient and her partner for these changes, recognize patients requiring more active intervention, and, in the event of perinatal loss, support the couple as they grieve and ultimately reorganize their lives.

## REFERENCES

Alder, E. M., and Cox, J. L.: Breastfeeding and postnatal depression. *J. Psychosom. Res.,* 27:139–144, 1983.

Borg, S., and Lasker, J.: *When Pregnancy Fails,* Beacon Press, Boston, 1981.

Bratfos, O., and Haug, J. O.: Puerperal mental disorders in manic–depressive females. *Acta Psychiat. Scand.,* 42:285–294, 1966.

Braverman, J., and Roux, J. F.: Screening for the patient at risk for postpartum depression. *Obstet. Gynecol.,* 52:731–735, 1978.

Brooten, D. A.; Brown, L. P.; Hollingsworth, A. O.; and Tanis, J. L.: A comparison of four treatments to prevent and control breast pain and engorgement in non-nursing mothers. *Nurs. Res.* 32:225–229, 1983.

Carter, S. M. B.; Reveley, M. A.; Sandler, M.; Dewhurst, Sir J.; Little, B. C.; Hayworth, J.; and Priest, R. G.: Decreased urinary output of conjugated tyramine is associated with lifetime vulnerability to depressive illness. *Psychol. Res.,* 3:13–21, 1980.

Clarke, M.: Depression in women after perinatal death. *Lancet,* 1:916–917, 1979.

Coppen, A.; Eccleston, E. G.; and Peet, M.: Total and free tryptophan concentration in the plasma of depressive patients. *Lancet,* 2:1415–1416, 1972.

Cox, J. L.; Connor, Y.; and Kendell, R. E.: Prospective study of the psychiatric disorders of childbirth. *Br. J. Psychiatry,* 140:111–117, 1982.

Crout, T. K.: Caring for the Mother of a Stillborn Baby, *Nurs. 80,* 10:70–73, 1980.

Dalton, K.: Prospective study into puerperal depression. *Br. J. Psychiatry,* 118:689–692, 1971.

Davidson, G. W.: *Understanding Death of the Wished for Child.* OGR Corporation, Springfield, Ill., 1979.

Donnelly, K. F.: *Recovering from the Loss of a Child.* Macmillan, New York, 1982.

Eheart, B. K., and Martel, S. K.: *The Fourth Trimester: On Becoming a Mother.* Appleton-Century-Crofts, Norwalk, Conn., 1983.

Furlong, R. M., and Hobbins, J. C.: Grief in the Perinatal Period, *Obstet. Gynecol.*, 61:497–500, 1983.

Furman, E. P.: The death of a newborn: Care of the parents. *Birth and the Family J.* 5:214–218, 1978.

George, A. J.; Copland, J. R. M.; and Wilson, K. C. M.: Prolactin secretion and the postpartum blues syndrome. *Br. J. Pharmacol.*, 70:102–104, 1980.

Handley, S. L.; Dunn, T. L.; Baker, J. M.; Cockshott, C.; and Gould, S.: Mood changes in puerperium and plasma tryptophan and cortisol concentration. *Br. Med. J.*, 2:18–20, 1977.

Handley, S. L.; Dunn, T. L.; Waldron, G. E.; Baker, J. M.: Tryptophan, cortisol and puerperal mood. *Br. J. Psychiatry*, 136:498–508, 1980.

Howells, J. G.: *Modern Perspectives in Psycho-Obstetrics.* Brunner/Mazel, New York, 1972.

Hullen, R. P.; Bailey, A. D.; McDonald, R.; Dransfield, G. A.; and Milne, H. B.: Variations in 11-hydroxycorticosteroids in depression and manic–depressive psychosis. *Br. J. Psychiatry*, 113:593–60, 1967.

Jansson, B.: Psychic insufficiencies associated with childbearing. *Acta Psychiatr. Scand.* (Suppl.), 40:172, 1964.

Johnson, S. H.: *High Risk Parenting.* Lippincott, Philadelphia, 1979.

Kaij, L., and Nilsson, A.: Emotional and psychotic illness following childbirth. In Howell, J. (ed.): *Modern Perspective in Psycho-Obstetrics.* Brunner/Mazel, New York, 1972.

Kaplan, H.: *The New Sex Therapy.* Brunner/Mazel, New York, 1974.

Karacan, I., and Williams, R. L.: Current advances in theory and practice relating to postpartum syndromes. *Psych. Med.*, 1:307–328, 1970.

Kendell, R. E.; McGuire, R. J.; Conner, Y.; and Cox, J. L.: Mood changes in the first three weeks after childbirth. *J. Affective Disord.* 3:317–326, 1981.

Kennell, J. J.; Slyter, H.; and Klaus, M.: The mourning response of parents to the death of a newborn, *N. Engl. J. Med.*, 283 (7):344–349, 1970.

Klaus, M. H., and Kennell, J. H.: *Maternal–Infant Bonding: The Impact of Early Separation or Loss on Family Development.* C. V. Mosby, St. Louis, 1976.

Kowalski, K.: Helping Mothers of Stillborn Infants to Grieve. *Matern. Child Nurs. J.*, 6:29–32, 1977.

Kubler-Ross, E.: *On Death and Dying.* Macmillan Publishing, New York, 1969.

Kuevi, V.; Causon, R.; Dixson, A. F.; Everard, D. M.; Hall, D.; Hales, S. A.; Whitehead, C. A.; Wilson, C. A.; and Wise, J. C. M.: Plasma amine and hormone changes in postpartum blues. *Clin. Endocrinol.*, 19:39–46, 1983.

Lake, M.; Knuppel, R. A.; Murphy, J.; and Johnson, T. M.: The role of a grief support team following stillbirth, *Obstet. Gynecol.*, 146:877–881, 1983.

Lesh, J. A.: Postpartum Depression. *Curr. Pract. Obstet. Gynecol. Nurs.*, 2:52–64, 1978.

Lewis, E.: The management of stillbirth coping with an unreality, *Lancet*, 2:619–620, 1976.

Metz, A.; Stump, K.; Cowen, P. J.; Elliott, J. M.; Gelder, M. G.; and Grahame-Smith, D. G.: Changes in platelet $\alpha_2$-adrenoreceptor binding postpartum: possible relationship to maternity blues. *Lancet*, 1:495–498, 1983.

Nott, P. N.; Franklin, M.; Armitage, C.; and Gelder, M. G.: Hormonal changes and mood in the puerperium. *Br. J. Psychiatry*, 128:379–383, 1976.

Oehler, J.: The frog family books: Color the pictures "sad" or "glad". *Matern. Child Nurs. J.*, 6:281–283, 1981.

Peppers, L. G., and Knapp, R. J.: *Motherhood and Mourning: Perinatal Death.* Praeger, New York, 1980.

Phillips, G. R.: Grief, *The Backside of Love.* Human Services Division, Springfield, Ill., 1981.

Pitt, B.: Atypical depression following childbirth. *Br. J. Psychiatry* 114:1325–1335, 1968.

Pitt, B.: The aftermath of childbirth. *Proc. R. Soc. Med.*, 68:223–224, 1975.

Pizer, H., and Palinski, C.: *Coping with a Miscarriage,* Dial Press, New York, 1980.

Playfair, H. R., and Gowers, J. I.: Depression following childbirth—A search for predictive signs. *J. R. Coll. Gen. Pract.*, 31:201–208, 1981.

Reich, T., and Winokur, G.: Postpartum psychoses in patients with manic-depressive disease. *J. Nerv. Ment. Dis.*, 151:60–68, 1970.

Sandler, M.; Carter, S. B.; Reveley, M. A.; Glover, V.; and Rein, G.: Further light on the tyramine test in depression. *Can. J. Neurol. Sci.*, 7:265–266, 1980.

Scrimshaw, S. C. M., and March, D. M. S.: I Had a Baby Sister but She Only Lasted One Day. *JAMA*, 251:732–733, 1984.

Speck, W. T., and Kennell, J. H.: Management of Perinatal Death, *Pediatrics Rev.*, 2:59–62, 1980.

Stein, G.; Milton, F.; Bebbington, P.; Wood, K.; and Coppen, A.: Relationship between mood disturbances and free and total plasma tryptophan in postpartum women. *Br. Med. J.*, 2:457, 1976.

Steiner, M.: Psychobiology of mental disorders associated with childbearing, *Acta Psychiat. Scand.*, 60:449–464, 1979.

Szybist, C.: *The Subsequent Child.* National Foundation for Sudden Infant Death, Chicago, 1973.

Tentoni, S. C., and High, K. A.: Culturally induced postpartum depression. *JOGN Nurs.*, 9:246–249, 1980.

Tod, E. D. M.: A prospective epidemiological study. *Lancet.* 1264, 1964.

Treadway, C. R.; Kane, F. J.; Jarrahi-Zadeh, A.; and Lipton, M. A.: Psychoendocrine study of pregnancy and puerperium. *Am. J. Psychiatry*, 125:1380–1386, 1969.

Trethowan, W. H.: The Couvade syndrome. In Howells, J. G.:(ed.): *Modern Perspectives in Psycho-Obstetrics.* Brunner/Mazel, New York, 1972.

Vandenberg, R. L.: Postpartum depression. *Clin. Obstet. Gynecol.*, 23:1105–1111, 1980.

Wainwright, W. H.: Fatherhood as a precipitant of mental illness, *Am. J. Psychiatry*, 123:40–44, 1966.

Willis, R. W.: Conceived but not cradled: Grieving the unsuccessful pregnancy. *Thanatos*, 7:10–12, 1982.

Wilson, A. L.; Fenton, L. J.; Stevens, D. C.; and Soule, D. J.: The death of a newborn twin: An analysis of parental bereavement. *Pediatrics*, 70:587–591, 1982.

Yalom, D. I.; Lunde, D. T.; Moos, R. H.; and Hamburg, D. A.: Postpartum blues syndrome. *Arch. Gen. Psychiatry.*, 18:16–27, 1968.

# UNIT III Pathophysiology of Human Sexuality in Major Medical and Surgical Disease

# CHAPTER 19 CARDIOVASCULAR DISEASE

*Marjorie Seltzer Stanek, M.D.*

## INTRODUCTION

Disease of the cardiovascular system often has a negative impact on the sexual functioning of its victims, particularly for postmyocardial infarction patients. A forbidden subject for years, sexual function in cardiovascular patients was not discussed by most physicians and patients themselves were reluctant to bring it up. Doctors were often embarrassed or felt that older patients were not interested in sex. Studies of postmyocardial infarction patients revealed that, frequently, a considerable change in the pattern of sexual behavior occurred after the acute cardiac event. A reduction in the quality as well as the quantity of sexual activity is seen in both male and female patients. Although there are many reasons for this behavioral change, the most common are fear and anxiety. In particular, patients fear coital death. Studies have been done to evaluate the energy needed for sexual activity, and counseling is seen as a way to allay these fears. Physical conditioning programs are often helpful. Vascular disease and resultant surgery of the aorta can also contribute to sexual dysfunction as well as certain cardiovascular drugs, in particular, the antihypertensives. These subjects will be discussed with the hope of finding solutions to some of these problems.

## CARDIAC DISEASE

Evaluation of the extent of the problem of sexual dysfunction after a myocardial infarction was carried out most often by the distribution of questionnaires. Tuttle, Cook, and Fitch (1964) studied male postmyocardial infarction patients and found that two-thirds of these patients had reduced their frequency of sexual activity. Ten percent of the men interviewed became impotent permanently. There appeared to be no relationship between this behavior and the extent or severity of the heart disease, which suggests a psychological reason for the sexual dysfunction. Singh and coworkers (1970), studied 100 patients postmyocardial infarction and found that 91 were sexually active. Of these patients, 23 complained of decreased libido after the infarct. Twenty-two patients abstained altogether. The reasons given were medical advice, symptoms of pain, shortness of breath, weakness or exhaustion and fear of recurrence of the infarction. Of 69 patients, 23 or 46.4 percent had a much decreased frequency of sexual relations.

Hellerstein and Friedman (1970) studied 91 male subjects; 48 with myocardial infarctions and 43 who were apparently healthy but coronary prone. The overall frequency of orgasms per week decreased in patients with atherosclerotic heart disease from 2.1 times per week one year before the attack to 1.6 times per week at six months after the acute event. This was attributed to change in sexual desire, the wife's decision, and fear of symptoms of coronary artery disease. Forty-three of the postmyocardial infarction patients did complain of one or more symptoms, most commonly excessively fast heart rate, although 20 percent of patients complained of chest pain. Hellerstein and Friedman also noted a decreased frequency of sexual activity due to age alone. From age 25 or the first year of marriage to 20 years later, the overall frequency of sex decreased from 4.4 times per week to 2.1 times in the patients with atherosclerotic heart disease. In the apparently healthy subjects, the frequency decreased from 4.1 to 1.9 times per week.

Dobson and coworkers (1971) studied 17 patients after cardiac arrest, 12 of whom had regular intercourse before the acute event. Two of these patients stopped having sexual intercourse completely after the arrest due to fear on the part of the patient and spouse. Six of these patients had less frequent sex, three patients described no change, and one patient had increased sex.

Bloch, Maeder, and Haissley (1975) studied 100 patients, 88 men and 12 women with a mean age of 58 years. The monthly frequency of sexual intercourse was 5.2 before the infarct and 2.7 after. All of these patients had resumed a normal active life in other ways. Bicycle tests also showed lack of correlation between work capacity and frequency of sexual intercourse. They found that some of the more physically fit patients had lower levels of sexual activity. Other patients, despite poor physical fitness continued to have frequent intercourse. Patients blamed the reduced sexual activity on decreased sexual desire, depression, anxiety, fear of relapse or sudden death, fatigue, angina, impotence, and spouse's decision.

Abramov (1976) studied frigidity in postmyocardial infarction women—100 patients, ages 40–60, were compared to age-matched controls. Sexual dissatisfaction and sexual frigidity were seen in 65 percent of the coronary patients compared to 24 percent of the controls. Stern and colleagues (1977) studied 68 patients; 20 percent of the patients noted a decrease in the frequency of sex. Anxiety or depression was seen in most of these patients, and they described a decrease in the quality of their sexual activity as well.

Stein (1977) studied female postmyocardial infarction patients and showed less of a return to sex (40 percent) at one year, compared to their male counterparts (93 percent). Women also took longer to return to sexual activity postmyocardial infarction, 11.5 weeks versus 6.1 weeks for men. It was felt that husbands withheld sex due to fear of a wife's death more than wives withheld sex from their husbands for the same reason.

Mehta and Krop (1979) gave a questionare to 100 married male patients. By six months after the infarct, 30 percent had not yet resumed sexual activity, most not having participated in any shared sexual activity such as petting or manual stimulation. Over all there was reduced sexual activity in 59 percent of the patients. Mehta and Krop noted that the frequency of masturbation did not change. Rahe and coworkers (1979) found a 53 percent reduction in sexual activity in his untrained group of postmyocardial infarction patients. Less of a decrease was seen in the trained or treatment groups.

Of 100 wives of postmyocardial infarction patients interviewed by Papadopoulos's study (Papadopoulos *et al.*, 1980), 76 had resumed regular sexual activity postmyocardial infarction, but only 22 maintained the precoronary frequency of sexual activity. Five couples had increased frequency, but 49 couples had reduced frequency. Twenty-four patients did not resume sexual intercourse, 10 never tried and 14 tried but were unsuccessful due to impotence. The reasons given for the decrease in sexual activity were fear, anxiety, and guilt.

Gupta and Singh (1982) evaluated 150 patients, ages 35–76 years, and demonstrated that sexual activity decreased with age and even more so after a myocardial infarction. At age 25 or the first year of marriage, the average number of orgasms per week was 3.49. This decreased to 1.94 times per week 20 years later (or prior to the myocardial infarction). One year postmyocardial infarction, the number was 1.72 times per week. A delay in the return to sexual activity was also seen. Reasons for the decreased frequency of orgasms and delayed return to sexual activity were fear, symptoms during sex, depression, wife's decision, change in sexual desire, and social changes.

Papadopoulos and colleagues (1983) studied 130 female patients, ages 38–65. Of the 84 patients who were sexually active prior to the myocardial infarction, 61 or 72.6 percent resumed sexual activity. The monthly frequency of coitus decreased from 8.8 times prior to the myocardial infarction to 5.6 times per month afterward. Thus patients had decreased frequency of sex and some did not resume sex at all. Of the 84 patients, 43 or 51 percent expressed fear. Patients feared chest pain, acute infarctions, and coital death. They also feared being unattractive to their partners and feared that sexual intercourse would be of poor quality. Some patients expressed fear of discovery of an illicit relationship they were involved in. For these women, 44 percent of their husbands expressed fear of resuming sex, and 23 of the 84 patients did not resume sex at all. Reasons given were loss of libido, fear, the sex was not enjoyable, husband's illness, fear of coital death causing exposure of illicit relationship, and lack of partner. Some patients also complained of symptoms of chest pain, palpitations, sweating, shortness of breath and fatigue during sex.

Johnston and coworkers (1978) studied the frequency of sexual intercourse in postmyocardial infarction patients and compared this to patients who had revascularization surgery. Of 87 patients, 68 were postmyocardial infarction and 19 were postsurgery. The average age of the patients was 54.5 years. In the postmyocardial infarction patients, sexual activity decreased from 6.4 times per month before to 4.6 times per month after the acute event. The patients who had revascularization surgery had sexual intercourse 8.36 times per month before and 7.57 times per month after surgery, which is not considered significantly different. Postmyocardial infarction patients also waited longer to resume coitus after the acute event as compared to revascularization patients (9.6 weeks versus 5.7 weeks).

## Cardiovascular Changes During Sexual Activity

In all of these studies, fear of coital death figured prominently in the decreased sexual activity. This fear is bolstered by reports of symptoms during sex and of actual cases of coital death made known to the public through the media, and articles have appeared in the medical literature suggesting a causal relationship (Beyer and Enos, 1977; Massie, 1969). Studies have been done to evaluate the energy costs of sexual activity. Masters and Johnson (1966) demonstrated heart rate increases up to 170 to 180 beats per minute during sex, and blood pressure increases of 40–100 mm Hg systolic and 20–50 mm Hg diastolic. However, these figures were obtained by monitoring subjects performing in a laboratory setting. These conditions can obviously lead to anxiety and emotional stress and to considerably higher heart rates than might be found in home settings.

Hellerstein and Friedman (1970) studied the heart rates during sexual activity by employing Holter monitors. Patients who were then participating in an exercise program were given instructions to perform their usual activities while wearing the Holter monitors. No special mention was made of sexual activity. Fourteen patients did engage in conjugal sexual activity, and although this is a small group, extrapolation to larger groups of people can probably be made. Heart rate and electrocardiogram changes associated with sexual activity were compared to those occurring during other daily activities. Hellerstein and Friedman were unable to measure blood pressure during sexual intercourse and felt that the blood pressure measured during a bicycle exercise test which corresponded to the patients' heart rates during sex were probably equivalent.

The heart rates on the Holter monitors were observed in the period prior to going to bed, during the phases of the sexual act, and afterward. Hellerstein and Friedman assumed that the maximum heart rate occurred during ejaculation and orgasm and was 10–15 sec in duration. In the following one to two minutes, a rapid decline to baseline heart rate was observed. Hellerstein and Friedman found that the mean maximum heart rate during orgasm was 117.4 beats per minute (range 90–144). The average heart rates two minutes and one minute before were 87 and 101.2 beats per minute (bpm). The average heart rates one and two minutes after were 96 and 85 beats per minute. It is important to recall that these heart rates were recorded in the privacy of the patients' homes without direct observation by investigators.

Comparison was made of the maximum heart rate during sexual activity and during work activity. The mean maximum heart rate during occupational or professional activities was 120.1 beats per minute (range 107–130). This rate is quite similar to the average heart rate during sexual activity, 117.4 beats per minute. Six subjects had a maximal heart rate that was higher during sex than during work (127 versus 117 bpm), and eight subjects had a lower maximum heart rate during sex (110 versus 122 bpm).

The equivalent oxygen cost of the average maximum heart rate during sexual activity was less than that of climbing two flights of steps or walking briskly. Hellerstein and Friedman's equivalent blood pressures were 162/89 during sex and 147/87.7 for the period before and after.

Holter monitoring also revealed electrocardiographic abnormalities of ST segment depression in four subjects who had angina at the time of sex. Ectopic beats were noted in 23 patients during sex. ST segment depression occurred during the work activity in four subjects (three of these had similar changes during coitus). Five patients had ectopic beats during work.

All of the patients in the above study were males who had been married to the same woman 20 or more years. It does not appear therefore that conjugal sexual activity is particularly stressful on the cardiovascular system when compared with other everyday physical activities. The energy cost is approximately six kilocalories per minute or 4 to 6 METS (a MET is defined as the energy expenditure at rest or approximately 3.5 ml $O_2$ per kg body weight per minute) at maximum which lasts only about 30 seconds.

These numbers could obviously change depending on the circumstances. Extramarital relationships are more stressful, especially if conducted after a heavy meal including alcohol or under secretive, anxiety-producing circumstances. In the Johnston study group, ten patients reported having sex with someone other than the regular partner and two of these patients felt that angina was more severe during the "other" relationship (Johnston et al., 1978). There are many people who feel that changing the position used during sex, for example man on top to man on bottom may decrease the energy requirements. Others, including Kavanagh and Shephard (1977), found that this position reduces the pleasure or quality of sex.

Nemec, Mansfield, and Kennedy (1976) studied the heart rate and blood pressure responses during sexual activity in presumably healthy males in order to compare the cardiovascular response of the male on top to the male on bottom position. Ten male patients, ages 24–40, monitored themselves during sexual intercourse with their wives of at least six years in the privacy of their own homes. All subjects were professionals involved in the medical field including five physicians. A Holter monitor was used to continuously measure the heart rate beginning one hour prior to sexual activity. Arm blood pressure was measured by ultrasonic Doppler device. The blood pressure was measured at rest, intromission, and orgasm, and 30, 60, and 120 sec after orgasm. The subjects monitored themselves during five episodes of sexual intercourse over a one-week period. The first use of the monitoring equipment was for orientation of the subjects. Then alternating male on top and male on bottom positions were used. By the end of the study, 16 male on top and 19 male on bottom positions were monitored. In the male on top position, the investigators found that the resting heart rate was $60 \pm 8$ beats per minute and increased to $92 \pm 13$ beats per minute at intromission and was $114 \pm 14$ beats per minute at orgasm. After orgasm the heart rate fell to $69 \pm 12$ beats per minute by 120 seconds. The heart rate response for the male on bottom position was quite similar with the peak at $117 \pm 4$ beats per minute during orgasm. Thus, no significant difference was noted when the two positions were compared. The average blood pressure response for the male on top position was 112/60 at rest, 148/79 at intromission, 163/81 during orgasm, and 118/69 20 sec later. The blood pressure for the male on bottom position was slightly less during intromission but was similar during the other phases. There thus appears to be no significant difference in the heart rate or blood pressure responses for sexual activity in these two positions. Except for premature atrial contractions, few changes were seen in these healthy subjects. These blood pressures compare favorably to the "equivalent" blood pressures of Hellerstein and Friedman.

In comparing these blood pressure responses to earlier studies (Masters and Johnson, 1966), it is clear that studies done in the home environment reduce the emotional factors which may lead to higher blood pressures. Further studies need to be done to evaluate the blood pressure response in patients with ischemic heart disease, hypertension, and in the over 40 age group. It thus appears that fear of coital death with one's long-time marital partner in a comfortable home setting is probably not necessary.

The mean peak heart rate during masturbation has been found to be 118 beats per minute (Sanderson, 1982). Previous studies (Wagner, 1975) found heart rates from 110 to 130 beats per minute and even earlier studies (Masters and Johnson, 1966) noted much higher heart rates. Cases of sudden death during masturbation have been reported.

Ueno (1963) reviewed 5559 autopsies in patients who died suddenly between 1959 and 1963. In 34 of those patients who died during coitus, the circumstances of death were determined. Most coition deaths occurred in males (28 cases) and were from cardiac causes (18 cases). Death occurred in hotels most frequently (18 cases) and in relations with lovers (16 cases). There was a higher frequency of deaths in men who were older than their female partners by an average of 20 years. The women who died were only three years younger than their male partners. A preceding drunken state was noted in 12 cases. Most patients died during intercourse (11 cases), eight patients died prior to intercourse, and four cases one hour afterward. In several cases, death occurred 18 hours after sex. Three deaths occurred during masturbation.

COUNSELING THE CARDIAC PATIENT

Based on all of the above studies, it appears that the problems of reduced or absent sexual activities in the postmyocardial infarction patients can be solved through counseling. Counseling in association with physical conditioning programs is particularly helpful; patients in physical conditioning programs describe improvement in the quality and quantity of sexual activity when compared to patients not enrolled in these programs.

At the time of the hospital discharge after the acute event, frequently physicians do not give instructions regarding sexual activity. Patients are told to watch their diets and "take it easy," but sexual activity is not discussed, and patients are often too embarrassed to bring up the subject themselves. Tuttle and coworkers (1964) showed that two-thirds of all the postmyocardial infarction patients they studied received no advice at all while one-third received vague and nonspecific advice. Mehta and Krop (1979) reported lack of discussions between the patient and the physician about sexual activity in 64 percent of patients.

The Papadopoulos study found that the

number of patients receiving instructions regarding sexual activity at the time of discharge was inadequate with only 48 percent of the total group and 62 percent of the sexually active group receiving instructions (Papadopoulos et al., 1983). Although fears were still present, sexual instructions appeared to be a factor encouraging patients to resume sexual activity. This study also showed that when instructions were given, 27 percent of the patients expressed fear as compared to 37 percent of the group not receiving advice. Papadopoulos and colleagues also found that a significantly higher percentage of wives of postmyocardial infarction patients who received instructions feared sexual activity. This fear may reflect either inadequate instructions or, by raising the question of risk, anxiety.

Advising the postmyocardial infarction patients must begin with a history of the previous level of sexual activity. Patients who had no sexual activity prior to the myocardial infarction may be perfectly happy and well-adjusted and there is no need to encourage any change. In fact, the resumption of sex after many years of abstinence can be as anxiety-producing as an extramartial relationship. Patients who already had sexual difficulties prior to the acute event were found by Scalzi (1982) to develop increased fears of further sex and often impotence as a result of these fears.

It is also important to evaluate the patient's general health and tolerance for exercise. The extent of the cardiac damage must be considered as well as the frequency and severity of symptoms. The spouse should be involved as much as possible in discussions of sexual activity. If each partner is still anxious about sex, mutual pleasuring techniques may be helpful as an interim activity with resumption of intercourse later (Grauer et al., 1983). Masturbation is also helpful in relieving the fear of impotence and patients may try this early after an infarct.

In general, certain guidelines are helpful for all postmyocardial infarction patients. Sexual activity should be avoided after meals (wait three hours), after alcohol, or in extreme temperature. At times of fatigue, sex should also be avoided. Actually the optimum time for coitus is in the morning following a night's rest. Furtive, emotionally stressful situations and time restrictions should be avoided and anginal pain that occurs during or after intercourse should be reported to the physician. Palpitations lasting 15 minutes or more after intercourse, marked fatigue during the day following intercourse, and sleeplessness caused by sexual exertion should also be reported to the physician.

Nitroglycerine prior to sexual activity can relieve symptoms as well as the fear of anticipating symptoms and is very helpful in patients with coronary artery disease. Physical fitness programs have been shown to improve sexual functioning. Hellerstein and Friedman (1970) found that 32 percent of patients in a physical conditioning program noted improvement in the frequency of sex and 39.5 percent noted improvement in the quality.

Stein (1977) studied coital heart rates in 22 men, aged 46–54, in a bicycle training program, which lasted 16 weeks. Patients were exercised to 75 percent of predicted maximum heart rate for age. The mean coital heart rate before training was 127 beats per minute (range 120–130) compared to 120 beats per minute (range 115–122) afterward which is a decline of 5.5 percent in peak coital heart rate. An untrained control group did not have a significant change. It thus appears that coital myocardial oxygen requirements will decline with improved fitness levels. This training is particularly useful to the patient who is limited by symptoms during coitus.

Hellerstein and Friedman (1970) reported that, after a conditioning program, 67 percent of initially symptomatic patients had few or no symptoms during sex. Stern and Cleary (1981) found an increased frequency in sexual activity from 5.6 to 6.5 times per month in patients in the National Exercise and Heart Disease Project conditioning program as well as an improvement in the quality of sex. Also, the patients in this exercise program reported fewer symptoms during coitus. Johnston and coworkers (1978) showed an increased frequency of sexual activity in patients in an exercise program and felt this was due to a positive self-image.

## VASCULAR DISEASE

Sexual dysfunction can be seen in other forms of vascular disease as well as in the cardiac patient. Aortic occlusive disease in particular is associated with sexual dysfunction. Patients with aortic vascular disease may develop impairment of ejaculation and erection. Disturbed ejaculation is a function of injury to the autonomic nervous system while impaired erection is a function of inadequate blood flow to the hypogastric arterial system. Leriche's syndrome, for example, which is described as thrombotic obliteration of the bifurcation of the aorta, causes loss of ability to maintain an erection due to poor blood flow to the penis. May, DeWeese, and Rob (1971) studied 44 patients who required surgery for aortoocclusive disease of the distal aorta and 26 patients who required resection and replacement of an abdominal aneurysm. In patients requiring a lengthy (aorta to femorals) vascular prosthesis of the aorta, 45 percent complained of impaired erection. If a short prothesis was used, or an aortoiliac-thromboendarterectomy was done, only 27 percent of the patients had loss of erection. Thus vascular reconstruction that terminated above the origins of the hypogastric arteries provided better blood flow to the external genitalia. When reconstruction of the aorta ended below these arteries, twice as many patients complained of impaired erection.

The May study also looked at abnormalities of ejaculation (May et al., 1971). It appeared that the extent of dissection about the aorta had the most profound effect on problems of ejaculation. Bypass grafting that required less dissection was associated with a 26 percent incidence of ejaculatory disturbances. Resection or thromboendarterectomy requiring more dissection was associated with a 68 percent incidence of these problems.

Abnormalities of ejaculation occur when there is bilateral resection of the first two lumbar ganglia or by section of the intermesenteric plexus, the presacral nerves, or the hypogastric nerves. Retrograde ejaculation into the bladder occurs with loss of internal bladder sphincter tone when there is resection of lumbar 3 to lumbar 5 of the sympathetic nerves. Lumbar sympathectomy can also cause paralysis of the seminal vesicles, but does not affect sexual function in women. It does not cause loss of libido or orgasm. When care was taken to maintain the integrity of the hypogastric plexus in surgery for aneurysms or claudication, postoperative problems with ejaculation were minimized (van Vroohoven, 1977). Thus for proper male sexual function, an intact arterial and nervous system are needed and vascular disease may play a role in the loss of these functions.

## DRUG-RELATED SEXUAL DYSFUNCTION

A major cause of sexual dysfunction in cardiovascular patients is iatrogenic. Antihypertensive drugs in particular (Medical Letter, 1980) are responsible for sexual dysfunction. This contributes to poor compliance and treatment dropout. According to Wartman (1983), when a patient complains of sexual dysfunction, it is always best to assume that drug therapy is at fault. Switching to another drug—even if it has similar side effects—is often helpful. Reducing the dosage of certain drugs such as INDERAL may also help as the side effects may be dose related. When beginning a new antihypertensive, however, it is better not to mention sexual dysfunction as a side effect since the anxiety provoked may itself cause impotence. The true incidence of these side effects is difficult to ascertain as patients are often too embarrassed to bring up the subject and most physicians do not pursue it.

Any antihypertensive drug that acts on the sympathetic nervous system can cause sexual dysfunction. Studies have also shown that hypertensive patients themselves have a higher incidence of sexual dysfunction. Sannerstedt (1979) showed that there was a 17 percent incidence of impotence in the untreated hypertensive male compared to 7 percent in normal controls. Failure of ejaculation was seen in 7 percent of untreated hypertensives compared to zero percent of normals.

Clinical research done to evaluate various drugs has many flaws. Single drugs should be evaluated by themselves rather than in combinations. Hormone levels should be obtained and nocturnal penile tumescence should be used in the evaluations of these drugs (Moss and Procci, 1981). The drug most implicated in sexual dysfunction is guanethidine, which causes the sympathetics to be blocked resulting in paralysis of the internal bladder sphincter and retrograde ejaculation. It can also cause impotence and can interfere with orgasm in females.

Methyldopa (ALDOMET) (Lipman, 1977) causes inability to maintain an erection by blocking the reflex arc that is part of the mechanism of blood flow to the penis (Scheingold and Wagner, 1974). It can also cause loss of libido through its sedative effects. Clonidine (Medical Letter, 1977) also causes loss of libido probably through its sedative effect. It also causes a centrally acting sympathetic effect with resultant erectile difficulties, retrograde ejaculation, and inability to achieve orgasm in females.

Beta-blockers can cause loss of libido and impotence in higher doses (Hogan et al., 1980) due to sedative effects and reduced tissue perfusion. With long-term use diuretics also cause impotence and ejaculation difficulties, and this is thought to be related to orthostatic hypotension and electrolyte disturbances. Spironolactone also causes impotence, but adds the problem of gynecomastia in men which can be psychologically damaging. Chlorthalidone (HYGROTON) has also been associated with impotence.

Reserpine causes depression which leads to loss of libido in males and females as well as impotence in males (Medical Letter, 1983). Digitalis toxicity has also been associated with sexual dysfunction. Although Hydralazine has been associated with impotence, it and prazosin hydrochloride (MINIPRESS) are thought to have the least number of side effects related to sexual dysfunction.

## CONCLUSION

Thus patients with cardiovascular diseases are at risk for the development of sexual dysfunction. This may occur because of the psychological effects of fear of coital death after a myocardial infarction or may be the result of vascular disease of the aorta and lower extremities, or even due to the drugs used to treat cardiovascular diseases.

An understanding of these causes of sexual dysfunction is the first step in their treatment.

## REFERENCES

Abramov, L.: Sexual life and sexual frigidity among women developing acute myocardial infarction. *Psychosom. Med.,* 38(6):418–425, 1976.

Beyer, J. C., and Enos, W. F.: Obscure causes of death during sexual activity. *Med. Aspects Hum. Sex.,* 88(Sept.):88–94, 1977.

Bloch, A.; Maeder, J. P.; and Haissly, J. C.: Sexual problems after myocardial infarction. *Am. Heart J.,* 90(4):536–537, 1975.

Dobson, M.; Tattersfield, A. E.; Adler, M. W.; and McNicol, M. W.: Attitudes and long-term adjustment of patients surviving cardiac arrest, *Br. Med. J.,* 3:207–212, 1971.

Grauer, K.; Curry, R. W. Jr.; Kosch, S. G.; Kravitz, L.; Moore, W.; and Stewart, W. L.: Exercise testing and coronary artery disease. *J. Fam. Pract.* 16(2):241–257, 1983.

Gupta, M. C., and Singh, M. M.: Post-infarction sexual activity. *J. Ind. Med. Assoc.,* 79(4):45–48, 1982.

Hellerstein, H. K., and Friedman, E. H.: Sexual activity and the postcoronary patient. *Arch. of Intern. Med.,* 125:987–999, 1970.

Hoffman, W. F.: The behavioral side effects of the antihypertensive agents. AFP, 23, 1981.

Hogan, M. J.; Wallin, J. D.; and Baer, R. M.: Antihypertensive therapy and male sexual dysfunction. *Psychosom.,* 21(3):234–237, 1980.

Johnston, B. L.; Cantwell, J. D.; Watt, E. W.; and Fletcher, G. F.: Sexual activity in exercising patients after myocardial infarction and revascularization. *Heart Lung,* 7(Nov./Dec.):1026–1031, 1978.

Kavanagh, T., and Shephard, R. J.: Sexual activity after myocardial infarction, *Can. Med. Assoc. J.,* 116:1250–1253, 1977.

Lipman, A. G.: Drugs associated with impotence. *Modern Medicine,* May 15:81–82, 1977.

Massie, E.: Sudden death during coitus—Fact or fiction?, *Med. Aspects Hum. Sex.*, June:22-26, 1969.

Masters, W. H., and Johnson, V. E.: *Human Sexual Response.* Little, Brown, Boston, 1966.

May, A. G.; DeWeese, J. A.; and Rob, C. G.: Sexual function in men after abdominal aortic surgery, *Med. Aspects Hum. Sex.*, April:181–195, 1971.

*The Medical Letter,* Clonidine (Catapres) and other drugs causing sexual dysfunction. 19(20):81–84, (Issue 489), 1977.

*The Medical Letter,* Drugs that cause sexual dysfunction. 22(25):107–110, 1980.

*The Medical Letter,* Drugs that cause sexual dysfunction. 25:73–76, (Issue 641), 1983.

Mehta, J., and Krop, H.: The effect of myocardial infarction on sexual functioning. *Sexuality and Disability,* 2(2):115–121, 1979.

Moss, H. B., and Procci, W. R.: Antihypertensive drugs and sexual dysfunction, *Psychosom. Med.*, 43(6):473–474, 1981.

Nemec, E. D.; Mansfield, L.; and Kennedy, J. W.: Heart rate and blood pressure responses during sexual activity in normal males, *Am. Heart J.*, 92(3):274–277, 1976.

Papadopoulos, C.; Beaumont, C.; Shelley, S. I.; and Larrimore, P.: Myocardial infarction and sexual activity of the female patient. *Arch. Intern. Med.*, 143(August):1528–1530, 1983.

Papadopoulos, C.; Larrimore, P.; Cardin, S.; and Shelley, S. I.: Sexual concerns and needs of the postcoronary patient's wife. *Arch. Intern. Med.*, 140:38–41, 1980.

Rahe, R. H.; Ward, H. W.; and Hayes, V.: Brief group therapy in myocardial infarction rehabilitation: Three-to-four-year follow-up of a controlled trial. *Psychosom. Med.*, 41(3):229–242, 1979.

Sanderson, M. O.; Held, J. P.; and Bohlen, J. G.: Heart rate during masturbation. *J. Cardiac Rehab.*, 2(7):542–546, 1982.

Sannerstedt, R.: Negative consequences of reduction of blood pressure—influence on sexual function. *Acta Med. Scand.* (Suppl), 628:93–94, 1979.

Scalzi, C. C.: Sexual counseling and sexual therapy for patients after myocardial infarction. *Cardiovascular Nursing,* 18(3):13–17, 1982.

Scheingold, L. D., and Wagner, N. N.: *Sound Sex and the Aging Heart.* Human Sciences Press, New York, 1974.

Singh, J.; Singh, S.; Singh, S.; Singh, A.; and Malhotra, R. P.: Sex life and psychiatric problems after myocardial infarction. *J. Assoc. Physicians India,* 18:503–507, 1970.

Stein, R. A.: The effect of exercise training on heart rate during coitus in the post-myocardial infarction patient. *Circulation,* 55(5):738–740, 1977.

Stern, M. J., and Cleary, P.: National Exercise and Heart Disease Project, Psychosocial changes observed during a low-level exercise program. *Arch. Intern. Med.*, 141:1463–1467, 1981.

Stern, M. J.; Pascale, L.; and Ackerman, A.: Life adjustment post-myocardial infarction. *Arch. Intern. Med.*, 137:1680–1685, 1977.

Tuttle, W. B.; Cook, W. L.; and Fitch, E.: Sexual behavior in post-myocardial infarction patients. *Am. J. Cardiol.*, 13:140, 1964.

Ueno, M.: The so-called coition death. *Japanese J of Legal Medicine,* 17:333–340, 1963.

van Vroonhoven, Th. M. V.: Sexual dysfunction after aorto-iliac surgery. *VASA,* Band 6, Heft 3:226–229, 1977.

Wagner, N. N.: Sexual Activity and the Cardiac Patient, In Green, R.: (ed.): *Human Sexuality A Health Practitioner's Text.* Williams and Wilkins, Baltimore, 1975.

Wartman, S. A.: Sexual side effects of antihypertensive drugs: Treatment strategies and strictures. *Postgrad. Med.*, 73(2):133–138, 1983.

# CHAPTER 20  IMPOTENCE: DIAGNOSIS AND TREATMENT

*Harris M. Nagler, M.D., Ralph deVere White, M.D., and Jerry G. Blaivas, M.D.*

## INTRODUCTION

Historical perspective tells us where we have been, where we are, and, perhaps, by extrapolation, where we might find ourselves in the future. Impotence has been with us throughout the ages and undoubtedly will continue to afflict, as well as vex, men in the future. What has perhaps changed is our ability to discuss this malady openly and to explore its origins. Whereas, as recently as 1959, 90 percent of impotence was ascribed to psychogenic factors (Wershub, 1959), now patients frequently are found thought to have organic or physical causes of their sexual dysfunction (Blaivas et al., 1980a; Montague et al., 1979; Schrom et al., 1979; Spark et al., 1980).

The physiology of the erection has recently engendered much research. However, large gaps still exist in our knowledge. Basically, erections depend on sufficient blood flow into the erectile bodies of the penis (*i.e.,* corpus cavernosum). This influx and the control of the egress of blood result in entrapment of the blood within the corporal bodies producing erections. Although the precise neuromechanisms of this control are still to be elucidated, it is clear that erections due to local tactile stimuli are mediated through the sacral spinal cord on a reflex basis; those due to cerebral and psychic phenomena are mediated via the thoracolumbar and sympathetic pathways. Though a certain endocrinologic environment seems necessary for maintenance of normal erectile function, the level at which its influence is exerted is not clear. Though the interrelationships of the neurological, vascular, local, and psychological systems have yet to be clarified, each of these components can be assessed independently.

The diagnosis of impotence is no longer based purely on conjectures or impressions, but rather on sophisticated techniques by which the adequacy of penile blood flow is measured (Jevitch, 1980; Kempczinski, 1979; Nagler et al., 1982; Velcek, 1980). The neural pathways are tested (Blaivas et al., 1980b; Karacan, 1980). Hormones are assayed (Braunstein, 1983; Nikitinskaja, 1982). Penile erectile capability is observed and calibrated (Ek et al., 1983; Fisher et al., 1979; Godec and Cass, 1981; Karacan, 1980; Marshall et al., 1981).

Therapy has progressed beyond ground-up rhinoceros horns to sophisticated techniques of sexual therapy/behavior modification (Kaplan, 1974; Masters and Johnson, 1966; Smith and Fischer, 1983; Wolpe, 1969) as well as various surgically implantable prosthetic devices that create artificial erections which are widely utilized. The therapy for erectile dysfunction has recently progressed into the realm of microsurgery (Crespo et al., 1982; Michal et al., 1973, 1980c). Though arterial abnormalities (vasculogenic) are well-accepted causes of sexual dysfunction, reconstructive revascularization procedures are still in an experimental stage (Goldstein et al., 1983; Leriche, 1923; Michal et al., 1978, 1980a). Initial attempts to improve blood flow to the penis involved direct anastomoses of an arterial supply to the corpora cavernosa (Michal et al., 1973). More recent work has involved direct microsurgical revascularization of the corporal arteries (Michal et al., 1980c). The therapy for erectile dysfunction has progressed from mystical medicines to microsurgical reconstruction and undoubtedly will continue to progress through uncharted territories.

Our approach and therapy are accelerating to the point that, as we write, we are outdated; *that* is the message of our historical perspective.

## DEFINITIONS

When dealing with sexual dysfunction, one must be certain that he or she gains a clear understanding of the patient's symptoms. The patient may complain of impotence because his wife has not become pregnant or because his period of latency following sexual intercourse has increased from 10 minutes to one hour. Impotence is the inability to obtain or maintain an erection that permits satisfactory intercourse. Masters and Johnson (1970) state that intercourse must occur in at least 75 percent of encounters otherwise a man is impotent. Care must be taken to differentiate impotence from problems of altered libido or premature ejaculation. Ejaculatory incompetence is often confused with erectile impotence.

## ESTABLISHING THE DIAGNOSIS

Although most people agree with the definition of impotence, establishing the diagnosis may be difficult and, perhaps, represents the most controversial aspect of dealing with erectile impotence. One of the most useful means of establishing a diagnosis is the patient interview. The interview should be somewhat structured in order to fully understand the nature of the patient's complaint. Is the patient complaining of true erectile impotence or is it a problem of premature ejaculation, anorgasmia, or increased latency?

### CHARACTERIZATION OF SEXUAL DYSFUNCTION

It is important that a complete characterization of the sexual dysfunction be carried out. A structured interview is the most effective way to understand the patient's complaint, as well as to frame for the patient his specific complaint, thus enhancing his understanding.

**The Onset.** Unless of traumatic nature (physical) organic impotence generally has a gradual onset. The patient may be aware of increasing difficulty in obtaining, as well as maintaining, an erection. When he states that one day, he had good erectile function and the following, he did not, the physician must suspect a psychogenic etiology. When one obtains a history of an abrupt alteration in sexual function, further careful discussion will often uncover a specific event of rejection or of sexual failure. These events will, at times, lead to a self-fulfilling prophecy of further deterioration of sexual function. Though a patient may be intelligent and sophisticated, often this insight is blocked until it is elicited by the physician.

**Inability to Achieve or Maintain.** Does the erectile dysfunction manifest itself with delayed ability to obtain an erection? Or, does it represent an inability to obtain a full erection at any time? If a full erection is obtained and is lost upon attempted intromission, is it during physical thrusting of sexual intercourse or just the approaching of the penis to the vaginal introitus that leads to loss of erection? If indeed, erection seems to be lost with active thrusting, does position or passiveness effect the ability to maintain the erection. In these conditions, does ejaculation occur prior to the loss of erection, with the loss of erection, or not at all?

**Ejaculation.** Ejaculation preceding the loss of erection may indicate a problem of premature ejaculation, whereas ejaculation occurring after loss of erection is more consistent with organic dysfunction. If ejaculation does occur prior to loss of erection, the diagnosis of premature ejaculation should be rendered. If loss of erection is accompanied by thrusting without ejaculation, than vasculogenic impotence must be considered.

**Quantification.** Further questioning is directed to the patient's quantification of the best quality of the present, compared to previous, erections. Patients find it easy to describe the quality of erection as a percentage or on a scale of 1–10. Most patients do not complain of complete loss of erectile capability, but rather describe a flaccid, floppy penis which approximates 50 to 60 percent of previous erections. A question to ask is: "When do you obtain your best erection?"

**Morning Erections.** Many patients are aware of nocturnal or morning erections but feel these are achieved by a different physiological mechanism and attribute them to a full urinary bladder. These patients will often tell you of these erections but pass over them in a matter-of-fact fashion. In general, these patients do not have a physiologic abnormality. It is also helpful to ask patients if they have attempted to utilize these morning erections for sexual intercourse and if so, with what results.

**Masturbation.** Questions regarding erectile capability with masturbation and extramarital affairs must be asked directly in a *nonjudgmental* fashion. *Not*—"*If* you masturbate, do you get an erection? Do you ejaculate?" but rather "*When* you masturbate . . . ." If a patient masturbates to orgasm and does not achieve an erection, an organic etiology is more likely than a psychogenic one.

**Libido.** Special attention should be directed to the patient's libido or sexual drive. Depressed libido may be the only reason the patient is seeking help—at the insistence of his sexual partner or as a result of his own concerns. Decreased libido may be associated with depression or overwhelming life stresses as well as hypogonadal states of various etiologies.

**Situations.** A history of situational impotence should be sought. The patient who has erectile dysfunction with one partner and not another may not have the insight to understand the genesis of this sort of sexual dysfunction. In this regard, care must be taken to assure the patient of the confidentiality of these questions especially when there is a sexual partner other than the spouse.

## RELIABILITY OF SEXUAL HISTORY

The sexual history has been the mainstay of the diagnostic criteria for distinguishing psychogenic from organic impotence. A recent report by Abel and colleagues (1982) emphasizes the fallibility of such an approach. After the initial interview, patients were categorized as psychogenic, organic, or undetermined. After nocturnal tumescence monitoring regimens, 50 percent had to be recategorized. This study went on to list seven sexual symptoms that differentiate organic from psychological impotence in diabetics. These symptoms were: continuous impotence, lack of morning erections, ejaculations, impotence, sex not oriented to sexual intercourse, decreased ejaculation, and failure to achieve erections (Abel et al., 1982).

## MEDICAL HISTORY

It is mandatory that the physician obtain a thorough general medical history at the time of the initial interview. This history must include a thorough review of the patient's past medical history with specific reference to hormonal abnormalities (thyroid dysfunction, diabetes mellitus, hyperprolactinemic state), neurologic disease (herniated discs, multiple sclerosis, diabetic neuropathy), vascular disease (aneurysms, peripheral vascular disease, hypertension), urologic disorders, and lastly, any major surgical procedures particularly pelvic surgery.

Often the most revealing part of the medical history is the drug history. This inventory should specifically address medications prescribed for treatment of medical maladies as well as drugs of abuse or "recreational drugs." We have found the term "recreational drugs" to be very effective in eliciting an accurate history in that it is an entirely nonjudgmental term. The drugs of abuse include alcohol, marijuana, stimulants, sedatives, and narcotics (Nagler and Olsson, 1983). Essentially all drugs used for the treatment of hypertension can cause adverse sexual effects (*Medical Letter*, 1980). However, it is important to keep in mind that hypertensive patients may develop sexual dysfunction that is unrelated to the administered therapy (Veteran Administration, 1977). Other cardiac drugs such as digitalis, disopyramide (Norpace) perhexiline (Texid) are associated with sexual dysfunction as well (Howard and Reese, 1976; McHaffie et al., 1977; Neri et al., 1980). The purpose of this chapter is not to review all the drugs that have been implicated in altering sexual function, however, the major categories of drugs that may affect sexual function include: the drugs of abuse, antihypertensives, diuretic agents, cardiac agents, prolactin-altering agents, hormones, anticholinergics, and miscellaneous agents such as Cimetidine (Adikan and Karim, 1979; Barber, 1979; Nagler and Olsson, 1983). In some instances, the mechanisms by which these agents alter sexual function are clear; in others the etiology is obscure. At times it is difficult to differentiate a drug's side effect from the results of the disease itself. Nevertheless, it is important to obtain a full exposure history in an attempt to relate it to the onset of sexual dysfunction in the patient. When possible, alterations of the drugs should be attempted to demonstrate a cause and effect phenomenon.

## Physical Examination

Physical examination should initially establish the general well-being of the patient. Signs of systemic illness (hepatic or renal failure) may be of etiologic significance in the patient's sexual dysfunction. Signs of endocrinological abnormalities should then be sought. Loss of body or facial hair, gynecomastia, testicular location and size may all give an indication of potential hormonal abnormalities. Genital examination might disclose abnormalities of the penile structure itself. Palpation of both corpora cavernosa is necessary to determine abnormal fibrosis (Peyronies's disease) which may give rise to abnormal sexual function. Signs of corporal asymmetry should also be noted. The scrotum and its contents should be examined as in any urologic examination.

Neurologic examination is initiated at the time of the rectal examination. The bulbocavernosus reflex is assessed by squeezing the glans penis and noting contraction of the anal sphincter or bulbocavernosus muscle. The sacral spinal segments are examined by testing perianal sensation (Sacral S2–S4), sphincter tone, and the bulbocavernosus reflex at the time of rectal examination (Blaivas et al., 1980b). The lower extremities should be checked for presence or absence of Babinski reflexes as well as the normalcy of the deep tendon reflexes. Sensation and proprioception are evaluated in the distal extremities at this time. Any abnormality requires further neurological evaluation.

The final phase is the clinical assessment of the vascular competency. Though the penile dorsal arteries can be palpated in many patients at the time of examination, we do not routinely search for their presence or absence at the time of physical examination. Their presence does not demonstrate adequate vascular supply and further evaluation of the penile vasculature is almost always carried out using Doppler studies (see following). An assessment of the peripheral vasculature of the patient is carried out by palpating distal pulses including the femoral, dorsalis pedis, and posterior tibialis vessels. Bruits should be sought as well as signs of vascular insufficiency such as loss of hair and thin fine skin in the lower extremities, vascular ulcers, and so on. In addition, symptoms of vascular insufficiency should be looked for.

At the completion of the sexual history, medical history, and physical examination, one often has made an initial assessment about the potential etiology of the sexual dysfunction. However, perhaps the most difficult issue to sort out is whether the impotence is due to organic or psychogenic factors. A patient with a multitude of organic etiologies may still have psychogenic impotence and a patient with apparent psychogenic impotence may have organic causes. A partial organic impairment may initiate a sexual dysfunction because of the patient's fear and anxiety.

## ESTABLISHING THE DIAGNOSIS OF ORGANIC IMPOTENCE

The diagnosis of impotence as discussed previously is often made on the basis of historical reporting by the patient. When the patient reports that he is unable to achieve intercourse satisfactorily due to inadequate penile turgidity, that patient is indeed impotent. The question then becomes not whether he is impotent, but whether he is impotent because of physical or psychological reasons.

### Nocturnal Tumescence Monitoring

The basis of nocturnal penile tumescence (NPT) monitoring is that while the awake patient may be, involuntarily, able to suppress erections for psychological reasons, the sleeping patient will not have the ability to suppress the normal nocturnal erectile events associated with sleep, occurring in association with rapid eye movement (REM). Normally, periodic erections occur during sleep approximately every 90 minutes in association with REM (Bohlen, 1981). Though the occurrence of nocturnal erections associated with sleep was first described in 1944, it was not until 1970 that Karacan proposed its use as a diagnostic tool in the evaluation of impotence (Karacan, 1970; Ohlmeyer et al., 1944). Much is known about the occurrence of nocturnal tumescence. Though nocturnal erections tend to occur in association with REM sleep, they do not coincide in a uniform fashion (Bohlen, 1981). REM sleep is associated with a Stage 1 electroencephlographic pattern, dreaming, and increased autonomic nervous and somatic activity (Aserinsky and Kleitman, 1953). Though there are differences in the number as well as the duration of erectile episodes during various stages of life and though there does seem to be a decrease in erections after puberty, a 65-year-old male will continue to have approximately 1½ h of sleep with erection (Karacan et al., 1972a). It is felt that penile erections are such an intergral part of sleep that they cannot be suppressed by psychological factors (Bohlen, 1981). In addition, it is important to note that the erection a patient may note upon awakening in the morning has no relationship to the need to urinate or the degree of sexual activity prior to sleep (Fisher et al., 1975; Karacan, 1970).

It is the apparent reliability of the nocturnal tumescence event in males of all ages with all degrees of sexual activity that makes it an appropriate tool for the assessment of the accuracy of a patient's perceptions and reports of sexual capability. However, it must be emphasized that there is no clear proof that severe psychogenic etiologies cannot suppress nocturnal erections. This fact is highlighted by the observation that NPT monitoring may demonstrate abnormal tumescence patterns due to unfamiliar surroundings and that on subsequent nights, these abnormalities may dissipate. This finding would indicate that psychogenic factors may indeed lead to abnormal nocturnal tumescence tracings. Approximately 15 to 20 percent of all patients tested will have abnormal NPT monitoring without a definite organic etiology (Fisher et al., 1979; Karacan, 1976). Though there can be no definitive statement as to whether these patients have undefined organic etiologies or indeed psychogenic impotence, most physicians dealing with such patients believe that abnormal NPT monitoring with documented normal REM sleep patterns represents organic sexual dysfunction.

One further caveat for issue of the validity of NPT monitoring as an indicator of organicity is highlighted by the challenge offered by Marshall and colleagues (1981). They question the basic assumption that nocturnal and sexually elicited erections do indeed occur by the same physiological mechanism. Theoretically, then, the erections associated with sleep can be intact whereas those elicited by sexual activity can be impaired. Another limitation of nocturnal tumescence is that it measures only increases in penile diameter and does not give an assessment of penile rigidity and therefore its adequacy for sexual function. Thus, a patient may have normal expansion but the penis may not be rigid enough for penetration. Though various techniques have been developed for dealing with this problem, none has met with widespread approval (Krane, 1983; Karacan et al., 1978; Wabrak, 1981; Zafar Kahn, 1980).

Though the imperfections of the NPT monitoring as a tool for the diagnosis of organic or psychogenic impotence are apparent, it does remain one of the more reliable modalities for making this differentiation. Sleep studies can vary in degrees of sophistication from simple stamp techniques to the use of formal sleep laboratories in which many parameters including electroencephalograms, electrooculargrams, and electromyograms can be measured (Barry et al., 1980; Karacan et al., 1978). Changes in penile circumference alterations can be measured with mercury loop strain gauges positioned around the base of the penis as well as just behind the coronal sulcus. The device developed by Karacan is the most widely used device for the measurement of alteration in penile girth (Karacan, 1969). These loops are positioned around the phallus and are secured to the patient in such a way as to prevent them from being dislodged and to minimize movement artifact. NPT monitoring should be carried out for a minimum of two nights and preferably three nights. If, of course, after the first night of monitoring, normal erectile capability is demonstrated no further measurements need be obtained. Various systems have been devised for home monitoring by different companies. The disadvantage of home monitoring is that it is difficult to assess patient compliance, the proper placement of the strain gauges, or the "adequacy" of sleep. In formal sleep studies where REM sleep is monitored, the validity of the nocturnal tumescence for diagnosing organic versus psychogenic impotence is enhanced. Additionally, sleep studies performed in a formal sleep laboratory allow the utilization of confrontational techniques in which a patient is awakened from sleep to observe and evaluate the erection. At times, this may afford a therapeutic approach for the patient with psychogenic impotence. If it is decided that confrontational techniques should not be utilized, videotape monitoring and direct observation may be equally useful.

Nocturnal tumescence monitoring continues to be one of the most useful tools in assessing psychogenic impotence. The greater the degree of sophistication of the study, the more reliable it is in making this differentiation (Marshall et al., 1983).

Provocative Stimulation Studies

The use of video stimulation (erotic movies) in an attempt to elicit erections has significant theoretical advantages over nocturnal tumescence monitoring. As stated, the basic assumption of NPT monitoring is that the same erectile mechanism is responsible for both nocturnal and sexually associated erections. This assumption—though intellectually reasonable—has no sound basis in fact. Therefore, the utilization of stimulation studies in an attempt to elicit erections has appeal. Thus far, these techniques have not been widely used clinically, although undoubtedly they will be in the future (Wagner, 1981).

Nocturnal tumescence monitoring, visual stimulation studies, and the history and physical examination will generally present the clinician with a reasonably clear picture of whether sexual dysfunction is organically or psychogenically based. From that point, further diagnostic studies can be carried out in an attempt to delineate the etiology of organically based sexual dysfunction. If nocturnal tumescence studies confirm the impression of psychogenic impotence, the patient is then referred for sexual therapy evaluation, which will be discussed in the therapeutic section following.

## THE SEARCH FOR A REMEDIAL ETIOLOGY

After the initial evaluation including history, physical exam, and, possibly, nocturnal tumescence monitoring, an initial diagnostic impression has been formulated by the physician. If the impression is one of organic sexual dysfunction, the next pursuit is to evaluate potential etiologies of this dysfunction. The ultimate goal is to identify a remedial etiology so that specific therapy can be recommended or, if a remedial etiology is not identified, at least to have a greater understanding of the mechanisms responsible for the patient's dysfunction. The evaluation of impotence is a difficult task. Although the physician knows there is an interrelationship between hormonal, neural, vascular, and phallic functioning, the intricacies of this interrelationship are elusive. Therefore, even if individual components are fully studied, the functional significance of the detected abnormalities is difficult to define.

### BLOOD STUDIES

The yield of an endocrinologic screen of impotence is small, that is, the efficiency of the test is low. Despite this fact, most physicians feel that the search for an endocrinologic abnormality is worthwhile because if an abnormality is uncovered, the therapeutic approach will be altered and therapy specifically directed. It is important to realize, as Van Arsdalen and Wein (1983) emphasize, that the discovery of an abnormality in blood chemistries, glucose tolerance tests, or endocrinologic studies does not establish a cause and effect relationship.

**Hypogonadal States.** Though testosterone is widely accepted to be necessary for normal male sexual function, it has been adequately documented that normal sexual function can exist with levels of testosterone clearly thought to be abnormal (Nagler and Blaivas, 1983). Therefore, a minimum level of testosterone necessary for maintenance of normal sexual function probably does not exist. Moreover, it is known that testosterone levels in prepubertal boys are quite low. However, young boys do have erections (Bohlen, 1981; Halverson, 1940). Nevertheless, by and large, testosterone is widely accepted as being necessary for normal maintenance of erectile capability and, for the impotent male, abnormalities in testosterone levels do warrant correction prior to administration of any other therapy.

Hypogonadal states, which may be congenital or acquired, may be due to either testicular failure or to hypothalamic-pituitary abnormalities. Physical examination, as well as laboratory examination, will often make this differential diagnosis apparent. Evaluation is usually initiated with a serum testosterone. If this is found to be within the normal limits, further endocrinologic studies may be unwarranted. If however, a low testosterone is noted, further studies with luteinizing hormone (LH), follicle-stimulating hormone (FSH), and prolactin are indicated. The results of these studies will indicate either hypothalamic-pituitary dysfunction or testicular dysfunction. Elevations in the gonadotropins indicate testicular failure, whereas low levels of the gonadotropins in association with decreased serum testosterone would indicate hypothalmic or pituitary abnormalities. When a hypothalamic-pituitary abnormality has been discovered, the evaluation then turns to the determination of the etiology of this dysfunction. If a hypogonadal state is discovered associated with increase in the gonadotropins (hypergonadotropic hypogonadism), this demonstrates gonadal dysfunction. Hypogonadal states are the most common endocrinologic cause of impotence, and endocrinologic causes of impotence have been reported to account for 5 to 35 percent of all cases of impotence (Spark et al., 1980). Our experience would indicate that less than 5 percent of impotence is due to endocrinologic abnormalities.

Other endocrinologic abnormalities that can account for impotence include diabetes, hyperprolactinemia, and thyroid dysfunction.

**Diabetes.** Diabetes is said to result in impotence in approximately 53 to 55 percent of men over the age of 60 years (Smith, 1981). This fact has persisted in spite of improved diabetic control. Although most patients have both vascular and neurological abnormalities, evidence suggests that all aspects of the physiology of normal erectile function are impaired. In the series reported by Goldstein and coworkers (1983) vascular abnormalities were detected in 79 percent of the diabetic impotent males, neurological abnormalities in 30 percent, and psychological abnormalities in 55 percent of cases studied. Diabetes has well-documented effects on the microcirculation as well as the macrocirculation (McMillen, 1975; Zannini, 1974). Penile vascular abnormalities have also been demonstrated in the presence of diabetes (Ruzbarsky and Michael, 1980). Many series have been reported in which noninvasive studies of penile vasculature were carried out with an incidence of vasculogenic abnormalities varying from 33 to 87 percent (Goldstein et al., 1983).

Diabetes can cause neurologic abnormalities which may be associated with impotence in the diabetic population. Neuropathy exists both in the autonomic and the somatic system in a large number of diabetics. The peripheral neuropathy associated with diabetes is well-known and is associated with decreased vibratory sensation as well as loss of deep tendon reflexes. Autonomic dysfunction may involve the viscera with abnormal blood pressure and bowel and bladder symptomatology (Bennett et al., 1977; Duchen et al., 1980). Evidence of parasympathetic abnormalities leading to erectile dysfunction in impotent diabetics has been offered by urodynamics investigations (Ellenberg, 1971). Evidence of somatic dysfunction is offered by sacral latency studies in the diabetic population (Blaivas et al., 1980b).

Possibly a presenting manifestation of diabetes may be impotence (Ellenberg, 1971; Rubin and Babbott, 1958). It is important not to fall into the trap of labeling a diabetic with impotence as organically impotent simply because he is a diabetic (Waxberg, 1978). Indeed using nocturnal tumescence studies, Abel and coworkers (1982) found that approximately 30 percent of diabetics complaining of impotence had psychogenic causes. The diabetic population is a special group that further emphasizes the complicated interrelationships of organic and psychic etiologies.

The screening for diabetes in the impotent patient is generally limited to random blood glucose determination, 2-hour postprandial determinations, and urine glucose determinations. If these studies are normal, glucose tolerance testing is not routinely carried out.

**Hyperprolactinemia.** Hyperprolactinemia can interfere with gonadal function and result in low serum testosterone. Testosterone levels of normal value in association with hyperprolactinemia may result in impotence. By alleviating the hyperprolactinemic state, sexual dysfunction can be cured (Carter et al., 1978). Though decreased serum testosterones may be found in the presence of hyperprolactinemia, hyperprolactinemia without the decreased serum testosterones may also lead to sexual dysfunction. It should be noted that the level of hyperprolactinemia leading to male sexual dysfunction is usually greater than that leading to reproductive dysfunction (Carter et al., 1978). The fact that many drugs, which are mood-altering in nature, will cause hyperprolactinemia makes it a potentially significant cause of male impotence. Because of the indications of these mood-altering drugs, differentiating between the organic side effects of the drug and the psychogenic contribution to the sexual dysfunction may be difficult. Drugs found to cause hyperprolactinemia include the phenothiazines, tricyclic antidepressants, meprobromate, haloperidol, amphetamines, and opiates (*Medical Letter,* 1980). In addition, drugs used for the treatment of hypertension, including reserpine and α-methyldopa, have similarly been implicated in iatrogenic hyperprolactinemia. Therefore, one must differentiate the effect of the hypertension from the side effect of the treatment. The treatment of hyperprolactinemia will be discussed in the section on therapeutic techniques.

**Thyroid Function.** Thyroid function studies are generally not performed in the evaluation of sexual dysfunction unless there are manifest signs of either hyper- or hypothyroidism. The relationship to sexual dysfunction in these situations is not clear but certainly apparent endocrinologic abnormalities need to be dealt with for the general well-being of the patient.

NEUROLOGIC EVALUATION

Neurologic abnormalities may lead to impotence via various mechanisms. With neurologic impotence, most physicians are concerned with abnormal neuroregulation of the penile blood flow into the corporal bodies. However, abnormal sexual function due to neurologic etiologies may be based in abnormal penile sensation (Herbert, 1973) or abnormal modulation of the erectile centers (Goldstein, 1983; Herbert, 1973).

Neurologic abnormalities may be suspected after obtaining a history and performing a physical examination. Obviously, any previous neurologic abnormalities or systemic diseases associated with neurologic abnormalities will require thorough neurological evaluation. The initial interview should establish the adequacy of cognitive and cerebral functions. The neurologic examination specifically assesses both sensation and motor strength in the lower extremities. Sensation should be differentiated into pinprick, soft touch, and proprioceptive aspects. Sensation of the perineal and penile area should also be assessed. Deep tendon reflexes in the lower extremity, as well as the assessment of the Babinski reflex, are an integral part of this examination. By assessing perianal sensation, the adequacy of sacral segments 2, 3, 4, and 5 are assessed. The bulbocavernosus reflex, anal spincter tone and control assesses the integrity of the S2, 3, 4 reflex arch (Sax, 1979). Any abnormalities uncovered during this evaluation require further examination by a neurologist.

Urodynamics studies evaluate the parasympathetic S2, 3, 4, and sympathetic segments. Reports using cystometrography indicate that if there is no evidence of neurologic disorder after initial evaluation, the cystometrograms will invariably be normal (Rydin, Lunetberg, and Bretlberg, 1981). We do not routinely utilize these diagnostic modalities to demonstrate parasympathetic (S2, 3, 4) abnormalities unless there is evidence of concomitant voiding dysfunction.

The bulbocavernosus reflex latency time is an electrophysiologic manifestation or representation of the bulbocavernousus reflex. This reflex involves pudendal afferents (somatic sacral cord segments S2, 3, 4), pudendal efferents, and the striated muscle of the bulbocavernosus muscle (Ertekin and Reel, 1976). The bulbocavernosus reflex time is assessed by placing a needle electrode into the bulbocavernosus muscle on either side of the median raphe. A surface-stimulating electrode is placed on the distal penis and repetitive stimulation of 0.5 to 1.0 pulses per second are applied with a rectangular pulse wave form of 0.1 mil msec. The voltage is increased to a maximum of 250 v or until a response is obtained. Supramaximal stimulations are then applied and the bulbocavernosus reflex time is determined by measuring the interval from the stimulation to the onset of the evoked action potential response. The normal range is approximately 30–40 seconds (Blaivas *et al.*, 1980). Electromyographic assessment includes not only the actual latency of the reflex arc, but also the assessment of the individual motor unit action potential configuration, the recruitment pattern, and the ability to voluntarily contract the bulbocavernosus muscle (Blaivas *et al.*, 1980b). Any abnormal finding within these studies requires evaluation by a neurologist.

Recently, additional tests which assess the entire cerebrogenital neurological system have been described (Haldman *et al.*, 1982). Penile skin receptors, afferent pudendals, dorsal root ganglia, ascending second order of fibers, thalamic and cerebral sensory areas in the interhemispheric fissure are all assessed (Chippa and Roper, 1982).

Abnormalities in any of these objective neurologic assessments or in the routine neurologic examination need to be evaluated thoroughly by a neurologist. This will prevent inappropriate therapy of erectile dysfunction, as well as avoid missing potentially serious neurologic diagnoses that may need further evaluation and/or therapy. Neurologic evaluation carried out by physical examination, as well as sacral latency studies, revealed an 11 percent incidence of neurologic abnormalities in 100 unselected impotent males presenting for evaluation (Blaivas, 1979). Though abnormalities may be determined using these studies, once again a direct cause and effect relationship between erectile impotence and neurologic disorders has not been established as Blaivas and colleagues (1980a) have emphasized.

## VASCULAR EVALUATION

The evaluation of vascular causes of impotence can be divided into two categories, noninvasive and invasive techniques. In looking for vascular causes of erectile dysfunction, history and physical examination will only give reason to suspect vascular abnormalities. The evaluation of vascular insufficiency requires either invasive or noninvasive studies.

The historical information leading one to suspect vascular abnormalities includes that which is normally associated with vascular disease. History of lower extremity claudication certainly raises suspicions of a vascular abnormality as would major pelvic trauma and/or surgery. A history of loss of erections associated with thrusting activity may be suggestive of a vasculogenic "Steal" phenomenon (Goldstein et al., 1982; Michal et al., 1978). Physical examination, including assessment of distal extremities, temperature, loss of distal pulses, and atrophic changes, are all suggestive of a vascular insufficiency which may be significant in the pathogenesis of the patient's impotence.

However, because these physical findings and historical characteristics are unreliable, diagnostic studies have been devised by which adequacy of vascular blood flow is assessed objectively, easily, and inexpensively.

**Noninvasive Studies.** Assessment of penile vasculature can be carried out noninvasively by penile pulse palpation, penile Doppler blood pressure studies, penile phlethysmography, and thermography.

We have not found palpation of the dorsal arteries to be helpful in the diagnosis of impotent males. Though normally the dorsal artery pulses are palpable, reliance on this method to assess the adequacy of penile blood flow seems imprudent. Still if one cannot feel the dorsal arteries, the likelihood of a vasculogenic abnormality is higher. We do not find that the appreciation of the dorsal penile pulses by palpation or the lack of appreciation will lead us to alter the evaluation of a male who we feel has organic impotence.

If vasculogenic impotence is suspected, we utilize *penile Doppler blood pressure* measurements to assess the adequacy of the blood flow. Doppler ultrasonography for obtaining penile blood pressure was introduced in 1975 (Abelson, 1975). The initial technique has been modified from one in which the Doppler ultrasound probe was placed within the blood pressure cuff to one where the blood pressure cuff is placed around the base of the penis and using a pencil probe Doppler transducer, measurements are made of the various penile arteries distally. Most authors will in some way compare the measurements of the separate penile arteries to the systemic blood pressure. The actual calculation by which these comparisons are made vary from author to author. Zorgniotti and coworkers (1980) established a penile brachial mean pressure in which the penile systolic pressure ± brachial pulse pressure over 3+ the brachial diastolic pressure equals the penile brachial mean pressure (PBMP). A PBMP of less than +14 is considered abnormal.

Penile brachial index is probably a more

widely used method of assessing the adequacy of the penile vasculature. In this, the penile systolic blood pressure is simply divided by the brachial systolic blood pressure arriving at a penile brachial index (Metz and Bengtsson, 1981; Nagler et al., 1982).

The penile brachial index (PBI) is the most widely used indicator of vascular insufficiency. A resting index of less than 0.6 indicates a high probability of vascular disease and warrants further evaluation if clinically indicated (Metz and Bengtsson, 1981). A PBI greater than 0.75 is indicative of normal vascular function (Kempczinski, 1959; Queral et al., 1979). Utilizing these criteria, the Doppler studies have a 95 percent accuracy rate when confirmed by penile arteriography (Jevitch, 1980). Nagler and coworkers (1982) have demonstrated that the utilization of the frenular arterial sound may be an accurate indicator of normalcy of the remaining penile vasculature and that if this is intact, a more thorough Doppler examination need not be carried out, whereas if this reading is abnormal or marginal, then complete Doppler examinations are warranted.

All studies in which the adequacy of penile vasculature is assessed in the laboratory have a disadvantage in that they utilize a resting state to assess the adequacy of vasculature for a dynamic state. In this regard, the pelvic steal phenomenon as described by Michal attempts to unmask relative vascular insufficiency, which may appear to be normal in the resting state. Therefore, penile adequacy must be assessed resting and following lower extremity exercise. An alteration in the PBI of greater than 0.5 is felt to be indicative of vasculature insufficiency (Goldstein et al., 1982; Michal et al., 1978).

*Penile plethysmography* has also been utilized to diagnose the adequacy of penile blood flow. A digital plethysmographic cuff is placed around the base of the penis and inflated in order to attain mean arterial pressure. Via a transducer, a permanent pressure volume recording is obtained. The rate of systolic upstroke, as well as the presence or absence of dicrotic notches are assessed to indicate the normalcy of the penile vascular blood flow.

As a diagnostic tool *thermography* has not been successful in differentiating a group of patients with abnormal or normal penile vasculature by arteriographic studies (Buvat et al., 1982).

**Invasive Diagnostic Studies.** The invasive tests for vasculature insufficiency should only be utilized when noninvasive studies have documented vascular abnormalities and the patient is a suitable candidate for vasculature surgery.

Penile arteriography is an invasive study in which the penile arterial system is selectively studied. Until recently, this technique required instillation of undiluted contrast media that caused severe penile pain and required general anesthesia in order to be carried out. The patient is usually placed in an oblique position, with the side being studied upward. A Foley catheter in the urethra may be helpful for orientation especially in the early stages of experience with penile arteriography. Newer techniques using digital subtraction arteriography may be able to diminish the concentration of the contrast material as well as the volume injected. Therefore, the need for general anesthesia may be obviated. Michal and coworkers (1980b) recommend the use of passive erection at the time of arteriography. They feel this provides a precise anatomical picture of the arterial bed as it is associated with functional loading as represented by the artificial erection. The interpretation of penile arteriography requires significant experience. More importantly, it should be used only in those patients who would otherwise be considered candidates for a vascular reconstructive procedure.

*Radioactive xenon penography* was introduced by Shirai and coworkers (1978). The basis of this study is that a known quantity of radioactivity will be washed out of a vascular space at a rate dependent on local blood flow. A known quantity of radioactive xenon is injected into the cavernous bodies and by semilogarithemic plotting of the counts per minute, the blood flow can be determined per unit time. While these studies may uncover abnormalities in blood flow to the penis associated with sexual stimulation, as well as abnormal loss of blood from the erectile bodies with sexual stimulation (Wagner, 1981), they have not found wide utilization due to their complexity as well as the small clinical applicability of the information which is generated.

*Infusion cavernosography,* initially introduced by Fitzpatrick (1973), has recently become more popular. It is used in postpriapism-induced erectile dysfunction to delineate the degree of corpora cavernosal involvement due to the fibrous replacement as well as the delineation of abnormal fistulization as a result of the therapeutic intervention for priapism (Wagner, 1981). By continuous infusion cavernosography, drainage of the dorsal veins can be visualized. In association with visual stimulation techniques, it can be seen that egress from the corporal bodies diminishes as tumescence occurs. If this drainage does not decrease with sexual stimulation, erection will not occur. Such abnormal competence of the regulation function of the venous drainage system may represent a significant cause of impotence (Wagner, 1981). Leaks in the corporal bodies can be identified by such techniques. These abnormalities may be iatrogenic in certain circumstances (*i.e.,* treated priapism) but may also be etiologic factors in primary impotence (Ebbho et al., 1979).

PENILE OR LOCAL DISORDERS

The history that the patient provides as well as the physical examination will uncover most local penile factors that may be implicated in sexual dysfunction. A previous history of Peyronie's disease or priapism should be sought. In the face of either of these entities, the presence of fibrosis or apparent obliteration of the corporal body would generally be readily apparent. Local penile trauma can be an inciting event for a fibrotic process obliterating a corporal body or of vascular insufficiency.

DIAGNOSTIC TESTS FOR PSYCHOGENIC IMPOTENCE

Nocturnal tumescence monitoring is currently the best technique for differentiating psychogenic from organic dysfunction. Video stimulation studies are also a very effective modality. The utilization of psychological screening tests such as the Minnesota Multiphasic Personality Inventory (MMPI), the California Personality Inventory (CPI), the Derogatis Sexual Functioning Inventory (DSFI) and the Walker Sex Forum (SF), though widely used by many practitioners, have not been found useful by many others. The major shortcoming of these diagnostic studies is the same as any of the other diagnostic modalities used to study the impotent male—an abnormal finding does not indicate that the abnormality is the etiology of the dysfunction and that no other etiology may exist concurrently. Studies by Schoenberg (1982) as well as Robiner and colleagues (1982) have not been able to cross-validate these personality inventories for their discriminatory ability. Rather than using one of the standard personality inventory studies, we utilized evaluation by a sex therapist in all patients prior to implantation with a penile prosthesis. Certainly, however, these diagnostic standardized tests can be helpful to avoid overt psychopathology for the practitioner who does not have the support of an experienced sex therapist.

## SPECIFIC THERAPY AVAILABLE FOR IDENTIFIABLE ETIOLOGIES

The evaluation undertaken so far attempts to differentiate between organic and psychogenic sexual dysfunction. Within these categorizations, further attempts are made to differentiate specific etiologies that might respond to specific treatment.

HORMONAL ABNORMALITIES AND THE SPECIFIC THERAPY

As stated, a hypogonadal state may be due to testicular failure or pituitary or hypothalamic dysfunction. Though hypothalamic abnormalities can be dealt with by administration of gonadotropin-releasing factor, presently this is not a clinically utilized tool due to difficult administration. Pituitary abnormalities (*i.e.*, failure to produce or to release gonadotropins) can be specifically dealt with by administration of gonadotropins in the form of human chorionic gonadotropin (HCG). HCG has LH-like activity and can stimulate the production of testosterone by Leydig cells. The utilization of HCG has the disadvantage of requiring injections several times a week. If the hypogonadal state is due to a hypothalamic abnormality FSH may also be diminished, but this does not need to be replaced unless reproductive function is desired.

Hypogonadism secondary to testicular failure will obviously not respond to administration of HCG and in this circumstance, administration of testosterone either in an injectable form or in an oral form may be utilized. Testosterone propionate 10–50 mg. intramuscularly every 1–3 days or testosterone enanthate or cypionate can be administered 200–400 mg. intramuscularly every 2–4 weeks. Other forms of testosterone are methyltestosterone, fluoxymesterone. These drugs are orally administered and are taken on a daily basis. However, these oral forms of testosterone are found to be ineffective.

The administration of either parenteral or oral testosterone regimens is contraindicated when fertility status is desired. Under these circumstances, stimulation must be achieved by administration of the gonadotropins directly or by stimulation of the hypothalamic-pituitary axis, utilizing drugs such as clomiphene citrate. Clomiphene citrate may be able to stimulate the release of the gonadotropins due to its antiestrogen effect at the hypothalamic level. The regimens in which increased testosterone levels are achieved have the potential of resulting in hypercalcemia, salt and water retention, gynecomastia, and liver dysfunction (Weiderman and Northcutt, 1981).

As discussed, it is mandatory that in the presence of an acquired hypogonadotropic hypogonadism, the possibility of pituitary or hypothalamic lesions be explored. Such evaluation may require CAT scanning, visual field determinations, clomid stimulation studies as well as determination of other endocrine parameters including T3, T4, and thyroid-stimulating hormone (TSH) levels. Obviously, if there is evidence of a space-occupying lesion, this needs to be dealt with by neurosurgical consultation.

*Hyperprolactinemia* as a specific endocrine abnormality leading to sexual dysfunction can be dealt with surgically or medically. Evaluation of hyperprolactinemia obviously must investigate the possibility of hypothyroidism or drug-induced etiologies. If these are not found, it is imperative that a CAT scan of the pituitary be carried out to discern the presence or absence of a prolactin-secreting tumor. In concert with this, visual field studies are generally obtained. Approximately, 50 percent of the hyperprolactinemia seen in men is not associated with a detectable pituitary tumor as evidenced by CAT scanning. Therapy may initially utilize bromocriptine, a dopamine agonist drug. Bromocriptine inhibits the release of prolactin in the specific lactotropic cells of the anterior pituitary (Bartsch and Scheiber, 1983). The usual starting dose is 1.25 mg daily with gradual increments until the hyperprolactinemia is controlled.

If pituitary adenomas are visualized on CAT scan, neurosurgical consultation is required to ascertain a need for surgical intervention. If a macroadenoma is seen, surgery is generally advisable, however, it is important to realize that virtually all patients continue to require some additional bromocriptine therapy (Bartsch and Scheiber, 1983). Disorders of thyroid metabolism should be appropriately diagnosed and corrected.

Diabetes, although a significant cause of impotence, is not a remediable cause of impotence. The appropriate medical management of diabetes does not lead to the resolution of the resultant sexual dysfunction. The etiology of the diabetic sexual dysfunction may be multifactorial and, indeed, hormonal abnormalities may be found which can respond to a specific management.

## SPECIFIC NEUROLOGICAL THERAPIES

Spinal cord compression due to lumbar disc disease can present with sexual dysfunction that may be due to both the pain of the syndrome as well as the neurologic impairment (La Bau, 1966; Shafer, 1969). Spinal cord tumors may also present with evidence of sexual dysfunction, and it is these two entities which underline the need for thorough neurologic evaluation as part of the routine assessment of the impotent male. Effective therapy is often associated with return of sexual function. Spinal cord injuries can cause impotence depending on the degree and level of the insult. Patients with cervical and thoracic lesions usually have reflexogenic erections, but generally are incapable of attaining erections from erotic nontactile stimulation. As the cervical region is approached, the likelihood of the reflex erection approaches 100 percent (Torrens, 1983). Patients with lower lumbar and sacral lesions usually lack reflexogenic erections but may retain psychogenic erections. Other spinal cord disorders associated with impotence include multiple sclerosis and myeloid dysplasia. Unfortunately, these have no specific therapy.

## SPECIFIC SURGICAL THERAPIES

Although hyperprolactinemia and hypogonadism may respond to medical management, the majority of new advances in the therapy of male sexual dysfunction are surgical in nature and most are nonspecific or empiric.

**Corporal Shunts.** Corporal shunts may be iatrogenic, primary, or acquired. Whatever the etiology, they have in common the finding that there is abnormal leakage of normally entrapped blood from the corporal spaces into the corpus spongiosum, the glans penis, or the corporal veins. This condition leads to rapid detumescence or inadequate erections. One will generally suspect these conditions from the history and cavernosography is carried out to delineate the abnormality Iatrogenic shunts are generally the result of surgery for priapism. Recently, the Winter shunt utilizing a Vim–Silverman biopsy needle to create a temporary shunt between the corpora cavernosa and the glans penis (corpora spongiosa) has become widely utilized for the treatment of priapism. The therapeutic goal of this procedure is to allow the abnormally sequestered blood associated with priapism to drain via the corpora spongiosa. On occasion this will result in a persistent shunt with resultant inability to achieve or maintain a satisfactory erection. These findings can be confirmed by cavernosography, and surgical closure of this iatrogenically created shunt may be completed. Similar findings have been reported to occur primarily with no history of previous trauma or surgery. The surgical approach to these abnormal communications is to circumscribe the penis at the coronal sulcus and dissect the glans penis from the distal end of the corporal cavernosa bodies. Utilizing indigocarmine or methylene blue infusion into the corpora cavernosa, these abnormal interconnections between the corpora cavernosa and corpus spongiosa can be outlined, divided, and suture ligated.

**Peyronie's Disease.** Peyronie's disease can cause impotence due to the extensive penile curvature. This prevents intromission or causes pain with secondary impotence ensuing. Also, partial erections may result because of incomplete filling of the distal corporal bodies beyond the Peyronie's plaque. In the first situation, various surgical approaches have been tried to deal with the severe penile deformity that may be seen associated with Peyronie's disease. These include primary excision and closure of the tunica albuginea fascial defect with tunica vaginalis grafts (Das and Amar, 1982), dermal patch graft (Wilde, 1979), and placement of synthetic graft such as dacron. These procedures may be combined with the insertion of a penile prosthesis at the time of corporal repair (see below).

**Vascular Insufficiency.** Vascular abnormalities must be clearly delineated by aortography and selective internal pudendal angiography prior to attempts at correction of vasculogenic impotence.

**Endarterectomy and Aorto-Iliac Bypass.** Michal and coworkers have demonstrated that aorto-iliac occlusive disease can be responsible for erectile dysfunction and that by a properly tailored surgical approach, including endarterectomy of the internal iliac arteries, improved blood supply can restore sexual function. In their series of 112 patients, 80 of whom had impaired sexual dysfunction, when surgery was carried out with the intent of improving internal iliac arterial blood flow either by endarterectomy or aorto-iliac bypass surgery, 63.8 percent of patients had distinct improvements in erectile capability for more than 1 year after surgery. This, clearly demonstrates the role of aorto-iliac occlusive disease in erectile impotence (Michal et al., 1980).

**Direct Corporal Revascularization.** Other attempts at improving vascular supply to the penis have involved direct corpora cavernosal revascularization by anastomosis of an arterial conduit into the corporal body. Techniques have involved utilization of saphenous vein bypasses from the femoral artery to the corporal body, saphenous vein bypass from the inferior epigastric artery into the corpora cavernosa, or direct anastomosis of the inferior epigastric artery into the corporal body.

Results of direct revascularization techniques have met almost universally with failure. Hawatameh and coworkers (1982) reported that all shunts using saphenous vein graft were occluded at 28 months postoperatively. Zorgniotti and colleagues (1980) reported on a group of 15 men who underwent 16 revascularization procedures. Their results were similarly disappointing. Only 5 of 15 patients were able to perform coitus on a short-term basis. In this series, the type of revascularization included direct inferior epigastric artery revascularization as well as saphenous vein interposition between inferior epigastric or femoral arteries to the corporal body. The Michal study performed 32 epigastricocavernosus anastomoses. In 17 of the patients, the anastomosis maintained patency as determined by physical examination or arteriorography. Four patients developed a permanent pulsatile erection. Of the 17 patients with patent epigastricocavernosus anastomoses, 13 noted an improvement in their erectile capability and 10 could resume sexual activity, for an overall success rate of 31 percent (Michal et al., 1980c). The long-term follow-up showed that between 3–11 months postoperatively, all patent anastomoses eventually became occluded. Of the 10 patients who initially reported resumption of sexual activity, 6 continued the ability to have erections but to a diminished degree after occlusion of the shunt.

Attempts at direct corporal revascularization have theoretical disadvantages and quoted results indicate that these theoretical disadvantages have correlates in reality. One cannot expect that by simply allowing unregulated influx of blood into an organ which is normally dependent on both modulation of influx and egress that the result will be normal erectile activity. The results with direct revascularization certainly confirm this supposition. The resultant priapism graphically highlights the effect of unmodulated blood flow into the corporal bodies.

### EPIGASTRIC-DORSAL ARTERY REVASCULARIZATION

In the epigastric-dorsal artery revascularization technique, the inferior epigastric artery is mobilized from beneath the rectus muscle and tunneled beneath the inguinal ligament, bringing the epigastric artery to the base of the dorsal artery. An end-to-side anastomosis is then carried out, utilizing microsurgical techniques. This technique is advantageous as compared to the direct corporal revascularization in that the blood supply is into the vascular channels as opposed to the corporal spaces. Michal's results of this technique are superior to that of the direct corporal vascularization.

At the time of his report, 10 patients, (mean follow-up of 6.1 months) continued to have a patent anastomosis. While all these patients noted improvement, 8 of them had normal sexual function (Michal et al., 1980c).

The direct corporal revascularization has subsequently been abandoned and replaced by various modifications of Michal's initial technique for revascularization of the dorsal artery. However, in spite of the theoretical advantages of these newer techniques, the results continue to be unreliable and less than satisfactory (Michal et al., 1980c).

Recent techniques in which the revascularization of the penis is brought about by direct arterial anastomosis of a saphenous vein graft directly to the deep cavernous arteries have the advantage of providing blood flow to the profunda corporal vessels and therefore would, theoretically, be a more physiological procedure. In this technique, autologous venous grafts are taken either from the dorsal veins of the hand, foot, or forearm. A bifurcated venous graft is utilized when interposition is contemplated to the dorsal, as well as the corporal, arteries. The corporal cavernosal artery is isolated by probing the cavernous space with a hook-like instrument which snares the artery. An arteriotomy is made and anastomosis carried to the autologous graft. The proximal end is then anastomosed to the femoral artery which is approached below the inguinal ligament. Of 45 patients treated with either 1, 2, or 3 bypass vessels (84 percent having 2 vessels bypassed), 78 percent of the patients were reported as being cured (Crespo et al., 1982).

Though these results are preliminary, they are certainly encouraging and the technique warrants further investigation as, in theory, it is a more physiological approach to the problem of vascular insufficiency in the impotent patient. The field of revascularization of penile vasculature is still in great flux and certainly cannot be considered a clinical tool at present. The most recent report by Crespo and coworkers (1982) is certainly encouraging, but it needs to be documented by other investigators.

## NONSPECIFIC THERAPY

If a specific identifiable etiology of organic impotence cannot be ascertained and attempts at sexual therapy have been unsuccessful, the patient should be offered an implantation of penile prosthesis. These devices are constructed in such a way as to give the patient an erection sufficient for intromission. There are two basic types of devices, either semirigid or inflatable, currently in use.

### SEMIRIGID PROSTHESES

**Small–Carrion Prosthesis.** The prototype of the semirigid prosthesis, the Small–Carrion process prosthesis, was introduced by Small, Carrion, and Gordon (Small et al., 1975; Small, 1983). The Small–Carrion prosthesis has the disadvantage that it maintains the penis in the permanently erect state. The device is made of medical grade silicone rubber with a silicone sponge core. This was the first satisfactory penile prosthesis and had a great impact in the realm of penile prosthetic devices for erectile impotence.

The device may be implanted by various approaches. Earlier reports emphasized implantation by the perineal approach. In this approach, the patient is placed in a lithotomy position and the corporal bodies are identified as they insert onto the ischial tuberosities. The corporal bodies were then entered and dilated, using Hegar dilators, both proximally and distally until they accepted the penile prosthesis. The device is available in lengths of 12–22 cm and diameters of 0.9, 1.1, and 1.3 cm. Though initially this device was the most widely used, it is being supplanted by other devices affording greater flexibility and a more natural appearance for the patient.

**The Surgitek Flexi-Rod Penile Prosthesis (the Finney Prosthesis).** another simple prosthetic device which offers the advantage over the Small–Carrion prosthesis in that it has a hinged area enabling the phallus to be placed in a dependent position when not being used for intercourse. The diameters range from 0.9 to 1.2 cm and lengths from 7–13 cm (Finney, 1977). This device has the additional advantage that it can be shortened in the operating room, so the exact size does not need to be determined preoperatively and inventory can be kept to a minimum.

**Jonas Prosthesis.** The Jonas prosthesis (Jonas, 1979; Jonas and Jacobi, 1980) has these same advantages. It was first introduced in 1978. The initial version of this prosthesis, currently called the standard version (SV), had a nonadjustable length and diameter which need to be fitted to the patient at the time of surgical implantation. The prosthesis varies in length from 16–24 cm with 3 diameters of 9.5, 11.0, and 13.0 mm. The advantage of this prosthesis is the malleability of the prosthesis allowing the penis to maintain a dependent position when not being used for intercourse, as well as an upright position for coitus. The surgical approaches for implantation can include a subcoronal, midshaft, penoscrotal, suprapubic approach as well as the initial perineal approach.

Initial results with this prosthesis have been excellent, however one problem is that a high degree of spring in the silver made it difficult to maintain a dependent position. In 1982, this defect was modified by a specific bending zone thus enhancing its malleability (Jonas, 1983). Recently, further developments in the Jonas prosthesis system have included a variable version (VV). This device has a main silicone cylinder as well as a silicone cover, which can be inserted over the prosthetic device. This enables one device to have two different diameters. There are also two different covers enabling the prosthesis to obtain final diameters of 10–12 mm or 13–14 mm depending on the degree to which the sheath is placed over the cylinder. Additionally, the variable version enables the exact length to be determined at the time of surgery and trimmed appropriately. The Jonas system now also includes a trimming tip version which enables 2 prostheses to meet requirements between 16 and 25 cm. The new Jonas devices have also been contoured to enable a more natural shape to the erect penis with a larger bulk towards the midshaft (Jonas, 1983). These improvements make the Jonas prosthesis a more flexible system giving the surgeon greater ability to have perfect patient "fit" without having a large inventory of various prosthetic devices.

**AMS Malleable Penile Prosthesis 600.** A new device, developed by the American Medical Systems, is the AMS malleable penile prosthesis 600. It utilizes a fabric wrapped stainless steel core which is alleged to provide greater malleability as well as stability as compared to the silver core of the Jonas prosthesis. The device has the advantage of enabling three pairs of prostheses to result in 30 sizes, which by removing a silicone jacket over the "basic prosthesis," converts a 13 cm size to an 11 cm size. Also, with utilization of rear-tip extenders, standard 12 cm, 16 cm, and 20 cm sizes can be extended appropriately. This device is relatively new and has yet to be proven, though it seems to offer advantages over other flexible prostheses by its greater versatility of sizing as well as positioning of the prosthesis (Product Information, American Medical Systems).

All these devices offer certain advantages. It is most important that the physician become acquainted with the device to be used and is comfortable with its insertion. All these devices can be placed via the various approaches described. Our preference is the subcoronal incision or the penoscrotal incision. These offer a simple incision which heals readily and with minimal pain. With the semirigid, since the erect state produced by the prosthesis can lead to a paraphimosis resulting in the need for emergency intervention, it is preferable that a circumcision be carried out in the uncircumcized patient at the time of implantation—if this is agreeable to the patient.

## INFLATABLE PROSTHESES

Since the inflatable penile prosthesis was first developed and described by Scott, Bradley, and Timm in 1973 (Scott et al., 1973), there have been multiple revisions of the initial design (Scott et al., 1983). The initial device consisted of an inflate pump, a deflate pump, a reservoir, and paired inflatable penile cylinders. Subsequent design modifications have enabled the inflate and deflate mechanisms to be combined into one mechanism, thus eliminating the need for two pumps and sundry redundant connection tubings. The initial device had 6 segments of silicone rubber tubing and the current prosthesis has only 3 segments. To the patient, the benefits of this device are that in the flaccid state, it is unrecognizable from a normal phallus and upon inflation, it becomes indistinguishable from a normal physiologic erection. Because the cylinders are expandable, they conform to the patient's own corporal anatomy adding to the natural quality of these erections. However, it is this expandable quality which results in one of the most common complications—aneurysm formation. Another advantage of the inflatable over the semirigid prosthesis is that due to its flaccidity in the nonerect state, transurethral surgery can be performed without difficulty and there is little likelihood of erosion of the prosthesis through the glans, which can occur in 2 percent of patients with semirigid prostheses (Jonas, 1983; Small, 1983).

The major disadvantage of the inflatable prosthesis is the high mechanical failure rate. Of the 55 prostheses that had been implanted by F. Brently Scott and coworkers (1979), 52 or 95 percent had mechanical failure. Of the 95 prostheses implanted in 1982, there was one mechanical failure for an incidence of 0.01 (Scott et al., 1983). These improved results are attributable to the evolution of the surgical technique as well as the prosthesis itself. Several of the recent innovations have included the replacement of the initial reservoir with a seamless spherical design. From February 1973 to August 1974, the reservoir accounted for a failure rate of 16 percent. (Failures divided by n.) In the most recent reservoir design (interval from September 1980 to April 1982), the incidence of failures due to reservoir leaks was 0.004 (Scott et al., 1983). In addition, the incorporation of rear-tip extenders, which has facilitated the sizing procedure, more importantly reduces the mechanical failures of the cylinders due to abrasion of cylinder tubing against the prosthesis. The newest prosthesis referred to as the IPP 700 has stronger, thicker cylinder walls. Long-term data are not yet available to indicate improved cylinder reliability. However, the use of rear-tip extenders has increased the chance of a cylinder surviving for 4.5 years to 93 percent ± 5 percent, from 81 percent ± 5 percent. The value of these rear-tip extenders is pointed out by Malloy's group (1982) who had a one percent failure rate with the utilization of the rear-tip extenders as opposed to an 8 percent failure rate in a group of men receiving inflatable prostheses without rear-tip extenders. Although these data were not statistically significant, and life-table analysis was not utilized, these data certainly seem to suggest that these innovations will decrease the problem of tube wear on the cylinders and resultant mechanical failure (Malloy et al., 1982). The scrotal approach as well as kink resistant tubing have also decreased the incidence of connection tubing kinking, which was previously a frequent complication via the suprapubic approach (Scott et al., 1983). Kinks have also been greatly reduced by the use of right-angle tube connectors between the cylinders and tubing (Kaufman et al., 1982). These advances in the mechanical design of the prosthesis, as well as its surgical implantation, have made the inflatable prosthesis a more reasonable alternative for the impotent male. The results of the newer prosthesis designs are not yet available to assess the true incidence of failure. However, with continued design modifications and further advances in surgical techniques it is likely that mechanical failure will be greatly diminished.

There are two basic surgical techniques for the implantation of the inflatable penile prosthesis. A full description of these approaches is beyond the realm of this chapter. Briefly, however, the suprapubic approach uses either a midline or transverse suprapubic incision. The rectus muscles are separated and the reservoir is placed beneath the rectus muscles. The tubing from the reservoir is then brought through a separate opening in the rectus fascia inferiority. The corporal bodies are then identified at the most inferior margin of the midline incision beyond the pubis. The corporal bodies so identified are then incised and, utilizing Hegar dilators, dilated both proximally and distally. The corporal length is then measured. The appropriate size prosthesis is selected and inserted and rear-tip extenders are used as necessary to bring the cylinder tubing exit directly from the corporal incision at a right-angle without lying on the portion of the prosthesis just distal to the tube exit. This will prevent the cylinder wear. With the prosthesis positioned, a scrotal pouch is made for the pump mechanism. The pump mechanism is positioned within the scrotum as far inferiorally as possible and all tubing connections are made. Care is taken during the procedure to assure that there are no air bubbles within the tubing and that all the components function normally at the time of insertion. A Foley catheter is in place during the procedure and is left in for 24 hours postoperatively. Perioperative antibiotic prophylaxis is given as with any prosthetic device.

A relatively new insertion technique involves utilizing a scrotal approach for placement of the entire prosthesis. The scrotal approach has the advantage of having no abdominal incision. The reservoir is placed via the scrotal incision into the external inguinal ring. At this point, using a Metzenbaum scissor or a special instrument for passage of the reservoir, the transversalis fascia forming the floor of the inguinal canal is perforated and the reservoir is placed in the retropubic space. The remainder of the procedure is similar to that of the suprapubic approach.

As for results, in the original publication by Scott et al., (1973), the reoperation rate was 41.6 percent of the patients (n=12). However, recently the reoperation rate (Scott, 1979) was only 17 percent. Furlow's (1979) results parallel those of Scott's with initial reoperation rate of 27 percent dropping to 6 percent more recently.

Other than mechanical failures, the major complication is infection of the prosthesis, which is reported to occur in up to 3 percent of the patients and necessitates complete removal of the prosthetic device. Erosion of the scrotal pump occurs in a similar number. Phimosis and scrotal hematoma occur less frequently, but may be significant complications. That the inflatable prosthesis is not likely to erode through the corporal bodies is indicated by the incidence of one in 1243 cases (Clinical experience from 1973–1979 compiled in 1979 by the American Medical Systems, Inc., 3312 Goram Avenue, Minneapolis, Minnesota, 55426).

The progress made with the inflatable prosthesis is significant and the utilization of the penile prosthesis for patients with organic impotence has become routine. The results of these newer devices are yet to become available, but they represent significant advancements. Patient selection for an inflatable penile prosthesis by virtue of its higher complication rate must be somewhat more discriminatory. The patient must be aware that there is a chance that a second surgical procedure may be necessary. Also, the inflatable prosthesis may cost the patient more. (The price of one complete inflatable prosthesis on a replacement basis is $1,980-American Medical Systems, domestic price list, August, 1982.) Certain patients are not bothered by these cautions and want this prosthesis, whereas others in different life circumstances are not interested in the prospect of further surgical intervention. There is no wrong or right approach in terms of which prosthesis is used. The physician must be aware of all options and, if not comfortable with the utilization of one of them, should refer the patient for therapy elsewhere.

## THERAPY FOR PSYCHOGENIC ERECTILE DYSFUNCTION

"SEX THERAPY"

The treatment of erectile dysfunction of psychogenic origin, no longer relies on traditional psychoanalytic therapies. This major advance is the result of the landmark work by Masters and Johnson (1970), whose work clearly demonstrated that patients with erectile problems suffer concerns and anxieties of a minor nature and that with a direct approach, these can be alleviated with satisfactory results (Hengeveld, 1983). The main elements of sex therapy are sexual information, reassurance, encouragement, and general psychological support.

The concept of performance anxiety is the cornerstone of sex therapy. The patient becomes fixated on his sexual performance and takes the role of an observer in sexuality. The essential component of the sex therapy as advanced by Masters and Johnson involves the sensate focus exercises. These are regimented exercises in which the patient and his partner are brought through degrees of sexual activity, initially avoiding intercourse. The aim is to enhance the sexual and erotic aspects of the sexual experience. This process consists of educational presentation, educational discussions and couple exercises. Though therapy was initially described as a 2-week period away from the home environment, this requirement has generally not been met by therapists and is carried out within the normal environmental setting (Hengeveld, 1983). The major goal in the Masters and Johnson approach is to avoid self-observation and evaluation during sexual activity (Masters and Johnson, 1970). The progressive exercise technique enables the patient to realize the normalcy of his sexual activity and remove the goal of achieving sexual intercourse. This non-goal-oriented approach is very successful in dealing with psychogenic sexual dysfunction.

The approach of Masters and Johnson has been modified by Kaplan (1974). In this approach, there is integration of the psychoanalytic therapy with traditional sex therapy. This emphasizes the treatment of underlying and intrapersonal, as well as interpersonal, conflicts, which often become apparent while utilizing sensate focus techniques.

### OTHER THERAPEUTIC APPROACHES

**Traditional Behavior Therapy.** Behavior therapy utilizes the systemic desensitization work as presented by Wolpe (1958). This more traditional desensitization therapy is one where a series of anxiety-provoking scenarios are listed and ranked in degree of increasing anxiety provocation. The patient then progresses through these scenes—from the least to the greatest anxiety-provoking. The patient learns to experience each scene without anxiety and progresses to the next level. These scenes must be visualized in a state of deep muscle relaxation which is incompatible with anxiety provocation.

The difference between the Masters and Johnson approach and that of Wolpe's systematic desensitization is that the sexual arousal is a response that competes with anxiety in the Masters and Johnson approach, whereas in Wolpe's approach, relaxation is the competing response (Osborne, 1981).

**Biofeedback Technique.** These methods have been attempted in the treatment of male sexual dysfunction and are based on the evidence that non-patient subjects may have some voluntary control over the erectile response (Jensen and Rubin, 1971). The results from the utilization of biofeedback techniques have not been encouraging (Reynolds, 1980), and this technique is not generally used for the therapy of sexual dysfunction.

**Individual Therapy.** The approaches that have been discussed thus far have focused on the couple as the therapeutic unit. Zilbergeld (1978) has described a behavior modification method that does not utilize a sexual partner. This program combines both the Masters and Johnson as well as the Wolpe techniques. The patient goes through a series of exercises beginning with masturbation without sexual fantasies and progressing through imaginary sexual activity, including intromission and orgasm (Zilbergeld, 1978).

## PREMATURE EJACULATION

Another problem that needs to be discussed when dealing with sexual dysfunction is treatment for premature ejaculation. The technique, commonly referred to as the *squeeze technique,* is based on heightening the man's awareness of his sexual cues. Rather than disassociating from the sexual act as is a natural reaction in most men with sexual dysfunction, the man is taught to fixate on the sexual awareness so that stimulation can be discontinued prior to ejaculation and the glans penis squeezed. This will inhibit the ejaculatory process. The feeling of inevitability will pass and intromission may resume. While initially espoused by Semans (1956), it was widely popularized by Masters and Johnson and evolved to become the squeeze technique.

The psychogenic etiology of impotence is difficult to ascertain. It is important to realize that individual psychiatric factors in and of themselves have little prognostic significance because the same factors that result in impotence can result from sexual dysfunction (Karacan and Illaria, 1978).

## CONCLUSION

Impotence has been defined and we have attempted to outline the techniques available for establishing its etiology. Initially, one must determine if the patient's sexual dysfunction is based on organic or psychogenic abnormalities. When this determination has been made, an investigation can be resumed for potential etiologies of sexual dysfunction. Many of the components of normal sexual function can be studied but their true relevance to the abnormal sexual function is yet to be established. We have many pieces of the jigsaw puzzle, but how they fit together is not clear. Occasionally, the search will identify what we consider a specific correctable cause of male sexual dysfunction and then the therapy may be directed in a specific fashion. Most often, we are left with a patient who is impotent on what we believe to be primarily a psychogenic or an organic basis but this differentiation can never be sharp. Psychological sequela follow sexual dysfunction even if it is organically based. We attempt to treat specifically but most often, our therapy is nonspecific. The modern penile prosthetic devices offer great relief to many patients who previously would have had no opportunity for cure. The patients diagnosed as having psychogenic impotence can now be treated more effectively with techniques directed specifically at correcting the dysfunction. Although we have made great progress in diagnostic and therapeutic modalities, there is still much that we do not understand concerning the regulation of *normal* sexual function and, therefore, our understanding of sexual dysfunction is even less clear.

## REFERENCES

Abel, G.; Becker, J. V.; Kunningham-Rathner, J.; Nittelman, M.; and Primack, M.: Differential diagnosis of impotence in diabetics: validity of sexual symptomatology. *Neurourol. Urodynam.*, 1:57, 1982.

Abelson, D.: Diagnostic value of penile pulse and blood pressure: a Doppler study of impotence in diabetes. *J. Urol.*, 113:636, 1975.

Adikan, P. G., and Karim, S. M.: Male sexual dysfunction during treatment with Cimetidine, *Br. Med. J.*, 1:1282, 1979.

American Medical Systems: *Clinical Experience* (1973–1979). American Medical Systems, Inc., Minneapolis, Minn. 1979.

Aserinsky, E., and Kleitman, N.: Regularly occurring periods of eye motility and concominant phenomena during sleep. *Science*, 188:273, 1953.

Barber, S. G.: Male sexual dysfunction and cimetidine. *Br. Med. J.*, 1:1147, 1979.

Barry, J. M.; Blank, B.; and Boileau, M.: Nocturnal penile tumescence monitoring with stamps. *Urology*, 15:171, 1980.

Bartsch, G., and Scheiber, K.: Endocrinologic aspects of disturbed potency. *World J. Urol.*, 1:197, 1983.

Bennett, T.; Evans, D. F.; and Hosking, D. J.: Physiologic investigation of male diabetics complaining of impotence. *J. Physiol.*, 272:190, 1977.

Blaivas, J. G.: The diagnosis and treatment of erectile dysfunction. In Krane, R. J.; Siroky, M. B.: (eds.): *Clinical Neurourology*. Little, Brown, Boston, 1979.

Blaivas, J. G.; O'Connell, T. F.; Gottlieb, P.; and Labib, K. B.: Comprehensive laboratory evaluation of impotent men. *J. Urol.*, 124:201, 1980a.

Blaivas, J. G.; O'Donnell, T. F.; Gottlieb, P.; and Libib, K. B.: Measurement of bulbocavernosus reflex latency time as part of a comprehensive evaluation of impotence. In Zorgniotti, A. W.; Rossi, G.: (eds.): *Vasculogenic Impotence*. C. C. Thomas, Springfield, Ill., 1980b.

Bohlen, J. G.: Sleep erection monitoring in the evaluation of male erectile dysfunction. *Urol. Clin. N. Am.*, (February) 8:119–134, 1981.

Bors, E., and Comarr, A. E.: *Neurological Urology*. S Karger, Basel, 1971.

Braunstein, G. D.: Endocrine causes of impotence. *Postgrad. Med.*, 74 (4):207–217, 1983.

Buvat, J.; Lemaire, A.; Bresson, P.; Dehane, J. L.; and Buvat-Herbrant, M.: Lack of correlations between penile thermography and pelvic arteriography in 29 cases of erectile impotence. *J. Urol.,* 128:298, 1982.

Carter, J. N.; Tyson, J. E.; and Tolis, G.: Prolactin secreting pituitary tumors and hypogonadism in 22 men. *N. Engl. J. Med.,* 299:852, 1978.

Chippa, K. H., and Ropper, A. H.: Evoked potentials in clinical medicine (Part II). *N. Engl. J. Med.* 306:1205, 1982.

Crespo, E.; Soltanik, E.; Ovbove, D.; and Farrell, G.: Treatment of vasculogenic sexual impotence by revascularizing cavernosus and/or dorsal arteries using microvascular techniques. *Urology,* 20:271, 1982.

Das, S., and Amar, A.: Peyronie's Disease: Excision of the plaque and grafting with tunica vaginalis. *Urol. Clin. N. Am.,* 9:1977, 1982.

Duchen, L. W.; Anjorim, A.; Watkins, P. J.; and Mackay, J. D.: Pathology of autonomic neuropathy and diabetes mellitus. *Ann. Intern. Med.,* 92:301, 1980.

Ebbho, J. J., and Wagner, G.: Insufficient penile erection due to abnormal drainage of cavernous bodies. *Urology,* 13:507, 1979.

Ek, A.; Bradley, W. E.; and Krane, R. J.: Nocturnal penile rigidity measured by the snap-gauge band. *J. Urol.,* 129:964–966, 1983.

Ellenberg, M.: Impotence in diabetes: the neurologic factor. *Ann. Intern. Med.,* 75:213, 1971.

Ertekin, C., and Reel, F.: Bulbocavernosus reflex in normal men in patients with neurogenic bladder and/or impotence. *J. Neurol. Sci.,* 28 1, 1976.

Finney, R. B.: New hinged silicone penile implant. *J. Urol.,* 118:585, 1977.

Fisher, C.; et al: The assessment of nocturnal erection in the differential diagnosis of sexual impotence. *J. Sex Marital Ther.,* 1:277, 1975.

Fisher, C.; Schiavi, R. C.; Edwards, A.; Davis, D. M.; Reitman, M.; and Fine, J.: Evaluation of nocturnal penile tumescence in the differential diagnosis of sexual impotence. A quantitative study. *Arch. Gen. Psychiatr.,* 36:431–437, 1979.

Fitzpatrick, T. J.: Spongiosograms and cavernosograms: A study of their value in priapism. *J. Urol.,* 109:843, 1973.

Furlow, W. L.: Inflatable penile prosthesis. Mayo Clinic Experience with 175 patients. *Urology,* 13:166, 1979.

Godec, C. J., and Cass, A. S.: Quantification of erection. *J. Urol,* 126:345–347, 1981.

Goldstein, I.: Neurologic impotence. In Krane, R. J.; Siroky, M. B.; Goldstein, I.: (eds.): *Male Sexual Dysfunction.* Little Brown, Boston, 1983.

Goldstein, I., Siroky, M. B., Krane, R. J.: Impotence in diabetes mellitus. In Krane, R. J.; Siroky, M. B.; Goldstein, I.: (eds.): *Male Sexual Dysfunction.* Little Brown, Boston, 1983.

Goldstein, I.; Siroky, M. B.; Nath, R. L.; McMillian, T. N.; Menzoian, J. O.; and Krane, R. J.: Vasculogenic impotence: Role of the pelvic steal test. *J. Urol.,* 128:300, 1982.

Haldman, S. et al: Pudendal evoked responses. *Arch. Neurol.,* 39:280, 1982.

Halverson, H. M.: Genital and sphincter behavior of the male infant. *J. Genet. Psychol.,* 56:95, 1940.

Hawatameh, I. S.; Houttuin, E. Gregory, J. G.; Blair, O. M.; and Purcell, N. J.: The diagnosis and surgical management of vasculogenic impotence. *J. Urol.,* 127:910–914, 1982.

Hengeveld, M. W.: Erectile dysfunction: a psychological and psychiatric review. *World J. Urol.,* 1:227–232, 1983.

Herbert, J.: The role of dorsal nerves in the penis and the sexual behavior of the male rhesus monkey. *Physiol. Behav.,* 10:293, 1973.

Henson, D., and Rubin, H. J.: Voluntary control of eroticism. *J. Appl. Behav. Anal.,* 4, 37–44, 1971.

Howard, D. J., and Reese, J. R.: Long-term perhexiline maleate and liver function. *Br. Med. J.,* 1:133, 1976.

Jevitch, M. J.: Importance of penile arterial pulse sound examination in impotence. *J. Urol.,* 124(6):820–824, 1980.

Jonas, U.,: Silikon-Silber-Penisprosthese, *Aktuel Urol.,* 9:179, 1979.

Jonas, U., and Jacobi, G. H.: Silicone-Silver penile prosthesis: description, operative approach, and results. *J. Urol.,* 123:865, 1980.

Jonas, U.: Five years experience with a silicone Silber penile prosthesis: improvements and new developments. *World J. Urol.,* 1:251, 1983.

Kaplan, H. S.: *The New Sex Therapy.* Brunnel/Mazel, New York, 1974.

Karacan, I.: A simple and inexpensive transducer for quantitative measurements of penile erection during sleep. *Behav. Res. Meth. Instrumen.* 1:251, 1969.

Karacan, I.: Clinical value of nocturnal erections in the prognosis and diagnosis of impotence. *Med. Aspects Human Sex.,* 4:27, 1970.

Karacan, I.: Impotence: Psyche vs Soma. *Med. World News,* 17:28, 1976.

Karacan, I.: Diagnosis of erectile impotence in diabetes melitus. An objective and specific method. *Ann. Intern. Med.,* 92:334–337, 1980.

Karacan, I., and Ilaria, R.: Diagnostic advances in impotence. *Encephle,* 4:6, 1978.

Karacan, I.; Hursch, C. J.; and Williams, R. L. Some characteristics of nocturnal penile tumescence in elderly males. *J. Gerontol.,* 27:39, 1972a.

Karacan. I.; A. Sallis, P. J.; and Williams, R. L.: The role of the sleep laboratory in the diagnosis of impotence. In Williams, R. L.; Karacan, I.; Frazier, S. H.: (eds.): *Sleep Disorders: Diagnosis and Treatment.* Wiley, New York, 1978.

Karacan, I.; Hursch, C. J.; Williams, R. L.; and Thornby, J. I.: Some characteristics of nocturnal penile tumescence in young adults. *Arch. Gen. Psychiatr.,* 26:351, 1972b.

Kaufmar, J. J.; Lindner, A.; and Raz, S.: Complications of penile prosthesis surgery for impotence. *J. Urol.,* 128:1192, 1982.

Kempczinski, R. F.: Role of the vascular diagnostic laboratory in the evaluation of male impotence. *Am. J Surg.,* 138:278–282, 1979.

Krane, R. J.; Ek, A.; Bradley, W. E.: Nocturnal penile rigidity measured by the snap gauge band. *J. Urol.,* 5:964–966, 1983.

LaBau, M. M.: Sexual impotence in men having low back syndrome. *Arch. Phys. Med.,* 47:715, 1966.

Malloy, T. R.; Wein, A. J.; and Carpinello, V. L: Improved mechanical survival with revised model inflatable penile prosthesis using rear tip extenders. *J. Urol.,* 128, 489, 1982.

Marshall, P.; Surridge, D.; and Delva, N.: The role of nocturnal penile tumescence and differentiating between organic and psychogenic impotence: The first stage of validation. *Arch. Sex. Behav.,* 10:1–10, 1981.

Masters, W. H., and Johnson, V. E.: *Human Sexual Response.* Little, Brown, Boston, 1966.

Masters, W. H., and Johnson, V. E.: *Human Sexual Inadequacy.* Little, Brown, Boston, 1970.

McHaffie, D. J.; Guz, A.; and Johnston, A.: Impotence in patients on Disopyramide. *Lancet,* 1:859, 1977.

McMillian, D. E.: Deterioration of the microcirculation in diabetes. *Diabetes,* 24:944, 1975.

*The Medical Letter.* Drugs that cause sexual dysfunction. 22:25, 1980.

Metz, P., and Bengtsson, J.: Penile blood pressure. *Scand. J. Urol. Nephrol.,* 15:161, 1981.

Michal, V. et al: Direct arterial anastomosis of corpora cavernosa penis in the therapy of erective impotence. *Rozhledy v Chirurgii* (Praha), 52:587, 1973.

Michal, V.; Kramar, R.; and Pospichal, J.: External illice steal syndrome. *J. Cardio. Vasc. Surg.* (Torino), 19:255, 1978.

Michal, V.; Kramar, R.; Hejhal, L.; and Firt, P.: Aorta illiac occlusive disease. In Zorgniotti, A. W.; Rossi, G.: (eds.): *Vasculogenic Impotence.* Charles C. Thomas, Springfield, Ill., 1980a.

Michal, V.; Pospichal, J.; and Blazkova, J.: Arteriography of the internal penile arteries and passive erection. In Zorgniotti, A. W.; Rossi, G.: (eds.): *Vasculogenic Impotence.* Charles C. Thomas, Springfield, Ill., 1980b.

Michal, V.; Kramar, R.; and Jhal, L.: Revascularization procedure in the cavernus bodies. In Zorgniotti, A. W.; Rossi, G.: (eds.): *Vasculogenic Impotence.* Charles C. Thomas, Springfield, Ill., 1980c.

Montague, D. K.; James, R. E.; Dewolfe, V. G.; and Martin, L. M.: Diagnostic evaluation classification and treatment of men with sexual dysfunction. *Urology,* 14:545, 1979.

Nagler, H. M., and Blaivas, J. G.: Castration and sexual dysfunction. *Med. Aspects Hum. Sex.,* 17:237–241, 1983.

Nagler, H. M.; Katz, P. G.; and deVere White, R.: Role of frenular penile-brachial index in the assessment of penile vasculature. *Neurourology Urodynamics,* 1:71–76, 1982.

Nagler, H. M., and Olsson, C. A.: Drug related male sexual dysfunction. In Krane, R. J.; Siroky, M. B.; Goldstein, I.: (eds.): *Male Sexual Dysfunction.* Little, Brown, Boston, 1983.

Neri, A.: Subjective assessment of sexual dysfunction of patients on long term administration of Digoxin. *Arch. Sex. Behav.,* 9:343, 1980.

Nikitinskaja, L. P.: The significance of dyshormonal changes in the hypothalamo hypothyseal gonadal system in the diagnosis of infertility and impotence in the male. *J. Urol. Nephrol.,* 75:789–792, 1982.

Ohlmeyer, P.; Brilmayer, H.; and Hullstrung, H.: Te:rodische vorgange im schlaf. *Pfluegers Arch.,* 248:559, 1944.

Osborne, D.: Psychological aspects of male sexual dysfunction. *Urol. Clin. N. Am.,* 8:135–142, 1981.

Queral, L. A.; Whitehouse, W. M.; Flinn, W. R.; Zarine, C. K.; Bergan, J. J.; and Yao, J. S. T.: Pelvic hemodynamics after aortoilliac reconstruction. *Surgery,* 86:799, 1979.

Reynolds, B.: Biofeedback and fascilitation erection in men with erectile dysfunction. *Arch. Sex. Behav.,* 9:101–114, 1980.

Robiner, W. M.; Godec, C. J.; Cass, A. S.; and Meyer, J. J.: The role of the Minnesota Multiphasic Personality Inventory in evaluation of erectile dysfunction. *J. Urol.,* 128:487, 1982.

Rubin, A., and Babbott, D.: Impotence in diabetes mellitus. *JAMA,* 168:498, 1958.

Ruzbarsky, V., and Michal, V.: Histologic changes in the penile arterial bed with aging and diabetes. In Zorgniotti, A. W.; Rossi, G.: (eds.): *Vasculogenic Impotence.* Charles C Thomas, Springfield, 1980, p. 113–119.

Rydin, E.; Lundberg, P. L.; and Brattberg, A.: Cystometry and mictometry as tools at diagnosing neurogenic impotence. *Acta Neuro. Scand.,* 63(3):181, 1981.

Sax, D. S.: The history and examination in neurourology. In Krane, R. J.; Siroky, M. D.: (eds.): *Clinical Neurourology.* Little, Brown, Boston, 1979.

Schoenberg, H. W.; Zarins, C. K.; and Segraves, R. T.: Analysis of 122 unselected impotent men subjected to multidisciplinary evaluation. *J. Urol.,* 127:445, 1982.

Schrom, S. H.; Lief, H. I.; and Wein, A. J.: Clinical profile of experience with 130 consecutive cases of impotent males. *Urology,* 8:511, 1979.

Scott, F. B.; Bradley, W. E.; and Timm, G.: Management of erectile impotence. Use of an implantable, inflatable prosthesis. *Urology,* 2:80, 1973.

Scott, F. B.; Bryd, G. J.; Karacon, I.; Olsson, P.; Beutler, L. E.; and Attia, L. L.: Erectile impotence treated with an implantable, inflatable prosthesis. *JAMA,* 241:2609, 1979.

Scott, F. B.; Fishman, I. J.; and Light, J. K.: A decade of experience with inflatable penile prosthesis. *World J. Urol.,* 1:244, 1983.

Semens, J. H.: Premature ejaculation: a new approach. *South. Med. J.,* 49:353, 357, 1956.

Shafer, N.: Occult lumbar disc causing impotency. *N.Y. State J. Med.,* 69:2465, 1969.

Shirai, M.; Ishii, N.; Mitsukawa, S.; Matsuda, S.; and Nakamura, M.: Human dynamic mechanism of erection in the human penis. *Arch. Androl.,* 1:345, 1978.

Small, M. P.; Carrion, H. M.; and Gordon, J. A.: Small–Carrion prosthesis: new implant for management for impotence. *Urology,* 5:479–486, 1975.

Small, M. P.: The Small–Carrion Penile Implant. In Krane, R. J.; Siroky, M. B.; Goldstein, I. G.: (eds.): *Male Sexual Dysfunction.* Little, Brown, Boston, 1983.

Smith, A. D.: Causes and classifications of impotence. *Urol. Clin. N. Am.,* Feb.: 119, 1981.

Smith, A. D., and Fischer, S. C.: Behavioral treatments of erectile insufficiency. In Krane, R. J.; Siroky, M. B.; Goldstein, I.: (eds.): *Male Sexual Dysfunction.* Little, Brown, Boston, 1983.

Spark, R. F.; White, R. A.; and Connolly, S.: Impotence is not always psychogenic. *JAMA,* 243:750, 1980.

Torrens, N. J.: Neurological and neurosurgical disorders associated with impotence. In Krane, R. J.; Siroky,

M. B.; Goldstein, I.: (eds.): *Male Sexual Dysfunction.* Little, Brown, Boston, 1983.

Van Arsdalen, K. N., and Wein, A. J.: A critical review of diagnostic tests used in the evaluation of the impotent male. *World J. Urol.,* 1:218–225, 1983.

Velcek, D.; Sniderman, K. W.; Vaughan E. D. Jr.; Sos, T. A.; and Muecke, E. C.: Penile flow index utilizing a Doppler pulse wave analysis to identify penile vascular insufficiency. *J. Urol.,* 123:669, 1980.

Veterans Administration Cooperative Study Group on Antihypertensive agents. Propanalol in the treatment of essential hypertension. *JAMA,* 237:2303, 1977.

Wabreck, A. J.: *Penile rigidity—Concepts and correlations.* Paper presented at the 5th World Congress of Sexology, Jerusalem, Israel, June 23, 1981.

Wagner, G.: Methods for differential diagnosis of psychogenic and organic erectile dysfunction. In Wagner, G.; Green, R.: (eds.): *Impotence, Physiological, Psychological, Surgical Diagnosis and Treatment.* Plenum Press, New York, 1981.

Waxberg, J. D.: Sexual therapy of diabetic impotence. *Conn. Med.,* 42:555, 1978.

Weiderman, C. L., and Northcutt, R. C.: Endocrine aspects of impotence. *Urol. Clin. N. Am.,* 8:143, 1981.

Wershub, L. B.: *Sexual Impotence in the Male.* Charles C. Thomas, Springfield, Ill., 1959.

Wild, R. M.; DeVine, C. J.; and Horton, C. E.: Dermal graft repair of Peyronie's disease: Survey of 50 patients. *J. Urol.,* 121:47, 1979.

Wolpe, J.: *Psychotherapy by Reciprocol Inhibition.* Stanford University Press, Stanford, Calif., 1953.

Wolpe, J.: *The Practice of Behavior Therapy.* Pergamon, New York, 1969.

Zafar Khan, Barry, J. M., Blank, B. and Boileau, M.: Nocturnal penile tumescence monitoring with stamps. *Urology,* 15:171, 1980.

Zannini, G.: Diabetic arteriopathy. *J. Cardiovasc. Surg.,* 15:68, 1974.

Zilbergeld, B.: *Male Sexuality.* Little, Brown, Boston, 1978.

Zorgniotti, A. W.; Rossi, G.; Padula, G.; and Makovisky, R. D.: Diagnosis and therapy of vasculogenic impotence. *J. Urol.,* 123:674, 1980.

# CHAPTER 21 NEUROLOGIC DISEASE AND SEXUAL FUNCTION

*Richard I. Katz, M.D.*

## INTRODUCTION

The area of human sexuality in medical practice has often received low priority compared to other psychological factors. Only in the last decade or so have issues of sexual health gained prominence as a subject worthy of scientific inquiry and one respectable enough to be admitted as a major consideration in health care. Diseases of the nervous system can interfere with sexual activity in diverse ways at many levels. In patients with well-defined brain, spinal cord, or neuromuscular deficits, the underlying anatomic or pathophysiologic basis of sexual dysfunction may be apparent, but psychological influences related to inevitable emotional responses by the patient or the partner complicate even the most simple problem. With notable exceptions, neurologists have avoided the issue of sexuality; it is our purpose to review current concepts of neuroanatomy, neurophysiology, diagnostic, clinical, and rehabilitative science as it relates to human sexuality.

## ANATOMY AND PHYSIOLOGY

The bulk of knowledge of the anatomy and physiology of neurologic structures responsible for sexual function relates to spinal cord and peripheral nerves. While the neuroendocrine basis of sexual behavior has focused on the hypothalamic-hypophysiogonadal axis, information regarding higher neural circuits has only recently been emphasized (Blumer and Walker, 1975).

In an effort to characterize the neural foundation of sex in the brain, Blumer and Walker (1975) provide an excellent review, exploring animal studies, experiences with humans, and the relationship of sex and epilepsy. The importance of the hypothalamus for the overt expression of sexual behavior has been documented and a hormone-dependent neuronal system initiating copulation has been localized in the preoptic-hypothalamic region in almost all species studied (Lisk, 1967b). Implants of estrogens or testosterone proprionate and electrical stimulation in the area elicit the copulatory response, while destructive lesions decrease or eliminate sexual behavior; this is not restored by exogenous hormone therapy. A second center exists in the median eminence region that regulates gonadotrophin release, and exogenous hormone replacement restores the mating ability in animals lesioned in this area. An inhibitory system regulating the level of sex drive is located in the territory of the ventral border of the diencephalon and mesencephalon and is based on observations of increased copulation after lesions of the posterior hypothalamus and mammilary bodies in the male rat (Lisk, 1967a). It has been postulated that the overt sexual behavior of both male and female depends on the balance of activity between a hormone-dependent integrative and facilitory system, probably located in the region of the mammilary bodies.

Although less amenable to unifying hypotheses, experiments in the monkey and rat cortex have demonstrated hypersexuality after removal of both temporal lobes, amygdala, and piriform cortex. Detailed stereotactic electrical stimulation of subcortical structures in the squirrel monkey has dramatized the biological basis for sexual expression and aggressive social behavior—at least in the monkey. The vast gap between animal and human sexual behavior is dramatized by the relative unimportance of cerebral cortex in maintenance of mating behavior in most female mammals, and Bard (1939) removed increasingly larger portions of the cortex in the cat until all of the neocortex, most of the rhinencephalon, and a large part of striatum and thalamus were destroyed—without eliminating estrous behavior in response to estrogen. In contrast, cortex has been found essential for the initiation of mating behavior in most male mammals, perhaps relating to the more complicated sequence of recognition, orientation, mounting, pelvic thrusting, intromission, and ejaculation involved in the performance of the complete copulatory response in the male as opposed to the more passive response in the (non-human) female (Blumer and Walker, 1975). Finally, the Kluver–Bucy syndrome (1937) in which wild, aggressive monkeys were subjected to bilateral temporal lobectomy, should be mentioned. Not only did the monkeys become more docile, but striking changes in sexual behavior occurred with spontaneous erection and/or presenting reactions occurring on the approach of a human observer, suggesting manifest hypersexuality.

Various aspects of human sexual behavior may be affected by focal, regional, or diffuse cortical and/or subcortical disease, but for the most part, neurologic studies have underscored the significant vulnerability of sexual function to cerebral injuries rather than specific localization of such functions (Blumer and Walker, 1975). It is of interest that human sexual arousal may be instantaneous and may occur independently of any change in sex hormones in the circulating blood. Threshold complements of androgen need to be present for normal sexual behavior in man and castration, use of antiandrogenic compounds, such as progesterone, or sectioning of the hypophyseal stalk can abolish male sexual arousal by abnormally lowering androgen levels (Blumer and Migeon, 1975).

The most compelling evidence reflecting a higher neural basis for sexual behavior in man is derived from observations in patients with partial complex (temporal lobe) epilepsy. (See Blumer, 1970; Blumer and Walker, 1975 for comprehensive review.) Kluver and Bucy (1937) initially reported dramatic alterations in sexual behavior—namely hypersexuality, following bilateral temporal lobectomies in rhesus monkeys. The hypersexuality coincided with a marked diminution of anger and fear and excessive tendency to notice and attend to all stimuli in sight ("hypermetamorphosis"), a continuous need to take everything to the mouth ("oral tendencies") and a continuous inability to recognize objects (psychic blindness). The so-called Kluver–Bucy syndrome (1939) engendered much interest in the relationship of the temporal lobes to behavior, and it became apparent that the limbic medial portion of the temporal lobe was responsible for the behavioral changes. In man, bilateral anterior temporal lobectomies can produce such hypersexuality, but after this radical operation had been performed in a few chronic debilitated schizophrenics and epileptics, its devastating effect on memory became apparent and, for neuropsychiatric as well as ethical reasons, the bilateral procedure was abandoned.

An equally dramatic aberration in human sexual behavior was reported in patients with partial complex (temporal lobe) epilepsy by Gastaut and Collomb (1954), who noted marked global hyposexuality in more than half of their patients with this seizure type. The authors reasoned that sexual change in temporal lobe epilepsy (hyposexuality) was, not surprisingly, the opposite of the change after bilateral temporal lobectomy (hypersexuality); the former was due to the continuous excessive activity of the medial temporal structures, while the latter resulted from lack of neural activity from the same area.

The relationship of sexuality and epilepsy has been examined in regard to interictal, ictal, and postictal sexuality. Understandably, the most abundant data is derived from observation of the interictal phase and it appears that sexual *normality* is the exception and that global hyposexuality predominates—perhaps in as many as 60 percent of subjects studied (Blumer and Walker, 1967). Since most study groups were patients with medically intractable epilepsy—many ultimately requiring seizure surgery—effects of chronic illness, polypharmacy, and more diffuse brain involvement probably contribute; but even in less severely affected subjects, such hyposexuality has been repeatedly documented and includes marked decrease in libido, diminished genital arousal as well as impotence (Blumer and Walker, 1975).

Although it has been known that selective lesions of the temporal lobe limbic complex causes hypogonadotrophic hypogonadism as well as hyperprolactinemia in animals, suggesting that the temporal lobe is important in modulating neuroendocrine function in animals, a comparable role has not been specifically defined for the human temporal lobe. Based on observations that individuals with temporal lobe epilepsy are often hyposexual, oligomenorrheic, infertile, and impotent, the diagnosis of previously unrecognized temporal lobe epilepsy has recently been reported in a group of hyposexual males with hypogonadism and hyperprolactinemia. In these men with neuroendocrine dysfunction and temporal lobe epilepsy, the most effective therapeutic sequence was first to treat the epilepsy with anticonvulsants and then to add appropriate neuroendocrine therapy. In half the patients, sexual function was restored on anticonvulsant therapy alone (Spark *et al.,* 1984).

The most convincing confirmation of the relationship of mesiotemporal seizure discharges and sexual arousal are findings in patients who were previously hyposexual but are completely free from any seizure activity after unilateral temporal lobectomy. Normalization of sexual desire and ability occurs and occasionally, a marked hypersexuality presents in the second postoperative month. Further, the hypersexuality is reversed if there is recurrence of temporal lobe seizures after surgery (Blumer and Walker, 1967).

The subject of ictal sexual manifestation has been reported mainly in complex partial seizures, usually relating to temporal or parietal seizure origin but occasionally frontal or other subcortical structures. A single report depicts absence (*petit mal*) status epilepticus manifest by compulsive masturbation (Jacome and Risko, 1983). Such manifestations may take the form of automatisms, emotionalism, or somatosensory phenomena in the genitals (defined as clinical mannerisms that encompass exhibitionism, masturbatory, or other sexual activity for which the patient is amnesic (Spencer *et al.,* 1983). Postictal sexual arousal, typically manifest by exhibitionism or confused undressing, occurs and occasionally, brief seemingly appropriate hypersexual episodes for which the patient is not amnesic, may follow a seizure (Blumer and Walker, 1975).

Homosexuality, particularly transvestism and fetishistic deviations, and, rarely, more apparent perversions may occur but like unprovoked rage in temporal lobe epilepsy, well-documented cases are quite rare. It must be noted that although abundant behavioral observations in temporal lobe epileptics reflect a relation to sexuality, the cellular-neuronal basis of the "cerebrocognitive" aspect of sexuality remains to be elucidated.

Recently, neuroendocrine observations have aided differential diagnosis of seizures as well as the traditional neuropsychiatric dilemma of distinguishing factitious (hysterical) from authentic seizures—a distinction which still carries a 30 to 50 percent error rate even with the aid of modern video electroencephalogram (EEG) monitoring in sophisticated epilepsy units. Many investigators have now confirmed that serum prolactin increases during seizures, especially after generalized epilepsy, but also with partial complex seizures (Dana-Haeri et al., 1983; Pritchard et al., 1983). Maximum increases are seen at 15–20 minutes, although elevations are apparent immediately after the seizure has occurred. Return to baseline takes place within one hour. Luteinizing hormone (LH) values also rise immediately, remain elevated at 20 minutes and, in contrast to prolactin levels, LH remains elevated one hour later. Follicle-stimulating hormone (FSH) changes have been less constant and are noted mainly in females (Dana-Haeri et al., 1983). Particularly in an emergency room or psychiatric setting, such observations have become remarkably helpful in diagnosis and initiation of appropriate therapy.

## HEADACHE

Although rarely related to well-defined central nervous system disease, headaches related to sexual activity may interfere with normal sexual function in otherwise healthy individuals. As reviewed by Lance (1976), the sudden appearance of headache during sexual intercourse, particularly at the time of orgasm may give rise to anxiety with thoughts of imminent death from cerebral hemorrhage, although subarachnoid bleeding precipitated by sexual intercourse is distinctly rare. Such headaches have been granted various rubrics including "benign orgasmic cephalalgia," "benign coital headache," "benign masturbatory cephalalgia," and the more inclusive term, "benign sex headache," has been suggested (Lana, 1976). The pathophysiology appears to relate to muscle contraction and/or vascular (migrainous) factors.

In the absence of associated history or other symptoms, it is probably fair to say that the development of headache during sexual activity, which is bilateral (particularly occipital) and accompanied by awareness of contraction of the neck and facial muscles, may be regarded as benign and may require no further investigation other than reassurance, explanation of the likely mechanism, and some direction about how to help the patient relax the involved muscles. Since such patients appear to be vulnerable to benign sex headaches on one occasion and not on another, the development of abrupt headache during sexual activity might be regarded as a warning to desist on that particular occasion, since orgasm usually aggravates headache.

## EFFECTS OF MEDICATION

Drugs may affect sexual function in diverse ways and often, effects of a disease process are difficult to separate from adverse effects of pharmacologic intervention, such as anticonvulsants for seizure disorder, antidepressants or neuroleptics for psychiatric disease, and cardiac medications. In such situations, temporary and often prolonged drug withdrawal may be necessary.

Undoubtedly because the cerebrocognitive aspects of sexuality remain so poorly understood, "central effects" are generally presented collectively, while more detail is applied to effects on sympathetic, parasympathetic, or skeletal neuromuscular function. Focusing primarily on problems with libido, erectile capacity, orgasm, ejaculation, and autonomic effects, systematic efforts and classification of drug effects have been made and with rare exception, include studies of males only. These studies present observations on antihypertensive, antidepressant, antipsychotic, anxiolytic, antiparkinsonian, and anticonvulsant agents as well as alcohol (Boller and Frank, 1982; DeLeo and Magni, 1983). Generally, such studies have lacked the use of control groups, proper statistical methodology, the exclusion of subjects with pre-existing sexual disturbances, the certainty that the drug is being regularly taken (measurement of blood levels of the drug or its metabolites), systematic records of the dose at which sexual disturbances arise, and adequate duration of the trial (De-

Leo and Magni, 1983). Nonetheless, the possibility that drugs may contribute to sexual dysfunction in the individual patient must be considered.

## NEUROANATOMY OF SPINAL CORD AND PERIPHERAL NERVE

The neuroanatomic substrate of sexual dysfunction secondary to disorders of spinal cord and peripheral nerve is better defined than for the cerebrocognitive syndromes. The drawings of Frank Netter, M.D. remain (CIBA Foundation, 1962) the touchstone for graphic depiction of sexual anatomy and its innervation, and a detailed exegesis including reproduction of these remarkable drawings is available (Verkuyl, 1976). Although the differential diagnosis of spinal cord syndromes in daily practice includes such diverse entities as compressive (spondylosis, tumor, hematoma), ischemic, metabolic, demyelinating, and congenital disorders, from an epidemiologic standpoint, the bulk of spinal cord dysfunction results from vehicular and related trauma and clinical rehabilitative approaches are characterized in relation to partial or complete myelopathy with efforts to define a segmental localization. Precise anatomy of ascending and descending spinal pathways remains poorly defined. Central afferent stimuli including olfactory, visual, auditory, and somesthetic stimuli to the cranial nerves reach the cerebral cortex, then the sympathetic and parasympathetic nuclei of the hypothalamus. Efferent spinal tracts include:

1. somatic efferents from the cerebral cortex; the pyramidal tract extending to the spinal anterior horn cells
2. visceral efferents from the hypothalamus
   a) to the thoracolumbar lateral horn sympathetic preganglionic cells;
   b) to the sacral parasympathetic preganglionic cells and;
   c) to the paraependymal fasciculus traveling to the lumbar and sacral cord.

The spinal segmental and peripheral innervation of sexual organs are best described together and a detailed, well-illustrated review is available (Boller and Frank, 1982). In the male, the sympathetic nervous system supplies fibers to the vas deferens, seminal vesicles, prostate, and testes. The cells of origin of the preganglionic fibers form a distinct group in the gray matter of the cord—the intermediolateral column. The sympathetic fibers innervating sexual organs are in the intermediolateral column of the lower thoracic (T10–T12) and upper lumbar (L1–L2) segments of the spinal cord, and these preganglionic fibers follow the presacral and hypogastric nerves ending on the hypogastric plexus or close to the structures they supply. The postganglionic fibers with which they synapse form a plexus near the smooth muscle of the end organs. From these organs comes an afferent (sensory) sympathetic system that follows in reverse the course of the sympathetic efferents and enter the spinal cord at the lower thoracic and upper lumbar (T10–L1) level.

The preganglionic parasympathetic fibers originate in the intermediolateral nucleus of the second sacral to fourth sacral spinal cord. The fibers travel in S2–S4 ventral roots and form the pelvic nerves, classically termed *nervi erigentes,* which join the hypogastric plexus and end in the erectile tissue of the corpus cavernosa and corpus spongeosum of the penis. Parasympathetic fibers also reach the prostate, seminal vesicles, vas deferens, and the ejaculatory ducts. An afferent parasympathetic system follows the same course, entering the spinal cord at the posterior roots of S2–S4.

The somatic (voluntary) innervation originates from anterior horn cells of S2–S4 and the fibers travel in the pudendal nerves, ending in the bulbocavernosus and ischiocavernosus muscles. The pudendal nerves also carry sensory fibers responsible for skin sensation over the S2–S5 dermatomes and this includes the so-called saddle area surrounding and including anus, scrotum, and penis. Boller and Frank (1982) have reviewed the sequence of neurologic events involved in sexual function in the male, which requires harmonious participation of the parasympathetic, sympathetic, and somatic divisions. Erection occurs as a result of vasocongestion within the sponge-like erectile tissue of the corpora cavernosum and corpora spongiosum of the penis. Stimulation of the pelvic parasympathetic nerves produces dilatation of the arteries and constriction of the veins of these spongy tissues, thus causing and maintaining erection. It is generally thought that sympathetic activity can also produce erection, although parasympathetic activity is primary (Bors and Turner, 1967). It has been postulated that the sacral (parasympathetic) erectile center is primarily responsible for reflexogenic erections (erections produced by direct physical stimulation of the genitalia) whereas the thoracolumbar (sympathetic) erectile center mediates psychogenic erection produced by mental stimuli. Ordinarily, both centers act synergistically and produce penile erection (Weiss, 1972).

The neurological basis of ejaculation appears to be more complex. For semen to be emitted, it must first be expelled into the prostatic urethra, a process dependent on the hypogastric sympathetic nerves. Emission and ejaculation are caused by the contraction of the bulbocavernosus and ischiocavernosus muscles modulated by the pudendal (somatic) nerve.

In the female, the ovaries are innervated by the sympathetic nervous system. The preganglionic fibers originate in the intermediolateral column of the lower thoracic (T10–T11) level and are part of the splanchnic nerves up to their synapse in the ovarian ganglion near the origin of the ovarian artery. The postganglionic fibers constitute the ovarian plexus which sends fibers to the ovary. It also supplies the fallopian tubes and broad ligament, which receive additional sympathetic supply from the hypogastric plexus and parasympathetic supply from the uterine plexus. The pattern of mixed sympathetic and parasympathetic supply applies also to the uterus and to the vagina and as in the male, parasympathetic supply derives from S2–S4 sacral segments and follows the pelvic nerves.

The somatic nervous supply to the female genital organs is provided by the pudendal nerve, which, as in the male, derives from S2–S4 spinal cord segments and passes to the lateral wall of the ischiorectal fossa, where it gives off the internal hemorrhoidal nerve and this divides into two terminal branches. The first is the perineal nerve that sends sensory fibers to the vulva and motor fibers to the superficial perineal muscles, the anal and vaginal sphincters, and levator ani. The other terminal branch is the dorsal nerve of the clitoris which is purely afferent (sensory); its sensory receptors are located in relation to the cavernous tissue which receives efferent (vasomotor) innervation of parasympathetic fibers to the cavernous plexus.

Most authors agree that the autonomic nervous system is not essential to fertility, since females with a denervated uterus can menstruate, become pregnant, and deliver normally. The role of the neural supply to the clitoris and other parts of the external genitalia is better defined. The parasympathetic nervous system contributes to the microscopic and, when present, macroscopic tumescence of the clitoris and produces increased vaginal secretion. As has been pointed out, tumescence of the clitoris has been equated to erection in the male but it has been noted that the clitoris is a unique organ limited in its physiologic function to initiating and elevating levels of sexual tension (Masters and Johnson, 1970). No such organ exists in the male. Although it appears that there is no event in the sexual function of the female that is the true counterpart of male ejaculation, some authors consider contraction of the smooth muscles of the uterine tubes and uterus to be equivalent to emission is the male, while the rhythmic contraction of the bulbospongiosus (vaginal sphincter) and ischiocavernosus muscle of the pelvic floor have been compared to ejaculation (Tarabulcy, 1972).

Precise correlation of the influence of the level and degree of spinal cord injury and sexual dysfunction has been summarized by Verkuyl. In the stage of spinal shock, voluntary control is abolished as descending messages from the brain are blocked at the point of transection. All reflex activity also ceases below the level of damage and all ascending afferent messages are blocked. This results in a loss of voluntary influence on erection, abolition of reflex erection and ejaculation, and loss of sensibility below the damaged area. It has been noted that in complete lesions, the penis becomes enlarged and more or less semi-erected. While this is often misinterpreted as priapism, it is in fact due to venous engorgement of the corpora cavernosa, due to paralytic vasodilitation, following interruption of the vasomotor fibers in the anterolateral tract of the spinal cord. Sometime after the acute spinal cord injury (variably days to many weeks), reflexes may return and it can be seen that the level and extension of damage influences the function of erection, coitus, and orgasm.

### Complete Cord Lesions in the Male

Following complete spinal cord lesions in the male, some general rules can be summarized:

- lesions at all levels with the exception of some forms of conus lesions—no orgasm
- lesions above the level of T11—no centrally and psychogenically induced erection; reflex erection available
- lesion between T11 and T12 and also between S2 and S4—possibility of psychogenically induced erection and reflex erections
- lesion between L2 and S2—erection reflex and seminal emission reflex are functional; no ejaculation reflex, resulting in dribbling of the seminal fluid
- damage of the conus-cauda equina—no erection reflex, no ejaculation reflex; emission reflexes available (dribbling); psychogenically induced erection and also some form of orgasm sometimes remain possible.

Erection is not the same as sustaining of the erection, and many spinal injured men may have erections, although coitus is not possible. The higher the lesion, the greater the possibility of erection; the lower the lesion, the greater the likelihood of ejaculation. Orgasm and ejaculation are more vulnerable than erection (Tarabulcy, 1972).

### Incomplete Cord Lesions in the Male

A great difference in sexual function exists between men with complete as compared with incomplete lesions. Given the level and state of the lesion, some prediction of the situation to expect may be made, but surprises and disappointments must be anticipated because neurological examination cannot always give adequate information for a firm prognosis about the extent of the lesion. In a series of 529 cases (Bors *et al.*, 1950), 26 percent of the men with complete, in contrast to 90 percent of the men with incomplete lower motor neuron lesions could achieve an erection. Ejaculation was possible in 18 percent and 70 percent respectively of these patients. In both incomplete and complete upper motor neuron lesions, the percentage of men who could achieve an erection was high. Ejaculation was possible in only 5 percent of patients with complete upper neuron lesions, whereas in patients with incomplete upper neuron lesions, this figure was 32 percent.

In incomplete lesions that only affect the motor function, there is no loss of pleasure of orgasm, but sometimes the spasticity may present mechanical difficulties. In incomplete lesions with "only" loss of sensibility (very rare), there is loss of both pleasure and orgasm. Given the complexity of the reflexes and neural pathways that are involved in erection, coitus, and orgasm, and the need for coordination of all these activities, one can understand that even when the lesions are incomplete, the hopes of many patients cannot be realized. In both flaccid and spastic paralysis, the man sometimes urinates during coitus and emptying of the bladder prior to sexual activity is to be recommended.

### Complete and Incomplete Lesions in the Female

A complete lesion appears to have no influence on menstruation, possibility of coitus, or fertility. However, regarding coitus, there is no sensation of touch, no pleasure, and no orgasm. In lesions that affect the sacral segments and where there is a flaccid paralysis of the bladder, the female often urinates during coitus. Emptying the bladder before the act is therefore necessary. If spastic paralysis is present, the same problem can arise, and therefore, emptying the bladder before coitus is necessary. Spastic or flaccid paralysis of the legs can, depending upon the height of the lesion, give problems with regard to positioning, creating "logistical" problems.

Females with incomplete cord lesions experience pleasure and orgasm more often than those with a complete lesion, but in many cases, spasticity gives rise to difficulty. Such difficulties as limb spasms and contractures, pressure sores, and a catheter infection can prohibit coitus. The immobility of the male or female partner with spastic or flaccid paralysis can impair the necessary movements and paralyzed arms are a great hindrance.

## SUMMARY

One can summarize these observations as follows:

1. Complete interruption of the continuity of the area of the cervical and middle thoracic cord results in loss of central voluntary influence on sexual function and on orgasm. Erection (insofar as this takes place by way of reflex), seminal discharge, and ejaculation are preserved but the coordination between the different reflexes is often disturbed. Therefore, proper normal ejaculation seldom occurs.
2. Complete lesions of the lower thoracic cord produce the same picture but there the centrally and psychogenically activated center (T11–L2) can be intact and influence erection.
3. Complete lesions in the area of the lumbar and sacral cord cause serious disturbance.
4. In conus-cauda equina lesions from S3 downwards, neither erection or ejaculation occur properly. Seminal discharge is not projectile (because of striated muscle paralysis), but dribbling in nature, the emissio seminis reflex being intact.
5. A practical rule could be: flaccid paralysis—no erection; spastic paralysis—erection possible (Verkuyl, 1976).

## DIAGNOSTIC CONSIDERATIONS

The clinical setting and nature of sexual dysfunction in the context of proven or suspect neurologic disease understandably determines the significance and yield of the neurologic approach. Methodical, comprehensive reviews of sexual dysfunction in disorders of brain, spinal cord, nerve, and muscle are available (Gastaut and Collomb, 1954; Kaplan, 1979), though are beyond the scope of this brief review. However, the clinical neurologic approach can be viewed in three settings. First, and most frequent, is the sexual dysfunction that attends or follows primary neurologic disease—stroke, traumatic injury to the brain and spinal cord, neuropathy, myopathy, and the like. Here, mechanical and functional defects are generally apparent and knowledge of the neurologic basis of sexual function become an integral aspect of comprehensive therapy, at times interventional, but most often a part of a broader rehabilitative effort.

A second setting is in partial neurologic disability such as could be seen in such varied chronic diseases as multiple sclerosis, parkinsonism, epilepsy or in systemic disease with neurologic complications—diabetes mellitus, systemic lupus erythematosus, chronic renal failure, to mention but a few. Again, the neurologic approach may contribute to the overall therapeutic effort.

Finally, and from a diagnostic and rehabilitative aspect, most challenging and critically important are the patients with unexplained sexual dysfunction with occult systemic or primary (undiagnosed) neurologic disease. Here, the diagnostic yield varies with the specific disease process. Thus, problems with libido could relate to a functional psychosocial or emotional etiology but organically determined cerebrocognitive or neuroendocrine deficits or more nonspecific indicators (such as depression as a presenting symptom of carcinoma of the pancreas, or altered sleep states in adrenal and thyroid disease) could obscure or delay diagnosis. Similarly, disorders of male potency could be due to any of the above but may be a presenting symptom in structural disease of brain, spinal cord, root, nerve, toxin drug, or metabolic disorder. Nevertheless, as in any diagnostic art, a comprehensive history and physical examination should determine a fruitful laboratory approach to delineate disease of the brain versus spinal cord or neuromuscular problems.

The introduction of noninvasive, relatively painless, low risk neuro-imaging techniques such as computerized tomography (CT) and magnetic resonance imaging (MRI) complement the standard electroencephalogram and myelogram for study of the brain and the spinal cord respectively. Remarkably, CT and MRI may diagnose as many as 80 to 90 percent of vascular, tumoral, demyelinative, or degenerative diseases of the central nervous system. Electromyography/nerve conduction studies, serum enzymes, and muscle/nerve histochemistry remain the standard of neuromuscular diagnosis.

Complementing the standard clinical and laboratory armamentarium, a plethora of conventional and more recently introduced approaches are available to assess sexual dysfunctions and, either directly or indirectly, their neurologic basis. Thus, since the genital organs and urinary tract share much of their innervation, tests of bladder function have a definite role in the evaluation of patients with sexual disorders. Specific tests such as cystourethroscopy, cystometry, and sphincter electromyography can provide accurate quantitative data. It should be cautioned, however, that although tests of bladder and related functions are important because of the close relationship between the innervation of the urinary tract and that of the genital organs, dysfunction in one of the systems is not necessarily accompanied by dysfunction of the other (Boller and Frank, 1982).

Complaints of impotence in the male can be assessed by penile tumescence studies, which are based on the observation that during sleep, males tend to have penile tumescence as part of the "autonomic storm" that accompanies REM sleep (Bohlen, 1981) (see Chapter 20). Changes in penile circumference can be recorded and may provide an objective index of a male's ability to obtain an erection. An objective way of analyzing female erotic response based on vaginal plethysmography (Sinthak and Geer, 1975) as well as male plethysmography has been described (Sinthak and Geer, 1975). Other specialized radiologic procedures including pelvic and internal pudendal arteriography and corporal cavernosography have also been reported. Pudendal nerve conduction as well as somatosensory evoked responses from the dorsal nerve of the penis and clitoris represent electrophysiologic approaches.

## REHABILITATION

Diseases of the nervous system can interfere with sexual activity at many levels and often there is an identifiable alteration of the underlying physiologic basis of sexual function. In addition, psychoemotional factors are operative not only in the individual patient but also in the sexual response of the partner. In some patients, cognition may be altered, resulting in diminished sexual activity. The emotional, cognitive, and physical aspects of sexuality are closely integrated and need to be considered concurrently for sexual education or counseling in neurologic rehabilitation (Ducharme and Ducharme, 1983). As often reiterated in this volume, it has only been in the past decade that health care professionals have begun to address the sexual concern of individuals with physical disabilities (Comarr, 1971; Kaplan, 1979). As recently as 1976, Bregman and Hadley reported that only 50 percent of rehabilitation patients received any information on sexuality during their hospitalization, despite the fact that the majority of the handicapped population continues to have sexual desire and strives to develop sexual relationships after the onset of disability. Thus, the endocrine, physiological and emotional aspects of sexuality as altered by disease and disability are important to all health care professionals. Sexuality is the driving force of life, and as long as life exists, attention to that aspect of the human condition must be acknowledged, encouraged, and treated.

## REFERENCES

Bard, P.: Central nervous mechanisms for emotional behavior patterns in animals. (Res. Publ. Assoc.) *Res. Nerv. Ment. Dis.*, (Proc) 19:190–218, 1939.

Blumer, D.: Hypersexual episodes in temporal lobe epilepsy. *Am. J. Psychiatry*, 126:1099–1106, 1970.

Blumer D., and Migeon, C.: Hormone and hormonal agents in the treatment of agression. *J. Nerv. Ment. Dis.*, 160:127–137, 1975.

Blumer, D., and Walker, A. E.: Sexual behavior in temporal lobe epilepsy. *Arch. Neurol.*, 16:37–43, 1967.

Blumer, D., and Walker, E. A. The neural basis of sexual behavior. In Benson, D. F.; Blumer, D.: (eds.): *Psychiatric Aspects of Neurologic Disease*. Grune and Stratton, New York, 199–217, 1975.

Bohlen, J. G.: Sleep erection monitoring in the evaluation of male erectile failure. In W. L. Furlow, (ed.): *Symposium on Male Sexual Dysfunction. Urol. Clin. N. Am.* 8:119–134, 1981.

Boller, F., and Frank E.: *Sexual Dysfunction in Neurological Disorders*. Raven Press, New York, 1982.

Bors, E.; Comarr, A. E.; and Moulton, S H.: The role of nerve blocks in management of traumatic cord bladders: Spinal anesthesia, subarachnoid alcohol injections, pudendal nerve anesthesia and vesical neck anesthesia. *J. Urol.*, 63:653–666, 1950.

Bors, E., and Turner, R. D.: History and physical examination in neurologic urology. In Boyersky, S.: (ed.): *The Neurogenic Bladder*. Williams and Wilkins, Baltimore, 1967.

Bregman, S., and Hadley, R.: Sexual adjustment and feminine attractiveness among spinal cord injured women. *Arch. Phys. Med. Rehab.*, 57:448–450, 1976.

Comarr, A.: Sexual concepts in traumatic cord and cauda equina lesions. *J. Urol.*, 106:375–378, 1971.

Dana-Haeri; Trimble, M. R.; and Oxley, J.: Prolactin and gonadotrophin changes following generalized and partial seizures. *J. Neurol. Neurosurg. Psychiatr.*, 46:331–335, 1983.

Ducharme, S. H., and Ducharme, J. D.: Sexual adaptation. *Seminars in Neurology, Rehabilitation of the Neurologically Impaired*, 3:135–140, 1983.

Gastaut, H., and Collomb, H.: Étude du comportment sexual chez lez épileptiques psychomoeurs. *Ann. Med. Psychol.*, (Paris) 2:657–696, 1954.

Jacome, D. E., and Risko, M. S.: Absence status manifested by compulsive masturbation. *Arch. Neurol.*, 40:523–524, 1983.

Kaplan, S.: Sexual counseling for persons with spinal cord injuries: A literature review. *J. Appl. Rehab. Couns.*, 10:200–203, 1979.

Kluver, H., and Bucy, P. C.: Psychic blindness and other symptoms following bilateral temporal lobectomy in rhesus monkeys. *Am. J. Physiol.*, 119:352–353, 1937.

Lance, J. W.: Headaches related to sexual activity. *J. Neurol. Neurosurg. Psychiatry*, 39:1226–1230, 1976.

Lisk, R.: Neural localization for androgen activation of copulatory behavior in the male rat. *Endocrinology*, 80:754–761, 1967a.

Lisk, R.: Sexual behavior: Hormonal control. In Martin, L.; Ganong, W. F.: (eds.): *Neuroendocrinology*, Vol. 2. Academic Press, New York, 1967b.

Masters, W. H., and Johnson, V. E.: *Human Sexual Response*. Little, Brown, Boston, 1970.

Pritchard, F. B.; Wannamaker, B. B.; Sagel, J.; Nair, R.; and DeVillier, C.: Endocrine function following complex partial seizures. *Ann. Neurol.*, 14:27–32, 1983.

Sinthak, G., and Geer, J. A.: A vaginal plethysmograph system. *Psychophysiology*, 12:113–115, 1975.

Spark, F. R.; Wills, C. A.; and Royal, H.: Hypogonadism, hyperprolactinemia and temporal lobe epilepsy in homosexual men. *Lancet*, 1:413–417, 1984.

Spencer, S. S.; Spencer, D. S.; Williamson, P. D.; and Mattson, R. H.: Sexual automatisms in complex partial seizures. *Neurology*, 33:527–533, 1983.

Tarabulcy, E.: Sexual function in the normal and in paraplegia. *Paraplegia*, 10:201–208, 1972.

Verkuyl, A.: Sexual function in paraplegia and tetraplegia. In Vinken, P. J.; Bruyn, G. W.: (eds.): *Handbook of Clinical Neurology*, Vol. 26. Part II: *Injuries of the Spine and Spinal Cord*. Elsevier, New York, 1976.

Weiss, H. D. The physiology of human penile erection. *Ann. Intern. Med.*, 76:792–799, 1972.

# UNIT IV Pathophysiology of Human Sexuality in Psychosocial Disease

# CHAPTER 22 DRUG ADDICTION

*Thomas Wolman, M.D.*

## INTRODUCTION

Substances of abuse elicit a wide spectrum of effects in users, ranging from the physiological to the psychosocial. Not surprisingly, among these effects are the many complex ways in which these substances influence sexual response. The same drug can act as a sexual enhancer in one situation and as a sexual inhibitor in another (Kaplan, 1974; Kolodny et al., 1979). Such opposite actions can occur between different individuals and with one individual at different times.

Simple pharmacologic parameters account for part of this variability. Dosage, absorption rate, rate of metabolism, body weight, excretion rate, chronicity of use, and interaction with other drugs all influence drug effect (Kolodny et al., 1979). The mode of action—central, peripheral nerve, vascular, local, or indirect—also is relevant (Kaplan, 1974). Many substances, particularly the central nervous system (CNS) depressants, act in such a way that a small amount produces an enhancing effect, a large amount an inhibiting effect (Freedman, 1975; Kaplan, 1974; Kolodny et al., 1979). Of course large, toxic amounts of any drug render sexual performance impossible. Drugs with a low therapeutic index require a high level of user experience to produce enhancing effects (Goode, 1972). User experience is also necessary to time sexual activity to drug effect. For example, drugs like cocaine may yield an enhancing effect on the rising side of the time-blood level curve, and a retarding effect on the descending slope (Gottheil and Weinstein, 1983).

It is never easy to predict how a drug will effect sexual performance in a given instance. Nonbiological factors such as user experience, situation variables, and mental state are often critical in determining the overall outcome. The difficulty of isolating the specific effects of many interacting factors has even led some investigators to conclude that alterations of sexuality are largely due to suggestability (Kolodny et al., 1979). Such a view tends to minimize not only the physiological, but also the more specific psychological parameters that affect sexual experience. With many substances, changes in sexuality arise as "side-effects" of complex interactions between biological, psychological, and sociological variables, in which positive and negative feedback play an important role.

To further complicate the field, investigators define human sexuality in different ways, leading to different judgments about drug effects. Biological studies assess changes in sexuality in terms of altered levels of circulating gonadatropins. Behavioral studies concentrate on erectile competence. Other researchers focus on interpersonal intimacy or erotic experience. These different approaches often lead to contradictory conclusions. Biological investigators may judge marijuana a sexual inhibitor because it reduces the level of circulating testosterone in men; others focusing on the perceived heightening of sexual experience, would label it an enhancer.

Additional sources of bias include political orientation (particularly relevant in marijuana studies) and the subjective distortion of experimental subjects (Winick, 1981). Most studies of the effects of substances on human sexual behavior have relied on anecdotal material, interviews, or questionnaires, which may be distorted by selective recall of the subjects and thus be of questionable reliability and validity. Political bias, by generating a climate of confrontation, may also distort the conclusions of research studies. Thus some investigators, reacting to an ideology that views both drugs and sexuality as necessary dissolvers of social barriers, may consciously or unconsciously emphasize those findings that tend to support their views.

Despite the many and complex problems involved in studying the effects of drugs on sexual responses, a good deal of work has been done and a considerable amount of information is available. In what follows, the effects on sexuality of one example of an enhancing drug, marijuana, and of one inhibiting drug, heroin, will be described and contrasted in considerable detail. Following this, the effects on sexual response of a variety of other commonly abused drugs will be reviewed more briefly.

## MARIJUANA

The protean effects of this "weed" have been well-described (Dawley et al., 1979; Freedman, 1975; Gay et al., 1982). Depending on the setting, subjects may report negative or positive experiences, and anything from vivid hallucinations to mild euphoria. In an attempt to make sense of the inconsistency and variety of reactions, it is postulated that the drug acts to intensify experience. In other words, any mental state, regardless of content, will be amplified and exaggeraged, not unlike the amplifying action of a "vacuum tube."

The specific qualities of the experience depend on the particular mental set of the user. Factors which contribute to "mental set" include user expectation, personality variables, and cultural norms. Recently the mass media have shaped the cultural context by portraying marijuana as a potent sexual enhancer. In the film *Annie Hall* the woman protagonist cannot enjoy sexual activity without marijuana. The message conveyed is that in an atmosphere of positive expectation, the drug will magnify mental states whose content includes sexual fantasy and will produce erotic enhancement.

In the literature, different dimensions of the marijuana experience are described that interact as intermediate variables, including a distortion of time sense, heightened sensory awareness, increased vividness of fantasy, and the reduction of sexual anxiety (Dawley et al., 1974; Kolodny et al., 1979; Ungerer et al., 1976; Winick, 1981). All may be viewed as contributing to the amplification of sexual experience. In addition, marijuana's psychologically disinhibiting effect may reflect positive group expectation, reinforced by the mass media.

Some individuals experience a negative, inhibiting effect on their sexual response. For example, a 22-year-old unmarried medical student consulted the clinic psychiatrist because he became frightened after an episode of "paranoia" following marijuana use. Although a virgin, he had recently been getting more intimate with his girlfriend. One evening the girlfriend suggested they smoke some marijuana, to which the man agreed. He later noticed his girlfriend was getting more and more amorous and sexually aggressive. He suddenly panicked and visualized a big man about to injure him. Since that night he worried ceaselessly that he was going crazy.

Mental set occurs at a key switch point in the flow diagram of sexual effects (Figure 22–1). A positive mental attitude directs the system on the track of amplified sexual enhancement; a negative mental attitude reroutes the flow toward a self-generating cycle and severe sexual inhibition (as in the previous example).

Two factors contribute to negative mental set in equal measure: user experience and personality variables. The former refers to a com-

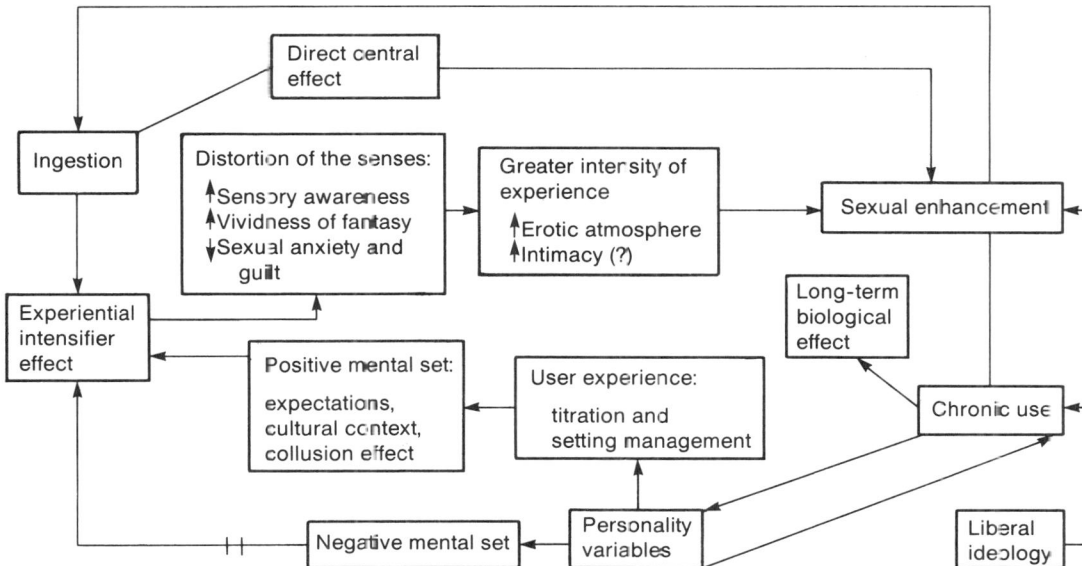

**FIGURE 22-1.** Marijuana enhancement of sexual response.

plex learning process during which the user becomes more aware of dosage, titrates his intake, and manages the physical and interpersonal setting, which involves matching drug-taking to an environment perceived as safe.

Investigators have found that sexual activity strongly correlates with user experience and belief in the sexual enhancement properties of the drug (Dawley et al., 1979; Goode, 1972) (although the relationship is not necessarily causal). Therefore, as user experience increases across the population, a powerful positive cycle will form. Group expectation, fueled by the media, facilitates more user experience. User experience in turn reinforces both sexual activity and positive belief. Possibly this mechanism accounts for the high prevalence of positive user expectation in the sexual realm and the relatively low incidence of negative, inhibitory effects in marijuana as compared with other drugs.

Personality variables can interfere with sexual enhancement in two ways. First, neurotic conflicts and sexual fears may lead to negative mental set especially when the environment mirrors the feared situation, as in the example. Second, certain well-defined personality patterns can contribute to the syndrome of chronic use with subsequent sexual inhibition. A person with pronounced schizoid traits, such as shallow interpersonal relationships and excess reliance on fantasy, will use marijuana for its potent intensifying effects. This individual will tend to exploit the drug-amplified fantasy life in the service of narcissism, masturbatory activity, and absorption in inner mental states. Consequently, this person will avoid efforts to seek new partners. Chronic use, in such circumstances may become self-reinforcing when long-term biological effects like reduction in circulating testosterone in men come into play (Kolodny et al., 1974).

In marijuana's overall enhancement effect, the experiential dimension seems critical, and behavioral and biological factors wane in importance. The level of interpersonal intimacy varies according to the narcissism of the users. Some investigators have suggested common factors—like liberal ideology—that generate both sexual activity and marijuana use. But perhaps liberal ideology shapes both users and investigators to focus for the most part on the experiential dimension of sexual activity.

It seems likely that in a safe, relaxing environment managed by experienced users who are capable of interpersonal intimacy, marijuana can have a positive, sexually enhancing effect.

## HEROIN

It is widely recognized that heroin use diminishes the user's interest in sexual activity (Cicero et al., 1975; Mintz et al., 1974). This sexual inhibiting effect occurs as a "side effect" of the complex interrelationships between heroin use, associated mental states, class and social factors, and biological states (Winick, 1981) (Figure 22–2). The final common pathway of this network is a massive deflection of energy away from the sexual arena. This displacement forms one corner of a triad that also includes intense substitute gratification and a mental set of finding the required amounts of the drug. We will examine each of these factors in turn.

Substitute gratification is, in part, the result of the intense mental states produced by ingestion. "Shooting-up" or ingestion by the intravenous route itself acquires a sexual meaning, especially when the user draws blood up and back into the syringe several times—a process called "boosting" (Winick, 1981). The immediate effects of heroin ingestion are so powerfully euphorogenic that they have been likened to orgasm (Chessick, 1960). Furthermore, IV administration produces sleep-like states akin to infantile satiation after a good feed (Winick, 1981). All these effects concentrate attention on inner states and drain off motivation needed for sexual activity. In many ways heroin ingestion seems analogous to contact with a fetish which effectively short circuits any attempt at intimacy. Both the fetish and the addiction provide an immediate, magical route to self-aggrandizement and self-repair that defeats efforts in support of the reality principle.

The possibility of instant gratification establishes a mind set of single-minded attention to finding the drug, the second line of the triad of sexual inhibition. The drug-finding orientation is maintained by two feedback cycles—one psychological, one sociological. Personality variables establish and reinforce mind set. Features of the addictive personality are foreshadowed in childhood by serious difficulties in the vulnerable individual's capacity to separate from the mother. Winnicott (1978) has described a defect in the child's ability to relate to a transitional object as antecedent to the development of addictive states. In such children the "bottle" becomes a magical means of denying rather than affirming (as in the case of the true transitional object) separateness. In later development, addictive individuals tend to relate to others as potential sources of "magical substance" rather than as love objects in themselves. The ability to manipulate people and other behavioral skills learned in the service of drug-finding, tend to reinforce the character patterns that gave rise to it.

In the social sphere, drug availability acts as a "switch" that initiates the "hustler" lifestyle. If availability is low, the individual is driven to hustle to sustain the drug habit (Mintz et al., 1974; Winick, 1981). All of the person's energies are deflected away from sexual and other pathways and fixated on the search for drugs. Such effort causes fatigue, malnutrition, and lack of sleep (Mintz et al., 1974; Winick, 1981), all of which contribute to sexual inhibition. Furthermore, drug-finding efforts lead to prostitution, and thereby helping to create an independent "subroutine" within the overall network of relationships (Winick, 1981; Winick and Kinsie, 1971). In women, prostitution, once chosen, promotes negative attitudes toward men as well as lowered self-esteem and an impaired sense of femininity. In both men and women, this defective self-image deflates enthusiasm for sexual activity and also narrows the affected person's range of life options, thus reinforcing the lifestyle of prostitution (Silbert et al., 1982). From another point of view, people entering prostitution may turn to drugs as a way of "anesthetizing" their painful existence (Winick, 1981). The presence of prostitution supports an illegal network of pimps and criminals, a network invested in maintaining the status quo.

In fact larger social networks also help to

perpetuate the hustler lifestyle. Organized crime, in as far as it partly controls the availability of drugs, requires a constant supply of users, ready to act as pushers. All of these factors stabilize the hustler lifestyle and form the final pathway toward the syndrome of chronic use. Long-term use may lead to biological effects that inhibit sexual responsiveness, such as reduced circulating testosterone in men and reduced gonadatropins in women (Cicero et al., 1975). When there is high drug availability as in methadone programs and among medical professionals, hustling becomes less necessary, and the loss of sexual function is less dramatic (Figure 22–2).

The combination of substitute gratification and a mind set of finding the drug brings about a massive displacement of energy and attention away from sexual activity. Heroin (and the opiates) depresses sexual functioning across the board; behavioral, biological, psychological, and sociological studies all demonstrate the impact.

Heroin ingestion (especially by hypodermic route) is so self-absorbing that it makes sexual activity superfluous. Many investigators have observed that efforts toward drug-finding leave little time and energy left for even the most minimal interpersonal relations, much less for sexual intimacy.

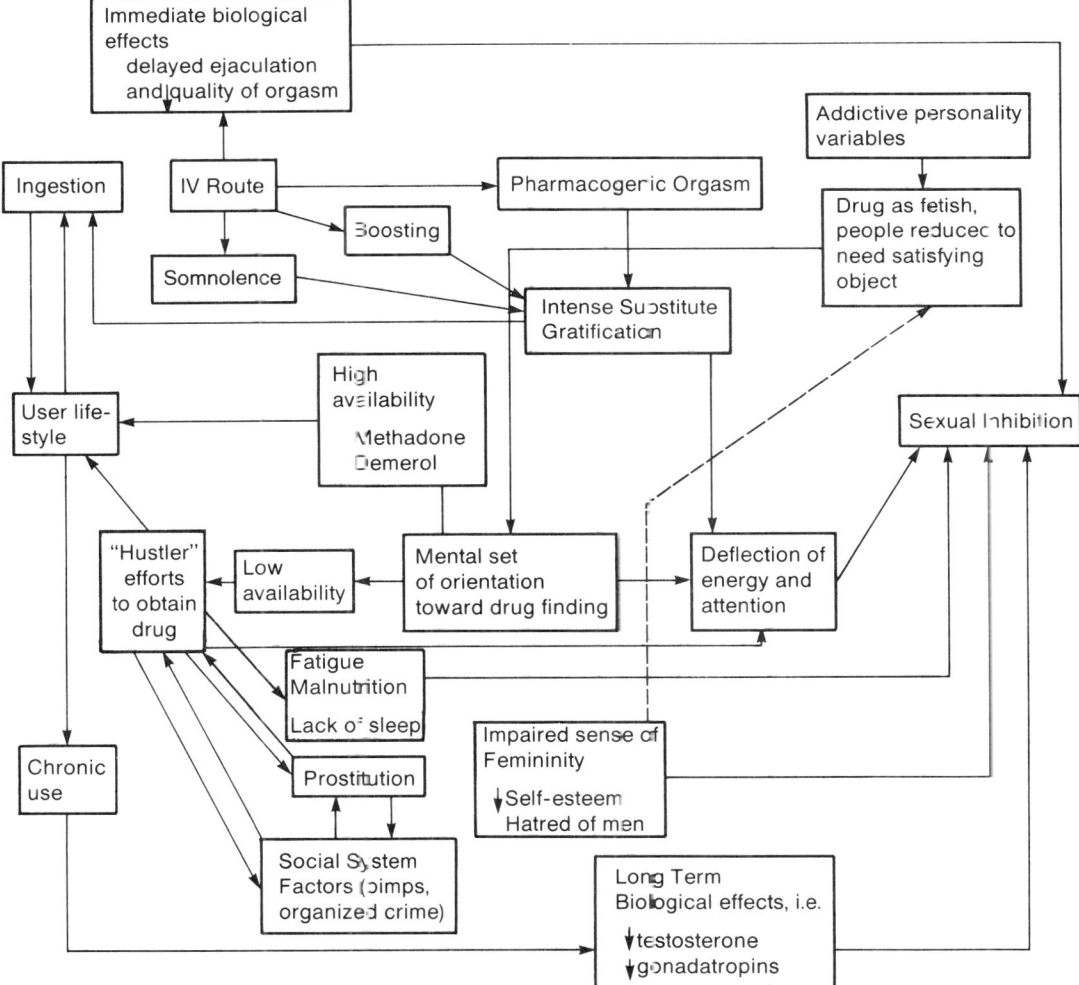

**FIGURE 22–2.** Effect of heroin on inhibiting sexual interest.

In both these substances, sexual effects are the result of complex multileveled networks of interacting variables. In both we see positive and negative feedback cycles as well as critical switch points. In neither substance are direct effects decisive: Research has failed to demonstrate a direct central, enhancing effect (marijuana) (Dawley et al., 1974) or a corresponding direct, central inhibiting effect (heroin) (Mintz et al., 1974).

Both networks reveal different basic mechanisms, however. Marijuana's intensifying effect depends on the context to supply the content. Heroin, on the other hand, creates an intense, direct experience that is considerably less bound by context. User experience plays a significant role in the former and a negligible role in the latter.

This difference allows us to classify drugs that affect human sexuality. For example, drugs like marijuana, LSD, and CNS depressants form a class whose effects vary with user experience. Direct effects apply to heroin, cocaine, the amphetamines, and nitrites. With many drug users learning is dose related: relevant at small doses, obliterated at high doses where direct effects take over. Most drugs have a threshhold beyond which meaningful sexual activity is impossible.

## OTHER DRUGS AFFECTING SEXUAL FUNCTION

### Aphrodisiacs

The dictionary defines aphrodisiac as any substance that provokes sexual desire. Most researchers use a narrow definition that denotes direct, physiologically activated sexual arousal (Benedek, 1971). One may also choose to accept a broader definition which allows for degrees of sexual enhancement within a context of other relevant factors. By the narrow definition of the word, there are no true aphrodisiacs. Many substances, like rhinoceros horn, possess a purely magical relationship to sexuality. Cantharides (spanish fly) do not affect the genitals directly, but act instead as a powerful irritant to the bladder and urethra, which in some individuals creates a pseudosexual excitement. This drug is reported to cause impotence and death (Winick, 1981). In a third class of drugs, which includes $d$-amphetamine, methadrine, Ritilin, and Preludin (all CNS stimulants) intravenous administration produces an orgasm-like effect (Winick, 1981).

### Alcohol

Alcohol and sexuality have been associated in the public mind since ancient times. Alcohol works to disinhibit sexual response at small doses and to depress at high doses. As Shakespeare writes in Macbeth (Act II, Scene 3) "It provokes and unprovokes: It provokes the desire but it takes away the performance." (See also Freedman, 1975; Kolodny et al., 1979). Disinhibition differs from the previously noted mechanisms of sexual alteration. Marijuana may produce disinhibition in small doses as a result of its amplifying effect coupled with user expectation. In alcohol the disinhibition is a direct effect, although user expectation may reinforce it. In the case of heroin, disinhibition is "erased" by CNS depression at relatively small doses.

All authorities agree that, at higher doses, alcohol causes pronounced loss of erectile and ejaculatory competence in men, presumably by interfering with reflex transmission of sexual arousal (Kolodny et al., 1979). Because the switch from disinhibition to depression is dose-related, user experience plays a key role. Winick (1981) reports that social learning variables are more significant in producing sexual alterations than any known physiological effect. Even the disinhibiting effect may be culturally determined to a degree (Horton, 1943). Apparently, in some non-Western societies imbibing does not lead to lowered inhibitions. In our culture, of course, drinking and sex are strongly associated. To some extent marijuana has usurped the role of "sexual lubricant," but not completely. As with marijuana, the user expectation that alcohol permits and facilitates sexual feelings plays a key role.

At higher doses, and in patterns of chronic

use, alcohol heavily inhibits sexual function. Alcoholism is the major cause of impotence in men (Wilson, 1977; Winick, 1981). Chronic drinkers enter a negative cycle in which high expectations are followed by failure and repeated bouts of drinking. Studies of women's response to alcohol are less well-documented, largely because reactions are less obvious and subjects more reticent. Available evidence does indicate that chronic drinking slows down vaginal lubrication (Winick, 1981). Furthermore, chronic use in either sex can lead to peripheral neuropathies which permanently impair sexual response.

## BARBITURATES

Barbituate substances operate directly on the CNS and have the same mechanism of action as alcohol. Moderate dosages disinhibit sexual behavior and excitement and reduce associated anxiety. Higher dosages reduce libido (Winick, 1981). A related drug, Methaquaalone (quaaludes) has gained popularity as a sexual enhancer, despite a low therapeutic index making it risky to all but the most experienced users (Freedman, 1975).

## AMPHETAMINES

Amphetamines produce a powerful, inner-directed "rush" that has sexual overtones. In men, intravenous injection may be associated with erection (Bell and Trethowan, 1961). It is not clear, however, if this effect is due to direct action, amplification, or disinhibition. It seems to bear some relationship to heroin's pharmacogenic orgasm: both experiences are intense, inner-directed, sexually tinged, and diffused throughout the body.

Use of these drugs as a sexual enhancer requires a high degree of user experience. Ingestion must be titrated and timed to coincide with the onset of sexual activity Apparently, amphetamines are an unreliable sexual enhancer, if popularity is any indication (Gay et al., 1982); high dosages produce a diffuse loss of coordination and restlessness, which interferes with any sexual response. Chronic users report a host of sexual difficulties including loss of libido (Bell and Trethowan, 1961).

## COCAINE

Exaggerated claims for the "champagne" of recreational drugs date back to its early discovery by Freud (1884/1963). His own self-experiment with the drug seduced him into viewing it as a panacea whose harmful effects were neglegible. Folklore and myth have consistently portrayed cocaine as an aphrodisiac: in slang cocaine and its effects are usually compared to a woman and her effects. It reportedly increases libido and enhances sexual performance at moderate dosages, sometimes producing multiple orgasms. Some users rub it on the head of the penis or clitoris to prolong thrusting, a practice which suggests partial anesthesia (Gay et al., 1982). These users exploit this effect to intensify the aggressive component of sexual activity, thus exposing themselves to genital injuries and infectious human bites (Gay et al., 1982).

As with many other substances, prolonged or heavy use of cocaine results in decline of sexual interest to which lack of coordination and excessive inner preoccupations both contribute.

## AMYL NITRITE

Nitrites act as powerful vasodilators, both systemically and intracerebrally (Israelstram et al., 1978; Winick, 1981). Generally the drug is "popped" just before orgasm (hence the term "popper" which refers to the sound of a glass vial breaking), and will produce a rush or high that lasts about one minute. Users report prolonged orgasm and delayed ejaculation (Isrealstram et al., 1978; Winick, 1981).

Recently nitrates have become very popular with homosexual men in association with sadomasochistic activities (Gay et al., 1982). If unavailable by prescription, users resort to butyl nitrite found in room deodorizers. Either nitrite can cause headaches, hypotension, tachycardia, and other serious cardiac effects (Kolodny et al., 1979).

## Tranquilizers

As is known, tranquilizers may be abused like barbiturates. They also disinhibit and reduce anxiety. Since they are safer than barbiturates, cause less sedation, and have a higher therapeutic index, sexual enhancement may be more reliable (Winick, 1981).

## LSD

Users report that lysergic acid diethylamide (LSD) markedly alters the perceived quality of sexual experience. They describe more "complex" experiences and a deeper orgasm (Kolodny et al., 1979). As with cocaine and amphetamines, LSD may impair coordination and concentration necessary for intercourse. User experience may facilitate a positive mental set that decreases the likelihood of "bad trips." LSD powerfully redirects attention inwards, away from externals. Such narcissistic focus may work against the interactive elements of sexual intercourse (Winick, 1981).

## PCP

Phencyclidine hydrochloride or PCP is a dissociative anesthetic with complex effects. At low dosage it produces disinhibition, perceptual distortion, and pain relief (Pupe et al., 1981), but not increased desire. Orgasm is not intensified yet is qualitatively altered. PCP is a preferred drug among homosexual men (as are amyl nitrite and quaaludes) and is used to reduce the pain and unfamiliarity of certain sexual practices like anal manual intercourse (Smith et al., 1980). In this population, smoking is the preferred route due to ease of titration.

Chronic and high dosage lead to ejaculatory failure. Adverse reactions are common in individuals with a pattern of chronic use and polydrug abuse (Gay et al., 1982; Smith et al., 1980).

## CONCLUSIONS

At least five mechanisms of sexual alteration have been proposed in the literature. They are as follows. (1) *Amplification:* Marijuana offers the purest example of this simple key to multiple effects. Its advantage lies in universal application. For instance, disinhibition occurs by amplifying an established sexually permissive mind set. Similarly, perceptual distortion results from magnifying normal attention to sight, sound, touch, and other sensory experience. Of course the simultaneous presence of other mechanisms can not be ruled out. (2) *Direct experiential flooding:* Heroin, amphetamines, and cocaine all provide an intense, inner-directed experience with sexual qualities. The striking shift in attention from outside to inside gratifies narcissistic wishes. (3) *Disinhibition–depression:* Many drugs including alcohol, barbiturates, and tranquilizers disinhibit at low doses and depress at high doses. In the case of heroin, the depressive effect comes into play so quickly that disinhibition ceases to be a factor. (4) *Perceptual distortion:* LSD, marijuana, and PCP alter the quality of sexual experience without necessarily increasing libido or intensifying orgasm. (5) *Pain control:* This recently discovered action applies to PCP, quaaludes, and cocaine in association with sadomasochistically tinged sexual activity.

These mechanisms can work alone or in combination. For example, amyl nitrite seems to elicit direct experience and also amplifies the intensity of orgasm. PCP causes perceptual distortion and pain relief.

To the author's knowledge, only a few of these mechanisms have been studied specifically. Disinhibition–depression seems to be the most substantiated (Kolodny et al., 1979). Several factors have contributed to the conceptual paucity and inconsistency of research in this area. Political bias (particularly with marijuana), a retrospective approach, and a biased sample have been mentioned. Most studies have been carried out on highly specific populations: college students, inner-city addicts (Mintz et al., 1974), Haight-Ashbury hippies (Gay et al., 1982), and homosexual men (Smith et al., 1980). In the past all populations were predominantly male, largely due to practical difficulties in measuring arousal in women. Of late the balance has been partly redressed with more studies in which women are included (Kolodny et al., 1979; Winick, 1981).

No one has attempted to study these populations in depth from an anthropological perspective as has been done with the Peyote Indian cults for example. Such study might reveal values common to both drug-taking and sexuality within a given population. These values might illuminate the phenomenon of the "fad" drugs that makes it hard to assess the prevalence and lifespan of a given substance–sexuality interaction.

Nor has there been much study of mediating psychological factors such as the effect of substitute sexual gratification. Rather, most studies pursue only direct effects by measuring single, well-defined, behavioral variables. Perhaps the future will witness a more systems-oriented approach to this interesting field.

## REFERENCES

Bell, D. S., and Trethowan, W. A.: Amphetamine addiction and disturbed sexuality. *Arch Gen. Psychiatr.,* 4:74–78, 1961.

Benedek, T. G.: Aphrodisiacs: Fact and fable. *Med. Aspects Hum. Sex.,* 5:42, 1971.

Chessick, R. D.: The "pharmacogenic orgasm" in the drug addict. *Arch. Gen. Psychiatr.,* 3:545–556, 1960.

Cicero, T. J.; Bell, R. D.; Wiest, W. G., et al: Function of the male sex organs in heroin and methadone users. *N. Engl. J. Med.,* 292:882–887, 1975.

Dawley, H. H.; Winstead, D. K.; Baxter, A. S.; and Gay, J. R.: An attitude survey of the effects of marijuana on sexual enjoyment. *J. Clin. Psychol.,* 35:212–217, 1979.

Freedman, D.: Drugs and sexual behavior. In Freedman, A.; Kaplan, H.; Sadock, B.: (eds.): *Comprehensive Textbook of Psychiatry,* Vol. 2, 2d ed. Williams and Wilkins, Baltimore, 1975.

Freud, S. (1884): *Uber Coca* (Reprinted Dunequin Press, 1963).

Gay, G. R.; NewMeyer, J. D.; Perry, M.; Johnson, G.; and Kurland, M.: Love and Haight: The sensuous hippie revisited. Drug/sex practices in San Francisco, 1980–1981. *J. Psychoactive Drugs,* 14:111–123, 1982.

Goode, E.: Drug use and sexual activity on a college campus. *Am. J. Psychiatry,* 128:1272–1276, 1972.

Gottheil, E., and Weinstein, S.: Cocaine: An emerging problem. In Akhtar, S.: (ed.): *New Psychiatric Syndromes.* Jason Aronson, New York, 1983.

Horton, D.: The function of alcohol in primitive societies: A cross-cultural study. *J. Stud. Alcohol,* 4:199, 1943.

Israelstram, S.; Lambert, S.; and Oki. G.: Poppers: A new recreational drug craze. *Can. Psychiatr. Assoc. J.,* 7:493–495, 1978.

Kaplan, H. S.: The effects on drugs on sexuality. In Kaplan, H. S.: *The New Sex Therapy,* Brunner/Mazel, New York, 1974.

Kolodny, R.; Masters, W.; and Johnson, V.: Drugs and sex. In Kolodny, R.; Masters, W.; and Johnson, V.: (eds.): *Textbook of Sexual Medicine,* 1st ed. Little, Brown, Boston, 1979.

Kolodny, R.; Masters, W.; Kolodner, R.; and Toro, G.: Depression of plasma testosterone levels after chronic intensive marijuana use. *N. Engl. J. Med.,* 290:872–874, 1974.

Mintz, J.; O'Hare, K.; O'Brien, L. P.; and Goldschmidt, J.: Sexual problems of heroin addicts. *Arch. Gen. Psychiatr.,* 31:700–703, 1974.

Pupe, H. G.; Ionescu-Pioggia, M.; and Cole, J. O.: Drug use and lifestyle among college undergraduates: Nine years later. *Arch. Gen. Psychiatr.,* 38:588–591, 1981.

Silbert, M.; Pines, D.; and Lynch, T.: Substance abuse and prostitution. *J. Psychoactive Drugs,* 14:193–197, 1982.

Smith, D. E.; Smith, M.; Baxton, M.; and Moser, C.: PCP and sexual dysfunction. *J. Psychoactive Drugs,* 12:269–272, 1980.

Ungerer, J. L.; Harford, R. J.; Brown, F. L.; and Kleber, A. D.: Sex/guilt and preferences for illegal drugs among drug abusers. *J. Clin. Psychol.,* 32:891–895, 1976.

Wilson, G. T.: Alcohol and human sexual behavior. *Behav. Res. Ther.,* 15:239–252, 1977.

Winick, C.: Substances of abuse and sexual behavior. In Lowinson, J. H.; Ruiz, P.: (eds.): *Substance Abuse: Clinical Problems and Perspectives.* Williams and Wilkins, Baltimore, 1981.

Winick, C., and Kinsie, P. M.: *The Lively Commerce: Prostitution in the United States.* Quadrangle Books, Chicago, 1971.

Winnicott, D. W.: Transitional objects and transitional phenomena. In Winnicott, D. W.: (ed.): *Through Paediatrics to Psychoanalysis.* Hogarth Press, London, 1978.

# CHAPTER 23 RAPE

*Elaine P. Bencivengo, M.A., and Joseph J. Romero, M.A.*

## INTRODUCTION

The purpose of this chapter is to explore the evidence of psychosexual dysfunction in the adult female subsequent to rape. The authors will use the current legal definition of rape from Bailey and Rothblatt (1973): a crime of a man against a woman that is forcible/without consent such that "the penis enters the labia of the female organ" (p. 276).

## BACKGROUND

Rape throughout the written history of humankind has referred to forced sexual intercourse between an adult male and adult female. Snelling (1975) reports that the Incan culture, as documented by the chronicles of the Spanish Conquistadores, regarded forced sexual contact as unacceptable behavior to be punished. Likewise, as noted by Brownmiller (1975), a proscription against rape can be found in Hebrew and Roman Law, as well as in Hammurabi's Code. Rape as a punishable crime also existed during colonial times in the United States as noted by Bienen (1976).

Although rape has been regarded as a crime throughout history, there were often variations in definition and application of the law. For example, in Roman law, rape as a crime could be committed against virgins only. In addition, there have also been variations in the assignment of guilt. In ancient Hebrew law, a married woman who was raped was punished to the same extent as the rapist and could only be saved by her husband. Today, in the United States rape laws specify that only a male can be the perpetrator, spell out penile–vaginal intercourse as the sexual act involved, and, if guilt is proven, provide guidelines for the punishment of the perpetrator.

In the United States, reported rapes increased 29 percent, from 63,020 reports in 1977 to 81,563 reports in 1981 according to the Federal Bureau of Investigation (FBI, 1978, 1982). Increased reporting may have been related to an increase in rape incidents or may be a reflection of the advocacy efforts of the women's rights movement for the provision of services to rape victims.

In summary, rape has been considered a breach of social conduct since the beginning of codification of human behavior and continues to be prosecuted in the United States today. Since rape continues to be a serious problem for our society, it requires our prevention efforts as well as our skills to treat those who have already been victimized.

## PSYCHOSEXUAL DYSFUNCTION IN THE ADULT FEMALE

We define human sexual dysfunction as the impaired functioning of the human sexual system. Since the writings of Freud the human sexual system has been considered to have a psychological and a biological component. The psychological component is thought to be learned and to give meaning to human sexual activities. Biological and psychological problems, either individually or jointly, can lead to a wide range of dysfunctions, including the inability to produce offspring and personal dissatisfaction with sexual activity. Lifetime sexual dysfunction may not be easily recognized by the individual, and sporadic dysfunction may go unattended. Significant changes in sexual functioning, however, are difficult to ignore and are more readily reported. When impaired sexual functioning cannot be attributed entirely to organic factors and a psychological factor is identified, it is termed a psychosexual dysfunction. For the adult female, psychosexual dysfunction can range from the avoidance of sexual contact to the inability to engage in heterosexual intercourse. Specific psychosexual dysfunctions of the adult female listed in the American Psychiatric Association's Diagnostic and Statistical Manual, Third Revision (DSM–III) are as follows:

| | |
|---|---|
| 302.71 | Inhibited sexual desire |
| 302.72 | Inhibited sexual excitement |
| 302.73 | Inhibited female orgasm |
| 302.76 | Functional dyspareunia (recurrent or persistent genital pain associated with coitus) |
| 306.51 | Functional vaginismus (involuntary spasm of the musculature of the outer third of the vagina which interferes with coitus). |

Kaplan (1974) notes that intense negative emotional states such as anger, fear, and depression, as well as chronic emotional disturbance, can lead to the disruption of sexual functioning. Following Kaplan's line of reasoning, it could be expected that a rape victim would manifest at least short-term psychosexual dysfunction. In the following section the Posttraumatic Stress Disorder is discussed as a reaction to rape and studies that address victims' psychosexual dysfunctions after the rape are reviewed.

## THE EFFECTS OF RAPE INCLUDING PSYCHOSEXUAL DYSFUNCTION

The victim's psychological reaction to rape is most frequently found to be an Acute Posttraumatic Stress Disorder. This reaction is identified as a psychiatric disorder in both the International Classification of Diseases, 9th Revision, Clinical Modification (1981), and the DSM–III. In the DSM–III acute (308.3) and chronic or delayed (309.81) Posttraumatic stress disorders are listed among the anxiety disorders. The DSM–III lists the diagnostic criteria for these disorders as follows:

A. Existence of a recognizable stressor that would evoke significant symptoms of distress in almost everyone.
B. Re-experiencing of the trauma as evidenced by at least one of the following:
   (1) recurrent and intrusive recollections of the event
   (2) recurrent dreams of the event
   (3) sudden acting or feeling as if the traumatic event were reoccurring, because of an association with an environmental or ideational stimulus
C. Numbing of responsiveness to or reduced involvement with the external world, beginning some time after the trauma, as shown by at least one of the following:
   (1) markedly diminished interest in one or more significant activities
   (2) feeling of detachment or estrangement from others
   (3) constricted affect
D. At least two of the following symptoms that were not present before the trauma:
   (1) hyperalertness or exaggerated startle response
   (2) sleep disturbance
   (3) guilt about surviving when others have not, or about behavior required for survival
   (4) memory impairment or trouble concentrating
   (5) avoidance of activities that arouse recollection of the traumatic event
   (6) intensification of symptoms by exposure to events that symbolize or resemble the traumatic event

The acute subtype is applicable when the symptoms appear within six months of the trauma and persist for not more than six months. With the chronic or delayed subtype, the symptoms either last longer than six months or appear more than six months after the trauma. [1981:238]

Sexual functioning may be impaired after any trauma but there are two diagnostic criteria which, when applied to sexual activities post-rape, could result specifically in psychosexual dysfunction. (1) Diminished interest and avoidance of activities which are reminiscent of the trauma could lead to a reduction of sexual interest or avoidance of sexual activities. (2) Exposure to situations which resemble the traumatic event could lead to an intensification of symptoms thereby interfering with sexual functioning.

The following studies document the short-term and long-term reactions of rape victims. For most victims, forcible rape is a traumatic experience resulting in a panic reaction with persistent increases in feelings of anxiety and fear. If sexual activities and feelings about men are examined, many victims report difficulties that would qualify as psychosexual dysfunction.

Sutherland and Scherl (1970) followed 13 rape victims for a 12-month period and reported three phases of adjustment:

*Phase One:* Acute Reaction—immediate reaction which can take many forms; victims may appear "agitated, incoherent and highly volatile" (p. 504)

*Phase Two:* Outward Adjustment—victim returns to pre-rape activity; often denies any problem and refuses psychiatric follow up treatment efforts

*Phase Three:* Integration and Resolution—superficial adjustment of Phase Two breaks down; re-emergence of concerns about rape often with anxiety, depression, and obsessive memories of the rape.

Similarly, Burgess and Holmstrom (1974) found that the adjustment period for 109 rape victims consisted of an acute phase of disorganization and a long-term reorganization phase. Notman and Nadelson (1976) in a theoretical discussion of the possible effects of rape suggested several long-term consequences which rape victims may experience. Two consequences that may impinge upon sexual functioning are: "mistrust of men with consequent avoidance or hesitation" and "a variety of sexual disturbances" (p. 412). To test these hypotheses Nadelson and colleagues (1982) interviewed 41 women 1–2½ years after the rape. More than half reported sexual difficulties, including 25 percent "who . . . described avoidance of any sexual relationship since the rape" (p. 1268). Burgess and Holmstrom also noted that many rape victims experienced a crisis in their sexual lives.

In follow-up studies conducted by Kilpatrick and coworkers (1979, 1981) rape victims (N=20) were compared to a non-victim group using objective psychological measures. Findings from the 1981 study indicated that victims continue to suffer from the effects of rape 12 months postassault. Victims had significantly greater scores on measures of fear and anxiety than non-victims. A large study conducted at Philadelphia General Hospital (see Krasner *et al.*, 1976; McCahill *et al.*, 1979; Peters, 1975) provided information regarding victim adjustment for the 11-month period following the sexual assault. McCahill and colleagues reported 11-month follow-up results for 213 victims of an initial population of 1401 victims. For the 213 victims, sexual difficulties were reported immediately after the sexual assault (46.6 percent) and 11 months after the assault (39 percent). It should be noted that not all of the victims were raped, but all were victims of some type of sexual assault. A study by the Marriage Council of Philadelphia (1979) of 43 victims and their partners found that sexual difficulties were a major problem post-rape. Using a scaling method for self-report, the Marriage Council found that "concerns about sex" represented the second most frequent category of response. In addition, it is reported that "over one-half of the victims had a diagnosable sexual dysfunction" (p.

4:32). The percentage of these dysfunctions which existed prior to the rape incident is unclear.

Feldman-Summers and coworkers (1979) asked 15 rape victims to rate retrospectively 23 sex-related activities pre- and post-rape. When the victim responses were compared to the responses of a non-raped sample, those women who were raped reported significantly ($p < .05$) less satisfaction with current sexual relations. Burgess and Holmstrom (1979) reinterviewed 81 rape victims four to six years post-rape. Of these, 63 victims were sexually active at the time of the follow-up interview: 38 percent reported being abstinent at least six months post rape; 33 percent reported a delay in resumption and a decrease of sexual activity; 19 percent reported no change in sexual frequency; and 10 percent reported increased sexual activity. Other findings indicated that a majority of the 63 victims reported flashbacks of the rape during sexual activities; 25 percent reported pain or physical discomfort when sexual relations resumed, and 41 percent reported orgasmic changes. Becker and colleagues (1982) interviewed 83 rape and/or incest victims from two months to more than three years after the assault. The findings showed that the majority of victims experienced sexual difficulties. It is further reported that "the vast majority of sexual dysfunctions resulting from rape fall into the DSM-III categorization of either fear of sex, arousal dysfunction, or desire dysfunction." (p. 73).

To explore the effects of rape upon sexual functioning in greater detail, the authors decided to re-examine available data collected on 790 victims from the Philadelphia Assault Victim Study. A sample of 105 cases was identified.

In order to be admitted to the sample the following requirements were applied:

- forcible penile–vaginal intercourse must have occurred
- victims must be over 18
- the rape must not have been the victim's first sexual experience
- all victims must have completed all four follow-up interviews
- all victims must be female

These restrictions were imposed so that the sample would provide the following:

- information concerning sexual adjustment of victims 11 months post-rape
- at least one non-rape experience of sexual intercourse prior to the rape which could establish a subjective standard for the estimate of change
- incidents which, at a minimum, fit the current legal definition of rape

## PHILADELPHIA ASSAULT VICTIM STUDY: RAPE VICTIM SAMPLE

The source of the data for the findings presented below is the Philadelphia Assault Victim Study. The Center for Rape Concern (CRC), now the Joseph J. Peters Institute, was funded in 1972 by the National Institute of Mental Health to conduct research on the social and psychological effects of sexual assault. During the years of the research, CRC was located in Philadelphia General Hospital (PGH), which was designated as the city-wide hospital to provide medical treatment to sexual assault victims. During the research period between April 1, 1973 and June 30, 1975, there were 1401 sexual assault victims of all ages examined at PGH.

### Study Design and Sample

The primary data collection technique used to assess the post-sexual assault adjustment was a standardized interview schedule. The interview was designed to collect information on the victim's behavioral, emotional, and social response following a sexual assault. This information was compared with the victim's pre-sexual assault level of functioning, and changes on a number of adjustment measures were computed. In addition, a portion of the interview focused on the particulars of the sexual assault incident, and on victim and offender background characteristics. Follow-up interviews were conducted by a female social worker at four time intervals: one immediately following the report of the sexual assault (usually within 5 days), and then at 3, 7, and 11 months after the assault. Four follow-up interviews were used so that victim adjustment could be examined at different periods after the sexual assault to see if her adjustment changed over time.

Table 23–1 provides demographic data and incident characteristics for the sample of 105 female rape victims.

TABLE 23–1 **Sample and Incident Characteristics (N = 105)**

*Race*
  Black—76%
  White—24%
*Age*
  Mean—30 years
  Mode—19 years
  Range—19 to 76 years
*Marital Status*
  Single—51%
  Married—22%
  Widowed/Divorced/Separated—27%
*Number of Prior Sexual Assaults*
  None—87%
  One—9%
  Two or more—4%
*Place of Rape*
  Victim's home—38%
  Rapist's home—11%
  Other's home—6%
  Automobile—11%
  Outside—9%
  Other—25%
*Type of Force Used**
  Coercion—69%
  Intimidation with object—52%
  Roughness—73%
  Brutal beating—35%
*Victim–Offender Relationship*
  Stranger—63%
  Relative stranger—12%
  Acquaintance—14%
  Friend—9%
  Family member—2%

* Total exceeds 100% due to multiple responses
Source: Based on data from Philadelphia Assault Victim Study, Final Report to the National Institute of Mental Health, Joseph J. Peters Institute, Philadelphia, June, 1976.

It is interesting to note that 14 victims (13 percent) had been previously sexually assaulted. Also, a majority of the rape incidents involved some type of physical force, with an object (gun, knife) used in 52 percent of the rapes.

Before presenting the findings, it is important to state a major limitation of the study sample. Almost all the victims in the Philadelphia Assault Victim Study chose to report the rape to the police and other official sources. There is considerable evidence that many rapes and/or sexual assaults go unreported. The characteristics of rape victims who choose not to report the assault may differ significantly from the characteristics and findings based on data collected from victims who report the assault. As a result, the findings presented below are not presumed to represent a complete profile of sexual adjustment problems experienced by rape victims.

RATINGS OF SEXUAL ADJUSTMENT

The impact of rape on sexual functioning was assessed by examining the victim's self-report of changes in feelings and sexual behavior comparing pre-rape functioning with post-rape functioning. For a variety of reasons not all responses are available for the sample of 105 victims.

As indicated in Table 23–2, a majority (68.4 percent) of victims reported negative feelings towards unknown men immediately after the rape. Feelings towards known men did not change for most victims, with 35 percent reporting an increase in negative feelings. The increase of negative feelings toward known and unknown men seems to be related to victim–offender relationship, note that 63 percent of the victims were raped by strangers.

For the other categories: heterosexual relations, husband/boyfriend relations, and sexual relations, more than 50 percent of the victims reported no change immediately after the rape. Of the victims, 25 percent reported improvement in their husband/boyfriend relations. Worsened heterosexual, husband/boyfriend, and overall sexual relations

TABLE 23-2  Ratings of Adjustment—Immediately After Rape

| Category | Response | | | Total Number of Respondents |
| --- | --- | --- | --- | --- |
| | Decreased | No Change | Increased | |
| Negative feelings toward known men | 1 (1.3%) | 51 (63.7%) | 28 (35.0%) | N = 80 |
| Negative feelings toward unknown men | (0.0%) | 25 (31.6%) | 54 (68.4%) | N = 79 |
| | Worsened | No Change | Improved | |
| Overall heterosexual relations | 35 (43.7%) | 44 (55.0%) | 1 (1.3%) | N = 80 |
| Change in husband/boyfriend relations | 14 (23.3%) | 31 (51.7%) | 15 (25.0%) | N = 60 |
| Change in sexual relations with partner | 24 (42.9%) | 31 (55.3%) | 1 (1.8%) | N = 56 |

Source: Based on data from Philacelphia Assault Victim Study, Final Report to the Institute of Mental Health, Joseph J. Peters Institute, Philadelphia, June, 1976.

immediately after the rape were reported by 44 percent, 23 percent, and 43 percent of the victims respectively.

The ratings of sexual adjustment at 11 months after the rape are presented in Table 23-3. Similar to the findings reported immediately after the rape, the data indicate that a portion of the victims reported at 11 months a persistence of increased negative feelings toward known (13 percent) and unknown men (24 percent) with the majority of victims reporting no change. In addition, 13 percent of the victims reported at 11 months after the rape a negative change in heterosexual relations, and 9 percent reported ongoing negative changes in relations with husband/boyfriend and sexual relations with partner. The ratings at 11 months show an improvement in sexual adjustment when compared with the ratings given immediately after the rape as indicated by a decrease in the percentage negative change responses. However, the persistence of sexual adjustment problems at 11 months following a rape indicates, that for a portion

TABLE 23-3  Ratings of Adjustments—11 Months After Rape

| Category | Response | | | Total Number of Respondents |
| --- | --- | --- | --- | --- |
| | Decreased | No Change | Increased | |
| Negative feelings toward known men | (0.0%) | 91 (87.5%) | 13 (12.5%) | N = 104 |
| Negative feelings toward unknown men | (0.0%) | 80 (76.2%) | 25 (23.8%) | N = 105 |
| | Worsened | No Change | Improved | |
| Overall heterosexual relations | 13 (12.5%) | 91 (87.5%) | (0.0%) | N = 104 |
| Change in husband/boyfriend relations | 8 (8.7%) | 77 (83.7%) | 7 (7.6%) | N = 92 |
| Change in sexual relations with partner | 8 (8.7%) | 82 (89.1%) | 2 (2.2%) | N = 92 |

Source: Based on data from Philadelphia Assault Victim Study, Final Report to the National Institute of Mental Health, Joseph J. Peters Institute, Philadelphia, June, 1976.

of the sample, rape results in long-term problems with sexual functioning.

## Predictors of Sexual Adjustment Problems

The information was further analyzed in order to identify situational factors which might be associated with negative changes in sexual functioning. The features of the rape situation itself were examined—type of force, type of sex act committed—for differences in adjustment outcome. Factors associated with short-term changes in sexual functioning will be presented first.

The relationship between the victim and the rapist was a significant predictor of short-term (immediately after the rape) differences in sexual adjustment outcome. The findings indicate that the closer the relationship the more likely the victim will report a negative change in sexual functioning. All six of the victims who reported that they were raped by friends had a negative change in overall heterosexual relations immediately following the rape.

Individuals who were raped by strangers are only half as likely to report a negative change in heterosexual relations immediately after the rape as those who were raped by non-strangers (Table 23-4).

Several situational factors were associated with long-term changes in the victim's sexual functioning. For example, when a weapon was used as part of a rape, respondents were almost seven times more likely to report negative changes in their sexual relations at 11 months after the rape (Table 23-5).

However, the use of roughness was significantly associated with lower rates of negative change in sexual functioning. It may be that the use of physical force in the rape situation is a factor associated with improved post-rape sexual adjustment.

In examining the relationship between sexual acts committed during the rape and the victim's sexual adjustment, a clear and consistent line of interpretation emerge. When cunnilingus was performed (Table 23-6), victims reported negative changes in their heterosexual relations at 11 months after the rape. Also, victims of repeated intercourse during the rape were significantly more likely to report a negative change in their heterosexual relations at 11 months after the rape.

## SUMMARY

A review of the literature found that many rape victims reported sexual difficulties immediately after being raped with fewer victims reporting persistent difficulties (up to 12 months). The most frequently noted sexual difficulty, which can be categorized as a psychosexual dysfunction, was the avoidance of heterosexual activity post-rape. This avoid-

TABLE 23-4 **Chi Square Analysis of Heterosexual Relations Immediately After the Rape by Victim–Offender Relationship**

| Raped by | Change in Overall Heterosexual Relations | | | |
|---|---|---|---|---|
| | Worsened | No Change | Improved | Total N |
| Friend/family | 16 (64.0%) | 9 (36.0%) | (0.0%) | 25 (31.6%) |
| Stranger | 19 (35.2%) | 34 (63.0%) | 1 (1.9%) | 54 (68.4%) |
| Totals | 35 (44.3%) | 43 (54.4%) | 1 (1.3%) | 79 (100.0%) |

Chi Square = 5.94
$df = 2$
$p = .05$

Source: Based on data from Philadelphia Assault Victim Study, Final Report of the National Institute of Mental Health, Joseph J. Peters Institute, Philadelphia, June, 1976.

TABLE 23-5  Chi Square Analysis of Sexual Relations with Partner at 11 Months After the Rape by Intimidation with an Object

| Intimidation with an Object | Sexual Relations with Partner | | | |
|---|---|---|---|---|
| | Worsened | No Change | Improved | Total N |
| No | 1 | 41 | 2 | 44 |
| | (2.3%) | (93.2%) | (4.5%) | (48.4%) |
| Yes | 7 | 40 | | 47 |
| | (14.9%) | (85.1%) | (0.0%) | (51.6%) |
| Totals | 8 | 81 | 2 | 91 |
| | (8.8%) | (89.0%) | (2.2%) | (100.0%) |

Chi Square = 6.42
$df = 2$
$p = .04$

Source: Based on data from Philadelphia Assault Victim Study, Final Report to the National Institute of Mental Health, Joseph J. Peters Institute, Philadelphia, June, 1976.

ance behavior may be understood as part of the rape victim's Posttraumatic stress disorder. The avoidance of sexual activities post-rape minimizes the possibility of re-experiencing the feelings of total helplessness and potential annihilation as felt by the victim during the traumatic event. In addition, an analysis of a subsample of rape victims ($N=105$) from the Philadelphia Assault Victim Study found similar proportions of victims reporting immediate and long-term sexual difficulties. A small number of the raped women were still bothered by debilitating psychosexual difficulties 11 months post-rape. Importantly, certain aspects of the rape incident were found to be predictors of acute and chronic sexual difficulties as noted:

Immediate sexual difficulties
• raped by friend(s)

Chronic sexual difficulties
• repeated sexual intercourse
• the addition of cunnilingus to penile–vaginal intercourse
• intimidation with an object.

While the findings indicated that the sexual functioning of some victims was impaired by the rape, the fact that not all rape victims report sexual difficulties post-rape may be due to any or all of the following reasons. (1) There may be the absence of specific incident factors which are associated with sexual difficulties. (2) Not all rape victims respond to the rape

TABLE 23-6  Chi Square Analysis of Heterosexual Relations at 11 Months After the Rape by Type of Sex Act

| Cunnilingus | Change in Overall Heterosexual Relations | | | |
|---|---|---|---|---|
| | Worsened | No Change | Improved | Total N |
| No | 10 | 88 | | 98 |
| | (10.2%) | (89.8%) | (0.0%) | (94.2%) |
| Yes | 3 | 3 | | 6 |
| | (50.0%) | (50.0%) | (0.0%) | (5.8%) |
| Totals | 13 | 91 | | 104 |
| | (12.5%) | (87.5%) | (0.0%) | (100.0%) |

Chi Square = 4.95
$df = 1$
$p = .03$

Source: Based on data from Philadelphia Assault Victim Study, Final Report to the Natioinal Institute of Mental Health, Joseph J. Peters Institute, Philadelphia, June, 1976.

with a Posttraumatic stress disorder. (3) For some victims, pseudo-adjustment efforts may result in the distortion of responses.

## CONCLUSION

The clinician, as well as the researcher, need to consider the following when evaluating psychosexual dysfunction in the adult female post-rape: (1) that the assessment of the nature and direction of sexual functioning requires the comparison of specific sexual behavior and their frequencies pre- and post-rape, and (2) that the details of the rape incident, such as, victim–offender relationship, type and degree of force, and type and frequency of forced sexual activity, should be obtained and their impact on psychosexual functioning should be explored.

## REFERENCES

American Psychiatric Association Committee on Nomenclature and Statistics: *Diagnostic and Statistical Manual of Mental Disorders,* 3d ed. (DSM–III). American Psychiatric Association, Washington, D.C., 1980.

Bailey, F., and Rothblatt, H.: *Crimes of Violence: Rape and Other Sex Crimes,* The Lawyers Co-operative Publishing Co., Rochester, New York, 1973.

Becker, J. V.; Skinner, L. J.; Abel, G. G.; and Treacy, E. C.: Incidence and types of sexual dysfunctions in rape and incest victims. *J. Sex Marital Ther.* 8:65–74, 1982.

Bienen, L.: Rape II. *Women's Law Rep.* Spring/Summer: 90–137, 1977.

Brownmiller, S.: *Against Our Will: Men, Women and Rape,* Bantam, New York, 1975.

Burgess, A. W., and Holmstrom, L. L.: Rape trauma syndrome. *Am. J. Psychiatry,* 131:981–86, 1974.

Burgess, A. W., and Holmstrom, L.: Rape: Sexual disruption and recovery. *Am. J. Orthopsychiatr.,* 49:648–657, 1979.

Federal Bureau of Investigation: *Uniform Crime Reports.* U.S. Department of Justice, Washington D.C., 1978.

Federal Bureau of Investigation: *Uniform Crime Reports.* U.S. Department of Justice, Washington D.C., 1982.

Feldman-Summers, S.; Gordon, P. E.; and Meagher, J. R.: The impact of rape on sexual satisfaction. *J. Abnorm. Psychol.,* 88:101–105, 1979.

Kaplan, H. S.: *The New Sex Therapy.* Bruner/Mazel, New York, 1974.

Kilpatrick, D.; Veronen, L.; and Resnick, P.: The aftermath of rape: Recent empirical findings. *Am. J. Orthopsychiatr.,* 49:658–669, 1979.

Kilpatrick, D.; Resnick P.; and Veronen, L.: Effects of a rape experience: A longitudinal study. *J. Soc. Issues.* 37:106–122, 1981.

Krasner, W.; Meyer, L. C.; and Carroll, N. E.: *Victims of Rape.* U.S. Government Printing Office, Washington, D.C. 1976.

Marriage Council of Philadelphia Inc.: *Marital Counseling for Rape Victims.* National Technical Information Service, U.S. Department of Commerce, Springfield, Va., 1979.

McCahill, T. W.; Meyer, L. C.; and Fischmann, A. M.: *The Aftermath of Rape.* Heath, Lexington, Mass., 1979.

Nadelson, C. C.; Notman, M. T.; Zackson, H.; and Gornick, J.: A follow-up study of rape victims. *Am. J. Psychiatry,* 139:1266–1270, 1982.

Notman, M. T., and Nadelson, C. C.: The rape victim: Psychodynamic considerations. *Am. J. Psychiatry,* 133:408–412, 1976.

Peters, J. J.: Social, legal and psychological effects of rape on the victim. *Penn. Med.,* 78:34–6, 1975.

Snelling, H. A.: What is rape?. In Schultz, L. G.: (ed.): *Rape Victimology.* C. C. Thomas, Springfield, Ill., 1975.

Sutherland, S., and Scherl, D. J.: Patterns of response among victims of rape. *Am. J. Orthopsychiatr.,* 40:503–510, 1970.

World Health Organization, U.S. National Center for Health Statistics: *The International Classification of Diseases, 9th Revision, Clinical Modification,* Vol. 1. Edwards Brothers, Ann Arbor, Mich., 1981.

# CHAPTER 24  GENDER IDENTITY DISORDERS

Ira B. Pauly, M.D.

## INTRODUCTION

Only within the last 30 years has there emerged a clear classification of gender identity disorders. This chapter deals with the spectrum of gender identity disorders, the most extreme of which is referred to as transsexualism or the gender dysphoria syndrome (Fisk, 1974). This psychiatric disorder is characterized by the individual's intense desire for transformation, by hormonal and/or surgical means, into the gender opposite to the individual's birth sex, and is based on the transsexuals complete identification with the gender role of the opposite sex. These individuals attempt to deny and reverse their original biological gender, and pass into and maintain the opposite gender role identification. Transsexuals emulate the characteristics of the opposite gender in behavior, dress, attitude, sexual preference, as well as in striving desperately to approximate the anatomical structure of the genitalia of the opposite sex. The so-called change of sex operation becomes the single theme and preoccupation of the transsexual's life, and these patients request sex reassignment surgery (SRS). Therefore they present to the surgeon not to the psychiatrist, and they seem to resent the implication that psychiatric referral is required, since they do not view their dilemma as a psychiatric problem, but as a matter of having been born into the wrong body. Thus, this syndrome is of interest to the surgeon, urologist, gynecologist, and plastic surgeon—as well as to the endocrinologist and psychiatrist. In an ironic sense, transsexualism may be considered iatrogenic, in that advances in surgical technique now permit the realization of fantasies of sexual metamorphosis. This fact is borne out by the response to the famous Christine Jorgenson case, where the reporting endocrinologist immediately received 465 letters from individuals requesting SRS (Hamburger, 1953). However, the decision to operate is an extremely complex one, made even more difficult by threats of suicide and self-mutilation by desperate gender dysphoric patients. The justification for SRS has been challenged vigorously from within the emerging subspecialty of gender dysphoria and from the larger medical community and the public. The final section of this chapter deals with follow-up studies that provide some data upon which to draw conclusions about the efficacy of SRS.

## HISTORICAL BACKGROUND

### EARLY LITERATURE

The concept of gender dysphoria and its specific forms of expression have been known since antiquity, and have been described in literature from Herodotus to Shakespeare (Green, 1966; Pauly, 1965). Well-known historical examples of preference for the opposite gender range from the Roman emperor Caligula to the French diplomat, Chevalier d'Eon

(Masson, 1935). In the medical literature the first mention of this problem came from Germany (Friedreich, 1830), while in 1838 Esquirol reported two cases of transvestism in the French literature. Westphal (1870) and Krafft-Ebing (1877) continued the German tradition describing cases of gender dysphoria in which ideas of sexual metamorphosis were thought to represent a form of paranoid psychosis. Excessive horseback riding, with presumed testicular atrophy, was postulated as an organic cause for gender reversal by de Montyel in 1877. Freud's term for this phenomenon was "psychosexual inversion," but he referred primarily to the reversal of sexual object choice or homosexuality (Freud, 1910). Marcuse (1916) underscored the intensity of the drive for change of sex or SRS. Magnus Hirschfeld (1910), the famous German sexologist, coined the term "transvestism," and indicated that cross-dressing represented only the most obvious aspect of the syndrome. Havelock Ellis (1936) used the term sexoesthetic inversion, and later eonism, stressing cross-gender living, and being accepted by society as a member of the opposite sex. German and French researchers (Binder, 1933; Masson, 1935) continued to contribute to this field through the 1930s. D. O. Cauldwell (1949), an American, first used the term "transsexualism," stressing its antisocial aspects by calling the syndrome *Psychopathia Transsexualis*. However, it was Dr. Harry Benjamin, (1953, 1966), sexologist from New York City, who popularized the term transsexualism and became the modern pioneer and major contributor to this field. In honor of his work and dedication to the cause of the transsexual, the International Gender Dysphoria Association was named after Dr. Benjamin. Currently research in this field has shifted from primarily German and French workers to American contributors.

## THE MODERN ERA OF THE GENDER IDENTITY MOVEMENT

The publicity surrounding the Christine Jorgenson case has ushered in the modern era of gender identity research. Certainly Christian Hamburger must be credited for initially bringing this syndrome to the attention of the public as well as to the medical profession (Hamburger et al., 1953). The surgical transformation from male to female of an American ex-army sergeant by a Danish plastic surgeon in Copenhagen was headline copy in newspapers all over the world in late 1952. However, it was not long before reprimands and criticism were leveled at the Danish team who evaluated and treated Jorgensen (Ostow, 1953; Wiedeman, 1953). This controversy continues to the present, since the removal of nondiseased organs, especially the genitalia, runs contrary to strongly held personal and professional beliefs.

Even though the Jorgenson case was not the first sex reassignment for a transsexual, the worldwide attention it received publicized that surgical technique had developed to the point where something could be done for the suffering transsexual (Pauly, 1965). Literally thousands of gender dysphoric individuals came forth requesting and demanding the so-called sex change operation. Many of these individuals were referred to Harry Benjamin in both New York and San Francisco, and he continued to provide evaluation and hormone treatment, while looking for medical centers to provide SRS in the United States, rather than having to send his patients abroad. He culminated years of research and treatment of gender dysphoric patients with the original and classic monograph *The Transsexual Phenomenon* (Benjamin, 1966).

With the help of the Erickson Educational Foundation, the Johns Hopkins Hospital initiated their Gender Identity Clinic in 1965 and performed their first SRS in 1966. In quick succession, gender identity programs developed in university medical centers at Minnesota, Stanford, Oregon, and Case Western Reserve, to name a few. Interdisciplinary teams, composed of psychiatrists, psychologists, surgeons (urologists, gynecologists, and plastic surgeons), endocrinologists, epidemiologists, formed as each specialist became interested in some aspect of the transsexual's evaluation and treatment. The very primitive speculations on gender identity formation, first promulgated by Freud, now were modified because of the study of these dramatic cases of gender misidentification (Pauly, 1974, 1980; Stroller, 1968).

Early theorists emerged in the gender identity movement (Pauly, 1983). John Money, the psychologist at the Johns Hopkins Gender Identity Clinic, was prominent in defining some basic concepts of gender identity formation, using data from children born with confusing external genitalia—pseudohermaphrodites (Money, et al., 1955). He has continued to be prolific in his writing, and in collaboration with Richard Green, edited the first definitive textbook in the field, *Transsexualism and Sex Reassignment* (Green and Money, 1969). Money's work on gender identity disorders culminated in the monograph, *Man and Woman: Boy and Girl* (Money and Ehrhardt, 1972).

The contributors to this new subspecialty are many and space does not permit more than cursory mention of a few. Robert Stroller from UCLA became a major theorist on gender formation, publishing his book, *Sex and Gender,* in 1968. This author began studying transsexualism in 1962, publishing articles in the medical literature over the next 20 years (Pauly, 1965, 1968, 1969a, b; 1974, 1980, 1981, 1983; Pauly and Lindgren, 1976). Richard Green emerged as an important researcher, furnishing the introduction to Benjamin's classic in 1966, coediting *Transsexualism and Sex Reassignment* in 1969, and establishing the journal *Archives of Sexual Behavior* in 1971 (Green, 1966; Green and Money, 1969). Later, Green published his own monograph on *Gender Identity Conflict in Children and Adults* (1974). Last but not least in this abbreviated list of early contributors is Jan Walinder from the University of Goteborg in Sweden. Since his doctoral thesis on *Transsexualism* (1967) to the present, Walinder has contributed significantly to the medical literature (Walinder, 1967, 1968, 1971; Walinder and Thuwe, 1975, 1976; Walinder et al., 1978, 1979). In particular, his epidemiological research has quite clearly defined the prevalence, incidence, and male to female ratio of transsexualism (Walinder, 1968, 1971; Walinder et al., 1979; Ross et al., 1981).

The number of publications on this topic has proliferated in the last 20 years (Pauly, 1981). This author collected 100 articles after an exhaustive review of the world literature on transsexualism through 1964 (Pauly, 1965). By 1969, Green and Money's textbook listed 381 references, 100 of which were previously mentioned by Pauly. Each year since 1970, there have been approximately 50 articles per year published on this subject, many of which appear in the monthly issue of the *Archives of Sexual Behavior.*

## TRANSSEXUALISM AND GENDER DYSPHORIA

The syndrome of transsexualism is characterized by a life-long preference for the opposite gender role, predicated on the conviction of belonging to the opposite sex. This conviction persists despite the painfully obvious fact of normal anatomy and genitalia, before and after puberty, and in the absence of delusional ideation or psychosis. Transsexuals are disgusted with the development of their primary and secondary sexual characteristics, and the penis in males and breasts in females, are perceived as the offensive organs and their removal becomes a preoccupation for transsexual individuals. In addition, these desperately unhappy people seek the anatomical status of the opposite gender, and the hallmark of this syndrome is the request for sex reassignment surgery.

Feeling they belong to the opposite sex, transsexuals feel "unnatural" in a love relationship with someone of the opposite biological sex, considering this to be homosexual. Perceiving themselves to be members of the opposite sex, they consider it appropriate to have a love relationship with an individual of the same biological sex but of the opposite gender identity. Some evidence suggests that the sexual activity *per se,* whether it be considered homosexual or heterogenderal, plays a minor or secondary role (Pauly, 1965, 1974). Certainly the primary goal of the transsexual is to pass successfully in society as a member of the opposite sex. Transsexuals are often sufficiently convincing in their ability to "pass" that some have lived for many years as members of the opposite sex, even without contrary hormone therapy or SRS. Other transsexuals are not so confident or fortunate and present to the physician requesting hormonal and surgical treatment in the hope that this will permit them to realize their goal of being accepted as members of the opposite sex. (The reader is referred to the original articles which describe in detail the adult manifestations of these syndromes in the male-to-female [Benjamin, 1966; Green and Money, 1969; Pauly, 1965, 1968, 1969a, b; Walinder, 1967] and female-to-male situation [Pauly, 1969; 1974; Lothstein, 1983].)

This syndrome has now been sufficiently described and accepted in the psychiatric literature that it became formally recognized in 1980 in the *Diagnostic and Statistical Manual* (DSM–III) of the American Psychiatric Association (APA, 1980). Under the section entitled Gender Identity Disorders are listed the following criteria for transsexualism, code number 302.8:

1. Sense of discomfort and inappropriateness about one's anatomic sex (feeling trapped in the wrong body).
2. Wish to be rid of one's own genitalia and to live as a member of the other sex (a request for hormone treatment and SRS in order to pass in society unnoticed as a member of the opposite sex).
3. Above has been continuous for at least 2 years (and usually present since earliest memory and persistent through childhood and adolescence).
4. Absence of physical intersex or genetic abnormalities (in other words, these patients are anatomically and genetically normal).
5. Not due to another mental disorder such as schizophrenia (in which case there may well be confused identity during an acute crisis). (pp. 263–264)

Thus, there are three positive and two negative criteria for the diagnosis of transsexualism. In addition, DSM–III lists the criteria for the diagnosis of childhood transsexualism in boys and girls (APA, 1980). These include a boy's persistent desire to be a girl and his insistence that he actually is a girl. Also, there is the repudiation of one's anatomical status and strong preference for the role, activities, dress, name, and social status of the opposite sex, all with their onset prior to puberty.

Spectrum of Gender Identity Disorders

Thus far we have emphasized the most extreme manifestation of gender identity misidentification, however, there is a continuum along which each and every individual might assume his or her place. The process of gender identification, as a normative development sequence, is only beginning to come under scientific scrutiny (Pauly, 1980). The nature/nurture and genetic/environmental dichotomies are still in contention when attempting to understand this normal developmental process, let alone problems that arise outside the norm. Certainly the very early onset (3–4 years) of strong preference for the gender role incongruent with the individual's normal biological sex, causes one to consider a biological force, either genetic or hormonal. Unfortunately, the promise of such an early genetic determinant of gender dysphoria, as determined by the H–Y antigen test (Eicher, 1981; Eicher et al., 1979), has been repudiated (Ciccarese et al., 1982; Pfafflin, 1981). The role of hormone imbalance, probably prenatal, influencing the central nervous system, has been suggested as an important predisposition towards contrary sex role behavior and gender identity (Money and Ehrhardt, 1972; Money, 1974). Money (1974) places transsexualism at the extreme end of the cross-gender identity spectrum, with transvestism and homosexuality as less extreme manifestations, all three having their origins in hormonal imbalance during some critical period of development. In contrast to this hormonal or biological view of the etiology of gender identity disorders are various social or intrafamilial forces which might explain this phenomenon. Pauly (1968, 1969a,b, 1974), Stoller (1968, 1972, 1980), and Lothstein (1983) have underscored the significance of intrafamily dynamics and relationships in the etiology of both male-to-female and female-to-male transsexualism. Finally, the influence of societal factors, especially the rigidity of society with reference to sex roles, sexual equality, and homosexuality, has been hypothesized as an etiological factor in the development of transsexualism (Ross et al., 1978). In fact, Ross and coworkers (1981) attempted to prove this hypothesis by comparing the frequency and sex ratio of transsexualism in two different cultures, Sweden and Australia. Although their results suggest significant societal factors bearing on the etiology and development of transsexualism, the authors are quick to point out the limitations of such research. Suffice it to say that hard data in this field have not emerged thus far. Therefore, the precise cause is far from clear. Multiple factors may operate in sequence, with a biological predisposition being augmented by intrafamily and social forces. In any event, further speculation on etiology is not warranted in this review.

Returning to the issue of the variability of human behavior, it is sometimes difficult to be sure when gender behavior is sufficiently atypical to warrant evaluation or treatment. Certainly gender roles are stereotyped and tend to be dimorphic in most Western cultures. In the extreme, pretranssexual boys and girls behave in a sufficiently cross-genderal fashion that their families have good reason for concern. These effeminate boys, often labeled "sissies" by their peers, receive much more abuse than their female counterparts, whose tomboyish behavior is better tolerated (Pauly, 1980). Even so, very young boys are brought to the physician for evaluation of their gender role behavior. Follow-up studies suggest these young boys with atypical gender role behavior grow up to demonstrate atypical gender role and/or atypical sexual preference as adults (Green, 1976; Lebovitz, 1972; Money and Russo, 1979; Zuger, 1966, 1984). Young girls are seen less often for atypical gender behavior, unless there is an extreme repudiation and denial of their femaleness. A broad range of gender behavior exists, and many aberrations are quite well tolerated by society, unless they become extremely pronounced. Although gender role behavior is dimorphic, it does overlap, which makes early detection of potential pathology quite difficult. Also, there appears to be a trend toward less rigidity and stereotyping and more acceptance It remains to be seen whether this unisex concept will develop to such an extent that individuals will feel less inclined to resort to SRS in order to feel comfortable.

As these children grow up into adolescents and adults, they identify themselves as feeling uncomfortable with their biological sex and prefer the opposite gender identity. Often they try to adjust to the gender expectations set by parents and society. However, at one point, the internal pressure to "be myself" intensifies and the individual makes the disclosure which usually results in professional evaluation. Clearly, not everyone who feels that a sex change operation is the solution to their problems is a good candidate for the procedure. The term "gender dysphoria syndrome" has emerged as the generic name for all those individuals who present with some form of gender identity difficulty (Fisk, 1974; Laub and Fisk, 1974). Under this umbrella of gender dysphoria fall other diagnostic categories, the common denominator of which is a person's displeasure with original genital anatomy and a desire or demand for SRS. Laub and Fisk (1974) list the following diagnostic possibilities:

1. Classic Transsexualism of Benjamin—lifelong history of desire to be a member of the gender opposite his/her biological sex.
2. Transvestism—cross-dresser who receives erotic stimulation from wearing female clothing as a prelude to heterosexual activity.
3. Effeminate Homosexuality (Male) or Masculine Lesbianism (Female)—erotically attracted to same biologically sexed individual, and gives history of enjoying the use of their genitalia in homosexual love making.

4. Psychosis—discomfort regarding one's gender identity in the face of a psychotic decompensation only, and does not endure when patient is over the acute episode.
5. Psychopathic or Sociopathic Personality—individuals who wish to achieve notoriety or financial gain from SRS, and who are not sincere or truthful in their protestations of cross-gender identification. (pp. 390)

The primary distinguishing characteristic of the above differential diagnoses is the age of onset and the persistence of the gender dysphoria, which is sometimes difficult to ascertain due to the patient's truthfulness and reliability as a historian. Also, most of the intelligent gender dysphoric individuals have become very familiar with literature on this topic and know what the criteria are considered to be. Person and Ovesy (1974) make a similar point by distinguishing primary from secondary transsexualism. In order to confirm the transsexual's history that their gender identity problem originated in early childhood, it is essential to have contact with the parents or other family members. For primary transsexuals, parents do confirm the patient's history that cross-gender identification has persisted since early childhood. However, when either the patient or family member reports that the individual had developed a comfortable gender identity that was congruent with biological sex, then one should begin to consider secondary forms of transsexualism or gender dysphoria (Stoller, 1980). Many authors have underscored the multiplicity of diagnostic and personality characteristics of those who request SRS (Levine and Lothstein, 1981; Meyer, 1974). The difficult question of evaluation and treatment will be considered in the following section.

## Epidemiology

Some difficulties arise in attempting to calculate the frequency (prevalence and incidence) of this condition. One problem has to do with the difficulties inherent in agreeing on the definition and diagnostic criteria, that is, distinguishing transsexualism from other types of gender dysphoria or distinguishing primary from secondary transsexualism. The other major problem is the issue of reporting cases—even if one were able to overcome the first problem of diagnostic criteria. Since there is no central clearing house or registry for reporting such information, it is difficult to collect these statistics. Different researchers have used different methods to determine prevalence. Also, some patients may not present to physicians for evaluation and treatment for a variety of reasons, and others may be treating themselves with illegally obtained contrary sex hormones. The following data are therefore considered to be only minimal estimates of the frequency with which transsexualism actually occurs.

In the first speculation on prevalence, the numbers of patients who presented themselves or were referred to the only university medical center in the state of Oregon were used (Pauly, 1968). These figures on the prevalence of transsexualism in the United States were 1 in 100,000 males and 1 in 400,000 females in the general population. At about the same time, Walinder published data from Sweden, in which he demonstrated a much higher prevalence, although some of this difference had to do with a difference in calculation; Walinder based his estimates on the population over the age of 15 years, rather than on the total population. In any event, Walinder's figures indicate a prevalence of 1 in 37,000, males and 1 in 103,000 females (Walinder, 1967, 1971; Walinder et al., 1979). Subsequent research from England and Wales, using Walinder's method, tends to confirm these higher prevalence figures (Hoenig and Kenna, 1974). Finally, more recent research from Australia suggests a somewhat higher prevalence for males, 1 in 24,000, but lower prevalence for females, 1 in 150,000 (Ross et al., 1981). This last research is weakened by the fact that only 30 percent of the psychiatrists returned the questionnaires which were sent out requesting information on the numbers of transsexuals seen. In any event, these figures would indicate that the estimates are less than the real prevalence.

In addition to calculations on prevalence—the total number of transsexuals at a given date—there are figures for incidence—the number of new cases each year. Clearly Walinder's work is the most accurate, since Swedish law now requires all transsexuals to apply to the authorities for sex reassignment (Walinder and Thuwe, 1976). Also, these figures are available for the years 1967–1978 (Walinder et al., 1979), and indicate an annual incidence of 0.17/100,000 inhabitants over age 15 years. On the other hand, more recent data from Australia indicates a much higher incidence, 0.58/100,000 over age 15 years (Ross et al., 1981).

Also of some interest is the male to female ratio. When Benjamin first reported figures on this ratio it was over an 8 to 1 male/female ratio. Since that time, more accurate estimates have revealed a 4 to 1 male/female preponderance (Pauly, 1968). However, the Swedish and British studies show a 2.8 to 1 and 3.2 to 1 preponderance of males over females, based on prevalence data. When looking at incidence data, that is, new cases each year since 1968, the Swedish data support an equal distribution of 1 to 1 male:female ratio (Walinder et al., 1979). The Australian data continue to show a marked male preponderance of about 5 to 1, based on incidence data. Ross and coworkers (1981) speculate that this marked difference reflects a social influence in the etiology of transsexualism. Briefly, they postulate that the more restrictive cultures are toward male homosexuality, the greater the number of males wishing to have SRS, so as to conceal their underlying homosexuality. They feel that only the male homosexuals are thus stigmatized and that female homosexuality is better accepted and tolerated. However, an alternative explanation may be that more female transsexuals live with their gender discomfort, without seeking medical attention, or perhaps they are aware that female to male surgery is less well-developed, than is male-to-female. In any event, it is difficult to conceive that the young child is sufficiently cognizant of society's negative bias toward homosexuality, so that it becomes a factor in early cross-gender behavior. If anything, most cultures continue to support the double standard, in which the male role is more valued than the female, which would support a cultural bias in favor of a greater prevalence for female transsexualism.

Transsexualism as DSM-III defines (APA, 1980) is clearly more prevalent than previously thought. At least 1 in 50,000 individuals over the age of 15 years is likely to be a transsexual. It would appear that the male/female ratio is probably close to 1 to 1 in most cultures. If a higher male preponderance is present, this could reflect a more negative basis in that culture toward male homosexuality. Or it could reflect a lack of availability in that culture for surgical sex reassignment for female-to-male transsexuals. Whatever the real statistics may turn out to be, this disorder carries more significance than the actual prevalence might suggest: perhaps there is some gender dysphoria in all of us, no matter how latent; certainly our culture is struggling with issues of women's equality. Most importantly, however, the study of the normative process of gender identification has been well served by our research into the etiology and prevalence of transsexualism.

## Transsexualism and Body Image

The concept of body image has particular relevance to the phenomenon of transsexualism and gender dysphoria (Lindgren and Pauly, 1975; Pauly and Lindgren, 1976). Body image has come to mean not only the way one perceives his or her own body, but also the way he or she feels about these perceptions. As such it is an important part of one's overall self-concept (Berscheid et al., 1973; Gorman, 1969; Kolb, 1959). The transsexual is unable to form a satisfactory body image because of the dissonance between anatomic sex and gender identity. Thus, the reality of the transsexual's body does not conform to the preferred or desired body image. The result is a disturbance in the formation of a complete and consistent self-concept.

The transsexual attempts to reduce this dissonance through a variety of means with the end result of bringing the physical body form in line with the preferred gender concept. The male transsexual cross-dresses, wears a wig, obtains electrolysis to remove facial hair or covers it up with make-up, uses a bra and padding, and so on, in an attempt to correct his body image dissatisfaction. In addition to these outward attempts to pass as a woman, the male transsexual assumes the preferred body image in fantasies and daydreams. Likewise, the female transsexual dresses in a masculine manner, cuts "his" hair short and in a masculine fashion, flattens "his" breasts, and pads "his" crotch to simulate the presence of a penis. Finally, however, the transsexual seeks the alteration of his or her actual body, through endocrinological and surgical means, to bring it into harmony with the preferred body image; hormone therapy and SRS are the hallmarks of the syndrome of transsexualism.

In 1975, Lindgren and Pauly introduced a Body Image Scale which they felt might help in the evaluation and treatment of transsexualism (Lindgren and Pauly, 1975). This 30-item list of body parts asks respondents to rate their feeling about that part of their body on a 5-point scale, from very satisfied (1) to very dissatisfied (5). Among other things, this research revealed that transsexuals invariably scored certain body parts as (5) or "very dissatisfied" and that these body parts were primary genderal characteristics (Lindgren and Pauly, 1975). For the male-to-female transsexual they are the penis, scrotum, testicles, facial hair, body hair, and breasts (lack of them). For the female-to-male transsexual the most hated parts of the anatomy are breasts, vagina, clitoris, ovaries–uterus, chest, voice, and facial hair (lack of it). This pattern of dissatisfaction is thought to be quite specific in identifying those gender dysphoric individuals who are correctly diagnosed as primary transsexuals. Also the Lindgren–Pauly Body Image Scale has been shown to be useful in following transsexuals from their initial pretreatment phase through hormone therapy and finally SRS. A statistically significant reduction in the overall score indicates that, in well-evaluated cases, this approach is successful in reducing the transsexual's negative body image. The body image scores come down as sex reassignment treatment continues, to closely approximate a normal control group's body image score (Pauly and Lindgren, 1976).

Body image is a useful parameter in the study and evaluation of individuals with a serious gender identity problem, allowing one to characterize the primary transsexual and distinguish this individual from the secondary transsexual, who would not be an appropriate candidate for sex reassignment. Using the Lindgren–Pauly Body Image Scale, a South African researcher has independently confirmed its usefulness in distinguishing "effectively between pre-operative transsexuals and homosexuals" (Theron, 1983, p. 6). Dutch workers have also used this instrument to follow transsexuals through hormone treatment and SRS; their work also confirms the body image scale as a useful objective measure of a transsexual's status while progressing through hormone treatment and SRS (Kuiper and Cohen-Kettenis, 1983).

## EVALUATION AND TREATMENT

Since transsexualism and gender dysphoria are considered psychiatric disorders, their evaluation requires a fully certified psychiatrist or psychologist. However, individuals requesting SRS do not necessarily agree that their condition is of psychogenic origin and usually present to a surgeon or internist. The nonpsychiatric physician should refer such gender dysphoric patients to a psychiatrist before recommending any form of treatment, although the physician might want to perform a medical evaluation, such as a physical examination, endocrinological studies that include testoterone and/or estrogen levels and the like. Even if the physician is convinced of the patient's sincerity and would like to alleviate the suffering, there are good reasons for not responding directly—not the least of which is that some patients have changed their minds, after hormone therapy and SRS, and have implicated their treating physicians in malpractice suits. Even if the physician is convinced that transsexualism is not a psychiatric, but rather an organic, disorder, some psychotic individuals do request SRS and the nonpsychiatrist physician should not attempt to make this distinction.

Once the individual comes to the psychiatrist, the evaluation process is similar to other clinical evaluations. A very careful past history is required, so that the intensity, duration, and stability of the gender dysphoria can be determined. Primary transsexualism is a lifelong identification with the gender role of the opposite biological sex. Since the patients are highly invested in the outcome of the evaluation, they may not be entirely candid or truthful. Transsexuals are usually well-read, and know what to reveal and what not to reveal to their evaluators. The standards of care recommend that such an evaluation extend over a significant period of time and that an independent source of information about the patient be sought (Walker et al., 1979). Obviously, it would help to interview the parents or other family members or friends who have known the patient for a long period of time. Unfortunately, this is not always possible because the patient may be estranged from his or her family. In these cases, a physician should have an even longer contact with the person requesting SRS.

A careful mental status examination is required, primarily to rule out the possibility of an underlying psychotic condition. It is important to inquire about delusions, auditory hallucinations, and other grandiose or bizarre ideation even though the patient may appear quite sane. Quite apart from the issues of psychosis, the evaluator needs to be alert to the issues of depression and suicidal ideation. Many gender dysphoric patients are quite desperate. They have experienced rejection and ridicule, and may regard this attempt at obtaining help as their "last chance." Many investigators have pointed out the prevalence of depression and suicidal ideation in the transsexual prior to their undergoing sex reassignment treatment (Lothstein, 1982; Pauly, 1965; 1974; Walinder, 1967). Obviously, the diagnosis of gender dysphoria or transsexualism need not be the only psychiatric diagnosis. Affective disorders, primarily depression, with or without psychotic features, may also be present. An accurate assessment of I.Q. is also important, since the evaluator must document that the patient has sufficient capacity and competence to understand the implications and consequences of SRS.

In addition to primary psychiatric diagnosis, there may be other, secondary, or Axis II diagnoses. Among other innovations, the DSM–III (APA, 1980) includes a multiaxial diagnostic formulation. Axis I is the primary psychiatric diagnosis—i.e., transsexualism. Major depression may also accompany transsexualism on Axis I. Personality disorders such as borderline personality have been suggested by the Case Western Reserve University Gender Identity program (Lothstein, 1983). Thus Axis II might include borderline personality, passive–dependent personality, or even sociopathic personality. In the final analysis, very few transsexuals are likely to be so well-adjusted, socially, as to be totally free of other psychopathology, especially depression. For this reason, in addition to the premise that this disorder is psychogenic in etiology, it is likely that the transsexual, primary or secondary, could benefit from psychiatric evaluation and from psychotherapy. This psychiatric evaluation and therapy is especially useful for the preoperative patient, although the postoperative transsexual may require support in adjusting to their new status even after SRS. However, psychotherapy is not effective in modifying the fixed gender misidentification that characterizes the primary transsexual. On the other hand, psychotherapy is compatible with the recommendation for hormone therapy or SRS. The role of psychotherapy in the treatment of gender dysphoria will be discussed later in this chapter.

It is clear that the evaluation process is an extended and extensive one. Unfortunately there are no objective laboratory tests which are of solid diagnostic value. Certainly a psychological consultation is useful. The Minnesota Multiphasic Personality Inventory (MMPI) with its M–F scale is helpful in confirming cross-gender identification and identifying other psychopathology. The Weschler Adult Intelligence Scale (WAIS) is useful in documenting adequate I.Q., and projective tests are helpful in ruling out psychosis. As mentioned, the Lindgren–Pauly body image scale has proven useful in distinguishing primary transsexuals from other gender dysphoric individuals for whom SRS would not be indicated (Lindgren and Pauly, 1975). Other instruments are being developed that offer promise in helping the clinician to make such discriminations, such as the Standardized Rating Format for the Evaluation of SRS (Hunt and Hampson, 1980). Also it is important to obtain peer review and have at least one other mental health professional perform an independent assessment of the patient *before* treatment is initiated. In fact, some 40 interdisciplinary teams, which are loosely designated as gender identity programs, have emerged in North America (Pauly, 1981; Walker et al., 1979). While none of these clinics are identical, the multidisciplinary composition underscores the importance of relying on different disciplines to collectively perform an adequate assessment. Clearly few treatment procedures are as dramatic and irreversible as SRS; it is not possible to undo the removal of the genitalia. Another function of this interdisciplinary composition is to remove the decision making from those clinicians who might be accused of standing to benefit financially from a decision in favor of SRS, that is, the surgeon performing the operation. Even among mental health professionals, subspecialists in gender dysphoria are emerging. On the other hand, this syndrome is now so widely described and included in the training of medical students, residents in psychiatry, and trainees in psychology, that well-trained mental health professionals are aware of transsexualism, even if they are not prepared to evaluate or treat this condition.

## STANDARDS OF CARE

In 1979, the Harry Benjamin Gender Dysphoria Association defined its standards of care (Walker et al., 1979), making clear that these were only "*minimal* requirements, and not to be construed as optimal standards of care." These standards define gender dysphoria as: "That psychological state whereby a person demonstrates dissatisfaction with their sex of birth and the role, as socially defined, which applies to that sex (of birth), and who requests hormonal and surgical sex-reassignment" (p. 2). The following are excerpts from these standards which help to clarify the evaluation and treatment process.

1. Hormone treatment and/or SRS on demand is contraindicated. It is herein professionally improper to . . . perform hormonal sex reassignment or SRS without careful evaluation of the patient's reason for requesting such services, and evaluation of the beliefs and attitudes upon which such reasons are based.
2. Hormone treatment and SRS must be preceded by a firm recommendation for such procedures made by a certified and licensed psychiatrist or psychologist who can justify making such a recommendation by appeal to training or professional experience in dealing with sexual disorders, especially the disorders of gender identity and role.
3. The psychiatrist or psychologist making the recommendation in favor of hormone treatment shall have:
   a) demonstrated the presence of gender dysphoria to have existed for at least two years.
   b) known the patient for at least three months.
   c) required the patient to have lived successfully for at least three months in the gender role opposite his/her biological sex.
   d) required the patient to receive a complete physical examination which includes liver function studies.
4. The psychologist or psychiatrist making a recommendation in favor of nongenital surgical reassignment (i.e., breast reduction or breast augmentation) shall have:
   a) required 3a, b, and d above, and

b) required the patient to have lived successfully for six months in the opposite gender role.
5. The psychiatrist or psychologist, prior to the recommendation in favor of genital SRS (penectomy, orchidectomy, and vaginoplasty in the male-to-female transsexual, and hysterectomy, oophorectomy, salpingectomy, vaginectomy, and phalloplasty in the female-to-male transsexual) shall have:
   a) required 3a, b, and d above.
   b) known the patient for at least six months before endorsing the patient's request for genital SRS.
   c) required the patient to be evaluated at least once by another psychologist or psychiatrist, who will also have recommended in favor of SRS. At least one of the two must be a psychiatrist.
   d) required the patient to have lived successfully in the opposite gender role for *at least* one year.
   e) required the patient to have an urological examination. (Walker et al., 1979)

## TRIAL OF CROSS-GENDER LIVING: THE REAL LIFE TEST

One of the requirements proposed above in the standards of care (Walker *et al.,* 1979) is the so-called real life test. Actually many primary transsexuals have already passed this test, since they may have lived for some time in the opposite gender role before seeking hormones or SRS. If this is the case, this fact is correlated positively with a favorable outcome from SRS. The fact that the individual had been able to pass successfully without hormone therapy speaks positively to the applicant's confidence in being able to pass in society in the gender role opposite to sex of birth and is particularly impressive when cross-gender living began when the individual was quite young. Quite often such individuals have formed close interpersonal relationships and are well-accepted by fellow workers as well as lovers. These relationships are not viewed by the participants as homosexual. The transsexual is perceived by his or her partner as belonging to the gender which the transsexual is portraying. In fact neither partner sees himself or herself or the other as homosexual. It is important to evaluate the transsexual and the partner.

For others, however, cross-gender living is only considered after the recommendation and support of the therapist. Despite the standards of care that advise cross-gender living for at least three months prior to recommendation for hormone therapy, some transsexuals require the additional help of hormones first. The author has found this trial important to the evaluator, but more important to the individual transsexual. Sometimes the fantasy is enjoyed more mentally than in reality. Anxiety over one's ability to pass convincingly must be confronted sooner or later. No matter how strong the opposite gender identification, not all transsexuals are able to pass. Whereas this difficulty may not deter some, for most gender dysphorics this painful reality forces them to consider some other alternative than SRS. Thus, experiencing the reality of living as a member of the opposite sex may or may not enhance the transsexual's motivation. In some cases, the person passes the real life test quite readily and thrives, feeling much happier being on the way to solving the gender problem.

For some, the real life test is a painful confrontation that cross-gender living is not really possible, if they are to enjoy any kind of meaningful social interaction. As painful as this confrontation may be, certainly it is better to appreciate it before any irreversible physical changes have occurred. Hopefully, the transsexual who is unsuccessful in this trial will have greater motivation to search for a psychotherapeutic approach to his or her gender dysphoria. Scattered cases of successful therapy with some gender dysphoric patients are beginning to be reported (Barlow *et al.,* 1973, 1979; Davenport and Harrison, 1977; Dellaert and Kunke, 1969; Kirkpatrick and Friedman, 1976). Lothstein and Levine (1981) summarized their experience in offering psychotherapy to the gender dysphoric patients who present to the Case Western Reserve Gender

Clinic: "Not all gender dysphoric patients are poor candidates for psychotherapy. Some seventy percent of our patients had a successful, non-surgical adaptation to their gender disorders. Although some patients will continue to receive and benefit from surgery, our current knowledge does not warrant its prescription as a panacea" (p. 112). Later, Levine (1983) goes on to explain that over the last decade some 300 patients have been seen for evaluation, psychotherapy, and postsurgical followup. "Prolonged individual and group therapies have been possible with approximately 20 percent of patients initially evaluated" (p. 6). Also, Levine states that "the patient who is considered normal apart from the gender problem has all but disappeared. It seems more clear that gender patients have a basic pervasive self pathology. Their preoccupation with gender issues masks the serious associated difficulties from themselves and for many years from professionals" (p. 7). However, a physician should explore all possible alternatives in the management of these patients before recommending SRS.

An underlying issue pertinent to any discussion about psychotherapy of these fundamental characterological issues is the theoretical orientation of the mental health professional. Fewer and fewer psychotherapists are committed to the long-term, intensive psychotherapy that Freud advocated. Psychologists and psychiatrists, who have neither the training nor inclination to treat, deep-seated characterological problems, refer these patients to dynamically oriented psychoanalysts. Eber (1980) has even suggested that "the transsexual patient may be avoided in psychotherapy because s/he is perceived as endangering the emotional equilibrium of the therapist by stirring up too much psychic pain in the therapist" (p. 36). (For a more thorough review of the status of psychotherapy in the treatment of gender dysphoria and transsexualism, see an excellent monograph by Lothstein (1983).

Returning to the real life test, some researchers recommend that it continue for at least two years (Money and Ambinder, 1978). For most true transsexuals, this period is often very rewarding, especially if the transsexual finds that he or she passes easily and well. Often the patient is supported through this period with hormone therapy, which helps to reduce negative body image problems and reassures the patient that progress is being made. During this time the clinician is able to ascertain if the individual is functioning better in the cross-gender role, with or without psychotherapy, or hormone therapy. This assessment should include some substantiation from sources other than the patient alone. In particular, it is important to document the person's ability to be gainfully employed. The individual's ability to relate socially and develop a support system is also important during this period. And finally, it is essential that the patient be able to cope with less anxiety and depression than before cross-gender living. If these hoped for changes do not occur during this trial of cross-gender living, the evaluator should be quite reluctant to recommend hormone therapy or SRS. Often the individual will become aware of the inadvisability of proceeding with SRS, and possibly elect to pursue a nonsurgical approach. Even if he or she is somewhat successful in the opposite gender role, the individual will realize that the reality of the situation is not as exciting as the fantasies about it. Second thoughts may arise forcing the individual to reconsider. It is important for the evaluator/therapist to take a neutral role of neither advocate or detractor during this process. The therapist should offer support and attempt to work through issues, but not be invested in prematurely determining for or against proceeding with SRS.

HORMONAL TREATMENT OF TRANSSEXUALS

The aim of endocrine treatment in the transsexual patient of either sex is dual: suppression of the existing sexual features (hormonal castration), and development and maintenance of sexual features belonging to the other sex—"paradoxical hormone therapy" (Hamburger, 1969). The recommended medications have not changed very much in the last 15 years (Benjamin, 1969): Estinyl$^R$ (ethinyl estradiol)

0.15–0.5 mg per day for the male-to-female transsexual. To this may be added Provera^R (medroxyprogesterone acetate) 10 mg per day. For the female-to-male transsexual, depotestosterone 200 mg by injections every two weeks is suggested. This hormone therapy reduces the dissonance between the transsexual's actual body configuration and their idealized body image. However, hormone therapy is recommended only after careful evaluation, requiring a minimum of three months contact with the patient, and preferably after a trial of cross-gender living. Since it is easy for the transsexual to have unrealistic expectations of what changes will occur, it is important for the physician to make it clear that a dramatic transformation will not be forthcoming. Again, hormone therapy, usually in conjunction with the real life test of cross-gender living, is a process of self-selection for the transsexual. Usually the transsexual passes this test; he or she is pleased with changes in the physical status which occur and is therefore encouraged by this improved self-perception. Also, it may give the transsexual the additional self-confidence to attempt passing, if he or she has not already done so. In some cases, however, the individual's fantasies of some dramatic sexual metamorphosis are not realized, and discouragement ensues.

When hormone therapy is successful, there is a significant reduction of the score on the Lindgren–Pauly Body Image Scale. Particularly in the male-to-female, the overall pretreatment scores are reduced from "dissatisfied" (3.76 of 5.0) to "satisfied" (2.26 of 5.0), which is significant at the .001 level (Pauly and Lindgren, 1976). Since the overall pretreatment score for the female-to-male transsexuals are not as "dissatisfied" to begin with (2.46 of 5.0), the change after hormone therapy (2.18 of 5.0) is not so significant ($p < .05$). Included in this overall improvement are specific changes that are very likely to follow hormone therapy. For biological males on estrogen therapy the most significant changes are breast development or gynecomastia. For some, this improvement falls short of what had been anticipated and the pre- to posttreatment comparison (reduction from 5.0 to 3.7) is barely significant ($p = 0.1$). Body hair is reduced to some extent, but beard growth continues and this obvious problem can only be addressed through electrolysis. Facial hair is particularly problematic if the male transsexual has a heavy, dark beard, which is not easily concealed by make-up. Several hundred hours of electrolysis are required for the successful removal of facial hair. Scalp hair may become fuller on estrogen therapy and this may or may not enable the transsexual to achieve the feminine hair style desired. If not, some individuals use wigs. It is not to be expected that hormone therapy would alter the other primary genderal characteristics such as penis, scrotum, or testicles. Obviously, these organs can only be removed through SRS. However, some of the secondary genderal characteristics are improved considerably, such as hips ($p = .02$), figure ($p = .05$) and waist ($p = .02$), while all the others are improved slightly (Lindgren and Pauly, 1975). Interestingly, even some body parts which are unresponsive to hormone therapy, such as feet, face, nose, height, eyebrows, seem to improve or are rated more positively by male transsexuals on hormone therapy. Therefore the overall sense of well-being that occurs for most primary transsexuals after initiation of estrogen therapy is reflected in a significant improvement in the overall body perception or body image even though many parts evaluated by this scale are not directly influenced by the hormone treatment. Undoubtedly, this is explained, to some extent, by the improvement in mood most transsexuals experience after hormone therapy and SRS. Although this body image scale has not been used on depressed patients, the author's clinical experience suggests that depressed patients would score more highly (more dissatisfied) when depressed as compared to the same respondent when not depressed.

Those males who self-select to discontinuing with hormone therapy show a different pattern from those who follow it. Their body image scores are usually very high to begin with, and do not show the pattern of improvement indicated above. Some attempt to go beyond the recommended doses prescribed. They feel they cannot attempt passing until their appearance is more convincing and this lack of self-confidence continues. Although hormone therapy should not be recommended lightly, especially in view of the possibility of irreversible testicular changes and sterility, once it has been recommended, it is a trial which can be either passed or failed. However, once the physician has embarked on this trial, it is very difficult to turn back, even though the physician may have made this possibility quite clear at the onset. Those within the subspecialty are becoming more and more conservative in recommending even hormone therapy, and certainly they insist on the minimal time requirements set forth in the standards of care. The self-assessment of the transsexual is very important in evaluating hormone therapy. The confrontation with reality which the transsexual has during hormone therapy may be painful, but certainly it is far better for this to happen before SRS rather than after: Any disappointment in passing, even after hormone therapy, may enable the gender dysphoric patient to consider a nonsurgical approach to his or her problem. Some transsexuals, primary or secondary, may elect to remain on hormone therapy indefinitely, in the hopes that eventually they will achieve the status of passability. Or they simply feel more content with whatever satisfaction they may have from slight breast development, softer skin, being less hairy, and having a more favorable distribution of fatty tissue and muscular tissue. Some elect, therefore, to remain on estrogen, but never go on to SRS.

For the female-to-male patient, the specific response to testosterone injections are marked improvement in voice, score lowers from 4.8 to 1.0 on a 5 point scale ($p = .02$), and satisfaction with the development of facial hair ($p = .05$). Also of great pleasure to the female transsexual is the discontinuation of menstruation, a monthly reminder of the female status. Other effects of testosterone therapy are the hypertrophy of the clitoris, associated with increased sensitivity and increased sexual drive or libido. Increased clitoral size can be quite significant such that the patient begins to perceive this organ as a penis. Indeed, some of the genital SRS procedures enhance this clitoral enlargement surgically and transfer the urethra through the enlarged clitoris to the tip, so the patient may stand to urinate (Durfee and Rowland, 1974). On the negative side, testosterone may cause some problems with acne and thinning of the scalp hair. As in the case with male transsexuals on hormone therapy, the primary genderal characteristics of breasts, vagina, ovaries–uterus, chest are unchanged by hormone therapy, and are still perceived as "very dissatisfied" and unwanted. Obviously, SRS is required for the removal of these parts. The secondary gender characteristics that are perceived more positively after testosterone therapy include appearance, muscles, biceps, body hair, and hips. Although the redistribution of fatty and muscular tissue is not as marked as female transsexuals might wish, they can enhance the effect of hormones on muscular development by weight lifting and body building. Since the female transsexual, as compared with the male, is not as dissatisfied to begin with, the improvement in the score is not so dramatic or significant ($p < .05$). However, in the author's experience, the female-to-male transsexuals, as a group, are more successful in passing, either before hormone therapy or after. They are less likely to conclude in their self-assessment that they can not make it, and it is a very unusual circumstance when hormone therapy or the trial in cross-gender living is not succeeded by SRS. Lothstein (1983) is not as positive in this regard. If there are delays in proceeding with surgery it is usually because of financial or practical reasons, not lack of motivation. In any event, at least one year, and preferably two is recommended before proceeding with SRS. Although there may be some reduction in breast size in some female transsexuals who have small breasts to begin with, this is usually not sufficient to preclude mastectomy. Often the request for breast removal is more urgent than genital surgery.

To summarize, hormone therapy is recommended only after careful evaluation, and not simply on request or on demand from the self-diagnosed transsexual. Certain irreversible changes, such as testicular atrophy in the male and permanent voice changes and clitoral enlargement in the female, should be explained in detail. A baseline endocrinological evaluation, together with baseline liver function studies, should precede hormone therapy. Administration of hormone therapy in adolescence should be avoided, especially in the female, where testosterone might prematurely close the epiphyses and prevent bone growth and attainment of the optimal height. However, once a careful evaluation and preliminary baseline studies have occurred, hormone therapy becomes the next step in the process of evaluation, after cross-gender living. Most genuine, primary transsexuals "pass" this test, are delighted with the physical changes that improve their body image, feel more self-confident in their ability to pass, and are encouraged with the progress they are making toward their goal. On the other hand, some self-select or are selected out of continuing toward SRS by their evaluators, for the variety of reasons mentioned.

## SEX REASSIGNMENT SURGERY FOR PRIMARY TRANSSEXUALS

Those gender dysphoric individuals who demonstrate a fixed and consistent cross-gender identification, using the previously listed criteria, are candidates for SRS. They establish themselves as primary transsexuals, and successfully pass the real life test of cross-gender living and hormone therapy for one to two years. Some are actively engaged in psychotherapy before and during this trial period, but they are all still involved in the evaluation process by a member of the mental health profession. Then, and only then, is it appropriate to recommend the patient to an experienced surgeon for SRS.

Even after this careful process of evaluation, some 10 to 15 percent of operated patients are thought to have had an unsatisfactory outcome from SRS (Pauly, 1981; Lundstrom, 1981; Lundstrom et al., 1984). As long as a single transsexual regrets having pursued this goal to its conclusion, and some 5 to 6 percent have, then the clinicians involved are obligated to exercise extreme caution in this decision making process (Dixen and Van Maasdam, 1983; Walinder and Thuwe, 1975).

Of 100 gender dysphoric individuals who may come to a gender identity clinic to request SRS, perhaps one-third to one-half will be considered appropriate candidates, using the criteria mentioned above. However, of those originally refused, some 23 percent (Lundstrom, 1981) to 40 percent (Meyer and Reter, 1979) are successful in obtaining SRS elsewhere. The majority of those refused continue to be interested in cross-gender living and their gender dysphoria persists. Only 10 to 14 percent of those refused gender dysphoric applicants give up their desire for SRS and continue their life without further pursuit of sex reassignment. Interestingly enough, none of the female transsexuals who were refused gave up their gender dysphoria. This tends to confirm the impression of several researchers that female transsexuals are a more homogenous diagnostic group, who are generally better candidates for SRS (Pauly, 1974; Lundstrom, 1981; Lundstrom et al., 1984). Only two published studies compare those accepted and treated with SRS and those refused. The study from Johns Hopkins Hospital concludes that "sex reassignment surgery confers no objective advantage in terms of social rehabilitation, although it remains subjectively satisfying to those who have rigorously pursued a trial period and who have undergone it (SRS)" (Meyer and Reter, 1979, p. 1015). The Swedish study concludes that those who were accepted and treated with SRS are more satisfied with their lives than those who were refused, and that this difference is statistically significant ($p<0.01$) (Lundstrom, 1981; Walinder and Thuwe, 1975). More information on outcome studies will be presented in the following section of this chapter.

Although the first published report of surgery for a transsexual patient came in 1931 from Germany (Abraham, 1931), the procedure for the creation of a neovagina goes back to the turn of the century (Baldwin, 1904). Thus, operations to correct cogenital absence or atresia of the vagina were developed and improved. These procedures utilized the McIndoe technique of utilizing a free, split-thickness skin graft (McIndoe, 1950). However, it was not until the early 1950s that SRS for transsexuals became well known. Paul Fogh-Anderson, a Danish plastic surgeon from Copenhagen, operated on Christine Jorgenson in late 1952, and thus initiated the modern era of SRS (Fogh-Anderson, 1956). Early on the surgical procedures were carried on in Vienna, Paris, and Casablanca (Burou, 1974; Edgerton, et al. 1983). It was not until the mid-1960s that U.S. centers became interested in SRS, through Benjamin's efforts to find competent surgeons for transsexuals. As previously mentioned, the first SRS in this country was at Johns Hopkins in 1966 (Edgerton et al., 1970; Edgerton and Bull, 1970; Jones et al., 1968). Early on there was a high incidence of complications, including rectovaginal fistulae, stenosed vaginae, or strictured urethrae. However, the procedures were modified in order to improve functional results and decrease complications (Laub and Fisk, 1974; Turner et al., 1978). The penile skin flap technique for vaginoplasty was introduced by Edgerton and Bull in 1970, and independently by Burou (Burou, 1974; Edgerton and Bull, 1970). Deepening the vagina by adding a skin graft to enlarge the penile flap at the neovaginal dome was introduced by Foerster in 1976 (Edgerton, 1983). Rudolfe Meyer, a Swiss surgeon, introduced a one stage penile island flap technique based on the transverse perineal arteries (Meyer, 1983; Meyer and Kesselring, 1980). Further refinements for constructing the labia and clitoris have been developed. By now various centers in the United States have performed hundreds of these SRS procedures (Laub, 1981; Laub and Fisk, 1974; Pauly, 1981). For a comprehensive review of the surgical techniques, the reader is referred to the surgical literature (Burou, 1974; Edgerton, 1974; Edgerton, 1983; Laub, 1974; Jones, 1969; Jones et al., 1968).

We have underscored the genital surgical procedure for the removal of the penis, scrotum, and testicles, and the creation of a functional neovagina. It should be emphasized that a successful outcome is largely dependent upon a good functional result. The ability to engage in sexual intercourse without pain or discomfort is highly correlated with postoperative satisfaction as judged by the transsexual (Edgerton, 1983; Satterfield, 1983). In addition, the breast enlargement secondary to estrogen therapy is usually not sufficient to preclude breast augmentation mammoplasty. This procedure is not essentially different from that requested by nontranssexual women who wish to enhance the size of their breasts. Other forms of plastic surgery are occasionally requested to improve the feminine appearance, such as facial surgery, rhinoplasty, and thyroid cartilage shave to reduce the size of the Adam's apple. When one compares the pretreatment male transsexual scores on the body image scale (3.76 of 5.0) with the postsurgical scores (1.46 of 5.0), one sees a significant improvement ($p = <.001$) (Pauly and Lindgren, 1976).

With reference to the female-to-male transsexuals, the surgical techniques are not as well-developed. Certainly it is easy enough to remove the breasts by mastectomy. These procedures can be accomplished through a small subareolar, key-hole incision in female transsexuals with small breasts. However, larger inframammary incisions are required for large-breasted female transsexuals (Hoopes, 1969). Usually, these postoperative female-to-male transsexuals are quite pleased with their flat chests, and thankful that they no longer have to resort to using bandages to wrap around their chests to minimize the size of their breasts. In the past, there have been some reports of unsightly scarring, especially in patients prone to keloid formation (Lothstein, 1983).

With reference to genital surgery in the female-to-male situation, total hysterectomy, salpingo-oophorectomy, and vaginectomy are performed initially. The creation of an artificial penis is a very complicated and multistaged procedure. The first report on total construction of a neophallus was in 1936 (Borgoras, 1936). The further evolution and development of this surgery has been reviewed by Hoopes (Hoopes, 1969). Subsequent authors report on the more recent development in the construction of a functional neophallus (Foerster and Reynolds, 1981; Hester et al., 1978; McGraw et al., 1976; Noe and Birdsell, 1974). A different approach to this challenge of creating a phallus was pioneered at the University of Oregon (Durfee and Rowland, 1974). This procedure takes advantage of the enlarged clitoris, and brings the urethra through to the tip so the patient may stand to urinate. Sexual function that allows penetration is not possible by this procedure. Often the female transsexual has already established a satisfactory sexual relationship with a partner with or without the use of a dildo (Pauly, 1974; Pierce et al., 1979). Emphasis is placed on obtaining surgical results that will: (1) allow the patient to stand to void; (2) permit sexual intercourse; (3) provide a presentable male appearance; and (4) be accomplished in a minimum number of operative steps (Edgerton et al., 1983). Although requests for SRS are currently coming equally from male and female patients, most of the surgical attention has been given to male-to-female transsexuals. Clearly the difficulties inherent in the surgical construction of a cosmetically and functionally satisfactory male-appearing perineum has not yet been perfected to the point where this is readily available. Until this has been accomplished, to the same degree as with the male-to-female transsexual, it will be difficult to achieve a completely favorable outcome from SRS for female transsexuals.

## Outcome of Sex Reassignment Surgery for Transsexuals

It is important to underscore the difficulties in reviewing the literature on the outcome of SRS. Only since the late 1960s are centers collecting systematic data on all patients treated. Previous reports gave highly selective follow-up data, authors feeling more inclined to publicize positive results than negative ones. Thus, early reports of outcome of SRS, in which very few unsatisfactory results are acknowledged, (Benjamin, 1966; Pauly, 1965, 1968) should be questioned, in the light of more recent studies. In the last few years, there have been three independent reviews of the literature on this topic (Lothstein, 1982; Lundstrom, 1981; Pauly, 1981). The results of Pauly's and Lundstrom's independent research were sufficiently similar to enable the data to be compared and reported in a subsequent report (Lundstrom et al., 1984). Lothstein concluded that it is almost impossible to make any firm conclusions regarding outcome from the literature available. The reasons for this include not only methodological problems, but uncertainties about whether the patients were primary or secondary transsexuals. Since each center may rely on different criteria for SRS, offers a different type of surgical procedure, and uses different criteria and instruments for assessing positive or negative results, Lothstein's reservations are well-founded (Lothstein, 1982, 1983).

Despite these somewhat detracting factors, it seems reasonable to report the data, given the above mentioned reservations (see Table 24–1). Pauly concluded that 71.4 percent of the male-to-female transsexuals reported in 11 follow-up studies, from 1969–1979, enjoyed a "satisfactory" result, 8.1 percent an "unsatisfactory" result, 2.1 percent committed suicide, leaving some 18.4 percent in the "uncertain" category. Lundstrom, reviewing 17 studies, concluded that 87.8 percent of male-to-female transsexuals having undergone SRS enjoyed a "satisfactory" result, 10.3 percent an "unsatisfactory" result, and 1.9 percent committed suicide. Since Lundstrom did not utilize the "uncertain" category, this fact may well explain most of the differences between the two studies. For the female-to-male transsexuals who underwent SRS, Pauly reported an 80.7 percent "satisfactory" outcome, 6.0 percent "unsatisfactory," and 13.3 percent in the "uncertain" category. Lundstrom's review reported 89.5 percent "satisfactory," 9.7 percent "unsatisfactory," and 0.8 percent in the

TABLE 24-1  **Literature Review of Outcome of Sex Reassignment**

|  | Number of Studies Reviewed | Number of Patients | Satisfactory | Unsatisfactory | Suicide | Uncertain |
|---|---|---|---|---|---|---|
| Pauly (1981) | | | | | | |
|   Males | 11 | 283 | 202 (71.4%) | 23 (8.1%) | 6 (2.1%) | 52 (18.4%) |
|   Females | 8 | 83 | 67 (80.7%) | 5 (6.0%) | 0 (0%) | 11 (13.3%) |
| Lundstrom (1981) | | | | | | |
|   Males | 17 | 368 | 323 (87.8%) | 38 (10.3%) | 7 (1.9%) | — |
|   Females | 12 | 124 | 111 (89.5%) | 12 ( 9.7%) | 1 (0.8%) | — |

suicide category. Rough conclusions from this study are as follows (Lundstrom et al., 1984):

1. An unsatisfactory result occurs in 10–15 percent of the gender dysphoric patients reported in the last 15 years. Stated more positively, the vast majority of patients having undergone SRS have enjoyed a satisfactory outcome.
2. Although the absolute percentage of favorable outcome in female-to-male patients is higher than in male-to-female transsexuals, this difference does not reach statistical significance.
3. Although the literature suggests that satisfactory outcome is to some degree dependent on good cosmetic and functional result from SRS, this relationship is complex, and other variables do affect the patient's perception of overall satisfaction.
4. Personal and social instability are correlated with unsatisfactory results. Supportive psychotherapy should be encouraged, both preoperatively and postoperatively, in order to insure the most favorable outcome.
5. There is an inverse relationship between age at the time of request for SRS, and favorable outcome. This probably reflects the larger number of secondary transsexuals in the older age group.
6. Secondary transsexuals have a higher frequency of unsatisfactory results from SRS than do true transsexuals. Evidence from other sources suggests that when these particular gender dysphoric patients are refused surgery, they seem to accept this decision and manage their life quite well, giving up their pursuit of SRS.
7. We conclude that sex reassignment surgery is the treatment of choice for carefully evaluated, genuine, primary transsexuals. SRS should not be offered patients with secondary gender dysphoria, those with unstable past histories, and patients over the age of 35. It is clear that the decision to offer SRS does not negate the clear indication for supportive psychotherapy before and after SRS. (Lundstrom et al., 1984, p. 293)

The relationship between homosexuality and gender dysphoria is an important issue. Most homosexuals are satisfied with their sexual preference and lifestyle, and like sexually contented heterosexuals, they would never dream of removing their genitalia through SRS, since they carry a positive body image and it is a source of pleasure. However, there are some, probably a very small, select group, whose primary homosexuality is so unacceptable, that they cannot accept this sexual orientation and lifestyle. It is interesting how frequently transsexuals state their strong aversion to homosexuality and deeply resent being cast in that mold. In any event, these self-stigmatized, ego-dystonic, homosexually oriented gender dysphoric patients see reassignment as a solution to their dilemma. Morgan (1978) states the problem this way: "It is becoming apparent that for both transsexual candidates and a good number of the physicians working with them, sex-reassignment surgery, as a concept, is more ego-syntonic than homosexuality" (p. 281). Some estimates indicate that as high as 30 to 35 percent of gender dysphoric applicants are self-stigmatized, homophobic homosexuals (Pauly, 1981). The Swedish study supports this view: "we ought to be very cautious with sex reassignment when the condition is difficult to differentiate from homosexuality, especially when the patient is very young" (Lundstrom, 1981, p. 112). For these patients, an attempt should be made to help them accept their homosexuality through psychotherapy. Obviously, the patient's chief complaint of desiring a sex change should never be taken at face value, and psychiatrists are familiar with patients attempting to camouflage other problems. In these situations there are indications that some success has been achieved through psychotherapy (Lothstein and Levine, 1981; Morgan, 1978).

Finally, a very few number of patients have regretted their decision to undergo SRS (Pauly, 1981). Walinder found five such patients from his review of 100 persons who applied for sex reassignment in Sweden up to 1972 (Walinder et al., 1978). The Stanford study revealed one of 20 male-to-female transsexuals, who underwent SRS, who regretted having done so, and none of the 30 female-to-male transsexuals regretted their decision (Dixen and Van Maasdam, 1983). The following factors were identified as being correlated with regret at having undergone SRS: increasing age at time of request, considerable heterosexual experience, interruption of hormone therapy, unstable personality, inability to support oneself, criminal activity, poor family support, and inability to pass readily as a member of the opposite sex (Walinder et al., 1978).

## CONCLUSION

As clinicians become more familiar with the gender dysphoria syndrome, they will be able to discriminate those who are indeed fixed in their cross-gender identification, have been stable and consistent in their pursuit of cross-gender living, and therefore, who would be expected to respond favorably to SRS, from those who do not meet the criteria discussed in this chapter. For this latter group, gender dysphorics for whom SRS is not indicated, psychotherapeutic measures have become increasingly successful in alleviating the unhappiness and gender dysphoria suffered. Of even greater significance is the information we have gained about the pathogenesis of this condition. Ultimately we may come to an understanding of the normative process of healthy gender identification. To whatever extent gender dysphoria may be caused by acquired postnatal, parental, or social factors, it may become possible to prevent it in the future. Despite the controversy associated with the diagnosis and treatment of this condition, certainly all would agree that transsexualism would be better prevented than treated, whether by SRS or psychotherapy.

## REFERENCES

Abraham, F.: Genitalumwandlung an swei maennlichen transvestiten. *Z. Sexualwiss.*, 18:223–226, 1931.
American Psychiatric Association (APA): *Diagnostic and Statistical Manual of Mental Disorders* (DSM-III), Washington, D.C., 1980.
Baldwin, F.: The formation of an artificial vagina by intestinal transplantation. *Ann. Surg.*, 40:398–404, 1904.
Barlow, D. H.; Abel, G. G.; and Blanchard, E. B.: Gender identity change in transsexuals: Follow-up and replications. *Arch. Gen. Psychiatr.*, 36:1001–1007, 1979.
Barlow, D. H.; Reynolds, E. J.; and Agras, S.: Gender identity change in a transsexual. *Arch. Gen. Psychiatr.* 28:569–579, 1973.
Benjamin, H.: Transvestism and transsexualism. *Int. J. Sexol.*, 7:12–14, 1953.
Benjamin, H.: *The Transsexual Phenomenon.* Julian Press, New York, 1966.
Benjamin, H.: For the practicing physician: Suggestions and guidelines for the management of transsexuals. In Green, R.; Money, J.: (eds.): *Transsexualism and Sex Reassignment.* Johns Hopkins Press, Baltimore, 1969, pp. 305–307.
Berscheid, E.; Walster, E.; and Bohrnstedt, C.: The happy American body: A survey report. *Psychology Today*, (November); 119–131, 1973.
Binder, H.: Das verlangen nach geschlechtsumwardlung. *Z. Neurol. Psychiat.*, 143:84–174, 1933.
Borgoras, N.: Über die volle plastische wiederherstellung eines zum koitus fahigen penis (penisplastica totolis). *Z. Chir.*, 63:1271–1276, 1936.
Burou, G.: Male to female transformation. In Laub, D.; Gandy, P.: (eds.): *Proceedings of the Second Interdis-*

ciplinary Symposium on Gender Dysphoria Syndrome, Edwards Brothers, Ann Arbor, Mich., 1974.
Cauldwell, D. O.: Psychopathia transsexualis. Sexology, 16:274–280, 1949.
Ciccarese, S.; Massari, S.; and Guanti, G.: Sexual behavior is independent of H-Y antigen constitution. Hum. Genet., 60:371–372, 1982.
Davenport, C. W., and Harrisson, S. I.: Gender identity change in a female adolescent transsexual. Arch. Sex. Behav., 6:327–341, 1977.
Dellaert, R., and Kunke, T.: Investigations on a case of male transsexualism. Psychother. Psychosom., 17:89–107, 1969.
De Montyel, M.: De la maladie des scythes, Ann. Med. Psychol., 1:161–184, 1877.
Dixen, J., and Van Maasdam, J.: The effectiveness of surgical sex reassignment as a treatment for gender dysphoria. In Proceedings of the 8th International Gender Dysphoria Association, Bordeaux, France, 1983.
Durfee, R., and Rowland, W.: Penile substitution with clitoral enlargement and urethral transfer. In Laub, D.; Gandy, P.: (eds.): Proceedings of the Second Interdisciplinary Symposium on Gender Dysphoria Syndrome, Edwards Brothers, Ann Arbor, Mich, 1974.
Eber, M.: Gender identity conflicts in male transsexualism. Bull. Menn. Clin., 44:31–38, 1980.
Edgerton, M. T.: A new male-to-female surgical technique. In Laub, D.; Gandy, P.: (eds.): Proceedings of the Second Interdisciplinary Symposium on Gender Dysphoria Syndrome, Edwards Brothers, Ann Arbor, Mich, 1974.
Edgerton, M. T.: The role of surgery in the treatment of transsexualism. In Proceedings of the 8th International Gender Dysphoria Association, Bordeaux, France, 1983.
Edgerton, M. T., and Bull, J.: Surgical construction of the vagina and labia in male transsexuals. Plast. Reconstr. Surg., 46:529–539, 1970.
Edgerton, M. T.; Knorr, N. J.; and Callison, J. R.: The surgical treatment of transsexual patients. Plast. Reconstr. Surg., 45:38–46, 1970.
Edgerton, M.; Gillenwater, J.; Kenney, J.; and Longman, M.: Further observations on surgical reassignment of female transsexuals. In Proceedings of the 8th International Gender Dysphoria Association, Bordeaux, France, 1983.
Eicher, W.: Transsexualism and H-Y antigen. In Pauly, I.: (ed.): Proceedings of the 7th International Gender Dysphoria Association, Lake Tahoe, Nevada, 1981.
Eicher, W.; Spoljar, M.; Clere, H.; Murken, J.; Richter, K.; and Stangel-Rutkowski, S.: H-Y antigen in transsexuality. Lancet, 2:1137–1138, 1979.
Ellis, H.: Eonism. Studies in Psychology of Sex, Vol. 2. Random House, New York, 1936.
Esquirol, E.: Mental maladies. In Hunt, E. K.: (ed.): Mental Maladies. Lea and Blanchard, Philadelphia, 1845.
Fisk, N.: Gender dysphoria syndrome. In Laub, D.; Gandy, P.: (eds.): Proceedings of the Second Interdisciplinary Symposium on Gender Dysphoria Syndrome, Edwards Brothers, Ann Arbor, Mich., 1974.
Foerster, D. W., and Reynolds, C. L.: Current development and progress in surgical conversion of female to male genitalia in the female transsexual. In Proceedings of the 7th International Gender Dysphoria Association, Lake Tahoe, Nevada, 1981.
Fogh-Anderson, P.: Transsexualism: Surgical treatment in a case of auto-castration. Acta Med. Leg. Soc., 9:33–42, 1956.
Freud, S.: Three Contributions to the Theory of Sex. Nervous & Mental Diseases Publishing Co., New York, 1910.
Friedreich, J.: Versuch Einer Literaturgeschichte der Pathologie and Therapie der Psychischen. Krankheiten, Würzburg, 1830.
Green, R.: Mythological, historical, and cross-cultural aspects of transsexualism. In Benjamin, H.: (ed.): The Transsexual Phenomenon. Julian Press, New York, 1966.
Green, R.: Sexual Identity Conflicts in Children and Adults. Basic Books, New York, 1974.
Green, R.: Atypical sex role behavior during childhood. In Sadock, B. I.; Kaplan, H. I.; Freedman, A. M.: (eds.): The Sexual Experience. Williams and Wilkins, Baltimore, 1976.
Green, R., and Money, J.: (eds.): Transsexualism and Sex Reassignment. Johns Hopkins Press, Baltimore, 1969.
Gorman, W.: Body Image and the Image of the Brain. Warren H. Green, St. Louis, 1969.
Hamburger, C.: Desire for change of sex as shown by personal letters from 465 men and women. Acta Endocrinol., 14:361–375, 1953.
Hamburger, C.: Endocrine treatment of male and female transsexualism. In Green, R.; Money, J.: (eds.): Transsexualism and Sex Reassignment. Johns Hopkins Press, Baltimore, 1969.
Hamburger, C.; Stürrup, G.; and Dahl-Iverson, E.: Transvestism. JAMA, 152:391–396, 1953.
Hester, T. R.; Hill, H. L.; and Jurkiewicz, M. J.: One-stage reconstruction of the penis. Br. J. Plast. Surg., 31:279–284, 1978
Hirschfeld, M.: Die Transvestiten: Eine Untersuchung Über den Erotischen Verkleidungstrieb. Alfred Pulvermacher, Berlin, 1910.
Hoenig, J.; and Kenna, J.: The prevalence of transsexualism in England and Wales. Br. J. Psychiatry, 124:181–190, 1974.
Hoopes, J.: Operative treatment of the female transsexual. In Green, R.; Money, J.: (eds.): Transsexualism and Sex Reassignment, Johns Hopkins Press, Baltimore, 1969.
Hunt, D. D., and Hampson, J. L.: Transsexualism: A standardized psychosocial rating format for the evaluation of results of sex reassignment surgery. Arch. Sex. Behav., 9:255–263, 1980.
Jones, H. W.: Operative treatment of the male transsexual. In Green, R.; Money, J.: (eds.): Transsexualism and Sex Reassignment, Johns Hopkins Press, Baltimore, 1969.
Jones, H. W.; Hoopes, J. E.; and Schirmer, H. K.: A fixed conversion operation for male transsexualism. Am. J. Ob. Gyn., 100:101–109, 1968.
Kirkpatrick, M., and Friedman, C.: Treatment of requests for sex-change surgery with psychotherapy. Am. J. Psychiatry, 133:1194–1196, 1976.
Kolb, L. C.: Disturbances of the body image. In Arieti, S.: (ed.): American Handbook of Psychiatry. Basic Books, New York, 1959.

Krafft-Ebing, R.: Über gewisse anomalien des geschlechtstriebes. *Arch. Psychiatry,* 7:291–312, 1877.

Kuiper, B., and Cohen-Kettenis, P.: *Ex post facto* study on the effects of the treatment of transsexualism. In *Proceedings of the 8th International Gender Dysphoria Association,* Bordeaux, France, 1983.

Laub, D.: Total management and responsibility for transsexual patients. In Laub, D.; Gandy, P. (eds.): *Proceedings of the Second Interdisciplinary Symposium on Gender Dysphoria Syndrome,* Edwards Brothers, Ann Arbor, Mich., 1974.

Laub, D.: The natural vagina. In *Proceedings of the 7th International Gender Dysphoria Association,* Lake Tahoe, Nevada, 1981.

Laub, D., and Fisk, N.: A rehabilitation program for gender dysphoria syndrome by surgical sex change. *Plast. Reconstr. Surg.,* 53:388–403, 1974.

Lebowitz, P.: Feminine behavior in boys: Aspects of its outcome. *Am. J. Psychiatry,* 128:1283–1291, 1972.

Levine, S.: Psychiatric diagnosis among gender patients: The value of perceiving gender dysphoria as a form of mental illness. In *Proceedings of the 8th International Gender Dysphoria Association,* Bordeaux, France, 1983.

Levine, S., and Lothstein, L.: Transsexualism or the gender dysphoria syndromes. *J. Sex. Marital Ther.,* 7:85–114, 1981.

Lindgren, T., and Pauly, I.: A body image scale for evaluating transsexuals. *Arch. Sex. Behav.,* 4:639–656, 1975.

Lothstein, L.: Sex reassignment surgery: Historical, bioethical, and theoretical issues. *Am. J. Psychiatry,* 139:417–426, 1982.

Lothstein, L.: *Female-to-Male Transsexualism.* Routledge and Kegan Paul, Boston, 1983.

Lothstein, L., and Levine, S.: Expressive psychotherapy with gender dysphoric patients. *Arch. Gen. Psychiatr.,* 38:924–929, 1981.

Lundstrom, B.: *Gender Dysphoria: A Social–Psychiatric Follow-Up Study of 31 Cases Not Accepted for Sex Reassignment.* Univ. of Göteborg Press, Sweden, 1981.

Lundstrom, B.; Pauly, I.; and Walinder, J.: Outcome of sex reassignment surgery. *Acta Psychiatr. Scand.,* 70:289–294, 1984.

Marcuse, M.: Ein fall von geschlechtsumwandlungstreib. *Z. Psychother. Med. Psychol.,* 6:176–185, 1916.

Masson, A.: *Le Transvestissement.* Ph.D. thesis, Le François, Paris, 1935.

McCraw, J.; Massey, F.; Shanklin, K.: Vaginal reconstruction using gracilis myocutaneous flaps. *Plast. Reconstr. Surg.,* 58:176–184, 1976.

McIndoe, A. H.: Treatment of congenital absence and obliterative conditions of the vagina. *Br. J. Plast. Surg.,* 2:254–261, 1950.

Meyer, J.: Clinical variants among applicants for sex reassignment. *Arch. Sex. Behav.,* 3:527–558, 1974.

Meyer, J., and Reter, D.: Sex reassignment. *Arch. Gen. Psychiatr.,* 36:1010–1015, 1979.

Meyer, R.: Ten years experience in 86 cases of male transsexualism with one-stage construction of vulva and vagina by means of penile skin flap. In *Proceedings of the 8th International Gender Dysphoria Association,* Bordeaux, France, 1983.

Meyer, R., and Kesselring, U. K.: One-stage reconstruction of the vagina with penile skin as an island flap in male transsexuals. *Plast. Reconstr Surg.,* 66:401–412, 1980.

Money, J.: Two names, two wardrobes, two personalities. *J. Homosex.,* 1:65–70, 1974.

Money, J., and Ambinder, R.: Two-year, real-life diagnostic test: Rehabilitation versus cure. In Brady, H.; Brody, J. (eds): *Controversy in Psychiatry.* W. B. Saunders, Philadelphia, 1978.

Money, J., and Ehrhardt, A.: *Man and Woman. Boy and Girl.* Johns Hopkins Press, Baltimore, 1972.

Money, J., and Russo, A.: Homosexual outcome of discordant gender identity/role in childhood: Longitudinal follow-up. *J. Pediatr. Psychol.,* 4:29–41, 1979.

Money, J. Hampson, J.; and Hampson, J.: Hermaphroditism: Recommendations concerning assignment of sex, change of sex, and psychological management. *Bull. Johns Hopkins Hosp.,* 97:284–300, 1955.

Morgan, A.: Psychotherapy for transsexual candidates screened out of surgery. *Arch. Sex. Behav.,* 7:273–283, 1978.

Noe, J. M., and Birdsell, D.: A surgical program for female to male transsexuals. In Laub, D.; Gandy, P. (eds.): *Proceedings of the Second Interdisciplinary Symposium on Gender Dysphoria Syndrome,* Edwards Brothers, Ann Arbor, Mich., 1974.

Ostow, M.: Transvestism. *JAMA,* 152:1553, 1953.

Pauly, I.: Male psychosexual inversion: Transsexualism. *Arch. Gen. Psychiatr.* 13:172–181, 1965.

Pauly, I.: The current status of the change of sex operation. *J. Nerv. Ment. Dis.,* 147:460–471, 1968.

Pauly, I.: Adult manifestations of male transsexualism. In Green, R.; Money, J.: (eds): *Transsexualism and Sex Reassignment.* Johns Hopkins Press, Baltimore, 1969a.

Pauly, I.: Adult manifestations of female transsexualism. In Green, R.; Money, J.: (eds): *Transsexualism and Sex Reassignment.* Johns Hopkins Press, Baltimore, 1969b.

Pauly, L: Female transsexualism: Parts I & II. *Arch. Sex. Behav.* 3:487–525, 1974.

Pauly, I : Sex and the life cycle. In Kaplan, H.; Freedman, A.; Sadock, B.: (eds.): *Comprehensive Textbook of Psychiatry,* Vol. 2, 3d ed., Williams and Wilkens, Baltimore, 1980.

Pauly, I : Outcome of sex reassignment surgery for transsexuals. *Aust. N. Z. J. Psych.,* 15:45–51, 1981.

Pauly, I.: History of the gender identity movement: Birth of a medical sub-specialty. In *Proceedings of the 8th International Gender Dysphoria Association,* Bordeaux, France, 1983.

Pauly, I., and Lindgren, T.: Body image and gender identity. *J. Homosex.,* 2:133–142, 1976.

Person, E.; and Ovesey, L.: The transsexual syndrome in males: Parts I and II. *Am. J. Psychother.,* 28:4–20; 174–193, 1974.

Pfafflin, F.: H-Y antigen in transsexualism. In Pauly, I : (ed.): *Proceedings of the 7th International Gender Dysphoria Association,* Lake Tahoe, Nevada, 1981.

Pierce, D.; Matarazzo, R.; and Pauly, I.: The adjustment of female transsexuals following hormonal and surgical sex reassignment. In *Proceedings of the 6th International Gender Dysphoria Association,* Coronado, California, 1979.

Ross, M. W.; Rogers, L. J.; and McCulloch, H.: Stigma,

sex, and society: A new look at gender differentiation and sexual variation. *J. Homosex.,* 3:315–330, 1978.

Ross, M. W.; Walinder, J.; Lundstrom, B.; and Thuwe, I.: Cross-cultural approaches to transsexualism: A comparison between Sweden and Australia. *Acta Psychiatr. Scand.,* 63:75–82, 1981.

Satterfield, S.: Follow-up of 25 transsexuals in the Minnesota program. In *Proceedings of the 8th International Gender Dysphoria Association,* Bordeaux, France, 1983.

Stoller, R.: *Sex and Gender.* Science House, New York, 1968.

Stoller, R.: Etiological factors in female transsexualism. *Arch. Sex. Behav.,* 2:47–64, 1972.

Stoller, R.: Gender identity disorders. In Kaplan, H.; Freedman, A.; Sadock, B.: (eds.): *Comprehensive Textbook of Psychiatry,* Vol. 2, 3d ed. Williams and Wilkens, Baltimore, 1980.

Theron, A.: Identification of male-to-female transsexuals. In *Proceedings of the 8th International Gender Dysphoria Association,* Bordeaux, France, 1983.

Turner, U.; Edlich, R.; and Edgerton, M.: Transsexualism: A review of genital surgical reconstruction. *Am. J. Obstet. Gynecol.,* 132:119–128, 1978.

Walinder, J.: *Transsexualism.* Scandinavian University Books, Akademiforlaget, Göteborg, Sweden, 1967.

Walinder, J.: Transsexualism: Definition, prevalence, and sex distribution. *Acta Psychiatr. Scand.* (Suppl.), 203:255–257, 1968.

Walinder, J.: Incidence and sex ration of transsexualism in Sweden. *Br. J. Psychiatry,* 119:195–196, 1971.

Walinder, J., and Thuwe, I.: *A Social–Psychiatric Follow-up Study of 24 Sex Reassigned Transsexuals.* Scandinavian University Books, Sweden, 1975.

Walinder, J., and Thuwe, I.: A law concerning sex reassignment of transsexuals in Sweden. *Arch. Sex. Behav.,* 5:255–258, 1976.

Walinder, J.; Lundstrom, B.; and Thuwe, I.: Prognostic factors in the assessment of male transsexuals for sex reassignment. *Br. J. Psychiatry,* 132:16–20, 1978.

Walinder, J.; Lundstrom, B.; Ross, M.; and Thuwe, I.: Transsexualism: Incidence, prevalence and sex ratio: Comments on three different studies. In *Proceedings of the 6th International Gender Dysphoria Association,* Coronado, California, 1979.

Walker, P.; Berger, J.; Green, R.; Laub, D.; Reynolds, C.; and Wollman, L.: *Standards of Care: The Hormonal and Surgical Sex Reassignment of Gender Dysphoric Persons.* H. Benjamin International Gender Dysphoria Association, San Francisco, 1979.

Westphal, C.: Die conträre sexualempfindung. *Arch. Psychiat. Nervenkr.* 2:73–108, 1870.

Wiedeman, G.: Transvestism. *JAMA,* 152:1167, 1953.

Zuger, B.: Effeminate behavior in boys present from early childhood. *J. Pediatr.,* 69:1098–1106, 1966.

Zuger, B.: Early effeminate behavior in boys. *J. Nerv. Ment. Dis.,* 172:90–97, 1984.

# INDEX

## A

Abdomen, pain and distention, in pelvic inflammatory disease, 162
Abdominal-pelvic mass, 104, 105, 107
Abortion. *See also* Miscarriage
    attitudes toward, historical perspective, 4
    fear of, sexual relations and, 65, 67–68
    habitual, psychologically-induced, 149–50
    juvenile, 36
Abstinence from sexual activity, 133–34
    during pregnancy, 56
        problems with recommending, 208–209
        prolonged, 56
    types, 133
Abstract thinking, 20, 24
Academic achievement, sex differences in, 33, 35
Acne, 13
Acting out, 20
Actinomycin D, effect on sexual receptivity, 116
Action-oriented behavior, in early adolescence, 24
Acton, W., 5
Acute salpingitis. *See* Pelvic inflammatory disease
Addictive personality, features, 280
Adenomyosis, 170
    sexual function and, 176
Adenosis, 193
Adnexal surgery, 109
Adnexitis, chronic, 163
Adolescence. *See* Puberty
Adoption, pregnancy following, 149
Adrenal androgens, increase in, 143
Adrenal androgen stimulating hormone, anovulatory process and, 143
Adrenal crisis, 88
Adrenal function, assessment of, 89
Adrenal hyperplasia, 88
    congenital, 89, 90
        treatment, 90
    congenital virilizing, 122–23
Adrenocorticotropic hormone (ACTH), anovulatory process and, 143
Adrenocorticotropic hormone (ACTH) stimulation test, 89

*f* = figure; *t* = table.

$\alpha$-Adrenoreceptors, platelet levels, in postpartum depression, 216
Aerocolpos, air embolism duct, 71–72
Afferent (sensory) sympathetic system, 268
Age, choice of contraception and, 132–33
    effect on sexual behavior, 130
    related to sexual activity during pregnancy, 65
Aging, 48
Aggression, 114, 265
    avoidance of expression, 19
    in early adolescence, 22, 23
Aggressive drives, force of, 21
Aggressive-instinctual impetus, 15
Air embolism, 204
    sexual activity during pregnancy and, 67, 71–72
Alcohol, effect on sexual dysfunction, 267, 282–83
Aldomet (methyldopa), 238
Aldosterone, 89
Amenorrhea and cryptomenorrhea, 98 *t*
    congenital vaginal agenesis, 98, 99–104
    hypothalamic hypogonatropic amenorrhea, 143
    psychogenic amenorrhea, 144
    congenital atresia of uterine cervix, 106–107
    imperforate hymen, 104–105
    partial vaginal agenesis, 103–104
    transverse vaginal septum, 104
Amniotic fluid, infection, 69, 247
Amphetamine(s), 247
    effect on sexual function, 282, 283, 284
d-Amphetamine, 282
Amplification, from drugs, 284
AMS malleable penile prosthesis, 256
Amyl nitrite, effect on sexual function, 283
Anal intercourse, 100
Anal-sadistic stage, 15
    conflicts in, 14
Anatomical differences, observation of, by child, 16
Ancient times, physician involvement in sexuality during, 3–4
Androgen(s), 124, 145
    fetal, 8
    influence on sexual behavior
        animal, 129
        human, 129
    production of, 11
        in congenital virilizing adrenal hyperplasia, 122
    threshold complements of, 265
Androgen insensitivity syndromes, 123

317

Androgenic treatments, side effects, 197
Androstenedione, 143
Androstenedione peak, 124
Animals, sexual activity of, 92
Anisomycin (ANI), 120
  effect on feminine reproductive behavior, 116–17, 118
Anomalous female genital duct development, 96, 109
  embryology, ovaries, 96–97
    uterus, fallopian tubes, cervix, vagina, 97
    symptomatic classification of paramesonephric duct anomalies. *See* Paramesonephric duct
Anovulation, 144, 146
Antepartum hemorrhage, sexual activity and, 67, 70
Anthropology, 43
Antihypertensives, 243, 267
  causing hyperprolactinemia, 247–48
  sexual dysfunction from, 237–38
Anxiety, during pregnancy, 210
  fetal affects, 202
  in rape victim, 288
Aortic occlusive disease, 237
Aortic vascular disease, 237
Aorto-iliac bypass, for impotence, 254
Aorto-iliac occlusive disease, impotence in, 254
Aphrodisiacs, effects of, 282
Apocrine metaplasia, 193
Arg-vasopressin (AVP), 120
Arteriography, penile, 250
Arteriotomy, 255
Artificial insemination, psychosexual problems from, 148–49
Atherosclerotic heart disease. *See also* Cardiovascular disease
  sexual activity in, 231–32
Autonomic nervous system, 269
  dysfunction, related to impotence, 247
Avoidance behavior, 120
Azospermia, 144–45

# B

Babinski reflex, 243, 248
Back lesions, dyspareunia in, 160
Backache, in uterine retrodisplacement, 164
Barbiturates, effect on sexual function, 283
Barrier method of contraception, 134
Bartholin's glands, 102
  occlusion of duct, 175
  swelling of, 169
Basal body temperature, infertility and, 147–48
Beard, G. M., 5
Behavior, in late puberty, 25
  problems, sex differences, 37
  sex-typed, influences on, 31–32
Behavior modification, 240
Behavioral therapy, 8
  for impotence, 259
"Benign coital headache," 267
"Benign masturbatory cephalalgia," 267
Benign neoplasia, 169
  human sexuality and, 175–76
  pelvic pain from, 170–72
    surgical treatment, 172–75
  vaginal bleeding from, 169–70

"Benign orgasmic cephalalgia," 267
Benign sex headache, 267
Benjamin, H., 296
Beta-blockers, 238
Biofeedback technique, for impotence, 259
Birth, fetal psychological problems associated with, 208
  socioemotional responses at, 45
Bisexuality, 91, 121
Bladder, function tests, 272
  retrograde ejaculation into, 237
"Blended families," 42
Blood pressure, during sexual activity, 234–35
Blood studies, for impotence, 246–48
Body, change, response to, 198
  stimulation, 8
Body image, change, in cancer patient, 180
  following mastectomy, 198
  transsexualism and, 301–302
Borneman, E., 8
Boys. *See also* Males
  effeminate behavior, 93
  pretranssexual, 299
Brachial index, penile, 249–50
Brain, deficits, 264
  estrogen receptors in, 114
  injury to, 271
  lesions, neuroendocrine function and, 114
  sex differences, 92
Breast(s), changes, during pregnancy, 58
  general cultural attitudes, 189–90
  medical definitions of, 189
  psychosocial definitions of, 189
Breast augmentation mammoplasty, 310
Breast-feeding, issues in, 190–91
  patterns, 192
  resistance, 191–92
Breast pathology, issues in, breast self-examination, resistance to, 195
  cancer anxiety, 194
  pain and discomfort: mastodynia and mastalgia, 193–94
  sexual concerns and importance of sexual history, 192–93
  management strategies, in benign disease, 196–97
  in malignant disease, 197–99
  reassurance and education, 195–96
Breast reconstruction, 194, 199
Breast self-examination (BSE), 194
  factors in resistance, 195
Briquet's somatization syndrome, 174
Bromocriptine, 196, 252
Buccal smear, 90
Bulbocavernosus muscle, 154, 155, 268, 269
Bulbocavernosus reflex, 248
  latency time, 248

# C

Calderone, M., 8
California Personality Inventory (CPI), 251
Calvinism, 4
Cancer. *See also* Cancer patient multidisciplinary approach, 185, 187
Cancer anxiety, 194

Cancer patient, stress in, 178–79, 186–87
   interventions, 184–86
   specific stress areas, 179
      follow-up phase, 183–84
      prediagnostic phase, 179
      recurrence phase, 184
      terminal phase, 184
      treatment phase, 180–83
Cantharides (spanish fly), 282
Cardiac arrest. See Cardiac disease
Cardiac disease, sexual activity in, 231–33, 238. See also Cardiovascular disease
   cardiovascular changes during, 233–35
   counseling of patient, 235–37
Cardiac drugs, sexual dysfunction from, 243
Cardiovascular changes, during sexual activity, 233–35
Cardiovascular disease, sexual dysfunction in, 231, 238. See also Cardiac disease
   drug-related, 237–38
   in vascular disease, 237
Career aspirations, female, relationship to prenatal hormone treatment, 34
Castration, 5
   hormonal, 306
Castration anxiety, 16
Catecholamine(s), blood levels, maternal sexual activity and, 202
   metabolism, 144
   secretion, relationship to postpartum mood disturbances, 215
   turnover, 143
Cathexis, 17
   narcissistic, 26
   outward movement of, 26
Cavernosography, 251, 253
Cellulitis, chronic, 163
Central nervous system, estrogen receptors in, 114
Central nervous system depressants, 277
Central nervous system stimulants, 282
Cerebral cortex, mating behavior and, 265
Cerebrocognitive aspect of sexuality, 266, 267
Cerebrocognitive deficits, in libido problems, 272
Cerebrogenital neurological system, assessment of, for impotence, 248–49
Cervical cancer, 179
Cervical cap, 134
Cervical os, external, cryptomenorrhea and menstrual egress per vagina in, 108
Cervicitis, 204
Cervix, absence of. See Rokitansky-Kuster-Hauser syndrome
   complete duplication of, cryptomenorrhea and menstrual egress per vagina, 107–108
   embryology, 96, 97
Cesarian section, 208
Chemotherapy, for breast cancer, 199
   sexual functioning following, 183
Child, children, interaction among, 31–32
   needs, in sibling death, 224–25
   self-help skills, 45
   sexual behavior of, 8–9, 92
   symbiosis with mother, 45
Child development, study of, 41
Child guidance, 41
Child psychology, 41

Child rearing, dissatisfaction during, 48
   gender identity and, 94
   phase of marriage, 47–48
Childbirth, psychological reactions to, 213
Childhood transsexualism, DSM-III criteria, 298
Childhood years: birth to infancy, psychological development during, 14–17
Childless period in marriage, 47
*Chlamydia trachomatis*, 161, 165
Chlamydial infections, 161, 162
Chlorthalidone (Hygroton), 238
Cholecystitis, 162
Cholelithiasis, 162–63
Choline acetylase, 115
Chorioamniotis, 210
   sexual activity and, 67, 69–70, 204
Christianity, ancient, view on marriage, 44
Chromosome study, 90
"Chronic cystic mastitis," 193
Chronic diseases, neurological disability and, 271
Circumcision, 3
Classic transsexualism of Benjamin, 299
Climacteric period, sexual behavior during, 124
Clitoral orgasm, 5
Clitoral reflex, 157
Clitoridectomy, 5
Clitoris, construction of, 310
   neural supply to, 269
Clomiphene citrate, 252
Clonidine, 238
Cocaine, effect on sexual function, 277, 282, 283
Cognitive aspects of sexuality, 272
Cognitive development, 11, 45
   in early adolescence, 19–20, 24
Coital death, 235
   fear of, 238
Coital-dependent methods of contraception, 133–34
Coital pain. See Dyspareunia
Coital position, during pregnancy, 201
Coital related contraception, effect on psychosexual function, 136
Coitus, 3
   in cardiac patient, 233, 236
   during pregnancy, 55, 56, 57, 74
      deleterious effects, 203–205
      frequency of, 61–63, 65, 66
      neonatal morbidity and, 71
      premature labor and, 68
   following SRS, 310
   frequency of, age and, 79
      decline in, 77
   premarital, 46
   spinal cord lesion and, 271
Common Era, view on marriage, 44
Communication, sexuality as, 6
Communication media, influence on choice of contraceptive, 133
Competence, development of, 32
   foundations of, 32
Concubines, 44
Conditioning, cultural, 48
Conditioning program, for cardiac disease, 236
Condom, 134
Conduct, rules of, 17
Congenital virilizing adrenal hyperplasia, 122–23

"Conspiracy of silence," 223
Consumerism, responsible, 52
Contraception, contraceptive, attitudes toward, historical perspective, 4
    development of, 7
    education on, 8
    influences affecting choice and use, 131–33, 137
    to juveniles, effects of, 36–37
    methods, 133
        coital-dependent, 133–34
        noncoital-dependent, 134–36
    psychosexual functioning and, 128, 136, 137
        coital related contraception and IUD, 136
        hormonal influences on sexual behavior and, 128–30
        of noncoital dependent methods, 136
        nonhormonal influences on sexual behavior, 130–31
        of postcoital contraception, 136–37
Contraceptive pill. *See* Oral contraceptive
Contraceptive sponge, 134
Conus-cauda equina, damage to, 270, 271
Conus lesions, 270
Corporal revascularization, direct, for impotence, 254, 255
Corporal shunt, for impotence, 253
Corpus luteum, 11
Cortisol, 122
    levels, depressive illness and, 214, 215
Counseling. *See* Sex therapy, Marital therapy
Courtship, 46
Couvade syndrome, 72–73
Crisis, impact on marriage, 50
Cross-gender identification, 313
Cross-gender living, real life test, 304–305, 307, 309
"Crushes," 22
"Cryptic nostalgia," 25
Cryptomenorrhea and menstrual egress per vagina, 98, 98 t, 108. *See also* Amenorrhea and cryptomenorrhea
    complete duplication of uterus and cervix, with noncommunicating uterine horn, 108–109
    with unilaterally imperforate external cervical os, 109
    with unilaterally imperforate vagina, 107–108
Culture, psychosexual development and, 7
    sexual practice and, 92
    transmission to young, 29–30
Cultural conditioning, discontinuity of, 48
"Cutaneous phase" of sexual development, 8–9
Cyclic nucleotides, 196
Cycloheximide, effect on reproductive behavior, 116
Cystine aminopeptidase, 115
Cystocele, vaginal relaxation associated with, 155, 156, 157–58

# D

Danazol, 196
Darwin, C., 41
Day-care centers, 32
de Laclos, C., 4
Death, coital, 235, 238
    fear of, 180
    perinatal. *See* Perinatal death
Deciduitis, 210

Defense mechanisms, 11
Dehydroepiandrosterone sulphate, 143
Delinquents, juvenile, 37
Denial, 179, 223
Dependence, in late puberty, 25, 26
Depo-medroxyprogesterone acetate (DMPA), 134–35
Depostesterone, 307
Depression, 284
    in cancer patient, 179
    hysterectomy and, 107, 173–74, 176
    in late puberty, 25–26
    postpartum, 213–14, 219
    related to infertility, 147
    in transsexualism and gender dysphoria, 303
Desensitization therapy, for impotence, 259
Deutsch, H., 7
Dexamethasone suppression test, 144
Diabetes, diabetes mellitus, 271
    impotence in, 247, 252–53
Diagnostic phase of cancer, stress in, 179–80, 185
Diaphragm, 134
    in relaxed vagina, 156
Dickinson, R., 6
Diderot, D., 4
Diencephalon, 264
Digitalis, 243
Digitalis toxicity, 238
Dihydrotestosterone, reduced levels, 94
Direct experiential flooding, 284
Disinhibition, 284
Disopyramide (Norpace), 243
Divorce, 40, 48, 50, 51. *See also* Remarriage
    historical perspective, 44
    rate of, 50, 51
Divorce mediation, 52
Dopamine, 55, 143, 144
    release, 143
Dopamine agonists, 196
Doppler blood pressure, penile, 249
Doppler studies, 243
    for vascular impotence, 249, 250
Dorsal artery, palpation, for impotence, 249
Dream content, during pregnancy, 60
"Dream orgasm," 209
Drug(s), drug addiction, affecting sexual activity, classification, 282
    causing hyperprolactinemia, 247–48
    effect on sexual function, 237–38, 243, 267–68, 277–78, 284–85
        alcohol, 282–83
        amphetamines, 283
        amyl nitrite, 283
        aphrodisiacs, 277
        barbiturates, 283
        cocaine, 283
        heroin, 280–82
        LSD, 284
        marijuana, 278–80
        mechanisms in, 284
        PCP, 284
        tranquilizers, 284
Drug-finding efforts, 280
Drug history, in impotence, 243
Drysdale, C., 5
Dunn, S., 6

Dysmenorrhea, 107, 145, 163, 171
  surgical treatment, 172-73
Dyspareunia, 146, 159. See also Pelvic pain
  etiologies, 160-61, 171
  psychogenic evaluation of, 159-60
  psychological causes, 165-67

# E

Early childhood education, sex differences in, 31-32
Early grades, sex differences in, 32-34
Economic insecurity, impact on marriage, 50
Ectopic pregnancy, in PID, 163-64
Education. See also Sex education
  in breast disease, 195-96
  expenditure on, 33
  for impotence, 259
  influence on contraceptive use and choice, 131-32
Educational career, effect on sexual behavior, 131
Educational groups, for perinatal loss, 225
Educational process, 28, 37-38
  psychosexual development and, 28-29
  public education, 29-31
  sex differences throughout, adolescence and high school, 34-37
    early childhood and preschool education, 31-32
    primary school and early grades, 32-34
Effeminate behavior, 93
Effeminate homosexual, 299
Efferent spinal tracts, 268
"Egalitarian," 42
Ego, function, 17
  in puberty, 10, 14, 25
Eighteenth century, physician involvement in sexuality during, 4
Einstein, A., 41
Ejaculation, 267. See also Premature ejaculation
  abnormalities, in vascular disease, 237
  during puberty, 13-14
  in impotence, 242
  onset of, 20
  in spinal cord lesion, 270, 271
Elderly. See also Menopause
  sexual behavior of, 77
Electrocardiogram, changes, during sexual activity, 233-34
Electrolyte study, in genital ambiguity, 89
Ellis, H. H., 5, 6, 296
Embryology, 96. See also Specific organ
Emotion(s), somatic reactions to, 166
Emotional aspects of sexuality, 272, 273
Emotional disturbance, infertility and, 142
Empathy, development of, 45
"Empty nest syndrome," 48, 81
Endarectomy, for impotence, 254
Endocrine changes, in prepubertal years, 18
Endocrine correlates, in feminine sexual behavior. See Feminine sexual behavior
Endocrine system, activation of, 12
Endocrine treatment, for transsexuals, 306-309
Endocrinologic studies, 246
  for transsexualism and gender dysphoria, 302, 309
Endocrinology of puberty, 11-12

Endometrial-vaginal communication, for congenital atresia of uterine cervix, 106, 107, 107 f,
Endometriosis, 146, 160, 169
  pelvic pain from, 170, 171
    hysterectomy for, 173. See also Hysterectomy
  polyps, vaginal bleeding from, 169, 170
  sexual function and, 176
  symptoms, 171
Endorphins, effect on behavioral patterns, 143
  release, 143
Enterocele, vaginal relaxation associated with, 155
Epididymis, cells of, 11
Epigastric-dorsal artery bypass, for impotence 254-55
Epilepsy, 264
  relationship to sexuality, 266-67
  temporal lobe. See Temporal lobe epilepsy
Epinephrine, plasma levels, relationship to postpartum mood disturbances, 215
Episiotomies, 155, 158
Erection, 267
  in infants, 92
  impaired, 78, 237. See also Impotence
  neurologic basis, 269
  nocturnal, monitoring of, 244-45
  physiology of, 240
  spinal cord lesions and, 270, 271
Erhardt, A., 8
Eroticism, in early adolescence, 22
  during pregnancy, 60, 61
  feminine, 7
Estradiol ($E_2$), 113, 120, 129
  functional correlates, 116-17
  induction of progestin receptors, 117
  plasma levels, during estrous cycle, 113
  secretion, 11
  spatial correlates, 114
  temporal correlates, 114-16
Estradiol benzoate, 115
Estrogen, 55, 57, 129, 135, 264
  activation of feminine sexual behavior by, 113, 114-18
  feedback of, 11
  influence, on animal sexual behavior, 128
    on human sexual behavior, 129-30
  levels, relationship to puerperium mood changes, 214, 215 t, 215, 216
  loss, physical consequences, 182
  production of, 11
Estrogen therapy, 77, 82, 182, 310
  for relaxed vagina, 157
  sexual relationship and, 82-83
  for transsexuals, 307
Estrone, 129
Estrous cycle, endocrine action during, 113
Exercise, for relaxed vagina, 157, 158
Experimentation, in late puberty, 25
Extended family, 42
  organization of, 42
External and sphincter, 154
  disruption of, 156
External genital ambiguity, 87, 94-95
  biologic components, 87-91
  physiologic components, 91-94
External urethral sphincter, 154
Extramarital relationships, 48, 234

# F

Fallopian tube(s), 269. *See also* Tubal ligation
  anomalous development of, 98, 109
  atresia, 109
    partial, 106
  in congenital vaginal agenesis, 99, 99 $f$, 100 $f$
  embryology, 96, 97
  infection, etiology, 165
  inflammation, 162, 163. *See also* Pelvic inflammatory disease
  obstruction, 161
  spasms, 144
Fallopius, 4
Family(ies), 42
  blended, 42
  defined, 42
  grouping of, functional prerequisites, 43
  size, choice of contraception and, 133
  western, historical perspective, 43–45
Family of orientation, 42, 45–47, 48
Family of procreation, 42, 47–49
Family therapy, 41, 51
  disciplines, 51
Fantasy(ies), 92
  during pregnancy, 56, 60
  during puberty, 14, 23
Fat, distribution, in males, 13
Father, identification with, 17
  interaction with infant, 31
Fatigue, posthysterectomy, 175
Fear(s), during pregnancy, 67–68, 73
    related to sexual activity, 59–60, 64
  in rape victim, 288
Fecal diversion, effect on sexual functioning, 181
Fellatio, during pregnancy, 66
Female(s). *See also* Girls
  anomalous genital duct development. *See* Anomalous female genital duct development
  brain, 92
  delinquents, 37
  education of, 32. *See also* Educational process, sex differences
  endocrinology of, 11–12
  factors, in sexual dysfunction in infertility, 143
  in genital stage of psychosexual development, 17
  hermaphroditism, 90, 122
  homosexual. *See* Lesbians, Homosexuality
  maturation, compared to males, 12, 37–38
    psychological, 17
  orientation, of public schools, 32
  premarital intercourse, 46
  prenatal hormone treatment, relationship to career aspirations, 34
  pseudohermaphroditism, 87, 88, 89 $f$
  psychosexual development of, 7
  psychosexual dysfunction in, 286–87
  puberty in, 12
  roles and self-identity, historical perspective, 43, 44–45
    related to childbirth, 217, 217 $f$, 218 $f$
  sexual attitudes, 49
  sexual behavior. *See* feminine sexual behavior
  spinal cord lesion, sexual function and, 270–71
  teachers, ratio to men, 30–31, 35

Female(s)—*Continued*
  transsexuals, 301
  virilized, 93
Female-to-male transsexual, 308
  surgical technique, 310–11
Feminine sexual behavior, endocrine correlates and ontogeny of, 113, 124
  activation, by estrogen and progesterone, 113, 114–18
  during climacteric period, 124
  during peripubertal period, 123
  during prenatal period, 121–23
  during reproductive period, 123–24
  modulation of, by luteinizing hormone-releasing hormone, 114, 118–19
    by opiate peptides, 119–20
    by prolactin, 120–21
    by vasopressin, 120
  ontogenetic tracing, 121
Feminity, 121
Fertility, 269
Fetal death. *See also* Perinatal death, Perinatal loss
  facilitating of grief process, 223–24
  sexual activity and, 67, 70–71
Fetal distress, sexual activity and, 67, 71
Fetus, development, hormonal stimulation and, 8
  effects of maternal anxiety on, 202, 202 $f$, 203
  influence of mother behavior and habits on, 31
  learning in utero, sexual activity and, 207
  maternal bonding with, 208
  personality, 207
  psychological problems associated with birth, 208
  responses in utero, 205–207
Fetishistic deviations, 266
Fibroid uterus, 169, 175
"Fibrocystic disease of the breast," 193
"Fibrous mastopathy," 193
Final stage of marriage, 48–49
Financial concerns, effect on marriage, 52
Financial counseling, 52
Finney prosthesis, for impotence, 255–56
Fitz-High-Curtis syndrome, 162–63
Flaccid paralysis, 271
Follicle stimulating hormone (FSH), 11, 122, 246, 252
  action of, 11
  levels, during seizure, 267
    increase in, 11
  release of, 119, 144
  secretion, 11
    effect of endorphins on, 143
Follicular atresia, 97
Follow-up phase of cancer treatment, stress in, 183–84
Formal education, 32
  during infancy, 32
"Foundations of competence, the," 32
Freed, C., 8
Freud, S., 5, 6, 7, 41
Frigidity, 167
  infertility and, 142

# G

Galen, 4
Gender assignment, delaying of, 89–90

Gender differentiation, 87. *See also* External genital ambiguity
Gender dimorphism, 91
Gender schemas, developing set of, 29
Gender-specific activities, development of, 92-93
Gender dysphoria syndrome, 94, 295, 299, 300, 313. *See also* Transsexualism
  body image and, 301-302
  diagnostic possibilities, 299-300
  evaluation and treatment, 302-305
    sex reassignment surgery, 309. *See also* Sex reassignment surgery
    trial of cross-gender living, 305-306
  relationship to homosexuality, 312-13
Gender identity, 92, 124
  confusion, 94
  contributors to, 94
  critical period, 93-94
  disorders, 295
    gender dysphoria syndrome. *See* Gender dysphoria syndrome
    spectrum of, 298-300
    transsexualism. *See* Transsexualism
  documentation of, 93
  feminine, in congenital virilizing adrenal hyperplasia, 122
Gender identity movement, 296-97
Gender identity programs, 304
Gender role, 92
  behavior, 299
  development of, 92-93
  historical perspective, 43, 44-45
Genital ambiguity. *See* External genital ambiguity
Genital duct(s), anomalous development *See* Anomalous female genital duct development
  duplication, 98
  embryology, 97
Genital examination, for impotence, 243
Genital herpes, pelvic pain from, 165
Genital organs, changes, during pregnancy, 58-59
Genital ridge, 96
Genital stage of psychosexual development, 16-17
Genital surgery, corrective, sexual functioning and, 93
Genitourogram, 90
Genetic/environmental dichotomies, related to transsexualism, 298
Geriatric years. *See* Climacteric period
Germ cell (oogania), 96
  embryology, 96-97
Girl(s), emotional response to puberty, 13
  pretranssexual, 299
Glucose tolerance tests, 246
Gonad(s), 96
  dysfunction. *See* Hypogonadal states
  function, assessment, 89
Gonadal dysgenesis, 88, 99, 100
Gonadectomy, for genital ambiguity, 91
Gonadostat, change in, 11
Gonadotropin, 143
  administration, for impotence, 252
  increase, 246
  release, regulation of, 264
  secretion of, 11, 114
Gonadotropin-releasing factor, for impotence, 252
Gonadotropin releasing hormone (GNRH), 55

Grades, sex-related patterns of, 36
Granulosa cells, 97
Greeks, ancient, scientific medicine and, 3-4
Green, R., 297
Grief, process, in perinatal death. *See* Perinatal death, grief process
  stages of, 223
Grieving period, 180-81
Growth, physical. *See* Physical growth
Guanosine monophosphate (GMP), 196
Guaracum, 4
Guilt, related to infertility, 146
Gynecologic malignancies. *See* Malignant neoplasia, Cancer patient
Gynecomastia, 13, 252

# H

H-Y antigen test, 298
Headache, related to sexual activity, 267
Health, sexual activity and, 79
Health care provider, influence on choice of contraception, 133
  role in facilitating grief process, in perinatal death, 223-25
Hearing, fetal, 205
Heart rate, during sexual activity, 233-34, 235, 236
Hebrews, ancient, laws on rape, 286
  view of marriage, 44
Hegar dilators, 258
Helman, L., 8
Helplessness feelings, in cancer patient, 179
Hematocolpos, 105
Hematuria, cyclic, 105
Hemorrhage, antepartum, 67, 70
Hermaphroditism, female, 122
  male sex assignment in, 90
  true, 88
Heroin, effect on sexual function, 280-82, 284
Heterosexual patterning, in adolescent, 46
Heterosexual relationships, in early adolescence, 24
  following rape, 291, 292, 293, 293 *t*
Heterosexuality, in late puberty, 26, 27
High-risk pregnancy, psychosomatic aspects, 208, 211
  sexual activity during, 209-10
    maternal support of in vitro development, 210
    recommendations, 210
High school educational process, sex differences, 34-37
Hippocrates, 3
Hippocratic Oath, 3, 4
Hirschfeld, M., 296
History *See also* Medical history, Sexual history
  for infertility, 147
  for pelvic relaxation, 158
Holding, desire for, during pregnancy, 66
Holidays, stress from, 50
Home economics, 41
Homoaffiliative behavior, of preadolescent, 46
Homosexuality, homosexual, 40, 92, 298, 299
  attitude towards, historical perspective, 5, 6
  in children, 92
  in early adolescence, 23
  relationship to gender dysphoria, 312-13
  sex reassignment surgery for, 301

Homosexuality—*Continued*
    in temporal lobe epilepsy, 266
    use of nitrites, 283
Honeymoon, 47
Hormonal castration, 306
Hormonal contraceptives, 134–35
Hormonal regimen for contraception
    effect on psychosexual function, 136
    postcoital, 135–36
Hormonal stimulation, fetal development and, 8
Hormonal system, in early adolescence, 19
Hormone(s), 243. *See also* Sex hormones
    abnormalities, 243
        in gender identity disorders, 298
        related to impotence, 251–53
    influence of sexual behavior on, 130
    influences of, on animal sexual behavior, 128–29
        on contraceptive choice and use, 131
        on human sexual behavior, 129–30
    levels, fetal and pubertal, gender identity and, 94
        relationship to mood changes in puerperium, 214–16
Hormone tests, for genital ambiguity, 89, 90
Hormone therapy, 264
    prenatal, relationship to career aspiration, 34
    for transsexualism, 298, 304, 306–309
"Hostile mucous," 147
Hot flashes, 82, 182
Human chorionic gonadotropin (hCG), 252
Human chorionic gonadotropin (hCG) stimulation test, 89
Human sexuality, research, twentieth century, 8–9
Humankind, distinguished from other mammalian, 43–44
Husband, fears, during pregnancy, 73
    infidelity, during pregnancy, 72
    response to pregnancy, 56
    symptomatic emotional problems, during pregnancy, 72–73
Hustler lifestyle, 281
Hydrocortisone, 90
Hydromucocolpos 103
17-Hydroxycorticosteroids, 89
11$\beta$-Hydroxylase, deficiency, 88
17$\alpha$-Hydroxylase, deficiency, 88
21-Hydroxylase, deficiency, 88, 89, 90
17-Hydroxyprogesterone, 89
    levels, in genital ambiguity, 89
3$\beta$-Hydroxysteroid dehydrogenase, deficiency, 88
Hygroton (chlorthalidone), 238
Hymen, 97
    imperforate, 98
        amenorrhea and cryptomenorrhea in, 103–105
    microperforate, 104, 104 *f*
Hyperandrogenism, 124
Hypergonadotropic hypogonadism, 246
Hypermenorrhea, 163
"Hypermetamorphosis," 265
Hyperprolactinemia, 266
    impotence and, 247–48, 252
    therapy for, 252
Hypersexuality, 265
    neurologic studies, 265, 266
Hypertension, sexual dysfunction in, 243
Hypnosis, for psychosexual dysfunction in infertility, 151

Hypochondriacal complaints, 19
Hypoestrogenic state, 143
Hypogonadal states, related to impotence, 246–47, 251–52
Hypogonadotropic hypogonadism, 252, 266
Hypomenorrhea, 104, 105
Hyposexuality, neurologic studies, 265–66
Hypothalamic hypogonadotropic amenorrhea, 143
Hypothalamic-hypophysiogonadal axis, 264
Hypothalamic-pituitary abnormalities, in impotence, 246
Hypothalamic-pituitary-gonadal system, 12
Hypothalamic-pituitary-testicular axis, 144
Hypothalamus, 264, 265
    biosynthetic events in, 115
    cells of, 11
    dysfunction, in impotence, 251–53
        sexual behavior and, 114
    estradiol levels in, 115
Hypothyroidism, 196
Hysterectomy, 173, 174, 176, 310
    for cancer, 181
    for congenital atresia of uterine cervix, 106, 107
    for genital ambiguity, 90, 91
    posthysterectomy depression, 107
    psychosexual impact of, 173–75
    sexual functioning following, 81–82, 176, 181
    surgical techniques for, 175
Hysteria, 173, 174
    historical perspective, 5, 6
Hysteroscopic resection, 176

# I

Ictal sexual manifestation, 266
Id, during puberty, 10
Identification, intrapsychic development of, 17
Identity seeking, in late puberty, 26
Iliococcygeus muscle, 154
Illegitimate births, 40
Impotence, 266
    assessment, 272
    diagnosis and treatment, 240–41, 259, 260
        characterization of sexual dysfunction, 241–42
        definitions, 241
        establishing diagnosis, 241
        for identifiable etiologies, 251–55
        medical history, 242–43
        nonspecific therapy, 255–58
        for organic impotence, 244–46
        physical examination, 243–44
        premature ejaculation, 259–60
        for psychogenic erectile dysfunction, 258–59
        reliability of sexual history, 242
        search for remedial etiology, 246–51
Impulse(s), control of, 14, 16
Impulsiveness, in early adolescence, 24
Incest taboo, 43
Incestual wishes, during early adolescence, 20, 21
Incorporation, in late puberty, 25
Independence, establishing of, 14
    in late puberty, 25, 26
Inderal, 237
Individual therapy, for impotence, 259
    for marital distress, 52

Individuation. *See* Separation-individuation process
Infant, acutely ill or dying, facilitation of grief process, 223
   behavior, sex differences in, 31
   discovery of self, 45
   formal education of, 32
   psychological development and, 14–15
   separation anxiety, 9
   sexual behavior, 92
Infection, during pregnancy, sexual activity and, 69–70
Infertility, 266
   evaluation, termination of, 152
   female, 161
   from psychological disorders, 167
   psychosexual dysfunction and, 141, 152
      effect of pregnancy success or failure, 152
      etiologies and mechanisms, 143
      female factors, 143–44
      habitual abortion, 149–50
      identification, 141–43
      incidence, 143
      male factors, 144–45
      physician and infertility workup, stress and, 146–48
      physician and therapy, stress and, 148–49
      psychosocial factors, 145–46
      therapeutic modalities for, 150–52
Inflatable prostheses, for impotence, 256–57
Infusion cavernosography, for impotence, 251
Intellectual development, failure in, 35
   impediment to, 36–37
Intelligence, development of, 15
Interaction, 41
Intrafamilial forces, in gender identity disorders, 298–99
Intrauterine device (IUD), 7, 134
   effect on psychosexual function, 136
   pelvic pain from, 165
Intrauterine fetal demise, sexual activity and, 67, 70–71
Ischiocavernosus muscles, 154, 268, 269
Isosexual, 87
IUD. *See* Intrauterine device

## J

Johnson, V. E., 8, 57–58
Jonas prosthesis, for impotence, 256
Jorgenson, C., 296, 310
Juvenile(s), sexual activity of, results of, 36–37
Juvenile delinquents, 37

## K

Kelly, H. A., 6
17-Ketosteroids, 89
Kinsey, A., 6–7
Klippel-Feil syndrome, 100
Knowlton, C., 5
Kroger, W., 8

## L

Labia, constructing of, 310
   during pregnancy, 58, 59

Labor, premature, sexual activity and, 67, 68
Lacerations, obstetrical, 155
Laparoscopy, 171
   for pelvic pain, 166
Latency, 18
Latency years, 19
Lay counseling, for perinatal loss, 225
Learning, problems, sex differences, 37
   processes of, 29
   skills, 17
Leiomyoma, 99 *f*
Leriche's syndrome, 237
Lesbianism, 93, 299
Levator-ani spasm syndrome, 164
Levator muscles, 155
Levatores ani, 154
Lewis, D., 6, 8
Leydig cells, 11
Libido, 55
   changes in, 145
   drug effects on, 267
   following hysterectomy, 175
   impotence and, 242
   problems in, 272
Lief, H., 7
Life style, choice of contraception and, 132
Lindgren-Pauly Body Image Scale, 307
Lipoid adrenal hyperplasia, congenital, 88
Liver, dysfunction, 252
Lordosis quotient scores, effect of vasopressin on, 120
Lordosis reflex, activation of, 114, 116, 119, 120
   effect of prolactin on, 120–21
Lower extremity, claudication, 249
LSD. *See* Lysergic acid diethylamide
Lumbar cord, lesions in, 271
Lumbar disc disease, 253
Lumbar sympathectomy, 237
Luteal phase, defects, 144, 147
   hormone levels during, 129
Luteinizing hormone (LH), 11, 122, 246
   action of, 11
   activation of feminine sexual behavior, 113
   increased response, 143
   influence of sexual behavior on, 130
   levels, during seizures, 267
      increase in, 11
   release of, 11, 118, 143, 144
   secretion, 11
      effect of endorphins on, 143
Luteinizing hormone-releasing hormone (LHRH), 11, 120
   action, 11
   effect of endorphins on, 143
   modulation of feminine sexual behavior by, 118–19
   release, 11, 119, 120
Lysergic acid diethylamide (LSD), effect on sexual function, 282, 284

## M

Macroadenoma, 252
Male(s). *See also* Boys, Husbands
   adolescent, 35
   aging, sexuality in, 77–78

Male(s)—*Continued*
   attitude toward, of rape victim, 288, 290
   brain, 92
   contraception, 132, 135
   delinquents, 37
   education of, 32. *See also* Educational process, sex differences
   emotional response to puberty, 13
   endocrinology of, 11
   factors in psychosexual dysfunction in infertility, 144–45
   in genital stage of psychosexual development, 17
   homosexuals. *See* Homosexuals
   maturation of, compared to females, 12, 37–38
   paramesonephric duct embryology, 97
   premarital intercourse, 46
   pseudohermaphroditism, 87, 88, 89 *f*
   puberty in, 12
   reproductive behavior, effect of opiate peptides on, 119
   roles, historical perspective, 44
   sexual arousal, neurologic studies, 265
   sexual attitudes, 49
   spinal cord lesion, sexual function in, 270
   teachers, ratio to female, 30–31, 35
   transsexuals, 301. *See also* Transsexualism
Malignant neoplasia, 178
   stress from. *See* Cancer patient, stress in
Mammalian, distinguishing of humans in, 43–44
   sexual behavior, 3
Mammary dysplasia, 193, 196
   treatment for, 196
Mammoplasty, 310
Marijuana, effect on sexual behavior, 277–78, 278–80, 282, 284
Marital therapy, 41, 51–52
   development of, 7–8
   disciplines, 51
   effectiveness of, 52
Marriage, 40–41, 49, 52. *See also* Remarriage
   defined, 40
   experimentation with, 42
   functional prerequisites of, 43
   future of, 40
   general theoretical considerations and definition, 41–43
      western marriage and family, historical perspective, 43–45
   life span overview of, 45
      premarital (family of orientation) stages, 45–47
      postmarital (family of procreation) stages, 47–49
   marital strain, divorce remediation, 49–52
   rate, decline in, 40
Married individual, social view of, 47
Masculinity, 121
Masochism, 7
Mastalgia, 193–94
   treatment for, 196
Mastectomy, 194, 197, 199
   issues in, 198
      external prosthesis and breast reconstruction, 199
      phantom breast syndrome, 198–99
   for transsexuals, 310
Masters, W. H., 8, 57–58
Mastitis, chronic cystic, 193
Mastodynia, 193–94

Mastopathy, fibrous, 193
Masturbation, 236
   age and, 78–79
   attitude toward, historical perspective, 4, 5, 6
   in children, 92
   during pregnancy, 66
   in early adolescence, 23
   in impotence, 242
   neurologic studies, 266
Maternal feelings, development of, 217
Maternal role, adaptation to, 217
Mathematics achievement, sex differences in, 35, 36
Maturation, processes of, 28
Maturity, early, 13
   late, 13
MBH-POA, 118
   progestin receptors in, 115, 116
Medical history, for impotence, 242–43
Medical practice, human sexuality in, 264
Medication. *See* Drugs
Medroxyprogesterone acetate (Provera), 307
Membranes, premature rupture of, sexual activity and, 67, 68–69
Menopause, 48. *See also* Hysterectomy
   sexuality and, 77, 78–80
      aging male and, 77–78
      menstrual cycle and, 80–81
      replacement therapy, 82–83
      sociological variables, 81
Menometrorrhagia, from benign neoplasia, 169–70. *See also* Vaginal bleeding
   sexual function in, 176
Menorrhagia, concern for safety and, 170
Menses, 13
   failure of, 98
Menstrual cycle, 11–12
   in infertility, 145
   phases, human sexual behavior during, 129–30
   sexuality and, 80–81, 124
Menstrual egress per vagina, 98, 104. *See also* Cryptomenorrhea and menstrual egress per vagina
Menstruation, 170
   during puberty, 13–14
   in fantasy, 14
   onset of, 20
Mental operations, development of, failure in, 35
Mental set, in heroin use, 280
   in marijuana use, 278, 279 *f*, 279
Mental status examination, for transsexualism and gender dysphoria, 303
Mesencephalon, 264
Mesenchymal cells, 97
Mesonephric ducts, 97
Mesonephros, 96
Mesiotemporal seizure discharges, sexual arousal and, 266
Met-enkephalin, 119–20
Metaplasia, apocrine, 193
Methadrine, 282
Methaqualone (quaaludes), 283
Methyldopa (Aldomet), 238
Methylxanthines, withdrawal of, 196
Metroplasty, 110
Middle Ages, physician involvement in sexuality during, 4
Midteens, psychosexual development during, 19, 24–26

Mind set. *See* Mental set
Minipress (prazosin hydrochloride), 238
Minnesota Multiphasic Personality Inventory (MMPI), 251, 304
Miscarriage, 221, *See also* Abortion
 reaction to, 222
Money, J., 8, 297
Monogamy, 42
 distinguished from polygamy, 42
 historical perspective, 44
 serial, 42
Mood disturbances, in puerperium. *See* Puerperium, mood disturbances
Moodiness, of adolescent, 21
Moos Menstrual Distress Questionnaire, 80
Moral taboos, sexual practice during pregnancy and, 56
Morning erections, impotence and, 242
Mother, identification with, 17
 interaction with infant, 31
 symbiosis with child, 45
Motivation, 41
Motor development, fetal, 206
Mullerian derivatives, 87
Myocardial infarction. *See* Cardiac disease
Myomata, sexual function and, 176
 uterine. *See* Uterine myomata
 vaginal bleeding from, 169–70
Myometrial hemostasis, 109

# N

Naloxone, 119, 143
 -induced LHRH release, 119
Narcissism, 24
 primary, 16
Narcissistic cathexis, 26
Nature/nurture dichotomies, related to transsexualism, 298
*Neisseria gonorrhoeae,* 161
Neonatal death, 221
 sexual activity and, 67, 71
Neonate, ambiguous genitalia in, 87, 88, 91, 91 *f*
 differential diagnosis, 88, 89
Neophallus, construction of, 311
Neoplasia, benign. *See* Benign neoplasia
 malignant. *See* Malignant neoplasia
Neovagina, creation of, procedures, 310
 in Rokitansky-Kuster-Hauser syndrome, 100, 101–103
 sexual function and, 181
Nervous system, diseases, 264. *See also* Neurologic disease
Neural basis of sexual behavior, 265
Neurasthenia, sexual, 5
Neuroendocrine basis of sexual behavior, 264
Neuroendocrine deficits, in libido problems, 272
Neuroendocrine function, modulation of, 266
Neurologic abnormalities, related to diabetes, 247
Neurologic development, fetal, 205–206
 rapid eye movement, 206–207
 real time *in utero,* ultrasonic studies, 206
Neurologic disease, sexual dysfunction and, 264
 anatomy and physiology related to, 264–67
 diagnostic considerations, 271–72

Neurologic disease—*Continued*
 effect of medication, 267–68
 headache, 267
 neuroanatomy of spinal cord and peripheral nerves. *See* Spinal cord, Peripheral nerves
 rehabilitation, 272–73
Neurologic evaluation, for impotence, 243, 248–49
Neurologic events, in male sexual function, 268–69
Neurologic studies, on sexual behavior, 264–67
Neurologic therapies, for impotence, 252
Neuromuscular deficits, 264
Newborn. *See* Neonate
Newlyweds, adaptation of, 49
Nineteenth century, physician involvement in sexuality during, 4–6
Nitroglycerine, 236
Nocturnal emissions, attitude toward, historical perspective, 5
Nocturnal tumescence monitoring (NPT), for impotence, 244–45, 251
Nomenclature, in fields of inquiry, 42
Noncoital dependent methods of contraception, 134–36
 effect on psychosexual function, 136
Noncoital sexual behavior, during pregnancy, 55, 56, 65–67, 201
Non-goal oriented approach to impotence, 259
Norepinephrine, 143
 plasma levels, relationship to postpartum mood disturbances, 215
Norpace (disopyramide), 243
Nostalgia, cryptic, 25
Nuclear family, 42
"Nurturant socialization," 43
 marriage function as, 48

# O

Object, constancy, establishment of, 17
 in late puberty, 26
 permanence, achievement of, 17
 during puberty, 10
 representations, 15
 formation of, 17
 self separation from, 20
Obstetrical trauma, pelvic relaxation from, 155
Obstetrician. *See also* Physician
 role during pregnancy, 56
Oedipal complex, 9, 17
 resolution of, 17
Oedipal conflict, in female, 17
Oligospermia, 144–45
Oocyte, 11, 96
Oogania. *See* Germ cells
Oophorectomy, 310
 for genital ambiguity, 90, 91
 psychological function following, 81, 82, 175
Opiate(s), 247
 exogenous, 211
Opiate peptides, effect on behavioral patterns, 143
 modulation of feminine sexual behavior by, 119–20
Oral contraceptives, 7, 134–35
 effect on psychosexual function, 136
Oral-libido impetus, in child, 15
Oral stage, 15

Orgasm, 4, 8, 267
    age and, 78–79, 82–83
    clitoral, 5
    during pregnancy, 55, 59, 63–64, 66
        deleterious effects, 203, 204 t
        fetal demise and, 70–71
        fetal distress and, 71
        premature labor and, 68
    menopause and, 79
    spinal cord lesions and, 270, 271
    vagina, 5, 157
Orgasmic dysfunction, in pelvic pain, 159
    in relaxed vagina, 156–57
Orgasmic intercourse, following hysterectomy, 175
Orgasmic platform, during pregnancy, 59
Orientation, family of, 42, 45–47, 48
"Original sin," 56
Orogenital sexual relations. See also Fellatio
    during pregnancy, 66
Osteoporosis, 82
Ovarian cancer, 179
Ovarian failure, from chemotherapy, 183
    radiation-induced, 182
Ovarian follicle, maturation of, 11
Ovarian plexus, 269
Ovary(ies), in congenital vaginal agenesis, 99, 99 f, 100 f
    embryology of, 96–97
    inflammation of, 162, 163. See also Pelvic inflammatory disease
    innervation of, 269
Ovulation, sexual activity at, 124
Ovulatory dysfunction, 145
Oxytocin, blood levels, maternal sexual activity and, 202
    release, breast-feeding and, 191–92

## P

Pain, control, from drugs, 284
    during intercourse, in pregnancy, 64
    pelvic. See Pelvic pain
Pain impulse, travel of, 172
Papanicolaou smear, 179
Papillomatosis, 193
"Paradoxical hormone therapy," 306
Paramedical personnel, in cancer treatment, 186
Paramesonephric duct, anomalies, symptomatic classification of, 96, 97–98, 98 t
    amenorrhea and cryptomenorrhea, 98–104
    asymptomatic, 110
    cryptomenorrhea and menstrual egress per vagina, 107
    reproductive failure, 109–10
    embryology, 97
Paranoia, in marijuana use, 278
Parasympathetic abnormalities, related to impotence, 247
Parasympathetic fibers, 268
Parent(s), separation from, 14. See also Separation-individuation process
    during early adolescence, 20–21, 22, 23, 26
    late puberty and, 26
Parental images, puberty and, 10
Parenting, social readiness for, 46
Partial abstinence, 133
Partner, influence on contraceptive choice and use, 132

Passivity, feminine, 7
PCP. See Phencyclidine hydrochloride
Peer group, influence on child behavior, 32
Peer relationships, in early adolescence, 22–23
    in late puberty, 25, 26
    during prepubertal period, 26
Pelvic abscess, 109
Pelvic congestion, 166, 210
    dyspareunia in, 160
Pelvic exenteration, effect on sexual functioning, 181–82
Pelvic inflammatory disease, 164, 166, 169
    diagnosis, 162
    dyspareunia in, 160
    etiology, 161–62, 165
    medical consequences, 163–64
    pelvic pain from, 168, 170, 171
        surgical treatment for, 172–73. See also Hysterectomy
    sequelae, 171 sexual function and, 164, 176
    symptoms, 162–63
Pelvic pain, 145, 159, 170, 176. See also Dyspareunia
    in absence of pathology, 171–72
    from benign neoplasia, surgical treatment, 172–75
    in cryptomenorrhea, 105
    cyclic, 98
    etiologies, 165, 175
        endometriosis, 171
        genital herpes, 165
        intrauterine device, 165
        pelvic inflammatory disease, 161–64, 171
        psychological, 165–67
        tubal ligation, 164
        uterine myomata, 170–71
        uterine retrodisplacement, 164–65
    postorgasmic, 210
Pelvic peritonitis, 162
Pelvic relaxation, 154, 158
    factors in, 155
    obstetrical trauma, 155
    sexual dysfunction and orgasmic failure in, 156–57
    studies on, 157
    support of vagina, 154–55
    symptoms, 155–56
    treatment, 157–58
Pelvic sonography, 107
Pelvic surgery, ultraradical, sexual functioning following, 181
Pelvis, lesions of, 160
Penile brachial index (PBI), 250
Penile disorders, in impotence, 251
Penile prosthesis, 251
Penile tumescence studies, 272
Penile vascular abnormalities, in diabetes, 247
Penile vasculature, assessment of, in impotence, 249–51
Penis, artificial, creation of, 310–11
    blood flow to, improvement in, 241
    removal of, 310
    revascularization of, 255
Penography, radioactive xenon, 250–51
Perceptual distortion, from drugs, 284
Performance anxiety, related to impotence, 259
Perhexiline (Texid), 243
Perianal sensation, assessment of, 248
Perimenstrual (early follicular) phase, hormone levels during, 129

Perinatal death, grief process, 222
　facilitation of, 223–25
　phases, 222–23
　problems concerning sexuality, 225
　support groups for, 225–26
　thoughts about another pregnancy, 226
Perinatal loss, 226
　coping with, 221
Perineal body, 154
Perineum, 154
Periodic abstinence, 133
Periovulatory phase, hormone levels during, 129
Peripartum period, psychosomatic aspects of, 210–11
Peripheral nerve, neuroanatomy, 268–70
Peritonitis, pelvic, 162
Personality, disorders, in transsexuals, 303
　organization of, in early adolescence, 20
　related to infertility, 142
　sexual satisfaction and, 160
　variables, in sexual enhancement by marijuana, 278
Peyronie's disease, 243
　impotence from, 253
　surgical therapy for, 253–54
Phallic correction, surgery for, 90
Phantom breast syndrome (PBS), 198–99
Phencyclidine hydrochloride (PCP), effect on sexual function, 284
Pheromones, influence on sexual behavior, in animals, 129
　in humans, 130
Philadelphia Assault Victim Study. *See* Rape, Philadelphia Assault Victim Study
Physical aspects of sexuality, 272, 273
Physical complaints, during prepubertal period, 18
Physical disabilities, sexual concerns in, 272–73
Physical examination, in impotence, 243–44
Physical force, in rape, related to sexual adjustment, 292
Physical growth, spurt in, 20
Physician. *See also* Health care provider
　input into sexuality during pregnancy, 73, 74
　involvement in sexual life and practices, 3
　　ancient times, 3–4
　　eighteenth and nineteenth centuries, 4–8
　　Middle Ages, 4
　　Renaissance, Reformation and Puritan period, 4
　recognition of sexual dysfunction by, 159
　stress related to infertility and,
　　in therapy, 148–49
　　in work-up, 146–48
Physiological changes, in aging, 82
Pituitary adenoma, 252
Pituitary dysfunction, 251
Place, F., 5
Placenta, leukocyte infiltration by, 69
Plasma volume, expansion, 209
Plateau phase of sexual stimulation, pregnancy and, 59
Plethysmography, penile, 250
Polycycstic ovary syndrome, 124, 144
Polygamy, 56
　distinguished from monogamy, 42
　historical perspective, 44
Polygyny. *See* Polygamy
Polyp(s), sexual function in, 176
　vaginal bleeding from, 169–70
Population Control Movement, 5

Pornography, 5
Postcoital method of contraception, 132, 135–36
　effect on psychosexual function, 136–37
Postcoital test, for infertility, 147
Postganglionic fibers, 268, 269
"Post-hysterectomy syndrome, the," 173, 174 175
Postictal sexual arousal, 266
Postmarital (family of procreation) stages, 47–49
Postpartum depression, 213–14
Posttraumatic stress disorder, DSM-III listing, 287–88
Potter's syndrome, 100
Prazosin hydrochloride (Minipress), 238
Prediagnostic phase of cancer, stress in, 179
Preganglionic fibers, 268
Pregnancy, 55. *See also* Fetus
　adjustment to, factors in, 56–57
　anxiety during, 201
　effect of sexual relations on, 67
　　abortion, 67–68
　　air embolism, 71–72
　　antepartum hemorrhage, 70
　　chorioamnionitis, 69–70
　　intrauterine fetal demise, 70–71
　　fetal distress, 71
　　neonatal morbidity, 71
　　premature labor, 68
　　premature rupture of membranes, 68–69
　effect on sexuality, 56–57, 67
　following perinatal death, 226
　high-risk. *See* High-risk pregnancy
　infidelity during, 72
　intrauterine, 161
　juvenile, 36
　marriage for, 50–51
　perception of sexuality during, 72–73
　physical changes associated with, 57
　physician input into sexuality during, 73, 74
　psychosomatic aspects of peripartum period, 210–11
　sexual abstinence during, problems with recommending, 208–209
　sexual activity during, 59–60, 201–202
　　fetal effects of, 202, 202 f, 203
　　frequency of sexual relations, 61–63
　　levels of sexual desire, 60–61
　　levels of sexual satisfaction, 63–65
　　maternal problems with, 203–205
　　noncoital sexual activity, 65–67
　sexual response during, 57–58
　　breast changes, 58
　　genital organ changes, 57–58
　success or failure, effect on psychosexual dynamics, 152
Pregnanetriol, 89
Pregnant women, behavior and habits, influences on fetus, 31
Preludin, 282
Premarin, 83
Premarital sexuality, 46
　social view of, 47
Premarital (family of orientation) stage, 45–47
Premature ejaculation, 242
　therapy for, 259–60
Premenstrual syndrome, 216
Prenatal period, female, androgen insensitivity syndromes, 123

Prenatal period—*Continued*
    androgenic exposure during, 121
    congenital virilizing adrenal hyperplasia, 122–23
    Turner's syndrome, 121–22
Preoccupations, 19
Preoptic area, lesions, sexual behavior and, 114
Prepuberty, homoaffiliative behavior, 46
    hormonal-behavioral relationships during, 123
    psychosexual development during, 17–18, 26
Presacral neurectomy, for pelvic pain from benign neoplasia, 172–73
Priapism, 270
"Primal castration, the," 202
Primary grades, sex differences in, 32–34
Primary transsexualism, 303
Problem children, 32
Procreation, family of, 42, 47–49
Professionally facilitated groups, for perinatal loss, 225–26
Progesterone (P), 11, 55, 57, 113, 120, 129, 265
    functional correlations, 118
    influence on sexual behavior, animal, 129
        human, 129–30
    levels, during estrous cycle, 113
        low or absent, 145
        relationship to puerperium mood changes, 214, 215 *t*, 215, 216
    sequential inhibition by, of reproductive behavior, 118
    spatial correlations, 117
    temporal correlations, 117–18
Progesterone-facilitated reproductive behavior, 114, 115
Progestin, 135
Progestin-concentrating neurons, 117
Progestin receptors, 115
    classes, 117
    estrogen-inducible, 115, 116, 117
Prolactin, 57, 144, 246
    levels, during seizure, 267
        increase, 143
        maternal sexual activity and, 202
        in puerperium, related to depression, 215–16
    modulation of feminine sexual behavior by, 120–21
    release, breast-feeding and, 191
    role in benign breast disease, 196
Prostaglandin, blood levels, maternal sexual activity and, 202
    semen, vaginal introduction to, 203
Prosthetic devices, for impotence, 240–41
    inflatable, 256–57
    semirigid, 255–56
Prostitution, 5, 280
Protestantism, view on marriage, 44–45
Provera (medroxyprogesterone acetate), 307
Provocative stimulation studies, for impotence, 245–46
Pseudohermaphroditism, distinguishing male from female, appearance of external genitalia, 88, 89 *f*
    female, 87, 88
    male, 87
        disorders resulting from, 87
        treatment, 91
Psyche, role in sexuality in menopause, 80
Psychiatric problems, from hysterectomy, 173–75

Psychic apparatus, disequilibrium of, in early adolescence, 19
Psychoemotional factors, in sexual dysfunction, 272
Psychogenic amenorrhea, 144
Psychogenic erection, 269
Psychogenic impotence, diagnostic tests, 251
Psychological development, 14
    childhood years: birth to latency, 14–17
    prepubertal years, 17–18
    puberty, 19–20
Psychological evaluation, for infertility, 142
    for transsexualism, 302, 303–304, 305
Psychological screening tests, for impotence, 251
Psychology, 43
    influence on contraceptive choice and use, 131–32
Psychopathic personality, 300
Psychosexual arousal, physiological response to, 129
Psychosexual counseling, for partial vaginal agenesis surgery, 105–106
Psychosexual development, educational process and, 28–29
    prepubertal. *See* Prepubertal years
    in puberty. *See* Puberty
    stages, Freud's theory, 5
"Psychosexual inversion," 296
Psychosexual medicine, history of, 3
    physician and sex, 3–8
    twentieth century research, 8–9
Psychosis, 300
    puerperal, 214
Psychosocial factors, effect on sexual behavior, 77, 131
    influencing infertility, 145–46
Psychosomatic disorders, 166
    following hysterectomy, 176
    pelvic symptoms, 166–67
Psychotherapy, for transsexuals, 306
Puberty (adolescent, adolescence), 10–11, 28
    age of onset, 35, 46
        intellectual development and, 36
        sex differences, 46
    defined, 46
    educational process, sex differences, 34–37
    endocrinology of, 11–12
    gender assignment and, 90
    heterosexual patterning in, 46
    hormone therapy during, 309
    period of, changes in, 34–35
    physical changes associated with, 12
        adaptation to, 14
        emotional reactions to, 12–14
    pregnancy, sexual activity in, 65
    psychosexual development during, 19, 26–27
        early adolescence, 19–24
        late puberty, 24–26
Public education, 29–30
    effect on psychosexual development, 28–29, 37
    environment, feminization in, 37
    public school system, 30–31
        female orientation in, 32
Public school teaching, feminization of, 35
Pubococcygeus muscle, 154, 155
    strengthening of, 157
Pudendal (somatic) nerve, 268, 269
Puerperal depression, 214
Puerperal psychosis, 214

Puerperium, 213, 226
 mood disturbance in, 213–14
  interventions, 219–21
  perinatal death and, 221–23
  perinatal loss and, 221
  physiological factors, 214–16
  psychosocial factors, 216–19
Pupil, ratio to teacher, 33
Puritan period, physician involvement in sexuality during, 4
Pus formation, in pelvic inflammatory disease, 162
Pyrexia, in pelvic inflammatory disease, 162
Pyosalpinx, 163

## Q

Quaaludes (methaquaalone), 283

## R

Race, choice of contraception and, 132
Radiation therapy, 178
 for cancer, 184–85
 for breast cancer, 199
 sexual functioning and, 182–83, 186
Radioactive xenon penography, 250–51
Radiologic studies, for external genital ambiguity, 90
Rape, 286
 background, 286
 effects, 287–89, 293, 294
 phase of adjustment, 288
 Philadelphia Assault Victim Study: Rape Victim Sample, 289, 290–92
  predictors of sexual adjustment problems, 292, 293 $t$, 294 $t$
  rating of sexual adjustment, 290–92
  study design and sample, 289–90
 psychosexual dysfunction following, 286–87, 294
  etiology, 293, 294
Rapid eye movement (REM) sleep, erection occurring with, 244, 245, 272
 fetal, 206–207
 sexual arousal in, 129
Rapprochment phase of psychological development, 15
Reassurance, in breast disease, 195–96
Real-life test, for transsexualism, 304–305, 307
Real time *in utero*, ultrasound studies, 206
Reciprocal interaction, conflicts in, 10–11
Reciprocation, sexual, 49
Reconstructive revascularization procedures, for impotence, 241
Recovery phase of grief process, 222–23
Rectocele, vaginal relaxation associated with, 155, 156, 157–58
Recurrence phase of cancer, stress in, 184
5α-Reductase, deficiency, 94
Reflex activity, cessation of, 269–70
Reflexogenic erections, 253, 269
Reformation, physician involvement in sexuality during, 4
Relationship, maturity of, choice of contraception and, 132

Religion, influence of, on contraceptive choice and use, 131, 132
 on sexual activity during pregnancy, 56
 on sexual behavior, 131
Remarriage, 40
 quality of life, 51
 statistics on, 51
Renaissance, physician involvement in sexuality during, 4
Renal agenesis, 99, 100, 107
Repression, intrapsychic development of, 17
Reproductive behavior, activation
  by estradiol, 115
  by progesterone, 114, 115
 effect of opiate peptides on, 119
Reproductive failure, 98 $t$
 complete or partial duplication of uterus, 109–10
 unicornuate uterus, 109
Reproductive hormones, cessation of, 78
Reproductive period, sexual behavior during, 123–24
Reproduction, 3–4, 113
Research on human sexuality, twentieth century, 8–9
Reserpine, 238, 247
Retirement, 48
Retroverted uterus, dyspareunia in, 160
Rhinoceros horn, 282
Ritilin, 282
Rock, J., 7
Rokitansky-Kuster-Hauser syndrome, 98, 103
 amenorrhea and, 98, 99–103
Role playing, in late puberty, 25
Romans, ancient, laws on rape, 286
 sex role designation and, 44
 sexual mores, 4
Romantic stage of marriage, 48
Romanticism, 4–5
"Round ligament pain," 210

## S

Sacral cord, lesions in, 271
Safety, concern for, menorrhagia and, 170
St. Augustine, 4
Salpingitis, acute. See Pelvic inflammatory disease
Salpingo-oophritis, swelling from, 163
Saphenous nerve bypass, for impotence, 254
Satisfaction, sexual, 49
Schizophrenics, 265
Scholastic Aptitude Test (SAT), scores, sex differences in, 35
School(s). *See also* Public education, 28
 sexual stereotyping in, 33
 social environment of, 36
School failures, sex differences, 37
School-grade placement, 28
Science achievement, sex differences in, 35, 35
Scientific medicine, history, 3
Scientific schema, 42
Scrotum, removal of, 310
Seasons, changing of, stress from, 50
Secondary infertility, therapy for, 151–52
Secondary sex characteristics, 11, 12
 in transsexuals, 307, 308

Sedimentation rate, in pelvic inflammatory disease, 162
Seizures. *See* Epilepsy
Self
  constancy of, establishment of, 17
  discovery of, 45
  during puberty, 10
Self-assessment, of transsexual, 308
Self-esteem, regulation of, 16
Self-gratification, wishes for, 21–22
Self-representation, 15
  formation of, 17
Self-stimulation, in infants, 92
Self-understanding, 41
Semen, analysis, 147
  emission, 12, 269
  in puberty, 13, 14
Semen prostaglandins, vaginal introduction to, 202
Semirigid prosthesis, for impotence, 255–56
Sensory-motor stage, 16
Separation anxiety, 9
Separation-individuation process, 15, 16, 17
  in prepubertal years, 18
  similarities in phases of, 21
"Sequential inhibition," 118
"Serial monogamy," 42
Serious illness, stages of dealing with, 178–79
Serotinin, 55
Sertoli cells, 11
Sex assignment, 94
Sex of assignment, 123
"Sex change" operations, 7. *See also* Sex reassignment surgery
Sex cleavage, 45–46
Sex cords, female, 96
Sex differences, awareness of, 29
  throughout education process. *See* Educational process, sex differences
Sex drive, inhibitory system regulating, 264
Sex education, effect on sexual behavior, 131
  historical perspective, 6
Sex hormones, change in, 265
  circulation of, 11
Sex of rearing, importance of, 94
Sex reassignment surgery (SRS), 295, 296, 298, 301, 304, 306, 313
  delays in, 308
  favorable outcome, 305
  individuals requesting, 302, 303
  for transsexuals, outcome of, 311–13
  for primary transsexual, 309–11
Sex roles. *See* Gender role
Sex steroids, regulation of sexual behavior by, 121
Sex therapy, counseling, 240
  development of, 7–8
  for impotence, 258–59
Sexes, segregation of, 18
Sexism, in education system, 33–34
Sexist, defined, 33
Sexoesthetic inversion, 296
Sexual abstinence. *See* Abstinence
Sexual activity, during pregnancy. *See* Pregnancy
  in elderly, 78, 79
  following perinatal loss, 225
  juvenile, results of, 36–37

Sexual adjustment, in rape victim, predictors of problems, 292, 293 *t*, 294 *t*
  ratings of, 290–92
Sexual affairs, 5
Sexual attitudes, contraception and, 7
Sexual behavior, 92
  animal, compared to human, 265
    influence of hormones on, 128–29
  feminine. *See* Feminine sexual behavior
  human compared to subhuman, 121
  influence on hormones, 130
  nonhormonal influences on, 130–31
  overt, 265
Sexual compatibility, 159, 167–68
Sexual concerns, in breast pathology, 192–93
Sexual desire, during pregnancy, 60–61
Sexual deviation, Freud's theory, 5
Sexual drives, force of, 21
Sexual dysfunction, in cardiovascular disease. *See* Cardiovascular disease
  human, defined, 286–87
  in impotence, characterization of, 241–42
  menopause and, 78
  in neurological disease. *See* Neurologic disease
  origins of, 159
  in pelvic relaxation. *See* Pelvic relaxation
  in relaxed vagina, 156–57
  treatment of, 8
Sexual expression. *See also* Sexual behavior
  biological basis, 265
Sexual fantasies. *See* Fantasy
Sexual frustration, 160
Sexual history, importance of, in breast pathology, 192–93, 195
  for impotence, reliability of, 242
Sexual identity, aspects of, 87, 88 *f*
  development of, research on, 8
Sexual inadequacy, feelings of, in vaginal agenesis, 103
Sexual incompatibility, 159
Sexual intercourse. *See* Coitus
Sexual lubricant, 282
Sexual neurasthenia, 5
Sexual organs, vasocongestion of, during pregnancy, 57, 58
Sexual practice(s), biological readiness vs. society, 46
  during pregnancy, 55
Sexual reciprocation, 49
Sexual relations, frequency of, during pregnancy, 61–63
Sexual response, during pregnancy. *See* Pregnancy
Sexual response cycle, breasts during, 191
Sexual satisfaction, 49, 55
  during pregnancy, 60, 63–65
  psychogenic factors in, 160
Sexual stimulation techniques, during pregnancy, 66
Sexuality, in aging male, 77–78
  avoidance of expression of, 19
  awareness of importance of, 49
  as communication, 6
  during pregnancy. *See* Pregnancy
  in early adolescence, 23
  effect of endocrines on, 55
  historical perspective, 44
  menopause and. *See* Menopause

Sexuality—*Continued*
  premarital, 47
  problems concerning, in perinatal loss, 225
  psychological aspects of, 91, 92
Sexually transmitted disease, 165, 204
  laboratory tests for, 162
  risk of acquiring, 168
Shock phase of grief process, 222
Silastic capsules, 115
Sinuvaginal bulbs, 97
Situational impotence, 242
Skeletal system, in congenital vaginal agenesis, 100
Sleep. *See also* Rapid eye movement during sleep
  erections occurring during, monitoring, 244–45, 272
  fetal, 207
Small-Carrion prosthesis, for impotence, 255
Social encounters, effect on sexual behavior, 130
Social influences, on etiology of transsexualism, 301
  in gender identity disorders, 298–99
Social rehabilitation, for transsexuals, 309
Social sciences, study of marriage and family within, 41–42
Social structure, in late puberty, 25
Social systems, processes governing, 28
Social work, 41
Socialization, 43
  nurturant, 48
Society, attitude toward sexuality, 18
  psychosexual development and, 7
  sexual activity during pregnancy and, 56
  status position in, 36
  view of married individuals, 47
Socioeconomic status, contraceptive choice and use and, 131, 132
  effect on sexual behavior, 130–31
  expenditures on education and, 33
  sex differences in education and, 31
  student, judgment of behavior and, 34
Sociological variables, related to menopause and sexuality, 81
Sociology, 43
Sociopathic personality, 300
Somatic dysfunction, related to diabetes, 247
Somatic (voluntary) innervation, 268
Somatic nerve, 269
Spanish fly (cantharides), 282
Spastic paralysis, 271
Spermatorrhea, 5
Spermatozoa, maturation of, 11
Spermicides, 134
Spinal cord, compression, impotence from, 253
  injury, related to sexual dysfunction, 269–70
  lesions, sexual function in, 271
    in female, 270–71
    in male, 270
  neuroanatomy, 268
  tumors, impotence from, 253
Spinal cord syndrome, 268
Spinal tract, efferent, 268
Spironolactone, 238
*Squeeze technique,* for premature ejaculation, 259–60
Status epilepticus, 266
Sterility. *See also* Infertility
  in uterine retrodisplacement, 164

Sterilization, 135
  effect on psychosexual function, 136
Steroid hormone, 7
Stillbirth, 221, 222. *See also* Perinatal death
  facilitation of grief process, 223–24
Stimulation studies, for impotence, 245–46
Stoma effect on sexual functioning, 181
Strassman technique, 109
Stress(es), in cancer patient. *See* Cancer patient, stress in
  emotional response to, 178
  impact on marriage, 50
  of pregnancy, 55, 56, 73, 210
    effect on fetus, 206, 207
  in puerperium, 218, 219
  related to infertility, 143, 144, 145, 146
    physician and work-up and, 146–48
    physician and therapy and, 148–49
  sources of, 50
Stress disorder, posttraumatic, DSM III listing of, 287–88
Stress urinary incontinence, 155
Stressors, marital, 49
Stroller, R., 297
Substitute gratification, 280
Suffering phase of grief process, 222
Suicidal ideation, in transsexualism and gender dysphoria, 303
Superego, constancy, 17
  definition of, 17
  function, 17
  in prepubertal years, 17, 18
  in puberty, 10, 14
    in late puberty, 26
Superficial transverse perineal muscles, 154
Support groups, for perinatal loss, 225–26
  for psychosexual dysfunction in infertility, 152
Support systems, during puerperium, 220
Supracervical hysterectomy, 175
Suprapubic approach, to inflatable penile prosthesis, 257–58
Surgery, for ambiguous genital assignment, 90–91
  for cancer, breast, 198. *See also* Mastectomy
    stress from, 180–82
  for impotence, 253–54
  for pelvic pain from benign neoplasia, 172–75
Surgitek Flexi-Rod penile prosthesis, 255–56
Swallowing, fetal, 205
Swelling, in pelvic inflammatory disease, 163
Sympathetic nervous system, 269
  male, 268
Syphilis, attitude toward, historical perspective, 4
Systemic desensitization, for impotence, 259

# T

Taste buds, fetal, 205
Teacher(s), discipline by, sex differences and, 34
  ratio to pupil, 33
  response to students, sex differences and, 34
  ratio of women to men, 30–31, 32–33, 35
Temporal lobe, 266
  limbic system, lesions of, 266

Temporal lobe epilepsy, relationship to sexuality, 265–66
Temporal lobectomy, 265
  effect on sexual behavior, 265
Teratogen, 99
Terminal phase of cancer, stress in, 184
Testes, testicles, 11
  removal of, 310
Testicular atrophy, 309
Testicular failure, 246, 251
Testicular feminization, 123
Testicular neoplasm, risk of, 91
Testosterone, 55, 124
  impaired biosynthesis, 89
  levels, for study of impotence, 246, 247
  secretion of, 11
Testosterone proprionate, 264
  for impotence, 252
Testosterone therapy, for congenital adrenal hyperplasia, 90
  for impotence, 252
  for transsexual, 308
Texid (perhexiline), 243
Thecal tunic, 97
Thelarche, 98
Thermography, for vascular impotence, 250
Thoracic cord, lesions, sexual function in, 271
Thyroid dysfunction, 144
Thyroid function, impotence and, 248
Thyroid hormone, 196
Thyroid metabolism, disorders, 252
Thyrotrophin-releasing hormone (TRH), 144
Tissot, S., 5
Tomboyishness, 93
  in congenital virilizing adrenal hyperplasia, 122
Toilet training, 45
Toileting behavior, cross-gender, 94
Tranquilizers, effect on sexual function, 284
Transcendental meditation (TM), for psychosexual dysfunction in infertility, 151
Transitory depression, 213–14
  hormonal changes in, 214, 215 t, 215
  in puerperium, 216, 218
Transsexualism, 295, 313. See also Gender dysphoria syndrome
  body image and, 301–302
  characteristics, 297–98
  criteria for, 298
  distinguishing primary from secondary, 300
  epidemiology, 300–301
  evaluation and treatment, 7, 302–305
    hormonal therapy, 306–309
    sex reassignment surgery, 309–11, 311–13
    trial of cross-gender living, 305–306
  historical background, 295–97
  spectrum of gender identity, 298–300
Transverse vaginal septum, amenorrhea and cryptomenorrhea in, 104–105
Transvestism, 6, 7, 93, 266, 296, 298, 299
Trauma, obstetrical, 155
  coitus and, 204–205
Treatment phase of cancer, stress in, 180–83
Tricyclic antidepressants, 247
  for pelvic pain, 172
Tryptophan, levels, related to puerperium depression, 216

Tubal ligation, 135
  pelvic pain from, 164
Turner's syndrome, 100, 121–22
Twentieth century, physician involvement in sexuality during, 6–8
  research in human sexuality during, 8–9
Tyramine loading test, 216

# U

Ullrich-Turner's syndrome, 88
Ultrasonography, 90
Unicornuate uterus, 98
  reproductive failure in, 109
United States, rape laws, 286
"Unruptured follicle syndrome," 144
Urethral intercourse, in vaginal agenesis, 100, 101
Urinary diversion, effect on sexual functioning, 181
Urinary incontinence, stress, 155
Urinary system, in vaginal agenesis, 99, 100
Urodynamic studies, for impotence, 248
Urogenital ducts, female, 96
Urogenital sinus, 97
User experience, in effects of marijuana, 279
Utah Infertility Reaction Scale, 145–46
Uterine cervix, congenital atresia in, 106–107
  double, 108 f
Uterine corpus, 97
Uterine horn, noncommunicating, cryptomenorrhea and menstrual egress per vagina in, 107
Uterine myomata, pelvic pain from, 170–71
Uterine retrodisplacement, pelvic pain from, 165–65, 166
Uterus, 269
  absence of, 99, 99 f. See also Rokitansky-Kuster-Hauser syndrome
  anomalies, 98
  during pregnancy, 58–59
  duplication of, 107, 108 f
    cryptomenorrhea and menstrual egress per vagina in, 107
    reproductive failure in, 109
  embryology of, 96, 97
  prolapse, vaginal relaxation associated with, 155, 156, 157–58
  retroverted, 160
  unicornuate, 98, 109
  unification, 109

# V

Vagina, 269
  absence of. See Vaginal agenesis, Rokitansky-Kuster-Hauser syndrome
  adenosis of, 104
  bacteria in, 68, 69
  creation of, See Neovagina, creation of
  embryology, 96, 97
  relaxation of. See Pelvic relaxation
  support of, 154–55
  unilaterally imperforate, cryptomenorrhea and menstrual egress per vagina and, 107

Vaginal agenesis, 105, 106, 123
  congenital, 98–104. *See also* Rokitansky-Kuster-Hauser syndrome
  partial, amenorrhea and cryptomenorrhea in, 107
Vaginal agglutination, 182
Vaginal atrophy, 78
Vaginal bleeding, from benign neoplasia, 169–70
Vaginal canal, 97
Vaginal laceration, 204
Vaginal lubrication, age and, 82
Vaginal orgasm, 5, 157
Vaginal outlet, symptoms, 155
Vaginal plate, 97
  cavitation of, 97
Vaginal septum, transverse, amenorrhea and cryptomenorrhea in, 104
Vaginismus, 146, 155, 161
Vaginitis, atrophic, 157
Vaginoplasty, penile skin flap technique, 310
Van de Velde, T., 6
Variable version (VV), 256
Variscosities, pelvic, 165
Vascular disease, sexual dysfunction in, 237
Vascular evaluation, for impotence, 243–44, 249–51
Vascular insufficiency, impotence from, surgical therapy for, 254
Vasculogenic impotence, 242, 249
Vasculogenic "Steal" phenomenon, 249
Vasectomy, 135

Vasomotor responses, 78
Vasopressin, modulation of feminine sexual behavior by, 120
Venereal disease. *See* Sexually transmitted disease
Ventromedial nucleus, 114
Victorian era, physician involvement in sexuality during, 5
Victorianism, 4
Video stimulation studies, for impotence, 245
Vision, fetal, 205
Visual stimulation studies, for impotence, 245–46
Vitamin E supplementation, for benign breast disease, 196
von Krafft-Ebing, R., 5–6
Vulvectomy, sexual functioning following, 181
Vulvular carcinoma, 179

# W

Walinder, J., 297
Weschler Adult Intelligence Scale (WAIS), 304
Western marriage and family, 42
  historical perspective, 43–45
Wife, emotional response to pregnancy, 56–57
Winter shunt, for impotence, 253
Withdrawal method of contraception, 133
Womanhood, core of, 7
Women. *See* Female, Girls, Wife

DATE DUE